Clinical Endocrinology
of Companion Animals

Clinical Endocrinology of Companion Animals

Edited by

Jacquie Rand

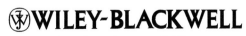

WILEY-BLACKWELL

A John Wiley & Sons, Inc., Publication

Wiley-Blackwell is an imprint of John Wiley & Sons, formed by the merger of Wiley's global Scientific, Technical and Medical business with Blackwell Publishing.

Editorial offices
2121 State Avenue, Ames, Iowa 50014-8300, USA
The Atrium, Southern Gate, Chichester, West Sussex, PO19 8SQ, UK
9600 Garsington Road, Oxford, OX4 2DQ, UK

For details of our global editorial offices, for customer services and for information about how to apply
for permission to reuse the copyright material in this book please see our website at www.wiley.com/wiley-blackwell.

Library of Congress Cataloging-in-Publication Data

Clinical endocrinology of companion animals / edited by Jacquie Rand.
    p. cm.
  Includes bibliographical references and index.
  ISBN 978-0-8138-0583-2 (pbk. : alk. paper) 1. Veterinary endocrinology. 2. Pets–Diseases. I. Rand, Jacquie.
  [DNLM: 1. Endocrine System Diseases–veterinary. 2. Endocrine Glands–physiopathology. 3. Endocrine System
Diseases–diagnosis. 4. Pets. SF 768.3]
  SF768.3.C55 2012
  636.089′64–dc23

2012014134

A catalogue record for this book is available from the British Library.

Cover design by Modern Alchemy LLC

Set in 9.5/11.5pt Sabon by SPi Publisher Services, Pondicherry, India

Printed in the UK

Dedication

This book is dedicated to the important people who shaped my life and goals.
My parents, Geoff and Moira, who inspired me to be the best I could be, to never accept mediocrity from myself, and to always remain optimistic about achieving my goals. They are not here to see the book published, but their legacy remains.
My husband, Tom, who is my greatest supporter, through the challenging times and the good times in life, always there, encouraging me to follow my dreams and be happy.
My daughter, Lisette, who reminds me to maintain a balance in my life and inspires me to be a better role model.
Merlin, our characterful Burmese cat, who has lived a full life despite many twists and turns—surrendered to a municipal animal facility and, on death row, acquired as one of my research cats, identified as insulin resistant and predisposed to diabetes, adopted into our family—and who sat beside me or on my desk as I wrote and edited chapters for this book.
Thank you all for your inspiration.

Contents

Contributors

Ellen N. Behrend, VMD, PhD, Dipl. ACVIM (Small Animal Internal Medicine)
Joezy Griffin Professor
Dept. Clinical Sciences
College of Veterinary Medicine
Auburn University
Auburn, Alabama, USA

Michelle L. Campbell-Ward, BSc, BVSc(Hons I), DZooMed(Mammalian), MRCVS
RCVS Specialist in Zoo and Wildlife Medicine
Taronga Conservation Society Australia
Taronga Western Plains Zoo—Wildlife Hospital
Dubbo, New South Wales, Australia

Patrick Carney, DVM, Dipl. ACVIM (Small Animal Internal Medicine)
Staff Internist
Tufts Veterinary Emergency Treatment & Specialties Walpole
MA Clinical Assistant Professor
Department of Clinical Sciences Cummings School of Veterinary Medicine
Tufts University
North Grafton, MA, USA

Sue Chen, DVM, DABVP – Avian Practice
Gulf Coast Avian and Exotics
Gulf Coast Veterinary Specialists
Houston, Texas, USA

Dennis Chew, DVM, Dipl. ACVIM (Small Animal Internal Medicine)
Professor, Emeritus
Center for Veterinary Medicine
Department of Veterinary Clinical Sciences
College of Veterinary Medicine
The Ohio State University
Columbus, Ohio, USA

David Church, BVSc, PhD, MACVSc, ILTM, MRCVS
Royal Veterinary College
University of London
London, United Kingdom

Kevin Eatwell, BVSc (hons), DZooMed (Reptilian), Dipl. ECZM (Herp), MRCVS
RCVS specialist in Zoo and Wildlife Medicine
European Recognised Veterinary Specialist in Zoological Medicine (Herpetological)
Lecturer in Exotic Animal and Wildlife Medicine
Royal (Dick) School of Veterinary Studies
University of Edinburgh
Hospital for Small Animals
Easter Bush Veterinary Centre
Roslin, Midlothian, United Kingdom

Linda Fleeman, BVSc, PhD, MANZVS
Animal Diabetes Australia
Rowville Veterinary Clinic, Rowville
Boronia Veterinary Clinic, Boronia
Lort Smith Animal Hospital, North Melbourne
Victoria, Australia

Danièlle Gunn-Moore, BSc, BVM&S, PhD, FHEA, MACVSc, MRCVS
RCVS Specialist in Feline Medicine
Professor of Feline Medicine and Director of Teaching Hospitals
Royal(Dick) School of Veterinary Studies and The Roslin Institute
The University of Edinburgh
Hospital for Small Animals
Easter Bush Veterinary Centre
Roslin, Midlothian, Scotland

Andrea M. Harvey, BVSc DSAM(Feline) Dipl. ECVIM-CA MRCVS
RCVS Specialist in Feline Medicine
European Veterinary Specialist in Internal Medicine
International Society of Feline Medicine
Wiltshire, United Kingdom

Rebecka S. Hess, DVM, Dipl. ACVIM (Small Animal Internal Medicine)
Associate Professor of Internal Medicine
Chief, Section of Medicine
Department of Clinical Studies-Philadelphia
School of Veterinary Medicine
University of Pennsylvania
Philadelphia, Pennsylvania, USA

Kate Hill, BVSc, MANZCVSc, Dipl. ACVIM (Small Animal Internal Medicine)
Senior Lecturer
Director Centre for Service and Working Dog Health
Institute of Veterinary, Animal and Biomedical Science
Massey University
New Zealand

Katherine M. James, DVM, PhD, Dipl. ACVIM (Small Animal Internal Medicine)
Veterinary Information Network
Davis, California, USA

Cheri A. Johnson, DVM, MS, Dipl. ACVIM (Small Animal Internal Medicine)
Professor and Chief of Staff
Small Animal Clinical Sciences
College of Veterinary Medicine
Michigan State University
East Lansing, Michigan, USA

John Keen, BSc, BVetMed, PhD CertEM (IntMed), Dipl. ECEIM MRCVS
RCVS and European Specialist in Equine Internal Medicine
Dick Vet Equine Hospital
Royal (Dick) School of Veterinary Studies
Easter Bush Veterinary Centre
Easter Bush
Roslin, Midlothian, United Kingdom

Hans S. Kooistra, DVM, PhD, Dipl. ECVIM-CA
Department of Clinical Sciences of Companion Animals
Faculty of Veterinary Medicine
Utrecht University
Utrecht, The Netherlands

Janice Sojka Kritchevsky, VMD, MS, Dipl. ACVIM (Large Animal
Internal Medicine)
Department of Veterinary Clinical Sciences
Purdue University College of Veterinary Medicine West
Lafayette, Indiana, USA

Patty Lathan, VMD, MS, Dipl. ACVIM (Small Animal Internal Medicine)
Assistant Professor
Department of Clinical Sciences
Mississippi State University College of Veterinary Medicine
Starkville, Mississippi, USA

Katharine F. Lunn, BVMS, MS, PhD, MRCVS, Dipl. ACVIM (Small Animal
Internal Medicine)
Associate Professor
Department of Clinical Sciences
College of Veterinary Medicine
North Carolina State University
Raleigh, North Carolina, USA

Linda Martin, DVM, MS, Dipl. ACVECC
Associate Professor, Emergency and Critical Care
Department of Clinical Sciences
College of Veterinary Medicine
Auburn University
Auburn, Alabama, USA

Catherine McGowan, BVSc, MACVSc, DEIM, Dipl. ECEIM, PhD, FHEA, MRCVS
Senior Lecturer in Equine Medicine and Director of Veterinary CPD
Institute of Ageing and Chronic Disease,
Faculty of Health and Life Sciences
University of Liverpool
Leahurst, United Kingdom

Carlos Melian, DVM, PhD
Director of Veterinary Teaching Hospital
Faculty of Veterinary Medicine
University of Las Palmas de Gran Canaria
Trasmontana s/n, 35416 Arucas, Las Palmas, Spain

Stijn J. M. Niessen, DVM, PhD, Dipl. ECVIM, PGCVetEd, FHEA, MRCVS
Lecturer Internal Medicine
Royal Veterinary College
University of London
Research Associate
Diabetes Research Group
Newcastle Medical School
United Kingdom

David Panciera, DVM, MS, Dipl. ACVIM (Small Animal Internal Medicine)
Professor
Department of Small Animal Clinical Sciences
Virginia-Maryland Regional College of Veterinary Medicine
Virginia Tech
Blacksburg, Virginia, USA

Mark E. Peterson, DVM, Dipl. ACVIM (Small Animal Internal Medicine)
Director of Endocrinology and Nuclear Medicine
Animal Endocrine Clinic
New York, New York, USA

Jacquie Rand, BVSc, DVSc, MACVS, Dipl. ACVIM (Small Animal Internal Medicine)
Professor of Companion Animal Health
Director, Centre for Companion Animal Health
School of Veterinary Science
The University of Queensland
Australia

Nicki Reed, BVM&S, Cert VR, DSAM (Feline), Dipl. ECVIM-CA, MRCVS
European Veterinary Specialist in Small Animal Medicine
Lecturer in Companion Animal Medicine
Head of the Feline Clinic
Royal (Dick) School of Veterinary Studies
The University of Edinburgh
Hospital for Small Animals
Easter Bush Veterinary Centre
Roslin, Midlothian, United Kingdom

Kent R. Refsal, DVM, PhD
Professor, Endocrine Section
Diagnostic Center for Population and Animal Health
Michigan State University
Lansing, Michigan, USA

Claudia E. Reusch, DVM, Dipl. ECVIM-CA
Professor
Head of Clinic for Small Animal Internal Medicine
Vetsuisse Faculty
University of Zurich
Zurich, Switzerland

Craig Ruaux, BVSc, PhD, Dipl. ACVIM (Small Animal Internal Medicine)
Assistant Professor
Department of Veterinary Clinical Sciences
Oregon State University
Corvallis, Oregon, USA

Patricia A. Schenck, DVM, PhD
Section Chief, Endocrine Diagnostic Section
Diagnostic Center for Population and Animal Health
Michigan State University
Lansing, Michigan, USA

Nico J. Schoemaker, DVM, PhD, Dipl. ECZM (Small Mammal and Avian),
Dipl. ABVP-avian
Division of Zoological Medicine
Department of Clinical Sciences of Companion Animals
Faculty of Veterinary Medicine, Utrecht University
Utrecht, The Netherlands

Kerry Simpson, BVM&S, Cert VC, PhD, FACVSc (Feline Medicine), MRCVS
RCVS Specialist in Feline Medicine
The Feline Expert
London, United Kingdom

Michael Stanford, BVSc, FRCVS
Birch Heath Veterinary Clinic
Birch Heath Road
Tarporley, Cheshire, United Kingdom

Annemarie M.W.Y. Voorbij, DVM, MS
Department of Clinical Sciences of Companion Animals
Faculty of Veterinary Medicine
Utrecht University
Utrecht, The Netherlands

Preface

The inspiration for the format of *Clinical Endocrinology of Companion Animals* was from teaching students in the clinic and consulting with busy veterinarians in busy practices. There was clearly a need for a quick reference guide that had detailed information, but in a format designed to easily find that information. My hope is that this book will provide valuable assistance for clinicians in diagnosing and managing endocrine cases in practice, as well as for students wishing to quickly find information to help with a case or learn in greater depth the details of diseases of the endocrine system. My aim is that this book be a quick reference book for practical use, to be referred to in the consulting room and in the field.

I thank the section editors, Ellen Behrend, Danielle Gunn-Moore, and Michelle Campbell-Ward, for their absolute dedication to making this a quality publication with the most current information known in veterinary science on endocrine diseases of the various companion animal species. I also thank the many contributors for the richness of their contributions, which represents the sum of many decades of combined knowledge.

I found it fascinating learning of the susceptibility of some exotic companion species to certain endocrine diseases. I hope you also enjoy and find useful the breadth of this book across the common, and not so common, companion animals that veterinarians see in practice.

CHAPTER 1

Hypoadrenocorticism in Dogs

Patty Lathan

Pathogenesis

- Primary hypoadrenocorticism results from the destruction of >90% of the adrenal cortex.
- Most cases are presumed to be due to an immune-mediated process.
- Combined glucocorticoid and mineralocorticoid deficiency occur most frequently, but isolated glucocorticoid deficiency ("atypical hypoadrenocorticism") is probably underdiagnosed.

Classical Signs

- Young to middle-age dogs are predisposed, as are poodles, West Highland White Terriers, and Great Danes.
- Addison's disease is known as the "Great Pretender" because nonspecific signs such as lethargy, decreased appetite, and weight loss predominate.
- Gastrointestinal signs such as vomiting and diarrhea are also common.
- Patients may present in hypovolemic shock or following collapse.

Diagnosis

- ACTH stimulation test demonstrates minimal cortisol response.

Treatment

- Glucocorticoid and mineralocorticoid supplementation, ± intravenous fluids and supportive therapy.

I. Pathogenesis
A. Pathophysiology:
   1. Most patients with naturally occurring hypoadrenocorticism ("Addison's disease") suffer from **combined glucocorticoid and mineralocorticoid deficiency:**

Clinical Endocrinology of Companion Animals, First Edition. Edited by Jacquie Rand.
© 2013 John Wiley & Sons, Inc. Published 2013 by John Wiley & Sons, Inc.

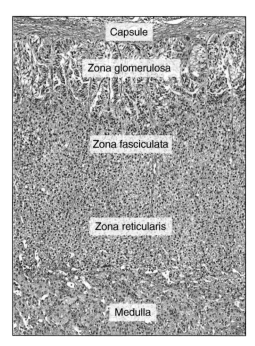

Figure 1.1   The adrenal cortex is made up of three layers—the zona glomerulosa, zona fasciculata, and zona reticularis. The zone glomerulosa is responsible for mineralocorticoid synthesis, whereas the inner two layers are responsible for glucocorticoid and sex hormone synthesis. (Image provided by Dr. Jim Cooley.)

    a. Aldosterone is a mineralocorticoid secreted in the outermost layer of the adrenal cortex, the zona glomerulosa (Figure 1.1). The major action of aldosterone is the conservation of sodium and water, and excretion of potassium and hydrogen ions (acid), from the distal renal tubule. In normal dogs, secretion of aldosterone is stimulated by hypovolemia and hyperkalemia and is primarily regulated by the renin-angiotensin-aldosterone system (RAAS). In patients with hypoadrenocorticism and subsequent **aldosterone deficiency, hyponatremia, hyperkalemia,** and **hypovolemia** are common.

    b. Cortisol is a glucocorticoid produced in the inner-most layers of the adrenal cortex, the zonae fasciculata and reticularis. Cortisol has activity in almost every cell in the body. Functions include stimulation of gluconeogenesis and erythropoiesis, maintenance of gastrointestinal mucosal integrity, and suppression of the inflammatory response. Additionally, cortisol has important roles in the maintenance of blood pressure and contractility of the heart. Cortisol requirements increase during times of stress. Cortisol release from the adrenal cortex is controlled by adrenocorticotropic hormone (ACTH) (Figure 1.2). Cortisol deficiency in dogs with hypoadrenocorticism may result in gastrointestinal signs, lethargy, hypoglycemia, hypotension, and anemia.

  2. Some patients with hypoadrenocorticism suffer from isolated glucocorticoid deficiency. In these cases, aldosterone secretion is preserved, and electrolyte abnormalities are **not** present. Patients with **isolated glucocorticoid deficiency** are often said to have "**atypical hypoadrenocorticism**" or "**atypical Addison's disease.**"

B. Etiology:

  1. Primary hypoadrenocorticism results from the destruction of greater than 90% of the adrenal cortex. Most cases of naturally occurring hypoadrenocorticism in dogs are idiopathic, most likely due to immune-mediated destruction of the adrenal cortex. Rarely, infiltration of the adrenal cortex by fungal disease, amyloidosis, or neoplasia has been reported. Trauma, hemorrhage, and infarction may also lead to hypoadrenocorticism.

  2. Drug-induced adrenocorticolysis can also result in hypoadrenocorticism in dogs being treated for hyperadrenocorticism:

(a)

(b)

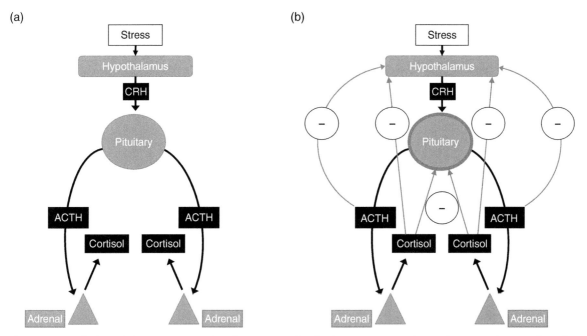

Figure 1.2 (a) The hypothalamic pituitary axis without negative feedback. Corticotropin-releasing hormone (CRH) is released by neurons in the hypothalamus and transported to the anterior pituitary by portal circulation. CRH then stimulates the release of ACTH from the pituitary gland into systemic circulation. ACTH then stimulates the synthesis and secretion of cortisol. (b) Negative feedback is the mechanism by which the endocrine system regulates secretion of its hormones. In the HPA-axis, ACTH feeds back to the hypothalamus to inhibit continued release of CRH, which then leads to decreased release of ACTH. Cortisol feeds back to both the hypothalamus to decrease CRH secretion, and to the pituitary gland to decrease ACTH release. By this mechanism, the HPA-axis is able to maintain the physiologically necessary concentration of cortisol in the bloodstream—not too much, nor too little.

    a. Adrenocortical necrosis caused by mitotane is usually selective to the zonae fasciculata and reticularis, resulting in decreased cortisol production. However, inadequate monitoring or use in a particularly sensitive patient may lead to destruction of the cells of the zona glomerulosa, resulting in aldosterone deficiency as well.

    b. The other commonly used medication to treat hyperadrenocorticism is trilostane. As an inhibitor of at least one enzyme involved in steroid synthesis (3β-hydroxysteroid dehydrogenase), trilostane overdose may lead to cortisol deficiency and, less frequently, aldosterone deficiency. Additionally, idiosyncratic adrenocortical necrosis has been reported to occur in some dogs taking trilostane, resulting in hypoadrenocorticism.

3. **Hypoadrenocorticism secondary to decreased ACTH production is characterized by isolated glucocorticoid deficiency since ACTH has little regulatory control of aldosterone production:**

    a. The most common form of secondary hypoadrenocorticism is iatrogenic, resulting from exogenous glucocorticoid administration (Figure 1.3). Exogenous glucocorticoids inhibit the release of adrenocorticotropic hormone (ACTH) from the pituitary gland. Adrenal gland atrophy then occurs, resulting in decreased secretion of cortisol. Following acute withdrawal of the exogenous glucocorticoid, a stressful event will cause increased release of ACTH, but the atrophied adrenal glands will be unable to respond by secreting an appropriate amount of cortisol, which may result in signs of cortisol deficiency. Chronic administration of glucocorticoids is more likely to result in hypoadrenocorticism than short-term use, and longer-acting reposital steroids (such as methylprednisolone acetate) are more potent suppressors of ACTH than shorter-acting glucocorticoids (such as oral prednisolone). Topical, otic, and ophthalmic preparations containing glucocorticoids may also lead to iatrogenic hypoadrenocorticism, particularly in smaller patients.

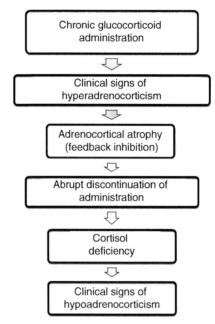

Figure 1.3 Diagrammatic representation of the relationship between iatrogenic hyperadrenocorticism and iatrogenic hypoadrenocorticism. Chronic glucocorticoid administration leads to clinical signs of glucocorticoid excess ("iatrogenic hyperadrenocorticism"). At the same time, the exogenous glucocorticoid provides feedback inhibition to the pituitary gland, decreasing the production of ACTH. Without ACTH, the dog's own adrenal glands atrophy. While the dog is still taking the exogenous glucocorticoids, the dog will appear to have hyperadrenocorticism. Upon abrupt withdrawal of the steroid, the dog's own atrophied adrenal gland will be unable secrete cortisol, potentially resulting in clinical signs of hypoadrenocorticism. Clinical signs may be seen more often following a stressful event in these patients.

   b. Naturally occurring causes of secondary hypoadrenocorticism include pituitary masses, trauma, or other lesions that inhibit ACTH release.
   4. At this time, the etiology of atypical hypoadrenocorticism (isolated glucocorticoid deficiency) is unknown. ACTH deficiency has been ruled out in many cases. It may be the result of partial immune-mediated destruction of the adrenal cortex, sparing the zona glomerulosa. Although some have hypothesized that atypical hypoadrenocorticism is simply an early manifestation of "typical" hypoadrenocorticism, many patients never lose their ability to secrete aldosterone.
C. Risk factors for hypoadrenocorticism:
   1. Dogs with other immune-mediated endocrinopathies, such as diabetes mellitus and hypothyroidism, may be at increased risk for hypoadrenocorticism.
   2. Dogs with the disease are more likely to have clinical signs during or following a stressful event.

II. Signalment
A. Any breed of dog may be afflicted with hypoadrenocorticism, including mixed-breeds. However, an increased prevalence of hypoadrenocorticism has been documented in all sizes of **poodles, West Highland white terriers, Great Danes, bearded collies, Portuguese water dogs, Leonbergers, Nova Scotia duck-tolling retrievers,** and possibly **Saint Bernards.**
B. A genetic basis has been proved in standard poodles, Bearded collies, and Nova Scotia duck-tolling retrievers.
C. **Young to middle-aged dogs** (2–5 years old) are predisposed. However, dogs of any age can be diagnosed with hypoadrenocorticism. Nova Scotia duck-tolling retrievers may be diagnosed at a younger age, as early as 2 months.

D. Females appear to be predisposed in some studies, while other studies reveal a more equal distribution between the sexes.

E. Dogs diagnosed with isolated glucocorticoid deficiency have a similar signalment to those with combined mineralocorticoid/glucocorticoid deficiency. As a population, however, dogs with atypical Addison's tend to be 2–3 years older at diagnosis compared to those with typical Addison's.

III. Clinical Signs

A. **The clinical manifestation of hypoadrenocorticism is highly variable in presenting complaint, chronicity, and severity.** Some dogs present for chronic clinical signs, whereas others present more acutely in "Addisonian crisis." Rigid rules differentiating acute from chronic hypoadrenocorticism do not exist; the pathophysiology is the same, and these presentations represent a continuum of disease progression. If not diagnosed and treated early in the course of the disease, many dogs with chronic signs will decompensate and present in crisis. However, they will be discussed separately, since initial treatment differs. Likewise, dogs with isolated cortisol deficiency (atypical hypoadrenocorticism) will also be discussed separately in order to highlight the contrasting features.

   1. **Chronic hypoadrenocorticism:**

      a. Addison's disease often causes vague, nonspecific clinical signs that can be confused with other diseases, thus earning it the moniker "The Great Pretender" (Table 1.1). Most patients experience **lethargy, decreased appetite,** and **weight loss** with varying severity. The owner may report that the patient just is not acting normally. A **waxing and waning pattern**, with improvement of clinical signs specifically noted following fluid or steroid administration, is common (Schaer and Chen 1983; Herrtage 2000).

      b. **Vomiting** and **diarrhea** are frequently reported, with or without concurrent **melena**. Rectal examination may also reveal melena previously unnoticed by owners. Dogs occasionally present with abdominal pain. These gastrointestinal signs are thought to occur due to loss of the "trophic" effects of cortisol on the gastrointestinal mucosa. Exacerbation of or onset of gastrointestinal signs following a stressful event is often noted in dogs later diagnosed with hypoadrenocorticism. Thus, it is critical that hypoadrenocorticism is considered in patients diagnosed with "stress colitis," particularly if the diarrhea is accompanied by melena, vomiting, and/or generalized lethargy and weakness.

      c. Patients may also exhibit **polyuria** and **polydipsia**. This is likely due to a combination of the decreased renal medullary concentration gradient resulting from hyponatremia, and decreased sodium (and, consequently, water) resorption in the collecting ducts of the kidney.

      d. Some dogs with hypoadrenocorticism present with **generalized or hindlimb weakness,** which may be the primary presenting complaint (Figure 1.4). Reflexes are generally normal in these dogs. The reason for this weakness is unclear. Generalized debility is a plausible explanation, but some of these dogs have hindlimb weakness only. Another hypothesis is that electrolyte abnormalities lead to aberrant neuromuscular function. Whatever the cause, hypoadrenocorticism should be considered in patients that are "down in the hindlimbs."

      e. Some dogs with hypoadrenocorticism have concurrent **megaesophagus.** Rarely, regurgitation is the major presenting complaint in dogs with hypoadrenocorticism. The severity of the megaesophagus is variable; **regurgitation** may be noted, but radiographic evidence without clinical signs is also possible. The esophageal dilation seems to be less severe than that seen in other cases of megaesophagus. Proposed explanations for this megaesophagus include disturbed neuromuscular function caused by electrolyte abnormalities and muscle weakness secondary to cortisol deficiency. Hypoadrenocorticism is one of the few underlying causes of megaesophagus in which appropriate treatment results in the resolution of esophageal abnormalities, so it should be ruled out in all cases of megaesophagus.

      f. **Muscle cramping** has been described in two Standard Poodles with hypoadrenocorticism. Again, aberrant electrolyte concentrations are hypothesized to cause an underlying neuron conduction abnormality.

   2. **Acute hypoadrenocorticism:**

      a. Approximately 30% of dogs with hypoadrenocorticism present in **hypovolemic shock.** Any of the clinical signs described for patients with chronic hypoadrenocorticism may be found in dogs with an

Table 1.1   Clinical signs and physical exam findings in dogs with hypoadrenocorticism.

Clinical signs and physical exam findings	Incidence (%)
Lethargy/depression	90
Decreased appetite/anorexia	80
Vomiting	80
Weakness	70
Weight loss	45
Diarrhea	40
Waxing/waning illness	40
Dehydration	40
Hypothermia	35
Shaking/shivering	30
Weak pulses	30
Polyuria/polydipsia	25
Melena	15
Painful abdomen	15

Data modified from Willard et al. (1982); Peterson et al. (1996); and Melian and Peterson (1996).

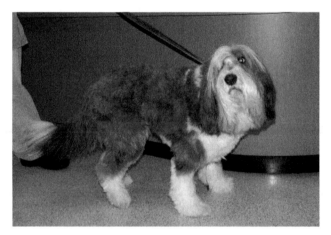

Figure 1.4   Hypoadrenocorticism is known as "The Great Pretender" because of the variety of presenting complaints and clinical signs seen in patients. This 8-year-old bearded collie presented for hindlimb weakness and collapse. Serum chemistry revealed hyperkalemia and hyponatremia, and ACTH stimulation confirmed hypoadrenocorticism.

acute presentation. History may reveal chronic gastrointestinal signs with acute presentation of vomiting and/or diarrhea. **Collapse** secondary to hypovolemia and/or generalized weakness is not uncommon.

b. Classic signs of hypovolemic shock are usually present, including **weak pulse, pale mucous membranes, and prolonged capillary refill time; hypothermia** occurs occasionally. Heart rate, however, is variable. Whereas most dogs in hypovolemic shock are tachycardic (>160 bpm), **patients in hypoadrenocortical crisis often have a normal to decreased heart rate.** This is due to the effects of hyperkalemia in lowering the heart rate. **Thus, the presence of a decreased or normal heart rate ("relative bradycardia") in a patient in hypovolemic shock should raise suspicion of hyperkalemia and hypoadrenocorticism.** Rapid treatment and correction of cardiac changes associated with hyperkalemia is critical for the survival of the patient.

c. **Melena** is frequently present in patients in Addisonian crisis, and may be severe enough to necessitate blood transfusion. Hematochezia is seen less frequently. Melena may be noted on initial exam, or may not be evident until after beginning therapy. Progressively decreasing hematocrit during treatment (more than by hemodilution alone) should increase suspicion of melena, and the possibility of melena should not be excluded due to its initial absence in feces or upon rectal examination. Ileus may decrease gastrointestinal (GI) transit enough to delay its appearance for 1–2 days. It is not uncommon for melena to appear 2–3 days into treatment. For this reason, hospitalization is recommended until the hematocrit stabilizes or increases.

d. Generalized muscle weakness results in **shaking** and/or **shivering** in some patients.

e. Rarely, severe hypoglycemia leads to **seizures** in dogs with Addison's disease.

3. **Atypical hypoadrenocorticism:**
   a. Dogs with isolated cortisol deficiency generally present with the same **nonspecific clinical signs** (lethargy, weight loss, and anorexia) as other dogs with hypoadrenocorticism.
   b. **Gastrointestinal signs** (vomiting and diarrhea) are also common, and **megaesophagus and seizures** (secondary to hypoglycemia) have been reported with atypical hypoadrenocorticism as well.
   c. **Atypical Addisonians infrequently present in acute crisis.** This is probably because **hyperkalemia and hyponatremia do not occur** in these dogs. **Hypotension** is **possible**, however, as a result of **decreased** vascular tone in the absence of cortisol. Acute collapse secondary to hypoglycemia and hemorrhagic shock secondary to GI hemorrhage has also been reported in this group of Addisonian patients.
   d. Patients with atypical Addison's disease have a slightly longer duration of clinical signs prior to diagnosis. This may be due to the fact that diagnosis is delayed because there are no electrolyte disturbances to stimulate the clinician's suspicion of hypoadrenocorticism.

IV. Diagnosis
A. Chronic hypoadrenocorticism:
   1. Most of the diagnostics performed in dogs with hypoadrenocorticism are done early in the workup, often prior to significant suspicion of hypoadrenocorticism. **A complete blood count, serum biochemistry analysis, and urinalysis should be performed in each patient with clinical signs consistent with hypoadrenocorticism** (Table 1.2). It is critical that electrolyte analysis is included in the biochemistry panel, as sodium and potassium abnormalities are often the first specific indicators of hypoadrenocorticism. Additionally, electrolyte disturbances are common in patients with gastrointestinal signs of any etiology, and need to be addressed during treatment:
      a. Serum biochemistry and urinalysis:
         1) Most dogs with "typical" hypoadrenocorticism are **hyperkalemic** (90%) and **hyponatremic** (85%) at diagnosis. Potassium concentration usually remains below 8 mEq/L, but may be as high as 11 mEq/L. Sodium concentrations are usually in the range of 120–140 mEq/L, but may be as low as 100 mEq/L. Some present with one abnormality without the other (e.g., hyperkalemia without hyponatremia). **Hypochloremia** often parallels hyponatremia and is seen in approximately half of the patients. Electrolyte disturbances are not always present early in the course of disease; they may appear when the patient's disease progresses, or not at all, as with atypical hypoadrenocorticism. Emphasis is sometimes placed on calculation of the **Na$^+$/K$^+$ ratio**. The lower the sodium and the higher the potassium concentration, the lower the ratio. The lower the ratio, the higher the likelihood that the patient has Addison's disease (Adler et al. 2007). However, a high ratio does not rule out hypoadrenocorticism, nor does a low ratio definitively diagnose it; thus, the utility of the ratio is debatable. Any dog with hyponatremia or hyperkalemia should be considered a suspect for hypoadrenocorticism, regardless of the ratio.

Table 1.2   Clinicopathologic abnormalities common with hypoadrenocorticism.

Clinicopathologic abnormalities associated with hypoadrenocorticism
Hyperkalemia
Hyponatremia
Hypochloremia
Azotemia
Isosthenuria
Hypoalbuminemia
Hypercalcemia
Hypocholesterolemia
Lymphocytosis
Lack of stress-related neutrophilia
Eosinophilia

2) **Azotemia** is a frequent finding, and is usually prerenal in nature. Both **creatinine** (increased in 65% of cases) and **blood urea nitrogen** (BUN) (increased in 90%) concentrations increase as a result of decreased renal perfusion due to hypovolemia; BUN may be further increased by GI blood loss. Phosphorus is also usually increased in azotemic patients (70% of all Addisonians):

a) Despite the **prerenal** nature of the azotemia, most dogs with hypoadrenocorticism also have a urine-specific gravity <1.030 (frequently <1.020). This is more dilute than would be expected in most patients with prerenal azotemia alone. For this reason, many of these patients are incorrectly thought to be in renal failure. It is imperative that clinicians **consider hypoadrenocorticism as a differential diagnosis in any azotemic dog**, particularly if the dog has a history of gastrointestinal signs.

3) Impaired excretion of acid (H+ions) in the distal tubule results in mild **metabolic acidosis** in half the canine Addisonians.

4) Approximately 15% of Addisonian dogs have **hypoalbuminemia**. Although the mechanism remains to be elucidated, it is likely due to loss through gastrointestinal hemorrhage, impaired gastrointestinal absorption, or decreased hepatic synthesis.

5) Although hypocortisolemia should result in decreased hepatic gluconeogenesis, **hypoglycemia occurs infrequently** (15%) in dogs with hypoadrenocorticism, and is usually subclinical. However, dogs with hypoadrenocorticism have been reported to present for hypoglycemic seizures. **Hypoadrenocorticism should always be a differential diagnosis for an adult dog with severe hypoglycemia.**

6) Total and ionized hypercalcemia occurs frequently, in approximately 30% of hypoadrenocortical dogs (Adamantos et al. 2008). Mild increases in calcium are most common, but severe hypercalcemia is possible. The reason for this hypercalcemia is unclear, but is likely related to decreased renal clearance. Hypoadrenocorticism accounts for anywhere from 5% to 25% of dogs with hypercalcemia; thus, **it should be considered a differential diagnosis in the workup of hypercalcemic dogs.**

7) Decreased hepatic production and gastrointestinal malabsorption are suspected to cause **hypocholesterolemia** in approximately 10% of Addisonian dogs.

8) Hepatic hypoperfusion and cholestasis may play a role in the mild **to moderate increases in alanine aminotransferase (ALT), alkaline phosphatase (ALP), and aspartate aminotransferase (AST)** seen in 20–30% of hypoadrenocortical dogs.

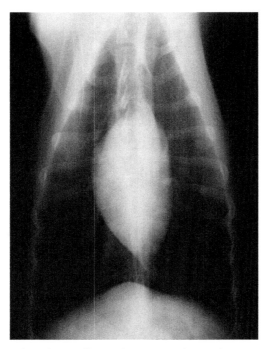

Figure 1.5 Microcardia is a nonspecific indicator of hypovolemia, and is frequently seen in dogs with hypoadrenocorticism.

   b. Complete blood count:
      1) Cortisol released during illness in dogs with normal adrenocortical function often results in the "stress leukogram" of neutrophilia, lymphopenia, monocytosis, and eosinopenia. These changes, particularly lymphopenia, are often absent in dogs with hypoadrenocorticism. Lymphocytosis and eosinophilia, part of the "reverse stress leukogram," are only present occasionally (10% of cases), while the final component, neutropenia, is rarely present. Despite the infrequent occurrence of the reverse stress leukogram, the **absence of a stress leukogram in a sick patient should heighten suspicion of hypoadrenocorticism.**
      2) Approximately 30% of dogs are **anemic** at diagnosis of hypoadrenocorticism, with the proportion increasing to approximately 70% following rehydration. The anemia is typically **normochromic, normocytic, nonregenerative,** and mild. Dogs with more severe anemia almost always have evidence of gastrointestinal blood loss, even if not evident at presentation.
2. Radiographs and ultrasound are often performed in patients that present for gastrointestinal signs, including most patients with hypoadrenocorticism. Although results are generally nonspecific, there are some findings commonly present in Addisonian dogs:
   a. Thoracic radiographs usually reveal nonspecific signs of hypovolemia, including **microcardia and decreased size of the caudal vena cava and pulmonary vessels** (**Figure** 1.5). Megaesophagus may also be seen, as discussed above.
   b. Abdominal radiographs and ultrasound may reveal microhepatica, consistent with hypovolemia. Adrenal gland length and thickness, on average, are lower in Addisonians than in normal dogs (Figure 1.6). However, there is significant overlap between values in normal and Addisonian dogs. One study reported that the length and thickness of the left adrenal in a small group of hypoadreno-cortical dogs was 10.0–19.7 mm (median, 13.1 mm) and 2.2–3.0 mm (median, 2.4 mm), respectively. The same measurements (length, thickness) of the left adrenal in a group of normal dogs were 13.2–26.3 mm (median, 17.4 mm) and 3.0–5.2 mm (median, 4.1 mm). Despite the trend in smaller adrenal gland measurements in hypoadrenocortical patients, the difference in values is not significant enough to definitively differentiate between normal and Addisonian patients.

(a)   (b)

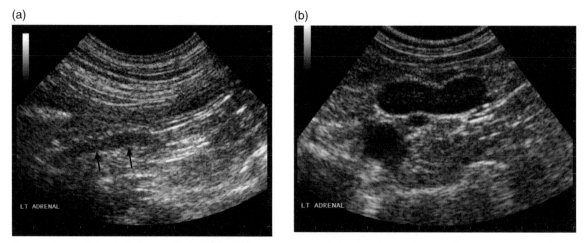

Figure 1.6   (a) Abdominal ultrasound often identifies very small adrenal glands in dogs with hypoadrenocorticism. Note how thin this left adrenal gland is (3.3 mm), compared to the one from a normal dog in (b). (b) Note the peanut shape and width (6.7 mm) of this normal left adrenal gland, compared to the gland from an Addisonian dog in (a). (Images provided by Drs. Erin Brinkman and Erica Baravik.)

3. Specific endocrine tests:
   a. The ACTH stimulation test is required for definitive diagnosis of hypoadrenocorticism. A supraphysiologic dose of ACTH is given to maximally stimulate the adrenal glands (Figure 1.7). In dogs with normally functioning adrenal glands, ACTH stimulation will result in a significant increase in cortisol concentration. In hypoadrenocortical dogs, minimal to no increase in cortisol concentration will occur:
      1) Protocol:
         a) A baseline blood sample is obtained.
         b) Synthetic ACTH (cosyntropin or tetracosactrin), 5 µg/kg (0.005 mg/kg) (up to a maximum of 250 µg/dog) is given, intravenously (Lathan et al. 2008).
         c) A 1 h post-ACTH blood sample is drawn.
         d) Pre- and post-ACTH samples are submitted for cortisol analysis.
         e) Due to inconsistent results, compounded ACTH gel is not recommended for the diagnosis of hypoadrenocorticism.
         f) In canine Addisonian suspects, intravenous administration of cosyntropin is recommended over intramuscular administration due to potentially altered intramuscular absorption in dehydrated and/or hypovolemic patients.
      2) Interpretation of the ACTH stimulation test is based on the value of the post-sample:
         a) **A post-sample of <2.0 µg/dL (55 nmol/L) is consistent with a clinical diagnosis of hypoadrenocorticism.** Lack of response to ACTH stimulation demonstrates that the adrenal cortex is incapable of secreting cortisol, even when stimulated with a much higher amount of ACTH than the body produces:
            i. **The ACTH stimulation test does not differentiate between primary adrenocortical failure and secondary hypoadrenocorticism due to decreased ACTH secretion.** Without the trophic effects of ACTH, the adrenal cortex atrophies, disabling a response to exogenous ACTH. Thus, dogs with primary and secondary hypoadrenocorticism both fail the ACTH stimulation test.
            ii. Patients with iatrogenic hypoadrenocorticism, resulting from acute withdrawal following prolonged administration of exogenous glucocorticoids, will also have a post-stimulation cortisol concentration <2.0 µg/kg (55 nmol/L). However, these patients should be easy to differentiate based on historical evidence of glucocorticoid administration.

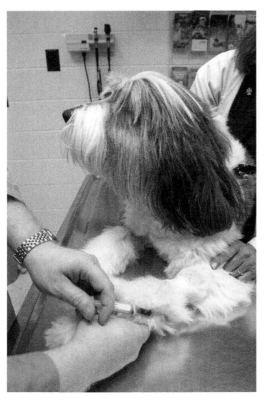

Figure 1.7 An ACTH stimulation test is required for definitive diagnosis of hypoadrenocorticism. In order to avoid problems with absorption, synthetic ACTH (cosyntropin) is given intravenously in Addison's disease suspects.

b) A post-sample >2 μg/dL (55 nmol/L) rules out the clinical diagnosis of hypoadrenocorticism in most patients.

c) Administration of glucocorticoids prior to the ACTH stimulation test can alter the test in two different ways:

i. Several synthetic glucocorticoids, including prednisone and methylprednisolone, cross-react with the cortisol assay. Thus, both the pre- and post-stimulation cortisol concentrations will be falsely elevated following administration of other glucocorticoids. To avoid this, the only glucocorticoids that should be given near the time of the test are dexamethasone and triamcinolone. Short-acting glucocorticoids, such as prednisone or methylprednisolone succinate, should be withheld for 12–24 h before the test. Longer-acting repositol steroids, such as methylprednisolone acetate, may cross-react with the assay for up to 4 weeks following administration. If glucocorticoid supplementation is necessary prior to completion of the ACTH stimulation test, dexamethasone or triamcinolone should be given.

ii. Short-term administration of glucocorticoids within a month of the test may lead to decreased response to ACTH, depending on patient sensitivity, dosage, and duration of treatment. Exogenous glucocorticoid administration (oral or topical) inhibits the release of endogenous ACTH, which causes atrophy of the adrenal cortex. Following removal of the source of exogenous glucocorticoid, the adrenocortical function slowly recovers. However, if an ACTH stimulation test is performed prior to full recovery, the post-stimulation cortisol may be below normal. A post-ACTH cortisol concentration between 2 μg/dL (55 nmol/L) and 5 μg/dL (138 nmol/L) is often the result of recent steroid administration as compared to spontaneous hypoadrenocorticism:

        i) Chronic administration of glucocorticoids may lead to suppression of the hypothalamic pituitary axis (HPA) and subsequent decreased response to ACTH for more than a month following discontinuation of the medication.

    3) For the diagnosis of hypoadrenocorticism, the use of synthetic ACTH (cosyntropin or tetracosactrin) is recommended. Compounded gel formulations are available, but testing results are not as consistent with the gels as they are with synthetic ACTH:

        a) If compounded ACTH gel must be used, it is recommended to obtain two post-stimulation cortisol samples at 1 and 2 h, due to inconsistent results from the use of the gel.

    4) After a 250 µg vial of cosyntropin or tetracosactrin is opened, it can be frozen in plastic syringes and stored for up to 6 months. ACTH binds to glass, so glass syringes should not be used. Freezing in 50 µg aliquots allows dosing for 10 kg dogs with each syringe and minimizes waste. Once thawed, cosyntropin should not be refrozen; a frost-free freezer should NOT be used because of the freeze/thaw cycles.

  b. **A baseline cortisol concentration is a relatively inexpensive way to rule out hypoadrenocorticism.** In almost all patients with hypoadrenocorticism, a baseline cortisol sample will be <2 µg/dL (55 nmol/L) (often <1 µg/mL (28 nmol/L)), so a baseline cortisol sample >2 µg/dL (55 nmol/L) rules out hypoadrenocorticism in a given patient. However, since normal dogs can have baseline cortisol samples <2 µg/dL (55 nmol/L), an ACTH stimulation test MUST be performed to confirm hypoadrenocorticism. **A baseline cortisol concentration can only be used to rule out hypoadrenocorticism— NOT to confirm it:**

    1) In rare cases, a patient with clinical hypoadrenocorticism may have pre- and post-stimulation cortisol values between 2 µg/dL (55 nmol/L) and 3 µg/dL (83 nmol/L). Therefore, strong clinical suspicion of hypoadrenocorticism would mandate an ACTH stimulation test in a dog with baseline values between 2 µg/dL (55 nmol/L) and 3 µg/dL (83 nmol/L).

B. Acute hypoadrenocorticism:

  1. Patients presenting in hypoadrenocortical crisis have similar diagnostic findings as patients with chronic clinical signs (see above). However, abnormalities are often more severe and can be immediately life-threatening (Figure 1.8):

    a. **Hyperkalemia and hyponatremia are often marked in patients in crisis.** Hyponatremia results in weakness, but severe hyperkalemia may be immediately life-threatening. Individual patients vary in susceptibility to the debilitating effects of hyperkalemia, but potassium concentrations less than 7.0 mEq/L generally cause few specific clinical signs. Values between 7.0 and 9 mEq/L result in weakness and moderate to severe cardiac dysfunction, and may be fatal. Values >9.0 mEq/L usually lead to severe cardiac dysfunction and are often fatal:

      1) Cardiac function in these patients should be monitored by electrocardiogram (ECG). Although ECG changes do not correlate exactly with specific potassium concentrations, they tend to appear in the following order, with increasing severity of hyperkalemia:

        a) Increased T-wave amplitude.
        b) Shortened Q–T interval.
        c) Decreased P-wave amplitude.
        d) Prolonged P–R interval.
        e) Absent P-wave (sinoatrial standstill).
        f) Severe bradycardia.
        g) Asystole.
        h) Bizarre QRS complexes, including paroxysmal ventricular tachycardia and ventricular fibrillation, may also be seen.

    b. **Most patients in Addisonian crisis will have significant prerenal azotemia** on presentation, which resolves upon correction of hypovolemia. Severe or prolonged hypovolemia, however, can result in ischemic renal damage secondary to hypoperfusion. If tubular epithelial damage results from the ischemia, renal azotemia may occur; however, with appropriate supportive care most patients fully recover renal function. Severe gastrointestinal blood loss is more common in patients in crisis, and may also lead to more severe azotemia (increased BUN).

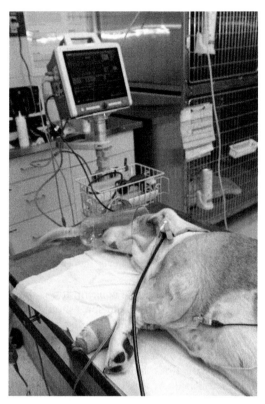

Figure 1.8 Stressful events often precipitate hypoadrenocortical crises. This 8-year-old Bassett hound underwent anesthesia for mass removal from a toe, and collapsed the next day. She presented nonresponsive, in severe hypovolemic shock. Electrocardiogram revealed spiked T-waves and flattened P-waves, the first evidence of hyperkalemia. Preanesthetic serum chemistry (2 days before presentation) revealed a potassium concentration at the high end of normal and normal sodium concentration. Following collapse, her potassium concentration was 8.3 mEq/L, and sodium concentration was still within reference range (143 mEq/L).

    c. Hemogram findings are similar between the chronic and acute presentation. Anemia may be more severe with the acute form due to gastrointestinal blood loss, and is often much more apparent following rehydration. Since patients in hypovolemic shock are severely stressed, **the absence of a stress leukogram in this situation should alert the clinician to consider hypoadrenocorticism.**

C. Atypical hypoadrenocorticism:
    1. Dogs with isolated glucocorticoid deficiency may have any of the same laboratory abnormalities as dogs with combined mineralocorticoid and glucocorticoid deficiency, with the exception of hyperkalemia, hyponatremia, and hypochloremia. However, there are some differences in the frequency and severity of these abnormalities:
        a. Since patients with atypical hypoadrenocorticism are much less likely to present in hypovolemic shock, fewer patients are azotemic. The degree of azotemia is usually less severe than that found in typical Addisonians.
        b. Anemia is more common in dogs with isolated cortisol deficiency. This is most likely because atypical Addisonians are less hemoconcentrated at presentation (when values are taken for use in comparative studies) than typical Addisonians. Atypical patients have lower serum albumin concentrations than typical patients, as well, supporting the hemoconcentration hypothesis.
        c. **Serum cholesterol concentrations are lower in dogs with atypical hypoadrenocorticism.** The explanation for this is not clear; it may reflect the more protracted course of disease prior to diagnosis.

2. Specific endocrine tests:

a. The ACTH stimulation test is required for definitive diagnosis of atypical hypoadrenocorticism; interpretation is the same as for typical hypoadrenocorticism.

b. Although atypical Addison's is an uncommon disease, treatment is simple and inexpensive. Because patients without mineralocorticoid deficiency do not have electrolyte abnormalities, atypical hypoadrenocorticism should be considered in most patients with unexplained gastrointestinal signs, lethargy, weight loss, and polyuria/polydipsia (PU/PD). **Measurement of the baseline cortisol concentration can be very helpful for ruling out hypoadrenocorticism in these patients.**

c. Patients with secondary hypoadrenocorticism and with atypical hypoadrenocorticism have similar clinical signs, due to their shared isolated cortisol deficiency. **Endogenous ACTH levels should be measured to differentiate between primary and secondary hypoadrenocorticism.** High levels indicate that the patient has primary hypoadrenocorticism (due to lack of negative feedback on the pituitary from cortisol), whereas low values are consistent with secondary hypoadrenocorticism. Since secondary hypoadrenocorticism is caused by a pituitary lesion, this information is helpful in directing further diagnostics, such as advanced imaging of the brain, in these cases. Additionally, patients with secondary hypoadrenocorticism should never acquire electrolyte abnormalities, whereas patients with atypical Addison's may.

d. Pre- and post-ACTH stimulation aldosterone concentrations may be measured to help confirm isolated cortisol deficiency. Dogs with atypical Addison's should exhibit an increase in aldosterone concentration following stimulation, while minimal to no increase in aldosterone concentration is suggestive of a combined mineralocorticoid and glucocorticoid deficiency:

1) Unfortunately, interpretation of post-stimulation aldosterone concentrations is not straightforward, as cut-off values between dogs that will develop electrolyte abnormalities and dogs that will not, have not been established. At this time, it appears that dogs with normal electrolyte concentrations, but minimal increase in aldosterone concentration following ACTH stimulation, may be at risk of developing electrolyte abnormalities in the near future.

V. Differential Diagnoses

A. Chronic and acute hypoadrenocorticism

The differential diagnoses for Addison's disease include conditions leading to **hyperkalemia** and **hyponatremia, gastrointestinal signs,** and **azotemia** (Table 1.3). Focusing on the causes of hyperkalemia and hyponatremia is usually most beneficial, as there are fewer rule-outs than for gastrointestinal disease and azotemia:

1. **Patients with Addison's disease are commonly misdiagnosed with acute renal failure (ARF) due to the overlap of clinical signs and diagnostic findings.** Gastrointestinal signs often accompany ARF due to the stimulation of the chemoreceptor trigger zone by uremic toxins. ARF may also result in hyponatremia and hyperkalemia in oliguric and anuric dogs. Azotemia is present in most patients with hypoadrenocorticism and all patients with ARF. Usually, prerenal causes of azotemia are differentiated from renal causes by evaluation of the urine-specific gravity. Dogs with renal azotemia lose the capacity to concentrate urine, so the urine is typically isosthenuric (1.008–1.012). In most dogs with prerenal azotemia, urine concentrating ability is maintained, and the urine specific gravity (USG) is >1.030, an appropriate response to dehydration.

In many dogs with Addison's disease, however, the USG is <1.020, despite the absence of underlying renal disease. Thus, clinicians may inadvertently believe that a dog with Addison's disease actually has ARF. Considering that the prognosis for a patient with hypoadrenocorticism is usually good, whereas prognosis for ARF is variable, misdiagnosis may not only delay appropriate treatment, but may sway the owners toward euthanasia.

There are several ways to differentiate the two diseases. The first is to perform an ACTH stimulation test; unfortunately, results are not generally available immediately or during emergency hours.

Practically speaking, **dogs with hypoadrenocorticism respond to fluid therapy much more quickly than dogs with renal failure.** Azotemia typically decreases within the first 12–24 h, and the dog's clinical

Table 1.3   Differential diagnoses.

Differential diagnoses for hyperkalemia and hyponatremia

Hypoadrenocorticism

Acute renal failure

Urinary tract obstruction/uroabdomen

Trichuriasis

Severe gastrointestinal disease

Peritoneal effusion

Chylothorax

Diabetic ketoacidosis

Congestive heart failure

Hepatic failure/cirrhosis

Primary polydipsia

Inappropriate anti-diuretic hormone (ADH) secretion

Mannitol administration

Hypothyroid myxedema

Massive tissue trauma

- Crush injury
- Aortic thromboembolism
- Rhabdomyolysis

Diuretic administration

- Furosemide
- Spironolactone

ACE-inhibitor administration

Metabolic acidosis

Pregnancy

Artifacts

- Erythrocyte lysis in Japanese breeds
- Marked thrombocytosis
- Marked leukocytosis

The conditions highlighted in gray represent the most common differential diagnoses in dogs with hyponatremia and hyperkalemia that are later diagnosed with hypoadrenocorticism.

condition often improves within the first 2 h. Additionally, hyperkalemia and hyponatremia rarely occur in dogs with ARF unless anuria or oliguria is present following rehydration. Thus, if the patient is producing an adequate amount of urine following rehydration, the hyperkalemia and hyponatremia are much less likely to be caused by ARF. Occasionally, oliguria or anuria is misdiagnosed in an Addisonian patient. The most common reason for this is failure to allow for adequate rehydration prior to determining whether urine output is adequate.

2. **Urinary tract obstruction** and **uroabdomen** often result in hyperkalemia, hyponatremia, and potentially abdominal pain, and should be ruled out in Addisonian suspects.

3. Dogs suffering from **whipworm infestation** may also have hyperkalemia, hyponatremia, vomiting, and diarrhea, in addition to melena ("pseudohypoadrenocorticism"). For this reason, all patients with suspected hypoadrenocorticism should have a fecal examination performed. It is also possible for a dog to have both hypoadrenocorticism and whipworm infection, causing more severe disease than either alone:

  a. **Severe gastrointestinal disease** from other causes (Ancylostomiasis, Coccidiosis, idiopathic hemorrhagic gastroenteritis) may also lead to pseudohypoadrenocorticism.

4. Other reported causes of concurrent hyperkalemia and hyponatremia include **peritoneal effusion, chylothorax, congestive heart failure, pregnancy, and severe acidosis**.

B. Atypical hypoadrenocorticism:

1. Most patients with atypical hypoadrenocorticism present for gastrointestinal signs, and may have hypocholesterolemia and hypoalbuminemia. Thus, other causes of GI disease with malabsorption, such as **inflammatory bowel disease** and **lymphangiectasia**, are often considered concurrently. Additionally, since signs are often exacerbated following a stressful event, dogs with hypoadrenocorticism may be thought to have **"stress colitis"** or **hemorrhagic gastroenteritis**. It is imperative that atypical Addison's disease be considered in these cases so that it is not missed.

2. Some dogs with **polyuria and polydipsia** are also eventually diagnosed with atypical hypoadrenocorticism, and PU/PD may be their only presenting complaint. The potential differential diagnoses are too extensive to list here, but hypoadrenocorticism should remain on the list of differential diagnoses for patients with polyuria and polydipsia.

VI. Treatment

A. Chronic hypoadrenocorticism:

1. Treatment of combined cortisol and aldosterone deficiency requires lifelong glucocorticoid and mineralocorticoid supplementation. Chronic therapy is started in patients that do not present in crisis, and following stabilization of those patients that do:

  a. Mineralocorticoids are given to control hyperkalemia, hyponatremia, and hypochloremia. Either a twice daily pill, fludrocortisone, or a monthly injection, desoxycorticosterone **pivalate** (DOCP), can be used for mineralocorticoid supplementation:

  1) DOCP is a long-acting injectable mineralocorticoid with no glucocorticoid activity. It is initially administered at a dose of 2.2 mg/kg, subcutaneously or intramuscularly, every 25 days:

   a) Adjustment of dose and dosing interval are based on electrolyte concentrations measured at specific times following administration:

   i. Electrolytes are first rechecked 2 weeks after the injection. Dosage of the FOLLOWING injection will be adjusted based on these values:

    i) If sodium and potassium concentrations are within the reference range, the dose remains the same.

    ii) If hyponatremia or hyperkalemia is present, dose should be increased by about 10%.

    iii) If hypernatremia or hypokalemia is present, dose should be decreased by about 10%.

    iv) In small patients (5 kg or less), doses may be adjusted by up to 25% at a time.

    v) If it is determined that the dose should be increased, measurement of electrolytes at day 25 is recommended to ensure that electrolyte values are not dangerously altered. However, adjustment of dose interval (see below) is postponed until after the following injection.

   ii. Dosing interval is determined by measurement of electrolytes on day 25:

    i) If sodium and potassium concentrations are within reference range, the dosing interval should remain the same, and the injection is to be given every 25 days.

    ii) If hyponatremia or hyperkalemia is present, the dosing interval should be decreased by 1–2 days, and the next injection should be given in 23–24 days.

iii) If hypernatremia or hypokalemia are present, the dosing interval should be increased by 1–2 days, and the next injection should be given in 26–27 days.

iv) Following each dosing interval change, the interval should be adjusted based on electrolyte concentrations measured prior to the next DOCP administration, as described above.

iii. Electrolytes should be rechecked at the above intervals each time the dose or dosing interval is changed, and then every 3–6 months thereafter.

iv. DOCP is an expensive medication, and owners will frequently ask for ways to decrease the cost. If electrolyte concentrations are normal on the day of the injection, the interval may be increased by 2 days, up until the interval is 30 days (or approximately once per month). This helps decrease expense and also helps owners remember the date of the next injection:

i) Although some dogs may only require injections every 6 weeks, monthly injections are recommended in order to help establish a consistent routine for the owner. Longer dose intervals are acceptable, but may result in decreased owner compliance.

v. Another way to decrease expense is to decrease the total dose. Some dogs do well on 1 mg/kg/month. However, the starting dose should be 2.2 mg/kg, and the dose decreased slowly (10% at a time) as long as electrolyte concentrations remain in the reference range immediately prior to the next injection. Use of this protocol saves money; however, using a lower dose leaves less room for error on the dosing interval. **It is imperative that owners wishing to use a lower dose adhere tightly to the dosing schedule.**

vi. The potential cost savings associated with prolonging the dose interval and/or decreasing the dose must be weighed against the expenses associated with the required monitoring following each adjustment. These adjustments are much more cost-effective for larger patients.

vii. Some owners will attempt to decrease cost by extending the dosing interval themselves. **Owners must be sternly warned that doing this increases the chances of their dog going into Addisonian crisis, which will most definitely be more costly, and potentially result in the death of their pet.**

b) Subcutaneous administration results in good control in most patients. However, there are occasional patients whose electrolyte values do not correct as expected. This may be due to an absorption problem. Most of these patients respond well to intramuscular injection.

c) There are few side effects of DOCP, although polyuria and polydipsia have been reported. It is less common with DOCP than with fludrocortisone, and may actually be due to the prednisone that the dog is on concurrently. However, if PU/PD are suspected to be due to the DOCP, decreasing the dose may decrease or eliminate this side effect.

d) All patients receiving DOCP will need additional daily glucocorticoid supplementation.

2) Fludrocortisone is a shorter-acting oral mineralocorticoid with some glucocorticoid activity. The initial dose is 0.02 mg/kg/day, divided:

a) The dose is adjusted based on weekly electrolyte concentrations, until the dose stabilizes:

i. If the patient's electrolyte values are within reference range, the dose is maintained.

ii. If hyperkalemia or hyponatremia is present, the dose is increased by 0.05–0.1 mg/day.

iii. If hypokalemia or hypernatremia is present, the dose is decreased by 0.05–0.1 mg/day.

iv. If mild hyponatremia is present without concurrent hyperkalemia, salting the food at a dose of 0.1 mg/kg/day may help. Salting is not usually necessary long term, however.

b) Once the dose has stabilized, electrolytes should be rechecked every 3–6 months. The dose frequently needs to be increased within the first 1.5 years of therapy.

c) Polyuria, polydipsia, and less frequently polyphagia, panting, and hair loss are reported in some dogs on fludrocortisone. These signs can usually be attributed to the glucocorticoid properties of fludrocortisone, and should resolve if the patient is switched to DOCP (with concurrent prednisone).

    b. Glucocorticoid supplementation usually controls the nonspecific and gastrointestinal signs of hypoadrenocorticism. Prednisone is the most frequently used glucocorticoid. The physiologic dosage of prednisone is 0.1–0.25 mg/kg/day:

      1) The prednisone dose is titrated "to effect," according to clinical signs. The dose is increased if lethargy, anorexia, vomiting, diarrhea, or melena occurs. The client is instructed to pay close attention to the dog's attitude, and the dose should be increased if the dog is not "acting herself." The dose is decreased if side effects of glucocorticoid excess are present, such as PU/PD, polyphagia, or panting.

      2) The prednisone dose needs to be increased by 2–10 times when the dog is in a stressful situation. This may include any trips to the veterinarian (such as to check electrolytes), new visitors in the home, a new addition to the household, vacation, etc. The increased dose is started the day or morning prior to the beginning of the stressful event, and continued for a day or two afterward. With time and guidance, the client should be able to determine the optimal dose for the patient in times of stress:

        i. Remember that **any unrelated illness places additional physiologic stress on the patient and will require additional glucocorticoid administration.**

        ii. It must also be noted that an **increase in clinical signs, such as vomiting or diarrhea, suggests that the prednisone dose needs to be increased.** Physiologic doses of prednisone should not cause gastric ulceration or other gastrointestinal side effects, so gastrointestinal signs usually mandate an increase in prednisone dose.

      3) Whereas fludrocortisone has some glucocorticoid activity, DOCP does not. Thus, **all patients on DOCP need daily glucocorticoid supplementation**, whereas about half of the patients on fludrocortisone do not:

        i. Dogs taking fludrocortisone should be started on 0.1 mg/kg/day of prednisone, divided BID or once daily. At the 1 week electrolyte recheck examination, the dose may be decreased by 50% if signs of cortisol deficiency (such as gastrointestinal signs or lethargy) are not present. It may be discontinued if these signs are still absent 1 week later. The dose should be increased at any point when signs of cortisol deficiency return, and the dose should be increased during stressful situations, as described above.

B. Acute hypoadrenocorticism:

    1. An Addisonian crisis is an immediately life-threatening condition that requires rapid intervention. **The initial goals of treatment are in order of importance to correct hypovolemia, hyperkalemia, and associated arrhythmias, hypoglycemia, acidosis, and hypercalcemia, if present:**

      a. **Aggressive intravenous fluid resuscitation is the first priority,** as it corrects hypovolemia, hyponatremia, hypochloremia, and most cases of hyperkalemia and metabolic acidosis. One-third to one-half of the shock volume (90 mL/kg) of an isotonic replacement crystalloid should be given initially. Response should be assessed based on heart rate, pulse quality/blood pressure, capillary refill time, and mental status. Additional fluids should then be given if necessary:

        1) Because of the high sodium and chloride content, and lack of potassium, 0.9% NaCl has traditionally been recommended as the fluid of choice for treating patients in adrenocortical crisis. However, Normosol-R and lactated Ringer's solution (LRS) are preferred by some clinicians. The low potassium content in these fluids still allows for correction of hyperkalemia, and they correct acidosis more quickly that 0.9% saline.

        2) Hetastarch (hydroxyethyl starch) may also be used for treatment of hypovolemic shock, particularly in hypoalbuminemic patients. A dose of 5–10 mL/kg is given as a bolus with the initial bolus of crystalloids for more rapid fluid resuscitation.

        3) **Care should be taken not to increase the sodium concentration more than 0.5 mEq/h (12 mEq/day) in patients with hyponatremia.** An abrupt change in extracellular sodium concentration (and subsequent osmolality) may lead to myelinolysis and neurologic signs. Hypertonic saline should NEVER be used to treat a patient in Addisonian crisis.

      b. If hypoglycemia is suspected or proven, an IV dose of 1 mL/kg of 25% dextrose in saline (a 1:1 mixture of 50% dextrose and 0.9% saline) should be administered. This should be followed by a

1.25–5% solution of dextrose in the patient's crystalloid fluids. Five percent dextrose (D5W) should not be given, as the fluid becomes hypotonic after the dextrose is metabolized, resulting in inadequate intravascular fluid expansion.

c. **Fluid therapy alone is usually adequate to treat the hyperkalemia.** However, in cases of severe hyperkalemia (>9.0 mEq/L) and/or life-threatening arrhythmias (severe bradycardia, absent P-wave, idioventricular rhythm), specific therapy is indicated:

    1) **Calcium gluconate is administered for its cardioprotective effects,** which are rapid and will often maintain the patient's life while allowing time for fluids and other therapies to take effect. It does not, however, decrease the potassium concentrations. 0.5–1.5 mL/kg of calcium gluconate is given slowly over 15 min, while monitoring the ECG for new arrhythmias (such as shortened Q-T interval) and further decreased heart rate due to calcium administration. Administration should be stopped if new arrhythmias occur.

    2) Intravenous regular insulin may also be given in concert with dextrose to drive potassium intracellularly. 0.2–0.5 U/kg of regular insulin is given, followed by 2 g of dextrose (diluted to 25% in an isotonic crystalloid) per unit of insulin administered. Blood glucose concentration should then be monitored and dextrose should be added to the replacement fluids to produce a 1.25–2.5% dextrose solution.

d. **Glucocorticoid deficiency may contribute to the hypotension seen in dogs in crisis,** and is also responsible for the hypoglycemia, gastrointestinal signs, and general debility. Supplementation should be implemented following initiation of therapy for hyperkalemia and hypovolemia. Dexamethasone sodium phosphate, at a dose of 0.25 mg/kg IV, is recommended. Since it has 7–8 times the glucocorticoid activity as prednisone, this is equivalent to 2 mg/kg of prednisone, or 10 times the physiologic dose:

    1) Other glucocorticoids, such as hydrocortisone sodium succinate (0.5 mg/kg/h) and prednisolone sodium succinate (2 mg/kg), have also been recommended. Hydrocortisone is an ester of cortisol, with equivalent glucocorticoid and mineralocorticoid activity:

        i. Most synthetic glucocorticoids, with the exception of dexamethasone and triamcinolone, interfere with the cortisol assay. Thus, only these glucocorticoids should be given prior to completing the ACTH stimulation test. This advantage and its availability make dexamethasone the author's glucocorticoid of choice for treating an Addisonian crisis.

        ii. Although dexamethasone and triamcinolone do not interfere with the cortisol assay, they do inhibit ACTH release, resulting in adrenocortical suppression. Administration of even a single dose of 0.1 mg/kg of dexamethasone can result in decreased cortisol response to ACTH administration for 3 or more days. However, post-stimulation cortisol concentrations should not be less than 2 μg/dL (55 nmol/L), as seen in clinical hypoadrenocorticism, following a single dose. Administration of multiple doses of dexamethasone, or chronic administration, will result in adrenocortical atrophy and decreased cortisol concentration following ACTH stimulation for a longer period of time, and could lead to iatrogenic hypoadrenocorticism.

e. Additional **supportive therapy** should be provided as necessary. For example, dogs with gastrointestinal signs (vomiting, diarrhea, and melena) are given **gastroprotectants**, including H_2-blockers and sucralfate. Due to the potential for bacterial translocation from the GI tract, the author also administers prophylactic ampicillin, although this is controversial. Some dogs have such severe GI blood loss that packed red blood cell or whole blood transfusion is necessary.

f. Following initial stabilization, frequent reassessment is necessary. Fluid rates should be adjusted to correct dehydration and azotemia, while keeping up with maintenance requirements and ongoing losses. Electrolyte values should be rechecked following fluid resuscitation, and then frequently (q 6–12 h) until the potassium and sodium concentrations stabilize. Too rapid correction of hyponatremia should be avoided.

g. Following definitive diagnosis of hypoadrenocorticism, mineralocorticoid supplementation should be provided. Intravenous therapy is continued until the dog is able to eat and maintain hydration on her own:

1) Since correcting hyponatremia too rapidly can result in myelinolysis, mineralocorticoid supplementation should be postponed until the sodium concentration is closer to normal (approximately 132 mEq/L) in patients with severe hyponatremia.

h. Dexamethasone or another parenteral glucocorticoid is continued at a dose of 0.2 mg/kg/day until prednisone is tolerated. Prednisone is then administered at 1 mg/kg divided BID until the patient leaves the hospital, after which it is slowly tapered to physiologic dose:

1) **Most patients respond quickly to therapy and dramatically improve within hours.** However, more debilitated patients, particularly the ones with severe hyperkalemia, may take 2–3 days to see great improvement. Dogs are usually hospitalized for 3–5 days following an Addisonian crisis.

C. Atypical hypoadrenocorticism:

1. Dogs with isolated cortisol deficiency require only glucocorticoid supplementation. Prednisone is initially given at 0.1–0.25 mg/kg/day. Dose titration is the same as described above. **The goal is to give enough prednisone to control the dog's clinical signs of hypoadrenocorticism, but not so much as to cause side effects of glucocorticoid supplementation.** Additional prednisone (2–10 times the normal dose) must be given prior to stressful events.

2. **Some dogs with atypical hypoadrenocorticism will develop mineralocorticoid deficiency following initial diagnosis.** In two studies (Lifton et al. 1996; Thompson et al. 2007), only 3 out of 29 dogs with isolated cortisol deficiency developed mineralocorticoid deficiency, from 3 weeks to 7 months following initial diagnosis. However, another case series suggests that over half of these dogs will develop mineralocorticoid deficiency at a later time. At this time, it is impossible to determine which dogs will do so. Thus, vigilant monitoring by the owner is imperative. Reevaluation of electrolytes at 1 and 3 months following initial diagnosis, and then every 6 months thereafter, seems prudent in these cases:

a. **Patients with secondary hypoadrenocorticism are glucocorticoid deficient only**, requiring prednisone administration as described above. Unlike dogs with atypical hypoadrenocorticism, these patients should never develop electrolyte abnormalities.

VII. Prognosis

A. With prompt diagnosis and appropriate treatment, the prognosis for patients with naturally occurring hypoadrenocorticism is excellent, and patients usually enjoy a good quality and normal span of life. The need for consistent treatment and patient monitoring must be stressed to owners, as skipping medication or prolonging the treatment interval for DOCP (without direction from a veterinarian) may lead to hypoadrenocortical crisis.

B. With prompt diagnosis and appropriate treatment, the prognosis for patients with iatrogenic hypoadrenocorticism is also excellent. The hypoadrenocorticism may be transient or permanent, depending on the cause.

VIII. Prevention

A. At this time, it is not possible to prevent idiopathic primary hypoadrenocorticism in most dogs. However, selective breeding may help decrease the prevalence in some breeds in which the mode of inheritance has been determined, such as the Standard Poodle, Portuguese water dog, and Nova Scotia Duck-tolling retriever.

References and Further Readings

Adamantos S, Boag A. Total and ionised calcium concentrations in dogs with hypoadrenocorticism. *Vet Rec* 2008; 163(1):25–26.

Adler JA, Drobatz KJ, Hess RS. Abnormalities of serum electrolyte concentrations in dogs with hypoadrenocorticism. *J Vet Intern Med* 2007;21:1168–1173.

Herrtage ME. Hypoadrenocorticism. In: Ettinger SJ, ed. *Textbook of Veterinary Internal Medicine*, 5th edn. Philadelphia: Saunders, 2000, pp. 1612–1622.

Lathan P, Moore GE, Zambon S, Scott-Moncrieff JC. Use of a low-dose ACTH stimulation test for diagnosis of hypoadrenocorticism in dogs. *JVIM* 2008;22:1070–1073.

Lifton SL, King LG, Zerbe CA. Glucocorticoid deficient hypoadrenocorticism in dogs: 18 cases (1986–1995). *JAVMA* 1996;209:2076–2081.

Melian C, Peterson ME. Diagnosis and treatment of naturally occurring hypoadrenocorticism in 42 dogs. *JSAP* 1996;37:268–275.

Peterson ME, Kintzer PP, Kass PH. Pretreatment clinical and laboratory findings in dogs with hypoadrenocorticism: 225 cases (1979–1993). *JAVMA* 1996;208(1):85–91.

Schaer M, Chen CL. A clinical survey of 48 dogs with adrenocortical hypofunction. JAAHA 1983;19:443–452.

Thompson AL, Scott-Moncrieff JC, Anderson JD. Comparison of classic hypoadrenocorticism with glucocorticoid-deficient hypoadrenocorticism in dogs: 46 cases (1985–2005). *JAVMA* 2007;230:1190–1194.

Willard MD, Schall WD, McCaw DE, Nachreiner RF. **Canine hypoadrenocorticism: Report of 37 cases and review of 39 previously reported cases.** *JAVMA* **1982;180:59–62.**

CHAPTER 2

Hypoadrenocorticism in Cats

Danièlle Gunn-Moore and Kerry Simpson

Pathogenesis

- Hypoadrenocorticism is caused by a deficiency of glucocorticoids and/or mineralocorticoids.

Classical Signs and Diagnosis

- Weakness, lethargy, depression, and anorexia.
- Hyperkalemia (Table 2.1), hyponatremia, abnormal Na:K ratio.
- Lack of response to ACTH stimulation, high endogenous ACTH concentration.

Treatment and Prognosis

- Supplementation with glucocorticoids and/or mineralocorticoids.
- Excellent prognosis.

I. Pathogenesis

A. **Overview of Hypoadrenocorticism**—The adrenal cortex is responsible for the production of **mineralocorticoids** (from the zona glomerulosa) and **glucocorticoids** (from the zonae fasciculata and reticularis):

    1. The secretion of aldosterone from the zona glomerulosa is a complex process, predominantly influenced by potassium and angiotensin II and to a lesser extent by sodium and circulating concentrations of adrenocorticotrophic hormone (ACTH), whereas glucocorticoid secretion is influenced almost exclusively by the release of ACTH. Glucocorticoids have an inhibitory influence on the release of ACTH, thereby regulating the plasma levels via negative feedback.

    2. **Hypoadrenocorticism** results from a **deficiency of glucocorticoids and/or mineralocorticoids**. This can occur as a result of either destruction of the adrenal cortex—**primary hypoadrenocorticism**—or a deficiency in the production of ACTH from the anterior pituitary, **secondary hypoadrenocorticism**.

B. **Primary hypoadrenocorticism arises from destruction of the adrenal cortex**. This is most commonly idiopathic or presumed to be immune mediated. Less common causes include infiltrative diseases such as lymphoma, amyloidosis or granulomatous disease, hemorrhagic infarction, and iatrogenic destruction:

    1. The lack of cortisol decreases the negative feedback on the pituitary, so the **circulating concentration of ACTH is increased**.

Clinical Endocrinology of Companion Animals, First Edition. Edited by Jacquie Rand.
© 2013 John Wiley & Sons, Inc. Published 2013 by John Wiley & Sons, Inc.

Table 2.1   Main differential diagnoses for hyperkalemia in the cat.

	Differential diagnosis
Hyperkalemia	**Decreased loss** Urethral obstruction Urinary tract rupture Anuric/oliguric renal failure Hypoadrenocorticism **Translocation from intracellular fluid** Reperfusion syndrome Acute acidosis Insulin deficiency Tumor lysis syndrome Hemolysis

2. For adrenal insufficiency to occur, it is believed that at least 90% of the adrenal cortex must be destroyed. As this is generally a gradual process, a partial insufficiency may initially occur, characterized by inadequate adrenal reserve. In such cases, basal hormone secretion may be adequate, but lack of adrenal reserve results in an inability to respond to stress.

3. The **lack of mineralocorticoid** results in an **inability to conserve sodium,** which can rapidly become deplete in animals which have decreased dietary intake due to anorexia or increased loss due to vomiting or diarrhea. Sodium depletion results in a **decreased circulating blood volume and hypotension.** In addition, the lack of aldosterone results in **potassium retention** and **myocardial hyperexcitability** (the resting membrane potential is shifted to a less negative value, closer to the threshold potential, and repolarization time is shortened). Concurrent hypoxia, acidosis, and hyponatremia further increase the myocardial irritability and the risk of arrhythmia.

4. **Glucocorticoid deficiency** results in impaired gluconeogenesis, hepatic glycogen depletion, impaired fat metabolism, and gastrointestinal signs including, vomiting, anorexia, and abdominal pain.

5. Typically, as all the layers of the adrenal cortex are affected, there are deficiencies of both mineralocorticoids and glucocorticoids. However, occasionally the zona glomerulosa function remains intact so the classical electrolyte alterations are not seen; this is known as "atypical" hypoadrenocorticism.

C. Secondary hypoadrenocorticism is most commonly associated with the **administration of drugs, such as corticosteroids or progestogens,** which suppress ACTH synthesis and/or release. However, it can also be the **result of an underlying hypothalamic-pituitary disorder** such as a tumor, trauma, or a congenital defect:

1. The **decreased ACTH production** results in decreased production of glucocorticoids and atrophy of the zonae reticularis and fasciculata. However, mineralocorticoid production is relatively unaffected as ACTH plays only a minor role in the production of aldosterone. Therefore, the clinical features of secondary hypoadrenocorticism are similar to those seen in "atypical" primary hypoadrenocorticism; that is, the electrolyte imbalances do not occur.

D. Hypoadrenocorticism in cats:

1. **Primary hypoadrenocorticism is a rare disorder in cats;** there have been fewer than 40 cases described as either case reports/series or in textbooks. **The majority have been idiopathic, although two were secondary to neoplastic infiltration of the adrenal glands and one occurred following trauma.**

2. **Iatrogenic cases of secondary hypoadrenocorticism have been described following the administration of either exogenous corticosteroids or megestrol acetate,** but no cases of naturally occurring secondary hypoadrenocorticism have been described. Typically, hypoadrenocorticism is evident based on ACTH stimulation testing, but clinical signs (lethargy, inappetence) are rarely reported; if clinical signs are present, they are more often referable to iatrogenic hyperadrenocorticism. Suppression of the adrenal cortex can be prolonged and requires as long as 4 months to recover from even one dose of long-acting steroid, for example, methylprednisolone.

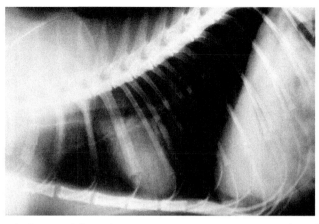

Figure 2.1   Thoracic radiograph of a cat with hypoadrenocorticism: Demonstrating microcardia and hypoperfusion. (From Tasker et al., 1999. With permission.)

II. Signalment

A. **In cats, primary hypoadrenocorticism** has been reported in a wide range of ages, **from 18 months to 14 years,** and the majority have been in either domestic short- or long-haired cats; one case has been described in a British short-haired cat. There appears to be no gender predisposition in cats, which is in marked contrast to dogs, where approximately 70% of cases occur in females.

III. Clinical Signs

A. Owners have reported that clinical signs have been present from as few as 1–2 days or as long as 3–4 months.

B. The most common clinical sings include **lethargy, depression, anorexia, and weight loss,** although, collapse, dysphagia, weakness, vomiting, polyuria, and polydipsia have also been reported. Clinical signs typically wax and wane, and often respond temporarily to symptomatic treatment with intravenous (IV) fluid therapy and/or corticosteroid administration.

IV. Diagnosis

A. **Hematological abnormalities** are not commonly reported, but have included mild normocytic normochromic nonregenerative anemia, lymphocytosis, and eosinophilia.

B. **Alterations in serum biochemistry** typically include azotemia and hyperphosphatemia, but occasionally involve mild increases in alanine aminotransferase, alkaline phosphatase, and total bilirubin:

  1. The **azotemia is generally prerenal in origin,** as a result of dehydration.

  2. However, **urine specific gravity is rarely above 1.030.** Although the inability to concentrate urine is not fully understood, it is thought to be the result of the hyponatremia, which leads to medullary wash-out and potentially interferes with the release of vasopressin.

  3. Approximately one third of cats tested have had a **decreased total CO_2** reflecting a metabolic acidosis, which is principally thought to result from the loss of the action of aldosterone on renal tubular hydrogen ion secretion.

  4. **Serum electrolyte alterations include hyponatremia, hyperkalemia, and abnormal serum sodium: potassium ratio.** Occasionally, hypochloremia and either hypo- or hypercalcemia have been reported.

C. **Thoracic radiography** may reveal **microcardia and hypoperfusion of the lungs** (Figure 2.1).

D. **Electrocardiographic (ECG) abnormalities** include **sinus bradycardia** and **atrial premature complexes.** However, these alterations have only been reported in a small number of cats:

  1. The **classical ECG alterations** associated with hyperkalemia (i.e., spiking of the T wave, shortening of the Q–T interval, prolongation of the P wave, PR interval and QRS complex) **have not been reported in cats with hypoadrenocorticism.** Why these changes have not been seen is unclear, but may reflect relatively mild hyperkalemia (the highest reported potassium level being 7.6 mmol/L).

Table 2.2   Testing cats with suspected hypoadrenocorticism.

Test	Protocol	Interpretation
IM test	Collect baseline blood sample for cortisol concentration. Inject ACTH gel (2.2 U/kg). Collect further samples at 1 h and 2 h	Low or low-normal baseline cortisol concentration with minimal response to ACTH gel administration
IV test	Collect baseline blood sample for cortisol concentration. Inject 125 µg of synthetic ACTH (cosyntropin or tetracosactrin). Collect further samples at 30 min and 1 h	Low or low-normal baseline cortisol concentration with minimal response to ACTH gel administration
ACTH conc.	Collect blood sample into EDTA; centrifuge and freeze plasma in plastic tube. Ship frozen	Demonstration of an elevated ACTH concentration in a cat with hypoadrenocorticism confirms primary disease

IM—intramuscular; IV—intravenous; ACTH conc.—endogenous ACTH concentration.

E. The **ACTH stimulation test** is the "gold standard" for diagnosis of hypoadrenocorticism in cats (Table 2.2). However, a range of protocols have been reported:

1. A study to compare the effect of administering cosyntropin by IV and intramuscular (IM) routes demonstrated higher peak levels of both ACTH and cortisol, and a longer duration of adrenocortical stimulation after IV administration. Peak cortisol concentration was obtained 60–90 min after IV administration.

2. A separate study assessed the effect of two synthetic corticotropin preparations (tetracosactrin and cosyntropin) in healthy cats; again mean plasma cortisol concentration reached a peak and plateaued between 60 and 120 min, then gradually decreased over 5 h.

3. This contrasts with a further study where IV tetracosactrin produced a significant rise in plasma cortisol level by 60 min, but the peak was not achieved until 180 min, and levels were still significantly elevated 5 h post injection.

4. It is unclear why these studies demonstrated such differing times to peak cortisol concentration, however, it remains that two studies demonstrated a significant increase in cortisol 60 min after corticotropin administration, although the time to peak response showed some variability between cats.

5. The dose–response relationship between cortisol and incremental doses of cosyntropin (1.25–125 µg IV) has also been evaluated in normal cats. These studies showed that while all doses produced a significant increase in plasma cortisol, this effect was prolonged at higher doses. Therefore, the **higher dose (125 µg) of cosyntropin** is recommended for cats.

6. A **synthetic ACTH gel preparation** (Repository Corticotropin Injection, USP, Organics/LaGrange Inc., Chicago, Illinois) has also been evaluated for use in cats. A dose of 2.2 mg/kg administered by IM injection resulted in a peak cortisol response within 1–2 h.

7. From these studies **two regimes for ACTH stimulation testing** have been proposed in cats, these are summarized in Table 2.1.

F. **Plasma endogenous ACTH:**

1. In cases of **primary hypoadrenocorticism**, plasma **ACTH is elevated**; of the cases reported, ACTH ranged from 500–8000 pg/mL (reference range: <10–125 pg/mL). Demonstration of an elevated ACTH in a cat with an inappropriate response to ACTH stimulation testing confirms destruction of the adrenal cortex. However, a **similar pattern** can be obtained from cases which are receiving drugs such as **ketoconazole**, which blocks the synthesis of cortisol.

2. Cats treated chronically with glucocorticoids or progestogens (such as megestrol acetate) can have low or undetectable cortisol levels at baseline and on stimulation. However, these drugs block the production of ACTH; hence **endogenous ACTH is low**, confirming **secondary hypoadrenocorticism**.

V. Differential Diagnosis

See Table 2.1 for the most common differential diagnoses for hyperkalemia in the cat which is the most consistent finding in cats with hypoadrenocorticism.

VI. Treatment

A. If a cat presents in a hypoadrenal crisis, the initial therapy should aim at restoring the circulating blood volume, providing a source of glucocorticoid and correcting serum electrolyte disturbances:

1. Aggressive IV administration of isotonic **fluid therapy** should be given; ideally with 0.9% sodium chloride. This is given at 40 mL/kg/h for the first 1–2 h until circulatory volume has been restored, then decreased to 60 mL/kg/q 24 h and tapered over the next few days as the electrolyte abnormalities resolve and the cat begins to maintain its own hydration.

2. **Glucocorticoid** deficits should be addressed by the administration of **IV dexamethasone** (0.1–2 mg/kg). Ideally, an ACTH stimulation test should be performed prior to the administration of any glucocorticoid; however, low doses of dexamethasone do not interfere with concurrent ACTH stimulation testing. Once the cat can swallow, glucocorticoid replacement can be given orally, as prednisolone (0.2 mg/kg/q 24 h).

3. **Mineralocorticoid replacement** with fludrocortisone acetate (0.05–0.1 mg/PO q 12–24 h) can be instigated once the cat can swallow. Alternatively, repositol desoxycorticosterone pivalate (DOCP) can be administered by IM injection to provide chronic mineralocorticoid support. Reported doses vary from 12.5 mg/cat every month or 2.2 mg/kg every 25 days. In some countries, desoxycorticosterone acetate (DOCA) is available in oil as a long-acting preparation (not to be confused with the short-acting preparation).

4. **Cats with hypoadrenocorticism typically respond more slowly to treatment than dogs**, with weakness, anorexia, and lethargy persisting for 3–5 days despite correct management.

5. Cats diagnosed with hypoadrenocorticism require **lifelong medication**. The dose of mineralocorticoid should be adjusted as necessary based on the results of serum electrolyte testing performed at 1–2 week intervals during the initial stabilization period. Glucocorticoid replacement is ideally provided as oral prednisolone (0.5–2 mg/q 24 h, divided q 12 h), however methylprednisolone acetate (Depo-Medrol; 10 mg/month IM) can be administered to cats which are difficult to pill. However, this protocol is not ideal and may predispose to the development of diabetes mellitus in the long term.

VII. Prognosis

A. **In cats surviving the initial hypoadrenal crisis, the prognosis is excellent**; in one report six of seven cats that survived the initial crisis were alive for a mean of 36 months and in one case that the author has treated was still alive 10 years after initial presentation.

VIII. Prevention

No known prevention.

References and Further Readings

Berger SL, Reed JR. Traumatically induced hypoadrenocorticism in a cat. *JAAHA* 1993;29:337–339.

Calsyn JDR, Green RA, Davis GJ, Reilly CM. Adrenal pheochromocytoma with contralateral adrenocortical adenoma in a cat. *JAAHA* 2010;46:36–42.

Feldman EC, Nelson RW. Hypoadrenocorticism in cats. In: Feldman EC, Nelson RW, eds. *Canine and Feline Endocrinology and Reproduction*, 3rd edn. Philadelphia: WB Saunders, 2004.

Feldman EC, Peterson ME. Hypoadrenocorticism. *Vet Clin N Am Small Anim Prac* 1984;14:751–766.

Ferasin L. Iatrogenic hyperadrenocorticism in a cat following a short therapeutic course of methylprednisolone. *JFMS* 2001;3:87–93.

Myers NC, Bruyette DS. Feline adrenocortical diseases: Part II—Hypoadrenocorticism. *Semin Vet Med Surg (Small Anim)* 1994;9:144–147.

Parnell NK, Powell LL, Hohenhaus AE, Patnaik AK, Peterson ME. Hypoadrenocorticism as the primary manifestation of lymphoma in two cats. *JAVMA* 1999;214:1208–1211.

Peterson ME, Greco DS, Orth DN. Primary hypoadrenocorticism in ten cats. *JVIM* 1989;3:55–58.

Peterson ME, Kemppainen RJ. Comparison of the immunoreactive plasma corticotrophin and cortisol responses to two synthetic corticotrophin preparations (tetracosactin and cosyntropin) in healthy cats. *AJVR* 1992a;53:1752–1755.

Peterson ME, Kemppainen RJ. Comparison of the intravenous and intramuscular routes of administering cosyntroopin for corticotropin stimulation testing in cats. *AJVR* 1992b;53:1392–1395.

Peterson ME, Kemppainen RJ. Dose-response relation between plasma concentrations of corticotropin and cortisol after administration of incremental doses of cosyntropin for corticotropin stimulation testing in cats. *AJVR* 1993;54:300–304.

Peterson ME, Kintzer PP, Foodman MS, Piccolie A, Quimby FW. Adrenal function in the cat: Comparision of the effects of cosyntropin (synthetic ACTH) and corticotrophin gel stimulation. *Res Vet Sci* 1984;37:331–333.

Smith MC, Feldman EC. Plasma enodgenous ACTH concentrations and plasma cortisol responses to synthetic ACTH and dexamethasone sodium phosphate in healthy cats. *Am J Vet Res* 1987;48:1717–1724.

Sparkes AH, Adams DT, Douthwaite JA, Gruffydd-Jones TJ. Assessment of adrenal function in cats: Responses to intravenous synthetic ACTH. *JSAP* 1990;31:2–5.

Tasker S, Mackay AD, Sparkes AH. A case of primary hypoadrenocorticism. *JFMS* 1999;1:257–260.

CHAPTER 3

Hypoadrenocorticism in Other Species
Michelle L. Campbell-Ward

Hypoadrenocorticism in Horses

Pathogenesis

- Primary hypoadrenocorticism may occur in critically ill adult horses due to damage to the adrenal glands.
- Relative adrenal insufficiency is common in septic and premature foals.
- Secondary hypoadrenocorticism may occur following abrupt cessation of corticosteroid or anabolic steroid therapy.

Classical Signs

- Vague and variable nonspecific signs including lethargy, poor hair coat, exercise intolerance, and weight loss.

Diagnosis

- Adrenocorticotrophic hormone (ACTH) stimulation test.

Treatment

- Electrolyte correction with fluid therapy.
- Glucocorticoid supplementation.

I. Pathogenesis

A. Hypoadrenocorticism results from an **inadequate production of glucocorticoids and/or mineralocorticoids by adrenocortical cells**:

    1. **Primary hypoadrenocorticism** occurs when there is **permanent damage** to (or removal of) more than 90% of the **adrenal cortices**:

Clinical Endocrinology of Companion Animals, First Edition. Edited by Jacquie Rand.
© 2013 John Wiley & Sons, Inc. Published 2013 by John Wiley & Sons, Inc.

a. This may occur in **critically ill horses** (e.g., those with colic, enterocolitis, endotoxemia, or sepsis) because the **adrenal gland is a shock organ** and adrenal hemorrhage, thrombosis, and cortical necrosis may lead to adrenal atrophy and dysfunction. In fact, adrenocortical hemorrhage and necrosis are common findings at necropsy in adult horses that succumb to acute severe gastrointestinal disease and endotoxic shock, although antemortem evidence of adrenocortical dysfunction is often lacking in such cases.

b. Classic hypoadrenocorticism (Addison's disease) resulting from immune-mediated adrenocortical destruction has not been described in the horse.

c. Irreversible adrenocortical tissue destruction may occur due to neoplastic infiltration or infectious organism presence in the adrenal gland/s but is rare.

2. **Secondary hypoadrenocorticism** is characterized by **deficient production and/or secretion of ACTH which leads to atrophy of the adrenal cortices.** Secondary hypoadrenocorticism can be caused by large nonfunctional tumors in the hypothalamus or pituitary or more commonly iatrogenically due to prolonged suppression of ACTH by drugs. In adult horses, secondary hypoadrenocorticism is **most commonly associated with discontinuation of long-term glucocorticoid or anabolic steroid treatment.**

B. A syndrome of adrenal exhaustion often referred to as "turnout" or "steroid letdown syndrome" characterized by lethargy, anorexia, and poor performance is anecdotally reported in racehorses. It has been attributed to adrenal insufficiency associated with chronic stress or long-term steroid administration. Laboratory tests, however, have failed to provide convincing evidence of adrenal insufficiency in such cases.

C. While **permanent adrenocortical insufficiency is rarely diagnosed** in equine practice, emerging evidence suggests that **transient reversible adrenocortical dysfunction resulting in cortisol insufficiency frequently develops during critical illness in horses and foals.** This syndrome is termed **relative adrenal insufficiency (RAI)** or **critical illness-related corticosteroid insufficiency (CIRCI)** and can contribute substantially to morbidity and mortality associated with the primary disease:

1. Research in human medicine suggests that RAI/CIRCI can result from temporary suppression of the hypothalamic–pituitary–adrenal (HPA) axis activity at one or more levels:
   a. Inhibition of corticotropin releasing hormone (CRH) and/or ACTH secretion.
   b. Decreased sensitivity to CRH or ACTH at their respective target tissues.
   c. Exhaustion of adrenocortical cortisol synthetic capacity.
   d. Impaired response to cortisol in the peripheral tissues.
2. The specific mechanisms leading to the development of RAI/CIRCI are poorly understood but may involve a combination of factors:
   a. Direct damage to the HPA axis components from the primary disease.
   b. Inhibition of hormone production by medications used to treat the primary disease.
   c. Suppression of activity of one or more components of the HPA axis by infectious organisms or the host's own immune and inflammatory responses.

D. Premature and septic foals appear to be particularly sensitive to adrenal insufficiency:

1. Compelling evidence suggests that **maturation** of the equine HPA axis occurs **much later** than in other species. The fetal foal's adrenal gland is incapable of synthesizing cortisol until very late in gestation and maturation of the system continues during the first few weeks/months of life:
   a. Premature foals have low baseline cortisol and concurrent high ACTH concentrations compared to term foals implying an impaired adrenocortical sensitivity to ACTH and/or a limited cortisol synthetic capacity (Table 3.1).
   b. By 12–24 h of age, mean basal cortisol concentrations are lower in healthy neonatal foals than reported mean concentrations in healthy adult horses despite the foals having comparable or higher concurrent ACTH concentrations.
2. The specific cause of the impaired cortisol responses of neonatal foals is unknown. However, the fetal and neonatal HPA axis immaturity may impair the foal's ability to respond to physiologic stress and disease during the neonatal period.
3. The mechanisms and management of RAI/CIRCI in critically ill foals require further investigation.

Table 3.1 Comparison of serum cortisol and endogenous ACTH concentrations in newborn premature and full-term foals.

	Time of sample collection	Premature foal	Full-term foal
Serum cortisol concentration (µg/dL)	120 min after birth	<3	12–14
Endogenous ACTH concentration (pg/mL)	30 min after birth	650	300

II. Signalment

A. Premature foals are predisposed to adrenal insufficiency.

III. Clinical Signs

A. Depression.
B. Anorexia.
C. Exercise intolerance.
D. Weight loss.
E. Poor hair coat.
F. Lameness.
G. Mild abdominal discomfort.
H. Dehydration.
I. Bradycardia/bradydysrhythmia.
J. Seizures.

IV. Diagnosis

A. **A complete history** must be obtained including performance, previous disease, drug administration, and potentially stressful conditions.

B. **Hematology and serum biochemistry** analysis may be supportive: results may be normal, or abnormalities such as anemia, hyponatremia, hypochloremia, hyperkalemia, and/or hypoglycemia may be present.

C. **Baseline cortisol and ACTH levels** as well as the **ACTH stimulation test** are critical to achieve a diagnosis. Note that cortisol levels feature daily fluctuations and single measurements do not provide sufficient diagnostic information on their own. **Horses with hypoadrenocorticism have low cortisol concentrations and do not or only minimally respond to ACTH administration:**

   1. ACTH stimulation test—adult horses:

     a. Obtain a baseline blood sample in heparinized or plain tubes immediately before ACTH administration.

     b. Give 1 IU/kg natural ACTH gel intramuscularly (IM) between 8 and 10 am; or 100 IU (1 mg) synthetic ACTH (cosyntropin) intravenously (IV) between 8 am and 12 noon.

     c. Obtain follow up blood samples 2 and 4 h after ACTH administration.

     d. Horses with a functional adrenal gland should have a 2–3-fold increase in plasma cortisol concentration after ACTH stimulation as compared with baseline values.

   2. Cosyntropin stimulation test—foals:

     a. Obtain a baseline blood sample for cortisol analysis.

     b. Administer 0.01–0.2 µg/kg (low-dose protocol) or 1–2 µg/kg (high-dose protocol) of cosyntropin IV. (The high-dose test may be less sensitive for the diagnosis of the transient reversible HPA axis suppression that occurs in RAI/CIRCI.)

     c. Collect additional blood samples at 30, 60, 90 and 120 min.

    d. With the low-dose protocol, cortisol should peak at a value twice the baseline at 30 min; with the high-dose protocol, cortisol should peak at 90 min at 2–3 times the baseline test. Time of day should not affect results. Results should be compared with age-matched controls or to values generated in the same laboratory.

    e. In one study, premature foals showed a blunted cortisol response to exogenous ACTH with only a 28% increase in plasma cortisol 30–60 min after stimulation compared with a 208% increase in normal-term foals.

    f. Poor response to cosyntropin and an elevated endogenous ACTH:cortisol ratio (compared with age-matched controls) is associated with a high probability of foal mortality.

D.   **Postmortem examination** findings may include adrenocortical hemorrhages and necrosis, as well as adrenal atrophy and fibrosis.

V.   Differential Diagnosis
A.   Primary gastrointestinal disease.
B.   Toxin ingestion.
C.   Renal disease.
D.   Pituitary pars intermedia dysfunction (see Chapter 11).
E.   Laminitis.
F.   Sepsis.

VI.   Treatment
A.   Rest and **supportive care**.
B.   Restore electrolyte balance with appropriate **fluid therapy**.
C.   **Glucocorticoid supplementation:**

    1. Prednisolone sodium succinate (up to 300 mg q 24 h IV or IM) is the initial treatment of choice for hypoadrenocorticism.

    2. Low doses of dexamethasone are the second option.

    3. Alternatively oral prednisolone (200–400 mg/horse) can be used and may be a consideration for longer term use.

    4. Prednisone (40 mg per os [PO] q 12 h or 50 mg IV) has been used to treat foals with adrenal insufficiency; however, the use of this drug orally in horses is questionable as it is poorly absorbed from the equine intestinal tract and the active metabolite, prednisolone, is rarely produced. In contrast, oral prednisolone has excellent bioavailability.

    5. Isoflupredone acetate (0.02 mg/kg q 24 h for 10 days) has been reported to ameliorate the clinical signs of secondary hypoadrenocorticism (due to abrupt cessation of an anabolic steroid) in a horse with preexisting pituitary pars intermedia dysfunction.

    6. Triamcinolone and prednisolone acetate should be avoided.

    7. If a prolonged course of glucocorticoid therapy is anticipated, gradual tapering of the dose is recommended before treatment is discontinued.

VII.   Prognosis
A.   Prognosis is fair for cases with iatrogenic hypoadrenocorticism.
B.   Guarded in cases with severe electrolyte aberrations (hyperkalemia, hypochloremia, and/or hyponatremia) or concurrent sepsis.
C.   Poor in premature foals.

VIII.   Prevention
A.   Judicious use of therapeutic corticosteroids/anabolic steroids in horses including prescription of gradual withdrawal regimens should minimize the risk of development of iatrogenic hypoadrenocorticism.

Hypoadrenocorticism in Ferrets

Pathogenesis

- Iatrogenic hypoadrenocorticism, an uncommon complication of subtotal or bilateral adrenalectomy.

Classical Signs

- Lethargy, weakness, and anorexia days to weeks after adrenal surgery.

Diagnosis

- Evaluation of serum electrolytes.

Treatment

- Glucocorticoid and/or mineralocorticoid supplementation.

I.   Pathogenesis
A.   **Iatrogenic hypoadrenocorticism** is an **uncommon complication of subtotal or bilateral adrenalectomy** carried out for the treatment of adrenal disease in ferrets (see Chapter 9). It may also occur following the use of mitotane. Signs occur days to weeks postoperatively.

II.   Signalment
A.   No sex predilections have been identified. Adrenal disease affects adults (generally >2–3 years of age).

III.   Clinical Signs
A.   Development of the following signs days to weeks following surgery:
   1. Lethargy/weakness.
   2. Anorexia.

IV.   Diagnosis
A.   **Evaluation of serum electrolytes:** Demonstration of abnormalities such as hyponatremia, hypochloremia, and hyperkalemia in postadrenalectomy patients warrants initiation of therapy.

V.   Differential Diagnosis
A.   Hypoglycemia, for example, if a concurrent insulinoma exists (see Chapter 23), or secondary to postsurgical anorexia.
B.   Metastases or cachexia associated with advanced adrenal neoplasia.
C.   Postsurgical infection/sepsis.
D.   Other systemic disease, for example, cardiac or hepatic dysfunction that may have been exacerbated by the surgery.

VI.   Treatment
A.   **Glucocorticoid** (if not already prescribed) **and/or mineralocorticoid supplementation** titrated to the individual and tapered to the lowest dosage interval to prevent clinical signs:
   1. Glucocorticoids: dexamethasone 0.5 mg/kg subcutaneously (SC), IM, or IV initially then prednisone 0.25 mg/kg PO q 12–24 h.
   2. Mineralocorticoids:
      a. Fludrocortisone acetate 0.05–0.1 mg/kg PO q 24 h or divided q 12 h.
      b. Deoxycorticosterone pivalate 2 mg/kg IM q 21 days.
B.   If critically ill, **fluid therapy** to correct electrolyte aberrations is indicated.
C.   **Monitor electrolytes carefully** and adjust the therapeutic regimen as required.

VII. Prognosis
A.   Fair if identified early and appropriate therapy instituted.
B.   Poor if severe electrolyte abnormalities are present.
C.   Recurrence of adrenal disease is common following surgery, especially if follow-up hormonal therapy is not given (see Chapter 9).

VIII. Prevention
A.   Judicious use of glucocorticoids (often long term) and regular electrolyte monitoring following subtotal or total bilateral adrenalectomy in ferrets.

Hypoadrenocorticism in Pet Birds

Pathogenesis

- Limited information exists regarding this condition in birds.

Classical Signs

- Dehydration, weakness, mild gastrointestinal signs, and/or feather loss.

Diagnosis

- No reports of antemortem diagnosis exist but measurement of serum electrolytes and the ACTH stimulation test may prove useful for suspected cases.

Treatment

- Based on limited anecdotal reports of glucocorticoid/mineralocorticoid supplementation.

I.   Pathogenesis
A.   Although there are **no appropriately documented cases of hypoadrenocorticism in pet birds**, it is likely that adrenal deficiency does occur in this group:
   1. As in other species, adrenal cell atrophy or necrosis may be induced by autoimmune diseases, neoplasia, inflammation, infectious diseases, amyloidosis, trauma, or drugs (e.g., mitotane, trilostane).
   2. **Rapid withdrawal of exogenous corticosteroids may result in iatrogenic hypoadrenocorticism.**

II.   Signalment
A.   Given the lack of documented cases, no information regarding sex, age, or species predisposition exists.

III.   Clinical Signs
A.   Dehydration.
B.   Episodes of weakness.
C.   Vague gastrointestinal signs, for example, anorexia, periodic diarrhea, and generalized abdominal tenderness.
D.   Feather loss.

IV.   Diagnosis
A.   There are **no clinical reports of antemortem diagnosis** of hypoadrenocorticism in birds.
B.   **Electrolyte abnormalities** such as hyperkalemia, hyponatremia, and a sodium to potassium ratio of <27:1 are highly suggestive of hypoadrenocorticism.
C.   Concurrent anemia and hypoglycemia may also be present.
D.   Low urine specific gravity may be identified.
E.   Confirmation of a clinical suspicion of adrenal insufficiency can be made by determining the **plasma corticosterone concentration before and after ACTH stimulation.** In all avian species tested, **corticosterone, not**

cortisol, is the main corticosteroid produced by the "adult" adrenal gland. Hypoadrenocorticism may exist even if the resting corticosterone level is normal. Extrapolating from other species, hypoadrenocorticism should be suspected when little or no increase in the corticosterone blood level is seen after ACTH administration:

1. **ACTH stimulation protocols** have been established in psittacines, raptors, chickens, and ducks:
    a. A baseline blood sample is collected.
    b. ACTH 16–50 IU is administered IM.
    c. A second blood sample is collected 1–2 h after ACTH administration.
    d. Quantification of corticosterone in both blood samples requires an assay specific to this hormone, for example, radioimmunoassay.
    e. In general, ACTH causes a peak corticosterone response within 30–60 min after injection with a return to baseline levels within 120–240 min. **Pre- and post-ACTH corticosterone concentrations vary significantly among avian species.** In healthy cockatoos, macaws, Amazon parrots, and lorikeets the mean post-ACTH corticosterone concentrations are 4–14 times the mean baseline concentration. The sensitivity and specificity of the test remains undetermined and further investigation is required in relation to interpretation of test results.

F.   The use of ACTH blood concentration to differentiate primary from secondary hypoadrenocorticism has not been investigated in birds.

G.   **Postmortem examination** may be required for definitive diagnosis. Adrenal degeneration histologically is characterized by swelling, vacuolation, and/or necrosis of adrenocortical cells and appears to be a relatively common finding in birds.

V.   Differential Diagnosis

A.   Renal disease.

B.   Gastrointestinal disease.

C.   Hepatic disease.

VI.   Treatment

A.   The following have been suggested as treatment protocols for psittacine birds:
    1. Fludrocortisone in the drinking water at a dose of 0.4 mg/L.
    2. Hydrocortisone 10 mg/kg IM q 24 h.

VII.   Prognosis

A.   No information is available regarding prognosis of this condition in birds.

VIII.   Prevention

A.   Corticosteroid treatment should be slowly tapered off to prevent the development of iatrogenic hypoadrenocorticism.

References and Further Readings

Couetil LL, Hoffman AM. Adrenal insufficiency in a neonatal foal. *J Am Vet Med Assoc* 1998;212:1594–1596.

de Matos R. Adrenal steroid metabolism in birds: Anatomy, physiology and clinical considerations. *Vet Clin North Am Exot Anim Pract* 2008;11:35–57.

Dowling PM, Williams MA, Clark TP. Adrenal insufficiency associated with long-term anabolic steroid administration in a horse. *J Am Vet Med Assoc* 1993;203:1166–1169.

Dybdal NO, McFarlane D. (2009) Adrenal glands. In: Smith BP, ed. *Large Animal Internal Medicine*, 4th edn. St Louis: Mosby, 2009, pp. 1345–1347.

Eiler H, Goble D, Oliver J. Adrenal gland function in the horse: Effects of cosyntropin (synthetic) and corticotropin (natural) stimulation. *Am J Vet Res* 1979;40:724–726.

Gold JR, Divers TJ, Barton MH, et al. Plasma adrenocorticotropin, cortisol and adrenocorticotropin/cortisol ratios in septic and normal-term foals. *J Vet Inter Med* 2007;21:791–796.

Hart KA, Barton MH. Adrenocortical insufficiency in horses and foals. *Vet Clin North Am Equine Pract* 2011;27:19–34.

Hart KA, Ferguson DC, Heusner GL, et al. Synthetic adrenocorticotropic hormone stimulation tests in healthy neonatal foals. *J Vet Intern Med* 2007;21:314–321.

Hurcombe SD, Toribio RE, Slovis N, et al. Blood arginine vasopressin, adrenocorticotropin hormone and cortisol concentrations at admission in septic and critically ill foals and their association with survival. *J Vet Intern Med* 2008;22:639–647.

Lothrop CD. Diseases of the endocrine system. In: Rosskopf WJ, Woerpel RW, eds. *Diseases of Cage and Aviary Birds.* Baltimore: Williams and Wilkins, 1996, pp. 368–379.

Lumeij JT. Endocrinology. In: Ritchie BW, Harrison GJ, Harrison LR, eds. *Avian Medicine—Principles and Application.* Lake Worth: Wingers, 1994, pp. 582–606.

Marik P. Critical illness related corticosteroid insufficiency. *Chest* 2009;135(1):181–193.

McGavin M, Zachary J. *Pathologic Basis of Veterinary Disease,* 4th edn. St. Louis: Mosby Elsevier, 2007.

Oglesbee BL. *The 5-Minute Veterinary Consult: Ferret and Rabbit.* Ames: Blackwell Publishing, 2006.

Onderka DK, Claffey FP. Adrenal degeneration associated with feather loss in a macaw. *Can Vet J* 1987;28(4):193–194.

Orsini JA, Donaldson MT, Koch C, et al. Iatrogenic secondary hypoadrenocorticism in a horse with pituitary pars intermedia dysfunction (equine Cushing's disease). *Equine Vet Edu* 2007;19(2):81–87.

Peroni DL, Stanley S, Kollias-Baker C, et al. Prednisone per os is likely to have limited efficacy in horses. *Equine Vet J* 2002;34:283–287.

Rae M. Avian endocrine disorders. In: Fudge AM, ed. *Laboratory Medicine—Avian and Exotic Pets.* Philadelphia: WB Saunders, 2000, pp. 76–89.

Rossdale P, Ousey J. Studies on equine prematurity 6: Guidelines for assessment of foal maturity. *Equine Vet J* 1984;16(4):300–302.

Rosskopf WJ, Woerpel RW, Howard EB, et al. Chronic endocrine disorder associated with inclusion body hepatitis in a sulfur-crested cockatoo. *J Am Vet Med Assoc* 1981;179(11):1273–1276.

Rosskopf WJ, Woerpel RW, Richkind M, et al. Pathogenesis, diagnosis and treatment of adrenal insufficiency in psittacine birds. *Calif Vet* 1982;5:26–30.

Silver M, Ousey J, Dudan F, et al. Studies on equine prematurity 2: Post natal adrenocortical activity in relation to plasma adrenocorticotrophic hormone and catecholamine levels in term and premature foals. *Equine Vet J* 1984;16(4):278–286.

Sojka JE, Levy M. Evaluation of endocrine function. *Vet Clin North Am Equine Pract* 1995;11:415–435.

Toribio RE. Adrenal glands. In: Reed SM, Bayly WM, Sellon DC, eds. *Equine Internal Medicine,* 3rd edn. St Louis: Saunders Elsevier, 2010, pp. 1248–1251.

Wong D, Vo D, Alcott C, et al. Adrenocorticotrophic hormone stimulation tests in healthy foals from birth to 12 weeks of age. *Can J Vet Res* 2009;73(1):65–72.

CHAPTER 4

Critical Illness-Related Corticosteroid Insufficiency (Previously Known as Relative Adrenal Insufficiency)

Linda Martin

Pathogenesis

- Critical illness-related corticosteroid insufficiency (CIRCI), previously known as relative adrenal insufficiency, is a syndrome that can occur in the critically ill; it does not occur in stable patients.
- Hypothalamic–pituitary–adrenal (HPA) dysfunction in CIRCI is relative and transient. The syndrome is characterized by an inadequate production of cortisol and/or ACTH in relation to an increased demand during periods of severe illness; HPA function normalizes after resolution of the critical illness.
- The pathogenesis of CIRCI in animals is unknown, but its development is most likely multifactorial, involving a complex interaction between the endocrine and immune systems.

Classical Signs

- Hypotension and hemodynamic instability that persists despite adequate fluid resuscitation and vasopressor therapy.
- Signs may be vague and nonspecific, such as depression, weakness, fever, vomiting, diarrhea, and abdominal pain.

Diagnosis

- CIRCI should be considered as a differential diagnosis in all critically ill patients requiring vasopressor support.
- No consensus exists regarding how to identify veterinary patients with CIRCI.
- Critically ill patients with CIRCI may have normal or elevated basal serum cortisol concentrations and a blunted response to ACTH stimulation.
- Hyponatremia and hyperkalemia are uncommon in CIRCI, unlike typical spontaneous hypoadrenocorticism.

Clinical Endocrinology of Companion Animals, First Edition. Edited by Jacquie Rand.
© 2013 John Wiley & Sons, Inc. Published 2013 by John Wiley & Sons, Inc.

Treatment

- Currently, no guidelines exist for the treatment of CIRCI in veterinary critically ill patients; however, it is reasonable to start corticosteroid therapy in volume-resuscitated, vasopressor-dependent animals after performing an ACTH stimulation test.
- The appropriate dosage, duration, and type of corticosteroid therapy is unknown in veterinary patients with CIRCI; however, it is reasonable to give supplemental doses of corticosteroids at physiological to supraphysiological dosages (0.25–1 mg/kg q 24 h of prednisone) until the results of an ACTH stimulation test are available.
- Corticosteroids can be continued in patients that have (1) a normal or elevated basal cortisol concentration and an ACTH-stimulated cortisol concentration less than the normal reference range; (2) a normal or elevated basal cortisol concentration and an ACTH-stimulated cortisol concentration that is <5% greater than the basal cortisol concentration (flat line response); (3) a delta cortisol concentration ≤3 µg/dL (83 nmol/L) where delta cortisol is the difference between basal and ACTH-stimulated cortisol concentrations; or (4) demonstrated a significant improvement in cardiovascular status within 24 h of starting corticosteroid therapy. Therapy can be discontinued in those that respond appropriately to ACTH.
- Because the HPA dysfunction in CIRCI is transient, lifelong therapy with corticosteroids is not required and is tapered and discontinued after resolution of the critical illness.

I. Pathogenesis

A. **CIRCI is increasingly being recognized in human critically ill patients with systemic inflammation** associated with sepsis, acute respiratory distress syndrome/acute lung injury, severe hepatic disease, trauma, acute myocardial infarction, or following cardiopulmonary bypass.

B. **Insufficient adrenal and/or pituitary function has been identified in dogs with sepsis/septic shock, trauma, gastric volvulus-dilatation, neoplasia** (i.e., lymphoma and several different types of nonhematopoietic tumors), **and genetic mutation of the multidrug resistance gene *ABCB1*** (formerly known as *MDR1*).

C. **Insufficient adrenal function has been identified in cats with neoplasia (i.e., lymphoma), trauma, and sepsis/septic shock.**

D. **Many illnesses have been associated with CIRCI; however, all human patients diagnosed with CIRCI are critically ill.** CIRCI has not been documented in stable patients with minor trauma, mild hepatopathy, or localized infections.

E. **HPA dysfunction in CIRCI is relative and transient.** The adrenal glands produce and secrete cortisol, but the quantity is inadequate for the degree of physiological stress or illness. Following recovery from critical illness, HPA dysfunction resolves.

F. **The pathogenesis of CIRCI in dogs is unknown,** but the development of this syndrome is most **likely multifactorial,** involving a **complex interaction between the endocrine and immune systems.**

G. Possible mechanisms for the development of CIRCI in humans and animals include:

1. **Proinflammatory cytokine (e.g., tumor necrosis factor-α)-mediated inhibition of CRH and ACTH secretion** resulting in decreased cortisol production.

2. **Proinflammatory cytokine (e.g., tumor necrosis factor-α and interleukin-1)-mediated glucocorticoid receptor dysfunction and reduction in receptor numbers.** A reduction in the activity or number of receptors would reduce the ability of cells to respond appropriately to cortisol.

3. **Corticostatin-mediated ACTH receptor antagonism.** Corticostatin, a peptide produced by immune cells, impairs adrenocortical function by competing with ACTH and binding to its receptor.

4. **Leptin-mediated inhibition of the HPA axis.** Leptin, an adipose-derived hormone, inhibits the HPA axis during stress or illness.

5. **Tissue resistance to the actions of glucocorticoids.** Several factors may be involved, including decreased access of cortisol to tissues secondary to a reduction of circulating cortisol-binding globulin concentrations and increased cytokine (i.e., interleukin-2, -4, and -13)-mediated conversion of cortisol (active) to

cortisone (inactive). Such mechanisms can account for decreased glucocorticoid activity while serum cortisol concentrations appear appropriate.

6. **Disruption of pituitary and/or adrenal gland function secondary to extensive tissue destruction** of these organs **by infection, infarction, hemorrhage, or thrombosis.**

7. ***ABCB1* gene mutation resulting in the lack of P-glycoprotein, the *ABCB1* gene product, at the blood–brain barrier:**

   a) P-glycoprotein normally restricts the entry of cortisol into the brain, limiting cortisol's feedback inhibition of CRH and ACTH.

   b) In *ABCB1* mutant dogs, P-glycoprotein is not present, **allowing greater concentrations of cortisol to be present within the brain, thus augmenting feedback inhibition of the HPA axis** and, ultimately, **impedance of sufficient cortisol secretion.**

   c) Thus, the mutation may lead to the inability to appropriately respond to critical illness and stress.

II. Signalment

A. Since CIRCI is caused by various serious illnesses, it can occur in dogs and cats of any breed, age, or sex.

B. Due to the ***ABCB1* gene mutation,** it is **possible** that there is a **genetic or breed predilection in canine CIRCI;** however, this has **yet to be proven.** The *ABCB1* mutation has been identified in herding breed dogs, such as **Collies, Shetland Sheepdogs, Old English Sheepdogs, and Australian Shepherds** and has been found at a higher frequency in sight hounds, such as **Long-haired Whippets** and **Silken Windhounds,** as well as in **McNabs.**

III. Clinical Signs

A. Clinical signs of CIRCI can be **vague and nonspecific,** such as depression, weakness, fever, vomiting, diarrhea, and abdominal pain. Additionally, **clinical signs of the underlying disease process** responsible for CIRCI (e.g., septic shock, hepatic disease, trauma, etc.) **can mask the clinical features of CIRCI.**

B. **The most common clinical abnormality** associated with CIRCI in human patients with septic shock is **hypotension that is refractory to fluid resuscitation, requiring vasopressor therapy.**

IV. Diagnosis

A. **CIRCI should be considered as a differential diagnosis in all critically ill patients requiring vasopressor support.**

B. Laboratory assessment of human critically ill patients with CIRCI **may demonstrate an eosinophilia and/or hypoglycemia.**

C. **Hyponatremia and hyperkalemia are uncommon** in humans with CIRCI, and to date, have not been reported in canine or feline critically ill patients with insufficient adrenal or pituitary function.

D. **Human patients with CIRCI typically have normal or elevated basal serum cortisol concentrations and a blunted response to ACTH stimulation.** Similar findings have been documented in critically ill dogs with sepsis/septic shock, trauma, and gastric dilatation-volvulus as well as in critically ill cats with sepsis/septic shock, trauma, and neoplasia.

E. **No consensus exists regarding the identification of patients with CIRCI in human or veterinary medicine.** A variety of tests have been advocated, including measurement of a random basal cortisol concentration, ACTH-stimulated cortisol concentration, delta cortisol concentration (i.e., the difference obtained when subtracting basal from ACTH-stimulated cortisol concentration), the ratio of cortisol concentration to that of endogenous ACTH, and combinations of these methods.

F. **The optimal way to identify critically ill veterinary patients with CIRCI has yet to be determined:**

   1. **Evaluation of adrenal function typically involves performance of an ACTH stimulation test:**

      a. The most commonly used protocol for ACTH stimulation testing in dogs involves the intravenous administration of 5 µg cosyntropin/kg up to a maximum of 250 µg.

      b. In cats, intravenous administration of 125 µg of cosyntropin/cat is commonly used.

      c. Serum or plasma is obtained for measurement of cortisol concentration before and 60 min after ACTH administration in both dogs and cats.

   2. **The standard doses of cosyntropin** (5 µg/kg in dogs and 125 µg/cat) currently used in ACTH stimulation testing **are greater than that necessary to produce maximal adrenocortical stimulation** in healthy small animals:

a. Doses as low as 0.5 μg/kg in healthy dogs and 5 μg/kg in healthy cats have been shown to induce maximal cortisol secretion by the adrenal glands.

b. The use of higher doses may be supraphysiologic and may mask subtle decreases in adrenal gland reserve and hinder identification of dogs and cats with CIRCI.

3. **Low-dose (0.5 μg/kg IV) ACTH stimulation testing** has been compared to standard-dose (5 μg/kg IV) ACTH stimulation testing in critically ill dogs:

a. In the study, every critically ill dog that was identified by the standard-dose ACTH stimulation test to have insufficient adrenal function (i.e., ACTH-stimulated serum cortisol concentration below the reference range or <5% greater than the basal cortisol concentration) was also identified by the low-dose test.

b. Additional dogs were identified with adrenal insufficiency by the low-dose ACTH stimulation test, which were not identified by the standard-dose test.

c. Thus, ACTH administered at a dose of 0.5 μg/kg IV appears to be at least as accurate in determining adrenal function in critically ill dogs as the IV administration of ACTH at 5 μg/kg. The low-dose ACTH stimulation test may even be a more sensitive diagnostic test in detecting patients with insufficient adrenal gland function than the standard-dose test.

4. Serum free cortisol concentration:

a. Assays that measure cortisol concentration typically measure total hormone concentration (i.e., serum free cortisol concentration plus a protein-bound fraction).

b. However, the **serum free cortisol fraction is believed to be responsible for the physiologic function of the hormone.** Therefore, serum free cortisol concentrations may be a more precise predictor of adrenal gland function.

c. **The relationship between free and total cortisol varies with serum protein concentration:**

1) In human critically ill patients, cortisol-binding globulin and albumin concentrations can decrease by approximately 50% due to catabolism at inflammatory sites and inhibition of hepatic synthesis via cytokine induction.

2) Therefore, serum total cortisol concentration may be falsely low in hypoproteinemic patients, resulting in overestimation of CIRCI.

3) **Serum free cortisol concentration is less likely to be altered in states of hypoproteinemia.** Consequently, **serum total cortisol concentrations may not accurately represent the biological activity of serum free cortisol during critical illness.**

d. Several human studies suggest that serum free cortisol concentrations are a more accurate measure of circulating glucocorticoid activity than total cortisol concentrations.

e. At this time, canine and feline studies are lacking and the ability to measure serum free cortisol concentration is not widely available:

1) Serum free and total cortisol concentrations have been compared in one study of critically ill dogs.

2) Fewer critically ill dogs with adrenal insufficiency (i.e., an ACTH-stimulated serum cortisol concentration below the reference range or <5% greater than the basal cortisol concentration) were identified by serum free cortisol concentration than serum total cortisol concentration. However, basal and ACTH-stimulated serum total cortisol concentrations were not lower in hypoproteinemic patients when compared to normoproteinemic patients.

3) The significance of this finding is unknown and warrants further investigation in veterinary patients.

5. The **delta cortisol concentration has been advocated as a method to identify critically ill patients with CIRCI in both human and veterinary medicine:**

a. A study in human patients with septic shock found that a basal cortisol concentration ≤34 μg/dL (938 nmol/L) combined with a delta cortisol concentration ≥9 μg/dL (250 nmol/L) in response to a 250 μg/person ACTH stimulation test were associated with a favorable prognosis:

1) Additionally, a basal cortisol concentration >34 μg/dL combined with a delta cortisol concentration <9 μg/dL were associated with a poor prognosis.

2) Since these values successfully predicted outcome, a delta cortisol concentration of <9 μg/dL is frequently used as a diagnostic criterion for CIRCI in human critically ill patients.

b. Veterinary studies have also assessed delta cortisol concentrations as a criterion for diagnosing CIRCI in critically ill patients:

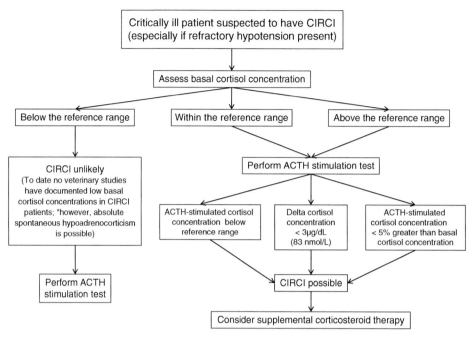

Figure 4.1 Strategy for diagnosis and treatment of critical illness-related corticosteroid insufficiency in dogs. *Low basal cortisol concentrations have been documented in dogs with neoplasia; however, these dogs were not critically ill and did not have clinical signs consistent with CIRCI.

1) One study found that septic dogs with delta cortisol concentrations ≤3 µg/dL (83 nmol/L) after a 250 µg/dog ACTH stimulation test were more likely to have systemic hypotension and decreased survival.

2) Additionally, another study investigating acutely ill dogs (i.e., dogs with sepsis, trauma, or gastric volvulus-dilatation) found that dogs with delta cortisol concentrations ≤3 µg/dL (83 nmol/L) after a 5 µg/kg ACTH stimulation test were more likely to require vasopressor therapy as part of their treatment plan.

3) Whether or not delta cortisol concentrations of ≤3 µg/dL (83 nmol/L) can be used as a criterion to diagnose all populations of veterinary critically ill patients with CIRCI has yet to be determined.

G. **Normal reference ranges do not exist for basal and ACTH-stimulated cortisol concentrations in critically ill dogs and cats.**

H. Based on the current veterinary literature, there are three scenarios which may indicate the presence of CIRCI in critically ill dogs (especially in the presence of refractory hypotension):

1. Dogs with a normal or elevated basal cortisol concentration and an ACTH-stimulated cortisol concentration less than the normal reference range.

2. Dogs with a normal or elevated basal cortisol concentration and an ACTH-stimulated cortisol concentration that is <5% greater than the basal cortisol concentration (flatline response).

3. Dogs with a delta cortisol concentration ≤3 µg/dL (83 nmol/L) (Figure 4.1).

I. Based on a few clinical studies and case reports, CIRCI appears to occur in cats. However, diagnostic criteria are undetermined at this time.

V. Differential Diagnosis

A. The following conditions may also produce hypotension that is poorly responsive to fluid and/or vasopressor therapy:

1. Sepsis/septic shock/systemic inflammatory response syndrome without the presence of CIRCI.

2. Absolute spontaneous hypoadrenocorticism.

3. Decompensated hypovolemic shock.

4. Cardiovascular disease:

   a. Cardiogenic shock.

   b. Overdose of vasodilator therapy.

  5. Hypermagnesemia.

  6. Diabetic ketoacidosis.

  7. Anaphylaxis.

VI. Treatment

A. **Human critically ill patients with CIRCI that are treated with supplemental doses of corticosteroids are more likely to be quickly weaned from vasopressor therapy and ventilatory support;** some treated populations of critically ill patients are **more likely to survive** than patients with CIRCI that do not receive corticosteroid supplementation:

  1. **The optimal dose and duration of treatment with corticosteroids in human patients with CIRCI is yet to be determined.**

  2. The dosages of corticosteroids used to treat human patients with CIRCI are referred to as supplemental, physiological, supraphysiological, low dose, or replacement.

  3. Most **human protocols** have used dosages of 200–300 mg IV q 24 h of **hydrocortisone** for an average 70 kg person (**2.9–4.3 mg/kg IV q 24 h**). The total daily dose is typically given as either a constant rate infusion or divided and given every 6 h.

  4. Hydrocortisone is one-fourth as potent as prednisone and one-thirtieth as potent as dexamethasone. Therefore, doses equivalent to that for hydrocortisone are **0.7–1 mg/kg q 24 h prednisone** or **0.1–0.4 mg/kg q 24 h dexamethasone.**

  5. **The hydrocortisone dose currently recommended for CIRCI in human patients is supraphysiological (the human physiological dose of hydrocortisone is 0.2–0.4 mg/kg q 24 h),** resulting in a serum cortisol concentration several times higher than that achieved by ACTH stimulation. This regimen was initially based on the maximum secretory rate of cortisol found in humans following major surgery.

B. Currently, there are **no guidelines for treatment of CIRCI in veterinary critically ill patients.**

C. It is reasonable to **start volume-resuscitated, vasopressor-dependent animals on corticosteroid therapy** after performing an ACTH stimulation test:

  1. When the test results are available, treatment can be withdrawn in animals that responded normally to the ACTH stimulation test.

  2. Corticosteroids can be continued in patients that have (a) a normal or elevated basal cortisol concentration and an ACTH-stimulated cortisol concentration less than the reference range; (b) a normal or elevated basal cortisol concentration and an ACTH-stimulated cortisol concentration that is <5% greater than the basal cortisol concentration (flat line response); (c) a delta cortisol concentration ≤3 µg/dL (83 nmol/L); or (d) demonstrated a significant improvement in cardiovascular status within 24 h of starting corticosteroid therapy.

D. **The appropriate dosage, duration, and type of corticosteroid therapy are unknown in veterinary patients with CIRCI:**

  1. It is reasonable to give supplemental doses of corticosteroids at physiological to supraphysiological dosages (**1–4.3 mg/kg IV q 24 h of hydrocortisone** [the total daily dose can be divided into four equal doses and given every 6 h or as a constant rate infusion], **0.25–1 mg/kg IV q 24 h of prednisone** [the total daily dose can be divided into two equal doses and given every 12 h], or **0.04–0.4 mg/kg IV q 24 h of dexamethasone**).

E. Because the **HPA dysfunction in CIRCI is transient, lifelong therapy with corticosteroids is not** thought to be **required** and is generally tapered after resolution of the critical illness. **The corticosteroid dose can be tapered by 25% per day following the resolution of the critical illness.** The ACTH stimulation test should be repeated following the resolution of critical illness and discontinuation of corticosteroid therapy to confirm the return of normal adrenocortical function.

VII. Prognosis

A. **Human critically ill patients with CIRCI have a worse prognosis than those with normal HPA function:**

  1. Nonsurvivors typically have low basal cortisol concentrations (<9 µg/dL), very high basal cortisol concentrations (>44 µg/dL or 1215 nmol/L), and/or a low cortisol response to ACTH stimulation (delta cortisol concentration <9 µg/dL).

2. Prior to corticosteroid therapy, a poor cortisol response to ACTH stimulation (delta cortisol concentration <9 μg/dL) is associated with poor response to vasopressor therapy.

3. In some patients, replacement therapy with corticosteroids (i.e., 200–300 mg hydrocortisone or equivalent per day) improved survival without causing overt harm (e.g., infection or gastrointestinal hemorrhage).

B. **Prognosis is not fully known for dogs with CIRCI:**

1. Delta cortisol concentrations ≤3 μg/dL after ACTH stimulation in septic dogs were associated with systemic hypotension and decreased survival.

2. Acutely ill dogs (i.e., had sepsis, trauma, or gastric volvulus-dilatation) with delta cortisol concentrations ≤3 μg/dL after ACTH stimulation were more likely to require vasopressor therapy.

3. Elevated basal serum cortisol and decreased basal serum thyroid concentrations at 24 and 48 h after hospital admission were associated with death in dogs with parvoviral enteritis.

4. Elevated basal serum cortisol and endogenous ACTH concentrations with decreased basal serum thyroid concentrations were associated with death in dogs suffering from *Babesia canis rossi* babesiosis.

VIII. Prevention

A. **Preemptive genotyping of dogs that come from breeds with a known high frequency of the *ABCB1* genetic mutation** may help identify animals with the genetic abnormality that may develop CIRCI if they become critically ill. *ABCB1* genotyping is available through the Veterinary Clinical Pharmacology Laboratory at Washington State University (www.vetmed.wsu.edu/depts-VCPL/).

B. CIRCI is not a primary disease; it develops secondary to critical illnesses. To prevent CIRCI, critical illnesses must also be prevented, which may not be possible in all cases.

References and Further Readings

Boozer AL, Behrend EN, Kemppainen RJ, et al. Pituitary-adrenal axis function in dogs with neoplasia. *Vet Comp Oncol* 2005;3(4):194–202.

Burkitt JM. Relative adrenal insufficiency. In: Silverstein DC, Hopper K. eds. *Small Animal Critical Care Medicine*, 1st edn. St. Louis, Missouri: Saunders Elsevier, 2009, pp. 318–320.

Burkitt JM, Haskins SC, Nelson RW, et al. Relative adrenal insufficiency in dogs with sepsis. *J Vet Intern Med* 2007;21(2):226–231.

Costello MF, Fletcher DJ, Silverstein DC, et al. Adrenal insufficiency in feline sepsis. In: Otto CM, ed. *American College of Veterinary Emergency and Critical Care Postgraduate Course 2006: Sepsis in Veterinary Medicine*, abstract 5. North Grafton, Massachusetts: American College of Veterinary Emergency and Critical Care, 2006, p. 41.

DeClue AE, Martin LG, Behrend EN, et al. Cortisol and aldosterone response to various doses of cosyntropin in healthy cats. *JAm Vet Med Assoc* 2011;238(2):176–182.

Durkan S, de Laforcade A, Rozanski E, et al. Suspected relative adrenal insufficiency in a critically ill cat. *J Vet Emerg Crit Care* 2007;17(2):197–201.

Foley C, Bracker K, Drellich S. Hypothalamic-pituitary axis deficiency following traumatic brain injury in a dog. *J Vet Emerg Crit Care* 2009;19(3):269–274.

Martin LG, Behrend EN, Holowaychuk MK, et al. Comparison of low-dose and standard-dose ACTH stimulation tests in critically ill dogs by assessment of serum total and free cortisol concentrations. *J Vet Intern Med* 2010;24(3):685–686.

Martin LG, Groman RP. Relative adrenal insufficiency in critical illness. *J Vet Emerg Crit Care* 2004;14(3):149–157.

Martin LG, Groman RP, Fletcher DJ, et al. Pituitary-adrenal function in dogs with acute critical illness. *J Am Vet Med Assoc* 2008;233(1):87–95.

Mealey KL, Gay JM, Martin LG, et al. Comparison of the hypothalamic-pituitary-adrenal axis in MDR1-1Δ and MDR1 wildtype dogs. *J Vet Emerg Crit Care* 2007;17(1):61–66.

Peyton JL, Burkitt JM. Critical illness-related corticosteroid insufficiency in a dog with septic shock. *J Vet Emerg Crit Care* 2009;19(3):262–268.

Prittie JE. Adrenal insufficiency in critical illness. In: Bonagura JB, Twedt DC, eds. *Kirk's Current Veterinary Therapy XIV*, 1st edn. St. Louis, Missouri: Saunders Elsevier, 2009, pp. 228–230.

Prittie JE, Barton LJ, Peterson ME, et al. Hypothalamo-pituitary-adrenal (HPA) axis function in critically ill cats. In: Hughes D, ed. *Proceedings of the 9th International Veterinary Emergency and Critical Care Symposium*, abstract 17. San Antonio, Texas: Veterinary Emergency and Critical Care Society, 2003, p. 771.

Schoeman JP, Goddard A, Herrtage ME. Serum cortisol and thyroxine concentrations as predictors of death in critically ill puppies with parvoviral diarrhea. *J Am Vet Med Assoc* 2007;231(10):1534–1539.

Schoeman JP, Rees P, Herrtage ME. Endocrine predictors of mortality in canine babesiosis caused by *Babesia canis rossi*. *Vet Parasitol* 2007;148(2):75–82.

CHAPTER 5

Hyperadrenocorticism in Dogs

Ellen N. Behrend and Carlos Melian

Pathogenesis

- The clinical signs of hyperadrenocorticism (HAC) result from chronically elevated serum cortisol concentrations.
- More than 80% of dogs with HAC have pituitary-dependent disease due to an adrenocorticotropic hormone (ACTH)-secreting adenoma; approximately 80% originate in the adenohypophysis (anterior pituitary) and 20% in the intermediate lobe.
- In 15–20% of cases, HAC is caused by a benign or malignant adrenal tumor.
- Ectopic ACTH secretion may occur but is extremely rare in dogs.
- Iatrogenic HAC can be caused by administration of exogenous glucocorticoids of any form.

Classical Signs

- Older, small breed dogs are predisposed to spontaneous HAC.
- Progressive polyuria/polydipsia is the most common clinical sign.
- Polyphagia, weight gain, abdominal distension, panting, weakness, and/or lethargy may occur.
- Dermatologic changes frequently exist, including alopecia, hyperpigmentation, comedones, and pyoderma.
- Iatrogenic HAC can occur in any dog; clinical signs are identical to the spontaneous disease.

Diagnosis

- Tests for spontaneous HAC are divided into screening tests, meant to determine if HAC is present, and differentiating tests, designed to ascertain whether the disease is pituitary- or adrenal-based.
- Screening tests include the ACTH stimulation test, low-dose dexamethasone suppression test and urine cortisol:creatinine ratio.
- Differentiating tests include measurement of endogenous ACTH concentration, high-dose dexamethasone suppression test and imaging, most commonly abdominal ultrasound.
- Choice of screening and differentiating tests depends on the situation.
- Iatrogenic HAC is diagnosed based on history and ACTH stimulation testing.

Clinical Endocrinology of Companion Animals, First Edition. Edited by Jacquie Rand.
© 2013 John Wiley & Sons, Inc. Published 2013 by John Wiley & Sons, Inc.

Treatment

- Mitotane is an adrenocorticolytic agent that is relatively specific for the adrenal zona fasciculata and zona reticularis.
- Trilostane is a synthetic steroid analogue that inhibits the secretion of adrenal steroid hormones.
- Ketoconazole also inhibits secretion of adrenal steroid hormones but is less effective.
- Selegiline inhibits the enzyme monoamine oxidase B and, as a result, increases hypothalamic dopamine concentrations, which, in turn, inhibit ACTH secretion from the intermediate lobe of the pituitary; it is effective in at most 20% of cases of pituitary-dependent HAC.
- Treatment for iatrogenic HAC consists of weaning the patient off the exogenous glucocorticoid.

I. Pathogenesis

A. The clinical signs of hyperadrenocorticism (HAC) result from **chronically elevated serum cortisol concentration.**

B. **Spontaneous HAC** in dogs can be caused by **excessive corticotropin (adrenocorticotropic hormone [ACTH]) secretion** or by a functional **adrenocortical tumor** that autonomously secretes cortisol:

    1. **The most common cause of ACTH hypersecretion is a pituitary tumor** leading to adrenocortical hyperplasia and excessive glucocorticoid secretion.

    2. Ectopic ACTH secretion or food-dependent hypercortisolemia has been reported rarely in dogs.

C. **Pituitary-dependent hyperadrenocorticism (PDH):**

    1. Around **80–85%** of dogs with spontaneous HAC have PDH.

    2. Most dogs with PDH have a **pituitary tumor,** but pituitary hyperplasia rarely causes HAC.

    3. **Approximately 80% of pituitary tumors causing PDH arise in the adenohypophysis (anterior pituitary);** the remainder originates in the intermediate lobe.

    4. The **most common type of pituitary tumor is a microadenoma** measuring <10 mm in height; larger pituitary tumors (macroadenomas) occur in 10–25% of patients.

    5. Pituitary **carcinoma** causing HAC is **rare.**

D. **Functional Adrenal Tumor (FAT):**

    1. In **15–20%** of dogs, the cause of HAC is a FAT that secretes excessive amounts of cortisol independent of pituitary control.

    2. Hypercortisolemia will suppress secretion of corticotropin-releasing hormone (CRH) and ACTH from the hypothalamus and pituitary, respectively, leading to **atrophy of normal adrenocortical tissue, including the whole cortex of the contralateral gland.**

    3. **Approximately 50% of FAT are adrenocortical adenomas and 50% adenocarcinomas.** They are usually unilateral but can present bilaterally.

    4. Occasionally FAT and PDH occur concurrently.

E. A report of the occurrence of PDH in a family of seven Dandie Dinmont terriers supports the role of genetic factors.

F. ACTH-independent HAC due to food-dependent hypercortisolemia was reported in a Vizsla dog with signs of hypercortisolemia. Testing indicated an increased morning urinary corticoid:creatinine ratio, which further increased (>100%) after a meal and the meal-induced increase was prevented with octreotide. Low plasma ACTH concentrations were present without evidence of an adrenal tumor. Based on similar cases in humans, it was proposed that there was ectopic expression of gastric inhibitory peptide (GIP) receptors coupled to steroidogenesis, which resulted in stimulation of cortisol secretion associated with eating.

II. Signalment

A. **Mean age at diagnosis is 9–11 years**; almost all dogs with HAC are older than 6 years.

B. **No sex predilection in dogs with PDH.** Although 60–65% of dogs with a FAT in one report were female, a sex predilection was not proven.

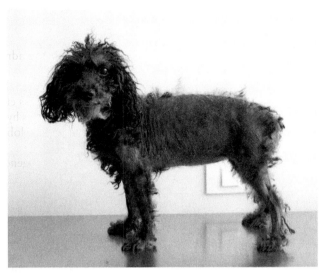

Figure 5.1 A 12-year-old female poodle with PDH showing bilateral alopecia, thin skin, superficial pyoderma, and muscle wasting.

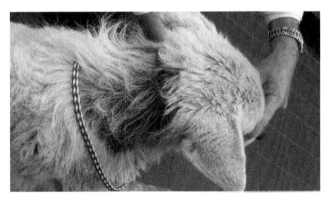

Figure 5.2 A 13-year-old spayed female mixed breed dog with PDH. Note the diffuse partial to complete alopecia with severe hyperpigmentation and loss of secondary hairs (undercoat) in the affected areas. (Photograph courtesy of Dr. Robert Kennis.)

C. **Poodles, dachshunds, various terrier breeds, German shepherd dogs, beagles, and boxers** appear to be at greater risk of developing HAC.

D. **PDH tends to occur in smaller dogs;** approximately 75% of dogs with PDH weigh <20 kg. In contrast, **almost 50% of dogs with FAT weigh >20 kg.**

III. Clinical Signs

A. **Common clinical signs:**

1. Earliest signs in most dogs are **polyuria and polydipsia;** eventually **affects 90%** of dogs with HAC by the time of diagnosis. Hypercortisolemia seems to interfere with the action and/or release of antidiuretic hormone.

2. **Alopecia,** usually truncal and bilaterally symmetrical, is common **(60–75%)** and in some dogs is the first sign noticed by the owners (Figure 5.1).

3. **Other common dermatologic signs** are a failure to regrow shaved hair; presence of thin, hypotonic skin; hyperpigmentation (Figure 5.2); pyoderma; and/or comedones, and increased susceptibility to bruising (Figure 5.3).

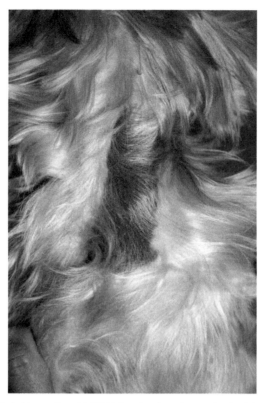

Figure 5.3   An 11-year-old male Yorkshire terrier with PDH that developed extensive bruising following jugular venipuncture.

4. Glucocorticoid excess appears to have a direct effect on appetite, causing **polyphagia and weight gain in most dogs (50–90%)**.

5. **Hepatomegaly** is present in **80–90%** of dogs. Redistribution of fat from various storage areas to the omentum, hepatomegaly, poor tone of abdominal wall musculature, and a distended urinary bladder usually cause a **distended or pendulous abdomen** (Figure 5.4), that is, a classic "pot-bellied appearance".

6. **Muscle weakness and lethargy** are often present (**50–85%**) and may be evidenced as reluctance or inability to jump; protein catabolism accounts for muscle wasting and, therefore, weakness.

7. **Panting** is often present, possibly due to many factors such as muscle weakness, pulmonary thromboembolism, abdominal enlargement, and bronchial calcification.

8. Hypercortisolism may decrease plasma concentration of follicle-stimulating hormone and luteinizing hormone causing **testicular atrophy and anestrus**.

B. **Less common clinical signs:**

1. If present, **calcinosis cutis** is highly suggestive of a diagnosis of HAC, but is not a common finding:
   a. The **lesions** consist of irregular plaques in or under the skin that feel firm or brittle (Figure 5.5).
   b. They are caused by dystrophic calcium deposition in the dermis and subcutis.

2. **Pseudomyotonia** is a myopathy characterized by persistent, active muscle contraction.
   a. It usually affects the pelvic limbs causing a stiff gait.
   b. Controversy exists as to whether pseudomyotonia is caused by HAC or is a comorbid condition worsened by HAC.

3. **Facial nerve paralysis**; cause in dogs with HAC not clear.

4. **Neurologic signs:**
   a. Occur due to the presence of a **pituitary macroadenoma**.
   b. **Initially behavioral changes** are noted; can progress to disorientation, listlessness, ataxia, aimless pacing, mental dullness, and stupor. **Seizures are rarely seen.**

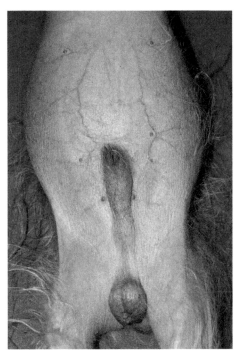

Figure 5.4 An 8-year-old male Yorkshire terrier with PDH. Note the abdominal distension, comedones, thin skin, and visible, prominent abdominal vessels.

(b)

(a)

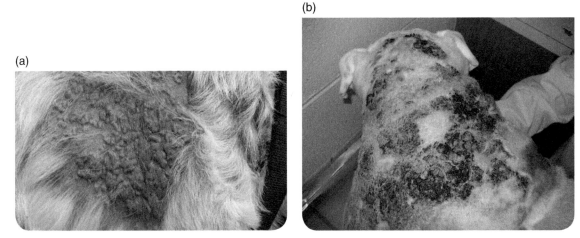

Figure 5.5 (a) A 10-year-old female spayed Labrador retriever with calcinosis cutis. Note the multifocal to coalescing, raised masses on the lateral aspect of the neck; the masses were palpably firm. Diffuse to patchy alopecia was present in the affected areas. (b) A 3.5-year-old male English bulldog with severe calcinosis cutis, presumed to be due to iatrogenic administration of glucocorticoids. The lesions were erythematous and alopecic with crusting due to excoriation and secondary bacterial infection. Note that the clinical signs of iatrogenic and spontaneous HAC are identical. (Photographs courtesy of Dr. Robert Kennis.)

    c. **Anorexia** is not common in HAC patients, but, **if present, strongly suggests the presence of a pituitary macroadenoma;** anorexia is likely due to increased intracranial pressure.
C. **Complications of HAC:**
    1. **Urinary tract infection** (UTI) is common in dogs with HAC due to the immunosuppressive effects of cortisol excess and urine retention. However, the anti-inflammatory effects of glucocorticoids may mask the clinical signs. **Recurrent infections** are possible elsewhere, **especially the skin.**

2. Dogs with HAC have increased urinary calcium excretion and a tenfold higher risk of developing **calcium-containing uroliths** compared to those without.

3. **More than 80%** of dogs with HAC have a systolic blood pressure >160 mm Hg and, thus, have **hypertension**.

4. Approximately **75% of dogs** with HAC are **proteinuric** with a urine protein:creatinine ratio >1.0 (reference range <0.5):

    a. May be related to blood pressure.

    b. The higher the blood pressure in one study, the greater the amount of protein lost in the urine and the more likely that glomerular damage was present.

5. **Pulmonary thromboembolic disease**, a rare complication of HAC, can cause moderate to severe respiratory distress.

6. As cortisol antagonizes the actions of insulin, approximately 5–10% of dogs with HAC have **diabetes mellitus**, typically with insulin resistance.

D. **Severity of clinical signs varies greatly between patients.**

E. Clinical signs of iatrogenic HAC:

    1. **Due to continued glucocorticoid administration** and are indistinguishable from those of spontaneous HAC.

    2. Alternatively, **signs of hypoadrenocorticism can be precipitated** by acute cessation of exogenous glucocorticoid administration or too rapid dose reduction.

IV. Diagnosis

A. Diagnosis of HAC can be difficult and **may require many steps. It should only be performed in dogs with appropriate clinical signs and laboratory abnormalities.**

B. Routine laboratory testing:

    1. CBC:

        a. **Stress leukogram,** which includes an elevated WBC count with **neutrophilia, monocytosis, lymphopenia, and/or eosinopenia,** is frequently present.

        b. Approximately 80% of dogs with HAC have eosinopenia and lymphopenia.

        c. Less common findings include thrombocytosis and mild erythrocytosis.

    2. Serum chemistry:

        a. Elevated liver enzyme activities most common abnormality; **alkaline phosphatase activity above the reference range in approximately 90%** and alkaline phosphatase (ALP) elevations are proportionately greater than that for alanine aminotransferase (ALT).

        b. **Cholesterol and total CO_2** may be elevated.

        c. **Hyperglycemia is common** but only about 10% of dogs with HAC have concurrent diabetes mellitus.

        d. **Blood urea nitrogen** may be decreased due to the polyuria/polydipsia.

    3. Urinalysis:

        a. Usually reveals **low specific gravity, that is, <1.015,** as 90% of patients with HAC have polyuria/polydipsia.

        b. **Proteinuria** is present in the majority; **usually low grade.**

        c. Due to the immunosuppressive effects of hypercortisolemia, UTI may be present. **Hematuria and bacteriuria may be noted;** even with infection **pyuria may or may not be present** since cortisol suppresses WBC function.

        d. Glycosuria is present if diabetes mellitus occurs concurrently.

C. **Endocrine testing:**

    1. It is **required** in dogs with history, clinical signs, and laboratory abnormalities suggestive of HAC to make the diagnosis.

    2. It is not recommended to perform testing for HAC in sick dogs until nonadrenal illness has been resolved, if possible.

    3. Endocrine testing is divided into screening and differentiating tests:

        a. **Screening tests are designed to determine if HAC present or not.**

        b. Once a diagnosis of HAC is made, **a differentiation test should be performed to determine if PDH or FAT is present.**

c. Differentiation provides information crucial to therapeutic decisions and an accurate prognosis.

d. **Differentiation tests should never be performed before a diagnosis of HAC is made via screening tests.**

4. **All cortisol concentrations below are used for illustration purposes; check with your own laboratory for its normal ranges and cutoff values.** To convert nmol/L to µg/dL, divide by 27.6.

5. Screening tests:

   a. **Urine cortisol:creatinine ratio (UC:CR):**

      1) **Protocol:** Have client **collect urine sample at home** when the pet is not stressed and bring to clinic; centrifuge sample and submit supernatant.

      2) **Principle:** Urine cortisol excretion increases as a reflection of augmented adrenal secretion of the hormone, whether PDH or FAT present; creatinine normalizes the reading for the urine concentration.

      3) **Interpretation:** An elevated UC:CR is consistent with the presence of HAC:

         a) It is a **sensitive** marker of HAC, and **present in 90–100% of affected dogs.**

         b) **False-positive results are common;** only about 20% of dogs with an elevated UC:CR have HAC.

         c) A normal ratio makes diagnosis of HAC very unlikely (≤ 10% chance).

         d) Since the chance of a false-positive result is great, an **ACTH stimulation test or low-dose dexamethasone suppression test must always be done to confirm the presence of HAC.**

   b. **Low-dose dexamethasone suppression test (LDDST):**

      1) **Protocol:**

         a) Collect a blood sample—check with your laboratory to see if plasma or serum needed.

         b) Administer **dexamethasone or dexamethasone sodium phosphate, 0.01–0.015 mg/kg IV or IM; IV preferred.**

         c) Draw blood samples 4 and 8 h after dexamethasone administration.

      2) **Principle:**

         a) In normal dogs, dexamethasone will feedback and turn off ACTH secretion from the pituitary, and, as a result, cortisol concentration will be low 4 and 8 h later, for example, < 30 nmol/L.

         b) With PDH, feedback does not work normally, so no or partial suppression of ACTH, and consequently cortisol, occurs.

         c) With FAT, the tumor secretes mainly or wholly autonomously of ACTH influence, so ACTH suppression has little to no effect on cortisol concentration.

      3) **Interpretation** (Figure 5.6a):

         a) Lack of suppression 8 h after an injection of a low dose of dexamethasone (e.g., cortisol > 30 nmol/L) is consistent with a diagnosis of HAC.

         b) **Highly sensitive; approximately 95%** of dogs with HAC are not suppressed 8 h post-dexamethasone.

         c) In dogs, there is a **relatively high chance of a false-positive result,** up to 50%, if nonadrenal illness is present.

         d) Lack of suppression at 4 h (e.g., > 30 nmol/L) but with full suppression at 8 h (e.g., < 30 nmol/L) is technically not consistent with HAC but is suspicious for its presence; further testing warranted.

         e) **With certain results, the LDDST may also serve as a differentiation test:**

            i. If the cortisol concentration in the 8 h sample is > 30 nmol/L, the result is consistent with HAC.

            ii. If, in addition, there is suppression at 4 h post-dexamethasone (i.e., an "escape" at 8 h post-dexamethasone) and/or the 4- and/or 8 h post-dexamethasone samples are < 50% of baseline, the results are consistent with PDH.

            iii. If criteria for PDH are not met, chances are still approximately 50/50 for PDH versus a FAT.

            iv. If the baseline cortisol concentration is close to 30 nmol/L or suppression is just at 50%, presence of PDH should be confirmed by other means.

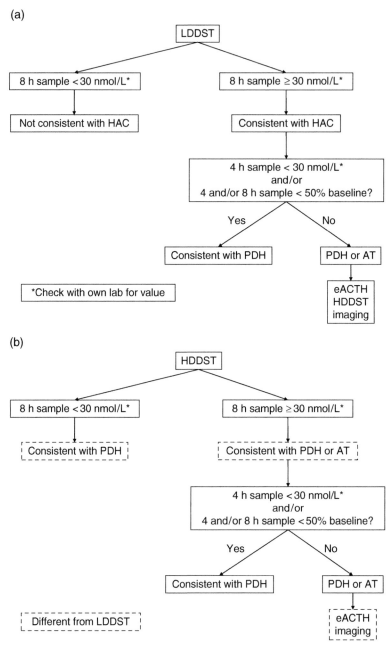

Figure 5.6 (a) Algorithm for interpretation of low-dose dexamethasone suppression test results for diagnosis of (screening for) HAC. (b) Algorithm for interpretation of high-dose dexamethasone suppression test results for differentiating between pituitary- and adrenal-dependent disease. *Check with your own laboratory for appropriate value.

   c. **ACTH stimulation test:**
     1) **Protocol:**
       a) Collect a blood sample—check with your laboratory to see if plasma or serum is needed.
       b) Administer cosyntropin at a dose of **5 μg/kg (maximal dose 250 μg/dog) IV or IM; IV preferred.**
       c) Collect a blood sample 60 min later.

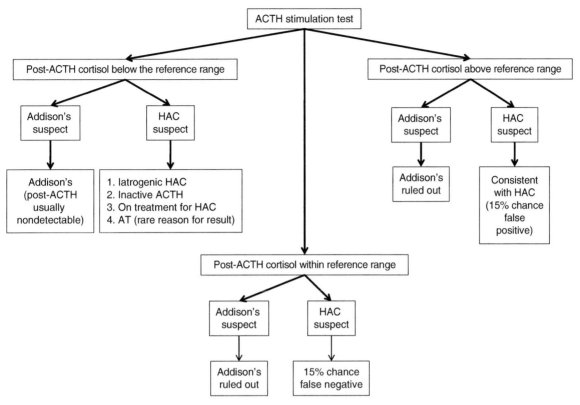

Figure 5.7 Algorithm for interpretation of ACTH stimulation test results for diagnosis of (screening for) HAC.

    d) **Compounded formulations may not work;** however if using, **collection of samples at both 60 and 120 min** after ACTH administration is recommended to ensure peak concentration measured.

2) **Principle:**
    a) ACTH stimulates adrenocortical cortisol secretion.
    b) Reserve capacity of adrenal cortex is increased either due to bilateral hyperplasia (PDH) or FAT.
    c) In iatrogenic HAC, ACTH secretion is chronically suppressed due to administration of exogenous glucocorticoids and as a result, bilateral adrenocortical atrophy occurs.

3) **Interpretation (Figure 5.7):**
    a) **Spontaneous HAC:**
       i. A **response greater than normal** is consistent with a diagnosis of spontaneous HAC.
       ii. **Overall sensitivity of the test is approximately 80%;** for PDH, sensitivity is approximately 87%, while for HAC due to a FAT, it is approximately 61%.
       iii. **Test is more specific in dogs than the LDDST;** there is only a 15% chance of a false-positive result in a dog with nonadrenal illness.
       iv. ACTH stimulation testing can never differentiate between PDH and FAT.
    b) **Iatrogenic HAC:**
       i. An **ACTH stimulation test is the only test that can diagnose iatrogenic HAC.**
       ii. **Basal and post-ACTH cortisol concentrations are typically low to unmeasurable.**
       iii. **Full diagnosis** is made with a **history of glucocorticoid exposure** by any route, presence of **consistent clinical signs** and a **post-ACTH cortisol concentration below the reference range.**

6. Differentiating tests:
   a. **High-dose dexamethasone suppression test (HDDST):**
      1) **Protocol:** Same as for LDDST, but dexamethasone dose is 0.1 mg/kg.
      2) **Principle:** Same as for LDDST; due to the higher dexamethasone dose used, more suppression of cortisol secretion may be seen in PDH cases than when a low dose is administered.
      3) Interpretation (Figure 5.6b):
         a) **Two responses are consistent with PDH:**
            i.   Complete suppression, for example, <30 nmol/L, at 4 and/or 8 h post-dexamethasone.
            ii. Concentrations are <50% of baseline 4 and/or 8 h post-dexamethasone.
         b) If baseline value is close to 30 nmol/L or suppression is just at 50%, presence of PDH should be confirmed by other means.
         c) **A HDDST can <u>never</u> confirm the presence of a FAT;** if criteria for diagnosis of PDH is not met, there is a 50/50 chance the patient has PDH or a FAT.
   b. **Endogenous ACTH (eACTH) concentration:**
      1) **Protocol:** Requires only a single blood sample but special handling is needed; check with your laboratory for instructions.
      2) **Principle:**
         a) With PDH, eACTH concentrations are inappropriately high due to secretion from the tumor.
         b) With FAT, the cortisol secreted from the tumor feeds back and turns off ACTH secretion so concentrations are low.
      3) Interpretation:
         a) In patients with PDH, eACTH concentration is normal to increased.
         b) With FAT, eACTH concentration is below normal.
         c) eACTH **can be used to confirm the presence of a FAT.**
         d) A gray zone exists in the results:
            i.   If the patient's eACTH concentration falls into this zone, results are not diagnostic.
            ii. With repeat testing when the original concentration measured is in the gray zone (**approximately 15% of cases**), approximately 96% have definitive differentiation.
            iii. There is **no way to predict when eACTH concentration will be in the gray zone.**
D. Imaging and Pathology:
   1. **Abdominal radiographs:**
      a. These may **differentiate PDH from FAT.**
      b. Approximately 40–50% canine FAT are able to be visualized; in dogs, presence of adrenal mineralization is highly suspicious for the existence of a FAT.
   2. **Chest radiographs** are indicated in patients with a FAT to check for metastases.
   3. **Ultrasonography:**
      a. Useful for differentiating PDH from FAT and staging FAT:
         1) **Bilateral adrenal enlargement is present in >90% of dogs with PDH.**
         2) **With FAT, typically the tumor is visualized on one side and atrophy of the contralateral gland** may be evident; atrophy can be difficult to assess with ultrasound and may not be apparent.
      b. Ultrasonography can **never be used as a screening test** as bilateral adrenal enlargement may be seen associated with chronic nonadrenal illness; **FAT can be small and difficult to see with ultrasonography.**
      c. Vena caval, hepatic, or renal invasion is an indicator of FAT malignancy.
   4. **CAT Scan (CT) and Magnetic Resonance Imaging (MR):**
      a. CT and MR are often useful for demonstrating pituitary macroadenomas.
      b. **Some authors advocate routine pituitary imaging in all dogs when PDH is diagnosed,** because radiation therapy (a treatment modality required for a pituitary macroadenoma) is more effective for smaller tumors. Follow-up and treatment recommendations vary depending on tumor size.
   5. **Adrenal biopsy** is usually performed on FAT obtained via adrenalectomy rather than biopsy and is often needed to differentiate benign versus malignant tumor.

6. Pathologic findings:
   a. PDH:
      1) Gross examination reveals a normal to enlarged pituitary and diffuse or nodular bilateral adrenocortical enlargement.
      2) Microscopically, any of the following may be observed: pituitary adenoma, adenocarcinoma, or corticotroph hyperplasia of anterior pituitary or intermediate lobe. Adrenocortical hyperplasia will be present.
   b. FAT:
      1) Gross examination reveals a variable-sized adrenal mass, atrophy of the contralateral gland (rarely bilateral tumors), and metastasis in some patients with adrenal carcinoma; invasion into vena cava or renal artery or vena caval thrombosis may be seen with malignant tumors.
      2) Microscopically, see adrenocortical adenoma, carcinoma, or, rarely, hyperplasia.
   c. With any form HAC, general changes of cortisol excess may be seen such as cutaneous atrophy, glomerulopathy, etc.

V. Differential Diagnoses
A. Differential diagnoses will depend on the organ systems affected.
B. **Polyuria/polydipsia:**
   1. Numerous differentials exist (see Chapter 42).
   2. Most common causes of polyuria/polydipsia in dogs, along with HAC, are **chronic renal failure and diabetes mellitus.**
C. **Polyphagia:**
   1. Numerous differentials exist.
   2. Polyphagia may be physiological, for example, pregnancy.
   3. Most common pathological differentials to consider are **diabetes mellitus, neoplasia, malassimilation syndromes, and administration of certain drugs,** especially glucocorticoids, progestins, anticonvulsants, and cyproheptadine.
D. Dermatological issues:
   1. **Differentials for bilaterally symmetrical alopecia** include hypothyroidism, sex hormone dermatoses, Alopecia X, and sex hormone–secreting adrenal tumors.
   2. **Differentials for recurrent pyoderma** include hypothyroidism, atopy, flea allergy, and food allergy.
E. **Enlarged abdomen:**
   1. In HAC, could be due to weight gain, hepatomegaly, fat redistribution, and/or weakening of the body wall.
   2. **Differentials for unexplained weight gain** include hypothyroidism, lack of activity, insulinoma, and acromegaly.
   3. **Differentials for increased abdominal circumference** include fluid accumulation, for example, ascites, tumor, organomegaly, and pyometra.
   4. **Differentials for hepatomegaly** include glucocorticoid administration, hepatic abscess, nonspecific glycogen deposition, primary hepatic tumor, diabetes mellitus, and acromegaly.

VI. Treatment
A. **General principles:**
   1. **Client education:**
      a. **If using medical therapy, lifelong therapy is required.**
      b. With mitotane and trilostane, **many follow-up visits will be required** in order to tailor the dose to the patient; serious side effects are possible with both medications.
      c. **If an adverse reaction to mitotane or trilostane occurs**—discontinue drug, give prednisone, and have a veterinarian reevaluate next day; if no response to prednisone is noted in a few hours, veterinarian should evaluate immediately.
   2. **Surgical considerations:**
      a. Surgery is the **treatment of choice in dogs with adrenocortical adenomas or nonmetastasized carcinoma** unless the patient is a poor surgical risk:

1) **Appropriate personnel and facilities are required,** as adrenalectomy is a technically demanding surgery and intensive postoperative management is required.

2) Removal of tumor and vena caval thrombi can be performed; surgery is not expected to be curative in such cases, but long-term survival can be achieved, for example, >1 year.

3) Depending on patient status, medical control of HAC may be desirable prior to surgery, if possible.

   b. **Hypophysectomy** has been described, but is generally not available in the United States.

   c. **Bilateral adrenalectomy is not used** for treatment of canine PDH.

3. **Response to treatment:**

   a. Timing of response is similar regardless of modality used:

      1) **Once control is achieved, certain signs resolve within 7–10 days;** initially, an increased activity level and decreased polyuria and polydipsia are noted.

      2) **Certain signs,** for example, dermatological, **may take several months** to completely resolve.

      3) Normalization of liver enzymes can take greater than 1 year and may never occur.

4. Special circumstances:

   a. Treatment of patients with a **pituitary macroadenoma:**

      1) Radiation therapy is required for local control of a pituitary macroadenoma.

      2) Since eACTH concentrations may take several months to decrease, the HAC should be controlled medically in the interim.

   b. Treatment of patients with **concurrent HAC and diabetes mellitus:**

      1) Treatment of diabetes must be initiated immediately to protect beta cells from glucose toxicity. However, tight glycemic control will likely not be achieved.

      2) **Control of HAC should be accomplished as soon as possible** to obviate glucocorticoid-induced insulin resistance.

      3) Careful monitoring of the diabetes needed; **insulin needs can decrease rapidly** with control of HAC.

      4) **Prednisone** administration (0.4 mg/kg once daily) has been **recommended** until medical control of HAC is achieved to ease the transition.

B. **Medical treatment of spontaneous HAC:**

   1. **Mitotane** (o,p′-DDD, Lysodren):

      a. **General info**

         1) **Destroys glucocorticoid-secreting cells of the adrenal cortex:**

            a) Zonae fasciculata and reticularis are targeted.

            b) Zona glomerulosa, that is, the zone that secretes aldosterone, is relatively spared but can be destroyed as well.

         2) Mitotane is one of two main drugs used for medical management of PDH in dogs.

         3) **May be drug of choice for medical management of FAT** since it may destroy tumor cells as well as control cortisol secretion.

         4) Used in **two treatment phases:**

            a) **Induction** (or loading) which consists of daily drug administration, ideally BID.

            b) **Maintenance,** in which the drug is dosed on a weekly basis; the dose is usually divided into two to three doses over the course of a week.

         5) **Should be given with food** to increase drug absorption.

         6) **Use with caution in patients with renal insufficiency and primary hepatic disease.**

      b. **Protocol for treating PDH:**

         1) **Induction** (Figure 5.8):

            a) Initial loading dose is **40–50 mg/kg, divided twice daily** if possible.

            b) Doses higher than 50 mg/kg/day increase the risk of complete cortisol deficiency.

            c) Loading should continue **until at least one endpoint is noted** (i.e., decreased appetite, vomiting, diarrhea, listlessness, or decreased water intake [<60 ml/kg/day; 1 cup = 240 mL and 1 oz = 30 mL]) or **maximum 8 days.**

            d) At that time, an **ACTH stimulation test** is performed.

            e) **Goal is for both basal and post-ACTH cortisol concentration to be in ideal range of approximately 30–150 nmol/L** (check with your own laboratory for ideal range).

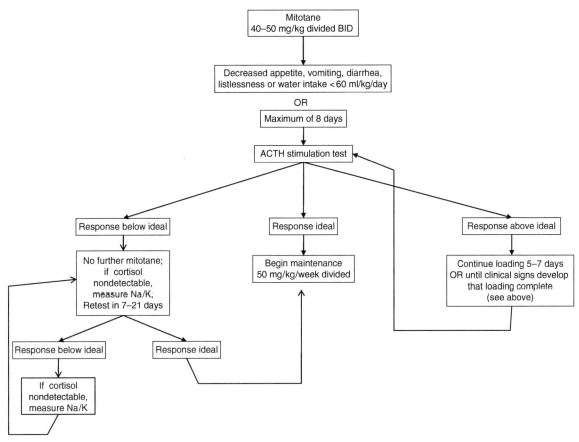

Figure 5.8 Algorithm for induction therapy using mitotane for PDH. Check with your reference laboratory for what is considered to be the "ideal range" for basal and ACTH-stimulated cortisol concentration; it is approximately 30–150 nmol/L or 1–5 µg/dL pre- and post-ACTH.

f) Induction is **continued with repeat testing as necessary until adequate response is seen**.

g) **Average length of induction** is 11 days.

h) **If a dog does not respond to the induction protocol after 14 days**, the following factors should be considered:

    i. The patient may have a FAT which are more resistant to mitotane.

    ii. The patient may be inherently resistant to mitotane; some dogs with PDH have required 30–60 days of daily therapy or high doses.

    iii. The induction dose is too low, that is, < 40 mg/kg/day.

    iv. The drug is not being absorbed well. Ensure the medication is given with food, preferably a fatty meal.

    v. The diagnosis may be incorrect or the patient is suffering from iatrogenic HAC.

    vi. Lack of owner compliance.

2) **Maintenance** (Figure 5.9):

a) **Once control is achieved, initiate maintenance therapy at 50 mg/kg/week divided into two to three doses** over the course of a week.

b) **First recheck ACTH stimulation test should be done 30 days after control is achieved**, then at 3 and 6 months and every 3–6 months thereafter or any time clinical signs return.

c) **All dosage adjustments should be based on ACTH stimulation testing** (maintain basal and post-ACTH cortisol levels within ideal range).

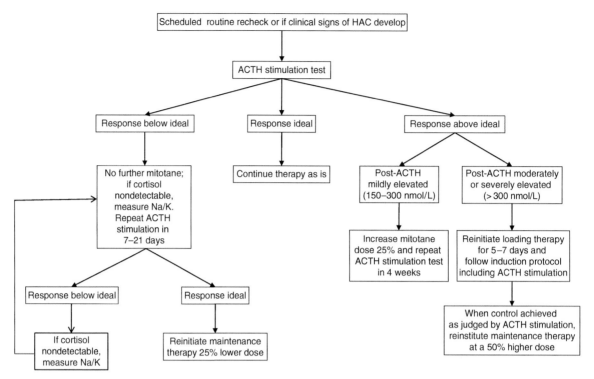

Figure 5.9   Algorithm for maintenance therapy using mitotane for PDH. Check with your reference laboratory for what is considered to be the "ideal range" for basal and ACTH-stimulated cortisol concentration; it is approximately 30–150 nmol/L or 1–5 µg/dL pre- and post-ACTH.

d) **If serum cortisol concentration pre- or post-ACTH is <30 nmol/L:**
   i.   **Stop administering mitotane and administer physiological doses of prednisone** (0.1 mg/kg BID).
   ii. Be aware that to obtain meaningful test results, do not **administer prednisone within 12 h before an ACTH stimulation test.**
   iii. Perform ACTH stimulation tests after 7 days initially; frequency of repeat testing will depend on whether cortisol concentrations increase at subsequent tests or not.
   iv. **Cortisol secretion usually recovers in weeks to a couple months** but can take longer.
   v.   Once cortisol concentration is in ideal range, discontinue prednisone and begin maintenance therapy.
   vi. **If dog had been on maintenance therapy when it became cortisol deficient,** once cortisol concentrations return to ideal range, restart maintenance at 25% lower dose.
e) **If relapse occurs** at any time while on maintenance therapy, as indicated by cortisol levels above ideal range:
   i.   **Dose adjustments are required.**
   ii. **If post-ACTH serum cortisol concentration 150–300 nmol/L,** increase maintenance dose 25% and re-evaluate with an ACTH stimulation test in 4 weeks.
   iii. **If post-ACTH serum cortisol concentration is >300 nmol/L:**
        i)   Reload for 5–7 days and do an ACTH stimulation test.
        ii) Continue loading until cortisol concentration is in ideal range, then reinitiate weekly maintenance dose at **approximately 50% higher dose.**
        iii) Retest with an ACTH stimulation test in 30 days.
   iv. One study determined the **chance of relapse to be approximately 60%** for dogs with PDH treated with mitotane; starting maintenance therapy at 50 mg/kg/week may decrease the relapse rate.

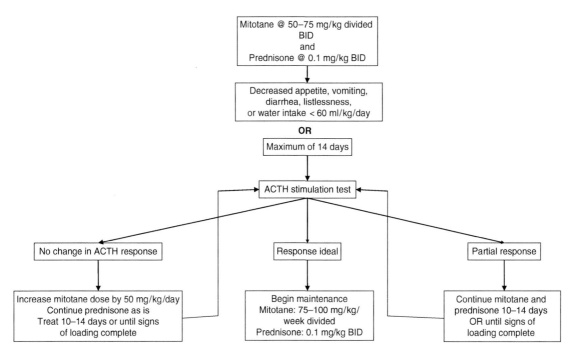

Figure 5.10   Algorithm for induction therapy using mitotane for FAT. "Ideal range" for cortisol basal and ACTH-stimulated cortisol concentration is approximately <30 nmol/L or <1 μg/dL pre- and post-ACTH; normal resting range is approximately 30–160 nmol/L or 1–5 μg/dL.

    f) The maintenance dose required may vary over time in an individual patient and is hugely variable between dogs.

  c. **Protocol for treating FAT**:

    1) **Induction** (Figure 5.10):

      a) Initial loading dose is **50–75 mg/kg, divided twice daily** if possible.

      b) Loading should continue **until at least one endpoint is noted** (i.e., decreased appetite, vomiting, diarrhea, listlessness, or decreased water intake [<60 mL/kg/day]) or **maximum 14 days**.

      c) At that time, an **ACTH stimulation test** is performed.

      d) **Goal is low-to-nondetectable (i.e., <30 nmol/L) basal and post-ACTH cortisol concentrations**:

        i. Dose should be increased by 50 mg/kg/day every 10–14 days if control has not been achieved as judged by an ACTH stimulation test.

        ii. If adverse effects develop due to mitotane, administration should continue at highest tolerable dose.

      e) Induction is **continued with repeat testing as necessary until adequate response is seen**.

      f) Since goal is to create glucocorticoid insufficiency, **give physiologic doses of prednisone during loading**.

      g) Induction **typically requires higher doses and is of longer duration than for treatment of PDH**; in one study of 32 dogs with a FAT, total induction time ranged from 10 days to 11 weeks with a mean of 24 days.

    2) **Maintenance** (Figure 5.11):

      a) Once control is achieved, maintenance therapy should begin at 75–100 mg/kg divided over the course of a week or at the highest tolerable dose.

      b) First recheck ACTH stimulation test should be done 30 days after control is achieved, then every 3 months thereafter or any time clinical signs return.

      c) All dosage adjustments should be based on ACTH stimulation testing.

      d) If cortisol levels pre- and post-ACTH rise into normal resting range (i.e., 10–160 nmol/L), increase maintenance dose 50% and recheck in 4 weeks.

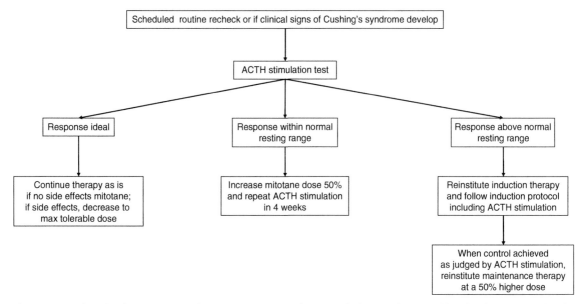

Figure 5.11 Algorithm for maintenance therapy using mitotane for FAT. "Ideal range" for cortisol basal and ACTH-stimulated cortisol concentration is approximately <30 nmol/L or <1 μg/dL pre- and post-ACTH; normal resting range is approximately 30–160 nmol/L or 1–5 μg/dL.

e) If cortisol levels rise above 160 nmol/L for pre- and post-ACTH, reload until control is achieved, then reinstitute weekly maintenance dose at a 50% higher dose.

f) As long as glucocorticoid insufficiency is present, give prednisone at 0.1 mg/kg q 12 h.

g) One study determined the chance of relapse is approximately 65% for dogs with FAT treated with mitotane.

d. **Adverse effects:**

1) Side effects of mitotane are **not uncommon:**

  a) **Occur in approximately 25% and 33% of dogs with PDH** on mitotane during the induction and maintenance phases, respectively.

  b) **Occur in approximately 60% of dogs with FAT** on mitotane; they are more common in dogs with FAT than with PDH due to the high doses of mitotane required.

2) **Side effects are mild in most dogs** and include lethargy, weakness, anorexia, vomiting, diarrhea, ataxia, disorientation, dullness, and iatrogenic hypoadrenocorticism; hepatopathy rarely reported.

3) **A CBC, biochemistry panel, and ACTH stimulation test** should be performed at every checkup and every time a dog on trilostane is ill.

4) If **vomiting, diarrhea, lethargy, weakness, and/or anorexia** occur in a dog on mitotane:

  a) It could be a direct adverse effect or due to hypocortisolemia.

  b) Mitotane administration should be stopped, physiological doses of prednisone administered, an ACTH stimulation test performed and serum electrolyte concentrations measured.

  c) **If the clinical signs are due either to hypocortisolemia or a direct effect of mitotane, they should resolve quickly with prednisone administration.** If the signs do not abate, presence of a nonadrenal illness should be suspected.

  d) **If the side effects are a direct toxicity,** mitotane dose reduction may be necessary or an alternate dosing scheme can be used, for example, divide the dose into smaller amounts to be given more frequently during the course of the week.

  e) If hypocortisolemia is present, prednisone therapy should be instituted; if aldosterone deficiency is suspected, mineralocorticoid replacement also required.

5) **If weakness, dullness, disorientation, and/or ataxia** occur in a dog on mitotane:
   a) **Could be due to direct drug toxicity or may suggest the presence of a pituitary macroadenoma.**
   b) If direct drug toxicity, signs should resolve in a few hours.
   c) CT or MRI is required to confirm the presence of a large tumor.
6) **Aldosterone deficiency is possible** secondary to mitotane therapy:
   a) Occurs in up to 10% of patients receiving mitotane therapy.
   b) Diagnosis is made on the basis of appropriate clinical signs and presence of cortisol deficiency as documented with ACTH stimulation testing, concurrent hyponatremia, and hyperkalemia.
   c) If it occurs, it is likely the patient will have permanent complete adrenocortical insufficiency; therefore, treatment for hypoadrenocorticism should be initiated (see Chapter 1).

2. Trilostane:
   a. Trilostane is a **synthetic steroid analogue that inhibits the synthesis and secretion of steroids in the adrenal cortex,** particularly cortisol and, to a lesser extent, aldosterone:
      1) It acts mainly as a **competitive inhibitor** of the 3β-hydroxysteroid dehydrogenase (3β-HSD) enzyme.
      2) Trilostane reaches peak blood concentrations at 1.5–2 h post-pill and concentrations return to baseline levels after 10–18 h.
      3) The **duration of cortisol suppression is variable,** but in most dogs, cortisol concentrations remain suppressed less than 13 h.
   b. It is recommended that trilostane be **administered with food** to enhance absorption.
   c. It is **not recommended in dogs with primary liver disease or chronic kidney disease.**
   d. Treatment protocol:
      1) Current starting dose recommended by the manufacturer is 3–6 mg/kg once daily (SID).
      2) **We recommend starting with a lower dose (1–2 mg/kg SID or 1 mg/kg BID).**
      3) **Adjustments will need to be made based on clinical signs and results of routine blood tests and ACTH stimulation testing** (Table 5.1).
      4) Even if duration of trilostane effect is shorter than 24 h, good control of the disease can be achieved with once-daily administration (Figure 5.12).
      5) Dogs that do not show significant clinical improvement despite adequate cortisol concentrations at peak effect will likely benefit from changing to twice-daily administration (Table 5.1).
      6) Initial reevaluation visits should be scheduled in **7–10 days, a month later, and every 3 months thereafter** once the dog is clinically doing well and the cortisol concentrations are acceptable. Until that time, ACTH stimulation tests should be performed 7–10 days after every dose adjustment.
      7) **A CBC, biochemistry panel, and ACTH stimulation test** should be performed at every checkup and every time a dog on trilostane is ill.
      8) **ACTH stimulating testing:**
         a) To interpret the ACTH stimulation test correctly, it **must be performed at a specific time post-pill** (i.e., started 4–6 h after trilostane is administered in order to evaluate peak effect; one author prefers doing the test closer to 4 h than 6 h); the optimal time for post-pill testing is not truly known.
         b) When using trilostane twice daily, the ACTH stimulation test can be performed as well 8–12 h post-pill to make sure cortisol is not suppressed just before trilostane administration.
         c) Performing the test 20–24 h post-pill can be useful to document short duration of trilostane action in a dog on SID treatment that is not responding clinically despite adequate cortisol concentration at peak trilostane action.
         d) Trilostane absorption is increased when given with a meal. Thus, if the pill is normally given with food, it should be given that way on the day of testing.
   e. Adverse effects:
      1) Trilostane is **well tolerated** in most dogs.
      2) Side effects (e.g., decreased appetite, lethargy, or hyperkalemia) are **usually mild** and can occur in **up to 25% of dogs.**

Table 5.1 Dose adjustment of trilostane treatment is based on clinical signs and results of routine blood and ACTH stimulation tests.

	Improvement or resolution of clinical signs	
Blood tests	**Results from ACTH stimulation test performed 2–4 h post-pill**	**Adjustment**
↓ Alkaline phosphatase	Post-ACTH cortisol: 50–200 nmol/L	Dose unchanged
↓ Alkaline phosphatase	Post-ACTH cortisol: <50 nmol/L	Discontinue trilostane administration for 5–7 days, then restart trilostane with a 25–50% dose reduction and retest in 2 weeks. If post-ACTH cortisol values remain <50 nmol/L with the reduced dose, discontinue trilostane indefinitely and retest in a month and every 3 months thereafter until recovery
↓ Alkaline phosphatase	Post-ACTH cortisol: >200 nmol/L	Dose unchanged, monitor clinical signs closely for recurrence
Mild hyperkalemia (K: 5.5–6.5 mEq/L)	Post-ACTH cortisol: 50–200 nmol/L	Dose unchanged

	Persistence of clinical signs of hyperadrenocorticism	
Blood tests	**Results from ACTH stimulation test performed 2–4 h post-pill**	**Adjustment**
↑ Alkaline phosphatase	Post-ACTH cortisol: >200 nmol/L	Increase the dose by 25–50% and retest in 2–4 weeks. Do not increase the dose in the first recheck to avoid increasing the risk of subsequent overdose!
↑ Alkaline phosphatase	Post-ACTH cortisol: 50–200 nmol/L	Consider short duration of trilostane action as a problem. Perform a 24-h post-trilostane ACTH stimulation test or a 24-h UC:CR to confirm short duration or change to BID administration starting with the same daily dose divided. Retest in 2–4 weeks

	Patient is ill	
Blood tests	**Results from ACTH stimulation test performed 2–4 h post-pill**	**Adjustment**
↓ Alkaline phosphatase	Post-ACTH cortisol: <50 nmol/L	Discontinue trilostane administration for 1 month, administer glucocorticoid as needed and retest with an ACTH stimulation test in a month. Then if dog has signs of HAC and the post-ACTH cortisol is >250 nmol/L, reinstitute trilostane treatment with a 25–50% dose reduction. If hypoadrenocorticism persists, adrenal necrosis is likely
Azotemia, ↑ K, ↓ Na	Post-ACTH cortisol: <50 nmol/L	Discontinue trilostane administration for 1 month; administer intravenous NaCl, glucocorticoids, and mineralocorticoids as needed and retest with an ACTH stimulation test in 1 month. Then if dog has signs of HAC and the post-ACTH cortisol is >250 nmol/L, reinstitute trilostane treatment with a 25–50% dose reduction. If hypoadrenocorticism persists, adrenal necrosis is likely

*CBC, biochemistry panel, and ACTH stimulation test should be performed at every scheduled checkup and every time a dog on trilostane is ill.
*Signs of HAC: increased appetite, polyuria/polydipsia, panting, distended abdomen, weakness
*Illness: decreased appetite, vomiting, trembling, dehydration, weakness
*If the ACTH stimulation test is performed 8–12 h post-pill, the ideal range for post-ACTH cortisol concentration is 50–250 nmol/L
*Dogs should be retested 2–4 weeks after any dose adjustment. Once good control of the disease is achieved, the patient should be evaluated every 3 months.

(Table adapted from: *Melian C, Perez-Alenza MD & Peterson ME. (2010) Hyperadrenocorticism in Dogs. In: Textbook of Veterinary Internal Medicine, Vol. 2, eds S.J. Ettinger and E.C. Feldman, 7th edn. pp. 1816–1840. Saunders, Philadelphia.***)**

(a)

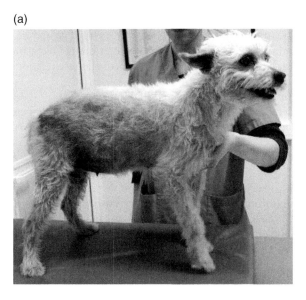

(b)

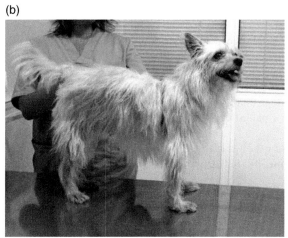

Figure 5.12   (a) An 8-year-old mixed breed dog with PDH showing alopecia and a distended abdomen. (b) Clinical signs of HAC resolved after treatment with trilostane. The dog is currently doing well after 33 months of treatment.

3) More serious side effects (e.g., depression, vomiting, shaking, or weight loss) are typically due to transient hypocortisolism and hypoaldosteronism and are uncommon, but can occur at any time during trilostane treatment.

4) **Adrenal function may remain suppressed for months or indefinitely** in dogs receiving trilostane treatment:

a) Prolonged hypoadrenocorticism was unexpected as an adverse effect since the drug is believed to act by inhibiting adrenocortical enzymes for <24 h.

b) Histological evaluation of the adrenal glands of dogs treated with trilostane has shown variable degrees of adrenocortical necrosis and hemorrhage, mostly in the zona fasciculata, but the zona glomerulosa may be affected as well.

5) **Considering** the potential serious complications, **it is extremely important to carefully monitor dogs receiving trilostane** and perform the recommended reevaluations, even if a dog is doing clinically well.

f. Trilostane **has been used successfully to treat FAT**, prolonging survival and improving quality of life, but is only suppressing cortisol secretion and not killing tumor cells.

3. L-Deprenyl (selegiline hydrochloride; Anipryl):
   a. **FDA approved** for treatment of PDH.
   b. **Mechanism of action**: Decreases pituitary ACTH secretion by increasing dopaminergic tone in the hypothalamic–pituitary axis, thus decreasing serum cortisol concentrations.
   c. **Uses**:
      1) **Indicated only for treating uncomplicated PDH.**
      2) Not recommended for dogs with concurrent illnesses such as diabetes mellitus.
      3) Since works by controlling ACTH secretion, **cannot be used to treat FAT.**
   d. **Protocol**:
      1) Initiate therapy with 1 mg/kg daily and increase to 2 mg/kg/day after 2 months if response inadequate.
      2) If higher dose also ineffective, switch to alternative therapy.
      3) **No objective monitoring;** assessment of efficacy based on subjective evaluation of remission of clinical signs.
   e. **Efficacy questionable;** one study found 20% efficacy and another judged L-deprenyl ineffective.
   f. **Adverse effects** such as anorexia, lethargy, vomiting, and diarrhea are **uncommon (<5% of dogs) and usually mild.**
   g. **Disadvantages** include poor efficacy, need for lifelong daily administration, and medication expense.
4. Ketoconazole:
   a. **Mechanism of action**:
      1) **Inhibits multiple adrenocortical enzymes** involved in hormone synthesis, including cortisol.
      2) May also block glucocorticoid receptors.
   b. **Indications**:
      1) Can be used to treat **PDH or FAT.**
      2) Can be used in dogs unable to tolerate mitotane.
      3) May be useful for palliation of clinical signs of HAC in dogs with FAT.
   c. **Protocol**:
      1) Dose is **10 mg/kg q 12 h initially;** up to 20 mg/kg q 12 h needed in some dogs.
      2) **Monitoring done by performance of ACTH stimulation tests** with same goals as for mitotane.
   d. **Efficacy approximately 50% or less.**
   e. **Adverse effects uncommon and usually mild but** include anorexia, vomiting, diarrhea, lethargy, thrombocytopenia, and idiosyncratic hepatopathy.
   f. **Use with caution** in patients with primary hepatic disease or thrombocytopenia; effect on breeding ability unknown.
5. Retinoic acid:
   a. **Mechanism of action**:
      1) May induce cellular differentiation and apoptosis.
      2) May decrease ACTH synthesis.
      3) May inhibit pituitary tumor development and proliferation.
   b. 9-*cis* retinoic acid has been used to treat a total of 27 dogs with PDH in two studies.
   c. Unfortunately, as ACTH stimulation tests were not used for monitoring, results difficult to interpret.
   d. Pituitary tumor size significantly decreased in 14 dogs that were treated for 180 days.
   e. Although results were promising, much more work needs to be done before retinoic acid therapy can be recommended.
   f. In addition, retinoic acid at the doses used in the study would likely be cost prohibitive to most owners.
6. Cabergoline:
   a. **Mechanism of action**: Cabergoline is a dopamine D2 receptor agonist; it decreases pituitary ACTH secretion by increasing dopaminergic tone in the hypothalamic–pituitary axis, thereby decreasing serum cortisol concentrations.

b. **Only limited use so far:**
1) One study reported with 42 dogs.
2) Long-term efficacy 42% (17/42 dogs); seven additional dogs responded transiently.
3) Unfortunately, as ACTH stimulation tests were not used for monitoring, results are difficult to interpret.
4) A significant reduction in tumor size was noted overall.
5) The only adverse effect noted was vomiting after the first one or two doses in some dogs.
6) The dogs that responded had significantly smaller tumors than those that did not.
c. Although results were promising, more work needs to be done before cabergoline therapy can be recommended.

C. **Treatment of iatrogenic HAC:**
1. The patient **needs to be tapered off glucocorticoid supplementation** until their adrenal gland function recovers.
2. **Protocol for tapering:**
a. The dose of glucocorticoid should be **decreased to physiological doses** of prednisone as quickly as possible; the tapering rate will depend on the disease being treated, the current dose, the chronicity of therapy, steroid administered, etc.
b. If adrenal suppression is secondary to topical glucocorticoid administration, **topical administration should be stopped and oral prednisone initiated** at physiological doses.
c. If a physiological dose is tolerated for a week without clinical signs of cortisol deficiency, the dosage should be reduced by administering the drug every other day.
d. After 2 additional weeks at the new dose, the dosage should be further reduced by giving the medication every third day.
e. After another 2–3 weeks, prednisone most likely can be discontinued. Ideally, however, **before discontinuation, an ACTH stimulation test should be performed** 12 h after the last dose of prednisone to ensure the patient has a normal adrenal reserve.
3. **If the glucocorticoid therapy must be maintained to treat a disease process and no alternative is available,** the dose should be decreased to the lowest dose possible of the least potent glucocorticoid to control the disease for which it is being administered; whether the clinical signs of iatrogenic HAC will abate depends on the final dose achieved.

D. **Drugs to avoid in dogs with HAC:**
1. Do not use **nonsteroidal anti-inflammatory agents** in dogs with uncontrolled HAC.
2. **Drugs that increase blood pressure or coagulation** should be used with caution.

VII. Prognosis
A. Untreated HAC is generally a progressive disorder with a poor prognosis.
B. **PDH due to a microadenoma:**
1. If treated, **usually a good prognosis**.
2. Median survival time with mitotane or trilostane treatment **approximately 2 years**; at least 10% survive 4 years.
3. Dogs living longer than 6 months **tend to die of causes unrelated to HAC.**
C. **PDH due to a macroadenoma:**
1. **Depends on presence of neurologic signs.**
2. With neurologic signs present, poor to grave prognosis.
3. With no or mild neurologic signs, fair to good prognosis with radiation and medical therapy.
D. **FAT:**
1. **Adrenal adenomas** usually have a good to excellent prognosis with removal.
2. **Small carcinomas (not metastasized)** have a fair to good prognosis overall, and a good to excellent prognosis with surgical resection.
3. **Large carcinomas and FAT with widespread metastasis** generally have a poor to fair prognosis, but impressive responses to high doses of mitotane are occasionally seen.

E.   **Iatrogenic HAC** has a good to excellent prognosis with ability to wean the patient from glucocorticoid therapy; if weaning not possible, decrease dose of exogenous glucocorticoid to absolute minimum required.

VIII. Prevention

A.   None known for spontaneous HAC.

B.   For **iatrogenic HAC, limit exogenous glucocorticoid use of any form** to the least potent form with the shortest duration of action at the lowest dose and for the shortest interval possible.

References and Further Readings

Alenza DP, Arenas C, Lopez ML, et al. Long-term efficacy of trilostane administered twice daily in dogs with pituitary-dependent hyperadrenocorticism. *J Am Anim Hosp Assoc* 2006;42(4):269–276.

Behrend EN, Kemppainen RJ. Diagnosis of canine hyperadrenocorticism. *Vet Clin North Am* 2001;31:985–1003.

Braddock JA, Church DB, Robertson ID, et al. Trilostane treatment in dogs with pituitary-dependent hyperadrenocorticism. *Aust Vet J* 2003;81:600–607.

Braddock JA, Church DB, Robertson ID, et al. Inefficacy of selegiline in treatment of canine pituitary-dependent hyperadrenocorticism. *Aust Vet J* 2004;82:272–277.

Castillo V, Giacomini D, Páez-Pereda M, et al. Retinoic acid as a novel medical therapy for Cushing's disease in dogs. *Endocrinology* 2006;147:4438–4444.

Castillo VA, Gomez NV, Lalia JC, et al. Cushing's disease in dogs: Cabergoline treatment. *Res Vet Sci* 2008;85:26–34.

Feldman EC, Nelson RW. Canine hyperadrenocorticism (Cushing's syndrome). In: Feldman EC, Nelson RW, eds. *Feline and Canine Endocrinology and Reproduction*, 3rd ed. Philadelphia: Saunders, 2004, pp. 252–357.

Kintzer PP, Peterson ME. Mitotane (o, p' -ddd) treatment of 200 dogs with pituitary-dependent hyperadrenocorticism. *J Vet Intern Med* 1991;5:182–190.

Kintzer PP, Peterson ME. Mitotane treatment of cortisol secreting adrenocortical neoplasia: 32 cases (1980–1992). *J Am Vet Med Assoc* 1994;205:54–61.

Galac S, Kars VJ, Voorhout G, et al. ACTH-independent hyperadrenocorticism due to food-dependent hypercortisolemnia in a dog. A case report. *Vet J* 2008;177:141–143.

Melian C, Perez-Alenza MD, Peterson ME. Hyperadrenocorticism in dogs. In: Ettinger SJ, Feldman EC, eds. *Textbook of Veterinary Internal Medicine*, Vol. 2, 7th edn. Philadelphia: Saunders, 2010, pp. 1816–1840.

Neiger R, Ramsey L, O'Connor J, et al. Trilostane treatment of 78 dogs with pituitary-dependent hyperadrenocorticism. *Vet Rec* 2002;150(26):799–804.

Ortega T, Feldman EC, Nelson RW, et al. Systemic arterial blood pressure and urine protein/creatinine ratio in dogs with hyperadrenocorticism. *J Am Vet Med Assoc* 1996;209(10):1724–1729.

Reusch CE, Sieber-Ruckstuhl N, Wenger M, et al. Histological evaluation of the adrenal glands of seven dogs with hyperadrenocorticism treated with trilostane. *Vet Rec* 2007;160(7):219–224.

Vaughan MA, Feldman EC, Hoar BR, et al. Evaluation of twice-daily, low-dose trilostane treatment administered orally in dogs with naturally occurring hyperadrenocorticism. *J Am Vet Med Assoc* 2008;232(9):1321–1328.

CHAPTER 6

Primary Functioning Adrenal Tumors Producing Signs Similar to Hyperadrenocorticism Including Atypical Syndromes in Dogs

Kate Hill

Pathogenesis

- Most adrenal tumors secrete cortisol, but oversecretion of other adrenal hormones is also possible.
- Adrenal tumors (particularly adenocarcinomas) may secrete adrenal sex hormones due to disruption of normal adrenal function.
- Progestins can act as glucocorticoid receptor agonists.
- Serum cortisol concentrations may be normal to subnormal in these cases.

Classical Signs

- Signs are the same as for hypercortisolism.
- Include polyuria, polydipsia, polyphagia, pendulous abdomen, excessive bruising, panting, alopecia, clitoral hypertrophy, testicular atrophy, anestrus, weakness/lethargy, exercise intolerance, muscle atrophy, and obesity.

Diagnosis

- Clinical signs of hypercortisolism, with serum cortisol concentrations below or within the reference range on ACTH stimulation or low-dose dexamethasone testing and elevated concentrations of adrenal sex hormones on ACTH stimulation testing.

Treatment

- Goal of treatment for functional adrenal tumors is resolution of clinical signs with surgical excision of the adrenal mass.
- If surgical excision is not possible or a tumor is not present, medical therapy may help with clinical signs, with mitotane being the drug of choice.

Clinical Endocrinology of Companion Animals, First Edition. Edited by Jacquie Rand.
© 2013 John Wiley & Sons, Inc. Published 2013 by John Wiley & Sons, Inc.

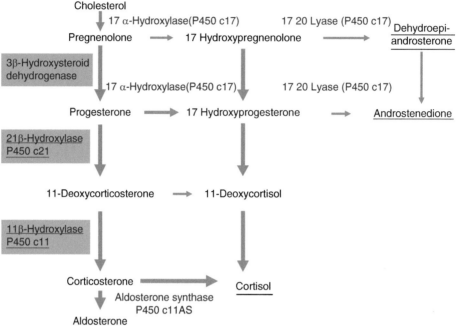

Cytochrome P450 enzymes present in the adrenal cortex

Figure 6.1 Cytochrome P450 enzymes present in the adrenal cortex.

I. Pathogenesis

A. Hyperadrenocorticism is defined as an excessive production of any of the adrenocortical hormones. Secretion of hormones other than cortisol has been well documented in humans with adrenal carcinomas. In the veterinary literature, a few case reports exist of dogs with **adrenal carcinomas** showing clinical signs of hyperadrenocorticism, but with normal cortisol concentrations, and that have **increased adrenal sex hormone and/or mineralocorticoid concentrations**. To date, the author is not aware of any cases of canine adrenal adenomas causing increases in adrenal hormones other than cortisol:

1. The exact pathogenesis and mechanism of increases in adrenal steroids other than cortisol in adrenal carcinomas is unclear. In humans, **aberrant biosynthetic pathways** resulting in a deficiency of the adrenal steroidogenic enzymes 21β-hydroxylase (P450 c21) and 11β-hydroxylase (P450 c11) have been well documented in adrenal carcinomas. The enzyme deficiencies result in an increased concentration and secretion of precursor steroids (Figure 6.1).

2. The invasion of malignant adrenal tissue into the adrenal cortex may disrupt or destroy enzymatic pathways, which can also result in increased steroid precursors.

3. **Progestins** (and possibly other steroid intermediates) can **displace cortisol** from its serum-binding protein, resulting in **elevated circulating concentrations of free cortisol**, the active form of cortisol. Elevations in free cortisol concentrations may then cause the associated clinical signs of hyperadrenocorticism.

4. Progestins can act as **glucocorticoid agonists**, and hence result in glucocorticoid activity.

5. Elevated secretion of mineralocorticoids alone should not cause signs similar to hypercortisolism (see Chapter 12).

B. A syndrome of "atypical hyperadrenocorticism" has been defined as the presence of clinical signs consistent with hyperadrenocorticism due to cortisol excess, but negative results on standard ACTH stimulation and/or low-dose dexamethasone testing. **Dogs with atypical hyperadrenocorticism** will have an **increase in adrenal sex hormones** (cortisol precursors):

(a)   (b)

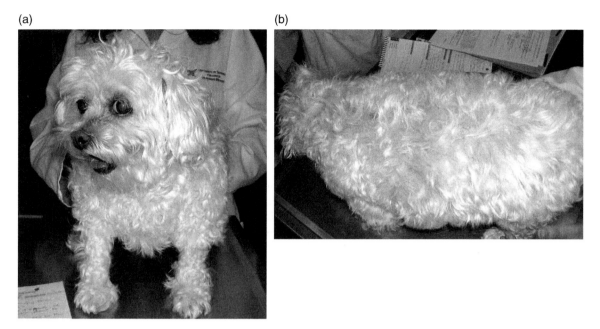

Figure 6.2   (a) A dog diagnosed with atypical hyperadrenocorticism. The dog presented for a thinning hair coat, polyphagia, and a perianal adenoma that was most likely induced from the increase in adrenocortical hormones. The cortisol testing was normal; however, ACTH-stimulated 17-hydroxyprogesterone concentration was increased (3.6 ng/mL; reference range 0.4–1.6 ng/mL). (b) Same dog as in (a); note the thinning hair coat on the dorsum.

1. Both pituitary- and adrenal-dependent forms (i.e., adrenal tumor) have been documented.
2. The exact pathophysiology of atypical hyperadrenocorticism has not been documented. It has been postulated that some of these may be early cases of hyperadrenocorticism where the cortisol concentrations have not increased enough to be detected.
3. Rarely, inadvertent exposure to hormone creams containing progestins can produce a syndrome consistent with typical hyperadrenocorticism. More often, these preparations are combined with estrogen and produce signs of hyperestrogenism.
4. Total cortisol concentrations, not free cortisol concentrations, are typically measured in standard ACTH stimulation tests and dexamethasone suppression tests. In cases of atypical pituitary-dependent HAC, since cortisol precursors may increase serum free cortisol concentrations, it is possible that total cortisol concentrations are within the reference range, but free cortisol concentrations are elevated.

II. Signalment
A. Middle-aged to older animals.
B. Currently no breed or sex predilection has been identified.

III. Clinical Signs
A. Clinical signs are similar to those of hypercortisolism in dogs (see Chapter 5).
B. Polyuria, polydipsia, polyphagia, and alopecia are predominantly reported.
C. Pendulous abdomen, excessive bruising, panting, alopecia, clitoral hypertrophy, testicular atrophy, anoestrus, weakness/lethargy, exercise intolerance, muscle atrophy, and obesity can also occur (Figure 6.2a and b).

IV. Diagnosis
A. This is a clinical disorder. Clinical signs consistent with hypercortisolemia must be present, but standard diagnostic testing for hyperadrenocorticism (ACTH stimulation test, low-dose dexamethasone suppression test, etc.) has resulted in subnormal, normal, or equivocal results.
B. CBC, serum chemistry, and urinalysis are usually consistent with hyperadrenocorticism (see Chapter 5).

C. Diagnosis is based on the ACTH stimulation test where assays are performed on an extended range of adrenal hormones. Elevations in the ACTH-stimulated hormone concentrations are considered diagnostic for the disease. Ideally cortisol, progesterone, and 17-hydroxy-progesterone concentrations are analyzed, with the possible addition of androstenedione and estradiol if ACTH-stimulated concentrations of cortisol and the progestins are within the reference ranges. Aldosterone and corticosterone concentrations may also be requested if mineralocorticoid excess is a possibility (e.g., hypernatremia, hypokalemia, clinical weakness, etc., are present).
D. It is important to realize that adrenal hormones can be increased in dogs with nonadrenal illness and also in dogs with adrenal medullary tumors. **Results must be interpreted along with the clinical signs of the dog.** Some dogs with nonadrenal disease, such as neoplasia, appear to have a proportionate increase in all of the adrenal hormone concentrations (which may include cortisol concentrations). One study of dogs with nonadrenal neoplasia showed that 32/35 (91%) had normal cortisol concentrations post-ACTH stimulation, but 11/35 (31%) had increased 17-hydroxy-progesterone concentrations after ACTH stimulation.
E. The sensitivity and specificity for adrenal hormone precursor concentrations for diagnosis of atypical hyperadrenocorticism have not been determined. The sensitivity and specificity of 17-α-hydroxy-progesterone concentrations in the diagnosis of typical hyperadrenocorticism was calculated at 71% when using a cut off of 2.5 ng/mL (8.5 nmol/L). When interpreting post-ACTH concentrations of 17-hydroxyprogesterone for atypical adrenocortical neoplasia, it has been suggested to interpret results below 5 ng/mL (16.5 nmol/L) with care. Post-ACTH stimulation reference ranges for 17-hydroxyprogesterone are usually in the range of 0.4–2.8 ng/mL (1.2–8.5 nmol/L).
F. Abdominal ultrasonography to examine the adrenal glands for the presence of unilateral or bilateral tumors is required as well as to investigate the potential for metastasis. Metastasis can be local or can be to the liver. Hepatomegaly is also common. Ultrasound can indicate the tumor is malignant if metastasis or vascular invasion is present; the absence of such findings, however, does not necessarily mean the tumor is benign.
G. *Three-view* thoracic radiographs should also be taken to ensure thoracic metastasis is not present.
H. Advanced imaging using CT or MRI may be required prior to surgery of the adrenal tumor to further identify metastasis or vascular invasion.
I. Histology of the tumor is required to differentiate adrenal adenoma from carcinoma. Biopsies are usually obtained surgically, but can be performed under ultrasound guidance or with laparoscopy.
J. Positron emission tomography (PET) CT, if available, may also help locate metastasis.
K. Repeated blood pressure measurements and a fundic examination are also recommended to ensure hypertension is not present. The presence of systolic blood pressure measurements greater than 160 mm Hg will most likely require therapy. Angiotensin-converting enzyme inhibitors (ACEI) such as benazepril (0.25–0.5 mg/kg q 24 h/os) or enalapril (0.25–0.5 mg/kg q 12–24 h/os) can be administered. Calcium-channel blockers such as amlodipine (0.1–0.4 mg/kg q 24 h/os) can also be used in conjunction with ACEI or alone.

V. Differential Diagnosis
A. Other causes of polyuria and polydipsia.
B. Other causes of polyphagia.
C. Other causes of bilaterally symmetrical nonpruritic alopecia.

VI. Treatment
A. **Adrenocortical neoplasia:**
   1. The primary therapy for adrenocortical neoplasia if possible is **surgical removal** of all neoplastic tissue (see Chapter 5). Adrenalectomy should be performed by an extremely experienced surgical team for the best results to be achieved.
   2. Medical management with **ketoconazole** (10–15 mg/kg/day) or trilostane (3–10 mg/kg/day) is recommended prior to surgery. Little information exists on the use of mitotane preoperatively in dogs; however, it could be used, starting at 25–37.5 mg/kg q 12 h PO. The goal of therapy is to minimize clinical signs prior to surgery. As cortisol concentrations are usually normal in affected dogs prior to medical therapy, cortisol concentrations should be monitored to ensure they do not decrease into the hypoadrenocortical range with presurgical treatment. Both the basal and the ACTH-stimulated cortisol concentration should be within the basal reference range prior to surgery. Residual tumor or metastasis should be treated with mitotane.

3. Medical therapy of adrenocortical tumors with **trilostane or mitotane** has been reported in dogs. Higher doses of mitotane are usually required for adrenocortical carcinomas and relapses occur in around 50% of cases treated medically. Mitotane can be adrenolytic and is the drug of choice (if available) when there are metastases or residual disease after surgery:

a. The induction dose of **mitotane** is 25–37.5 mg/kg PO q 12 h for 7–10 days (mean dose required in one study was 46 mg/kg/day for 14 days followed by an ACTH stimulation test every 10–14 days. **Prednisone** (0.2 mg/kg/day) should be dispensed for administration as the goal of therapy for adrenocortical tumors is to create cortisol deficiency, that is, nondetectable basal and ACTH-stimulated cortisol concentrations. If there is still a response to the ACTH stimulation test, mitotane is increased in 50 mg/kg/week increments. Once control is achieved, maintenance therapy should be initiated at 75–100 mg/kg/week divided into two to four treatment doses. The maintenance dose after a mean treatment time of 13.2 months in 30 dogs with cortisol-secreting adrenal tumors ranged from 35–1273 mg/kg/week. ACTH stimulation tests are performed every 3 months (see Chapter 5).

b. **Trilostane therapy** (3–10 mg/kg/day PO) has provided a palliative response and prolongs life but will not stop tumor growth or metastasis. The aim is to have an ACTH-stimulated cortisol concentration of less than 5 μg/dL (150 nmol/L). ACTH stimulation tests should be performed 4 h post pill administration.

B. Atypical hyperadrenocorticism:

1. Medical management alone using trilostane or mitotane has been used successfully to treat both typical and atypical cases of hyperadrenocorticism at routine dose rates. Trilostane appears to increase 17-hydroxyprogesterone concentrations; therefore, mitotane may be the preferred treatment. Cortisol concentrations need to be monitored with an ACTH stimulation test.

2. Therapy with **melatonin** (3 mg twice daily by mouth for dogs <30 lb [13.5 kg] or 6 mg twice daily for dogs >30 lb) has been suggested.

3. A combination of melatonin (3–6 mg) and mitotane has been used to treat dogs with alopecia and sex hormone imbalance (Alopecia X). Partial or complete hair growth occurred in 60% of dogs (Frank et al. 2004b).

4. Other drugs that have been suggested to treat atypical hyperadrenocorticism include **lignan** and ketoconazole.

VII. Prognosis

A. The prognosis for adrenal carcinomas is good if surgical excision can be performed and metastasis is not present. Median survival of dogs with surgery if no metastasis is present is 17.5–36 months.

B. Prognosis is poor if metastasis or local vascular invasion is present.

C. For adrenal tumors treated with mitotane, in one study mean survival was 16.4 months (median 11.5 months, range 20 days to 5.1 years).

D. In three dogs with adrenal tumors treated medically with trilostane, survival ranged from 9–16 months.

E. Dogs with atypical hyperadrenocorticism have a good prognosis if the clinical signs can be controlled with medical therapy.

VIII. Prevention

A. There is no known prevention for this condition. Anecdotally, some cases of atypical hyperadrenocorticism have been iatrogenic, with the owners exposing pets to hormone creams that contain progestins.

References and Further Readings

Anderson CR, Birchard SJ, Powers BE, Belandria GA, Kuntz CA, Withrow SJ. Surgical treatment of adrenocortical tumors: 21 cases (1990–1996). *J Am Anim Hosp Assoc* 2001;37:93–97.

Behrend EN, Kemppainen RJ, Boozer AL, Whitley EM, Smith AN, Busch KA. Serum 17-alpha-hydroxyprogesterone and corticosterone concentrations in dogs with nonadrenal neoplasia and dogs with suspected hyperadrenocorticism. *J Am Vet Med Assoc* 2005a;227:1762–1767.

Behrend EN, Weigand CM, Whitley EM, Refsal KR, Young DW, Kemppainen RJ. Corticosterone- and aldosterone-secreting adrenocortical tumor in a dog. *J Am Vet Med Assoc* 2005b;226:1662–1666.

Benchekroun G, De Fornel-Thibaud P, Lafarge S, Gomez E, Begon D, Delisle F, Moraillon R, Heripret D, Maurey C, Rosenberg D. Trilostane therapy for hyperadrenocorticism in three dogs with adrenocortical metastasis. *Vet Rec* 2008;163:190–192.

Benitah NM, Feldman EC, Kass PH, Nelson RW. Evaluation of serum 17-hydroxyprogesterone concentration after administration of ACTH in dogs with hyperadrenocorticism. *J Am Vet Med Assoc* 2005;227:1095–1101.

Brown CG, Graves TK. Hyperadrenocorticism: Treating dogs. *Compend Contin Educ Vet* 2007;29:132–144.

Chapman PS, Mooney CI, Ede J, Evans H, O'Connor J, Pfeiffer DU, Neiger R. Evaluation of the basal and post-adrenocorticotrophic hormone serum concentrations of 17-hydroxyprogesterone for the diagnosis of hyperadrenocorticism in dogs. *Vet Rec* 2003;153:771–775.

Eastwood JM, Elwood CM, Hurley KJ. Trilostane treatment of a dog with functional adrenocortical neoplasia. *J Small Anim Pract* 2003;44:126–131.

Frank LA, Davis JA, Oliver JW. Serum concentrations of cortisol, sex hormones of adrenal origin, and adrenocortical steroid intermediates in healthy dogs following stimulation wfth two doses of cosyntropin. *Am J Vet Res* 2004a;65:1631–1633.

Frank LA, Hnilica KA, Oliver JW. Adrenal steroid hormone concentrations in dogs with hair cycle arrest (Alopecia X) before and during treatment with melatonin and mitotane. *Vet Dermatol* 2004b;15:278–284.

Hill KE, Scott-Moncrieff JCR, Koshko MA, Glickman LT, Glickman NW, Nelson RW, Blevins WE, Oliver JW. Secretion of sex hormones in dogs with adrenal dysfunction. *J Am Vet Med Assoc* 2005;226:556–561.

Kintzer PP, Peterson ME. Mitotane treatment of 32 dogs with cortisol-secreting adrenocortical neoplasms. *J Am Vet Med Assoc* 1994;205:54–61.

Kyles AE, Feldman EC, De Cock HEV, Kass PH, Mathews KG, Hardie EM, Nelson RW, Ilkiw JE, Gregory CR. Surgical management of adrenal gland tumors with and without associated tumor thrombi in dogs: 40 cases (1994–2001). *J Am Vet Med Assoc* 2003;223:654–662.

Norman EJ, Thompson H, Mooney CT. Dynamic adrenal function testing in eight dogs with hyperadrenocorticism associated with adrenocortical neoplasia. *Vet Rec* 1999;144:551–554.

Oliver JW. Treatment option considerations steroid profiles in the diagnosis of atypical hyperadrenocorticism [Online]. 2010. Available at: http://www.vet.utk.edu/diagnostic/endocrinology/pdf/TreatmentInfoAtypicalCushingsRevised201001.pdf (accessed on February 26, 2010).

Ristic JME, Ramsey IK, Heath FM, Evans HJ, Herrtage ME. The use of 17-hydroxyprogesterone in the diagnosis of canine hyperadrenocorticism. *J Vet Intern Med* 2002;16:433–439.

Samuels MH, Loriaux DL. Cushings-syndrome and the nodular adrenal-gland. *Endocrinol Metab Clin North Am* 1994;23:555–569.

Scavelli TD, Peterson ME, Matthiesen DT. Results of surgical-treatment for hyperadrenocorticism caused by adrenocortical neoplasia in the dog—25 cases (1980–1984). *J Am Vet Med Assoc* 1986;189:1360–1364.

Schwartz P, Kovak JR, Koprowski A, Ludwig LL, Monette S, Bergman PJ. Evaluation of prognostic factors in the surgical treatment of adrenal gland tumors in dogs: 41 cases (1999–2005). *J Am Vet Med Assoc* 2008;232:77–84.

Syme HM, Scott-Moncrieff JC, Treadwell NG, Thompson MF, Snyder PW, White MR, Oliver JW. Hyperadrenocorticism associated with excessive sex hormone production by an adrenocortical tumor in two dogs. *J Am Vet Med Assoc* 2001;219:1725–1728.

CHAPTER 7

Hyperadrenocorticism in Cats

Danièlle Gunn-Moore and Kerry Simpson

Pathogenesis

- Excess cortisol as a result of a pituitary or adrenal tumor.
- Frequently results in insulin resistance and secondary diabetes mellitus.
- Iatrogenic hyperadrenocorticism is rare in the cat.

Classical Signs

- Most cats are middle aged to old.
- Moderate to severe polyuria and polydipsia (often secondary to diabetes), poor coat, fragile skin syndrome, pot belly.

Diagnosis

- Low-dose dexamethasone suppression test is the screening test of choice; but needs to be used in combination with other tests.

Treatment

- Medical therapy with trilostane and/or surgical removal of one or both adrenal glands.

I. Pathogenesis

A. **Naturally occurring hyperadrenocorticism is a relatively uncommon disease in the cat;** approximately 70 cases have been published. Iatrogenic hyperadrenocorticism has been seen only occasionally as **cats appear to be relatively resistant to the deleterious effects of exogenous corticosteroids.** The paucity of primary hyperadrenocorticoid cases may stem from the cats' ability to remain asymptomatic despite large doses of corticosteroids:

1. However, the incidence in cats is not dissimilar to that reported in humans, whereas dogs seem to be predisposed to the development of this condition.

B. **Approximately 80% of feline primary hyperadrenocorticism are caused by an adrenocorticotropin (ACTH)-secreting pituitary tumor.** The high circulating levels of ACTH result in bilateral adrenal hyperplasia

Clinical Endocrinology of Companion Animals, First Edition. Edited by Jacquie Rand.
© 2013 John Wiley & Sons, Inc. Published 2013 by John Wiley & Sons, Inc.

Table 7.1 Differential diagnoses for insulin-resistant diabetes mellitus (DM) and skin fragility in cats.

	Differential diagnosis
Insulin-resistant DM (see Chapter 16)	Obesity
	Infection
	Inflammatory process
	Neoplasia
	Drug administration
	Acromegaly
	Hyperadrenocorticism
	Hyperthyroidism
	Sex hormone–producing tumors
Skin fragility	Hyperadrenocorticism
	Diabetes mellitus
	Chronic disease especially liver disease
	Excessive exogenous glucocorticoids
	Pancreatic carcinomas
	Cutaneous neoplasms
	Sex hormone–secreting neoplasms
	Ehlers–Danlos syndrome

(i.e., **pituitary-dependent hyperadrenocorticism; PDH**). The majority of these tumors are adenomas, with 50% being large enough to visualize on CT or MRI.

C. **Approximately 20% of cases are caused by functional adrenal tumors (adrenal-dependent hyperadreno-corticism; ADH)** that autonomously secrete cortisol or occasionally other steroid hormones; 50% of these tumors are benign adenomas, and 50% are malignant adenocarcinomas.

II. Signalment

A. Hyperadrenocorticism is generally a disease of middle-aged to old cats (range 4–16 years, **mean ~11 years**). There appears to be no breed predisposition (the majority of cases have been domestic short- or long-haired cats), and there appears to be no gender bias.

III. Clinical Signs

A. **In general, clinical signs are not detected in cats until they develop diabetes mellitus** (as a result of insulin antagonism by the elevated cortisol concentration). Therefore, the majority of cats diagnosed with hyperadrenocorticism (approximately 80%) have concurrent diabetes mellitus, and many of the clinical signs can be attributed to this disease (Table 7.1):

1. The most commonly reported **clinical signs include polyuria, polydipsia, polyphagia, weight loss,** generalized **muscle loss, weakness,** and **lethargy**. Affected cats often have **poor coat condition**, with spontaneous **alopecia** or failure of hair regrowth after clipping, and **fragile thin inelastic skin that bruises easily and is prone to tearing** (i.e., fragile skin syndrome).

2. Cats frequently have a **potbellied appearance** which is thought to result from the catabolic effects of cortisol weakening the abdominal muscles and alterations in fat distribution leading to an accumulation of mesenteric fat.

B. The most commonly reported **abnormalities on physical examination are abdominal enlargement, muscle atrophy, thin skin, and an unkept hair coat or hair loss** (Figure 7.1). **Hepatomegaly** has been reported in approximately 20% of cases, although this is not an uncommon finding in cats with diabetes mellitus. Less frequently seen clinical signs include generalized skin tears, calcinosis cutis, plantigrade stance (which is thought to result from diabetic neuropathy), bruising, seborrhea, or occasionally a palpable abdominal mass.

IV. Diagnosis
A. **Clinical pathology changes are highly variable,** with the classic changes reported in dogs not generally being reliable indicators of hyperadrenocorticism in cats:
   1. Abnormalities detected on **routine hematology** may include a stress leukogram (neutrophilia and/or lymphopenia) or, occasionally, a mild variably regenerative anemia.
   2. **Serum biochemistry** may demonstrate increases in liver enzymes, although these alterations are present far less frequently in feline hyperadrenocorticism than they are in the canine form of the disease:
      a. Cats do not have a "steroid-induced" isoenzyme of serum alkaline phosphatase (AP) and therefore **AP is rarely elevated.** Serum alanine aminotransferase (**ALT**) activity **is increased slightly more frequently,** but many cats with elevations in this enzyme have concurrent hepatic disease.
      b. Since hyperadrenocorticism is frequently associated with **diabetes mellitus,** serum biochemistry and urinalysis often reveal persistent hyperglycemia and glucosuria, but very rarely show ketonuria. Hypercholesterolemia may be seen, but only in cats with concurrent diabetes mellitus.
      c. Azotemia is not an uncommon finding; however, whether or not this is related to the disease process, concurrent diabetes mellitus, or intrinsic renal insufficiency is unclear.
      d. Urinalysis generally reveals a specific gravity >1.020. However, the assessment of urine specific gravity is inaccurate in the face of significant glucosuria, and as no studies have assessed urine osmolality, no inferences can be made regarding the renal function in these cats.
      e. Other less common findings may include hypokalemia, hyperglobulinemia, and hypothyroxinemia.
B. **Endocrine screening** in cats includes the urine cortisol to creatinine ratio (UC:CR), low-dose dexamethasone suppression (screening) test (LDDST), and adrenocorticotropic hormone (ACTH) stimulation test (Table 7.2):
   1. **Urine cortisol to creatinine ratio (UC:CR):**
      a. The "Gold-standard" endocrine screen for hyperadrenocorticism in people is the repeated assessment of urinary excretion of cortisol over several 24 h periods which reflects secretion from the adrenal glands. Because secretion can be pulsatile, 24 h collection in a relaxed environment increases the reliability of this test.
      b. In cats, 24 h urine sample collection is problematic and the hospital environment leads to stress and increased cortisol levels. Therefore, a "shortcut" method is to assess the cortisol concentration in a randomly collected sample, and then calculate the ratio of the concentration of cortisol to creatinine.
      c. **Protocol:** Collect a urine sample, centrifuge it, and submit the supernatant.
      d. The test is **very sensitive** so a normal ratio ($<1.3 \times 10^5$ after the results have been converted into US units) almost always rules out hyperadrenocorticism, whereas a ratio $>3.6 \times 10^5$ may be suggestive of hyperadrenocorticism. Unfortunately, the test is **not very specific** as an increased ratio can also be associated with nonadrenal illness, especially diabetes mellitus and hyperthyroidism. The test is more reliable if the sample is collected at home since that cat is less likely to be stressed.
   2. **Low-dose dexamethasone suppression (screening) test (LDDST):**
      a. Dexamethasone suppresses the hypothalamic synthesis and secretion of corticotrophin. Decreased corticotrophin then decreases the production and release of ACTH and therefore the stimulus for the adrenal glands to produce cortisol. Dexamethasone also directly suppresses ACTH production from the pituitary.
      b. However, if a cortisol-producing adrenal tumor is present, ACTH is already suppressed (due to the autonomous secretion of cortisol, and its negative feedback on the production and release of ACTH). Therefore, administration of dexamethasone will have no/minimal influence on the already decreased ACTH release, and autonomous cortisol production will be unaltered.

(a)

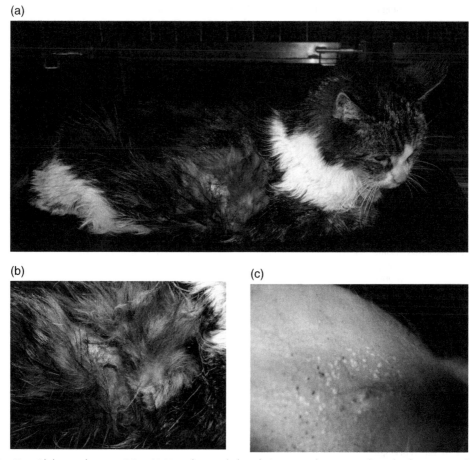

(b)   (c)

Figure 7.1   Cat with hyperadrenocorticism (a) Note the poorly kept hair coat and poor muscling; (b) skin tear. (c) The ventrum demonstrates alopecia, comedones, and calcium deposits within the skin, and the blood vessels can be clearly visualized.

c. Similarly, in individuals with a pituitary tumor that is producing ACTH; corticotrophin production is already reduced and the administration of dexamethasone will not influence the serum cortisol concentration.

d. **Protocol**: Collect a baseline blood sample, then give dexamethasone (**0.1 mg/kg IV**) and collect further blood samples after 4–8 h. The dose of dexamethasone used in cats is higher than the 0.01 mg/kg used in dogs. This is because the lower dose has been found to be less sensitive in cats, where 10–15% of normal cats and some cats with nonadrenal illness failed to suppress.

e. Normal cats should have a serum cortisol concentration of <1.4 μg/dL (<38 nmol/L) or less than 50% of the predexamethasone level at both 4 h and 8 h. Most cats with hyperadrenocorticism (80–95%) fail to suppress at 8 h, (while suppression at 4 h but not at 8 h is consistent with PDH).

f. Although false negatives may occur in mild cases of hyperadrenocorticism, this test is **sensitive and a very good screening test** for hyperadrenocorticism.

3. **Adrenocorticotropic hormone (ACTH—corticotropin) stimulation test:**

a. Administration of synthetic ACTH will stimulate cortisol production from the adrenal glands. However, in cases with adrenocortical hyperplasia (as occurs in pituitary dependant hyperadrenocorticism) or those with adrenal cortisol–producing tumors, this stimulation will be excessive.

b. There are various protocols which have been reported including both IV and IM routes of administration. However, the IV route is generally preferred because it gives a more marked and prolonged elevation in cortisol, with the peak occurring between 60–240 min after injection of synthetic corticotrophin.

Table 7.2 Screening test for the diagnosis of hyperadrenocorticism in cats.

Test	Protocol	Interpretation	Usefulness
UC:CR	Collect urine sample, centrifuge, and submit supernant	Normal ratio (US units) <1.3×10^5 ratio >3.6×10^5; highly suggestive HAC	Good sensitivity; but not very specific—can be improved by performing in home environment
LDDST	Collect baseline blood sample for cortisol concentration. Inject 0.1 mg/kg dexamethasone IV. Collect further samples at 4 h and 8 h	Normal cats cortisol concentration <1.4 µg/dL (38 nmol/L), or less than 50% of baseline value at 4 and 8 h. No suppression at 8 h is suggestive of HAC; suppression at 4 h but not 8 h suggestive of PDH	Good screening test, good sensitivity
ACTH stim.	Collect baseline blood sample for cortisol concentration. Inject 0.125–0.25 mg of synthetic ACTH IV. Collect further samples at 1 h and 2 h	Normal basal cortisol level is 0–5 µg/dL (0–138 nmol/L). At 1–2 h, this should increase to 5–15 µg/dL (138–414 nmol/L). Cats with HAC increase to >19 µg/dL (>525 nmol/L)	Poor sensitivity, fair specificity. Good from differentiating iatrogenic HAC from primary HAC

UC:CR—urinary cortisol to creatine ratio; HAC—hyperadrenocorticism; LDDST—low-dose dexamethasone suppression test; PDH—pituitary-dependant hyperadrenocorticism; ACTH stim.—ACTH stimulation test.

c. **Protocol**: Collect a baseline blood sample, give 0.125–0.25 mg of synthetic ACTH IV, then collect further blood samples after 1 ± 2 h.

d. The normal basal serum cortisol concentration should be 0–5 µg/dL (0–138 nmol/L); 1 h and/or 2 h after ACTH, the cortisol concentration in a normal cat should be 5–15 µg/dL (138–414 nmol/L), but will be >19 µg/dL (>525 nmol/L) in most cats with hyperadrenocorticism.

e. **Unfortunately, ACTH stimulation tests are not a sensitive screening test** for feline hyperadrenocorticism, with false negatives reported in a significant percentage (30–40%) of cats, and false positives can also occur. For this reason, the UC:CR and LDDST are preferred screening tests in cats. However, **ACTH stimulation testing is useful in differentiating between cases of iatrogenic hyperadrenocorticism and primary hyperadrenocorticism**, as cats with iatrogenic disease do not stimulate.

C. **Differentiating PDH from ADH**—Additional tests are used to try to differentiate PDH from adrenal neoplasia (Table 7.2):

1. **High-dose dexamethasone suppression test (HDDST)**:

   a. This works in a similar manner to the LDDST, with the exception that a high dose of dexamethasone is given. The autonomous production of cortisol by an adrenal tumor will remain unaltered. However, some pituitary neoplasms retain some sensitivity to ACTH, and therefore large doses of dexamethasone can result in suppression in PDH.

   b. **Protocol**: This test is performed as for the LDDST except that the cat is given 1.0 mg/kg IV of dexamethasone. A >50% decrease in plasma cortisol concentration at either 4 or 8 h, or a plasma cortisol concentration <1.4 µg/dL (38 nmol/L) at either 4 or 8 h is suggestive of PDH; whereas failure to meet any of these criteria is inconclusive.

   c. **An alternative "at home" protocol** has gained favor as it is easy to perform and interpret, gives more consistent results than the standard HDDST, reduces the stress to the cat, and reduces the risk of bruising.

  d. **Protocol**: The owner collects a urine sample from the cat on the morning of day 1 and day 2, and then gives three oral doses of dexamethasone (0.1 mg/kg/dose) at 8 h intervals at 8 am, 4 pm and 12 pm, or 2 doses at 4 pm and 12 pm, then collects a third urine sample on the morning of day 3. They then deliver all three samples to the veterinarian for submission for UC:CR assessment.

  e. The mean of the first 2 UC:CRs gives the "basal value" and acts as a screening test, confirming the presence of hyperadrenocorticism. The cat is then described as having suppressed if the UC:CR on day 3 is <50% of the "basal value." Cats with PDH may or may not suppress, while cats with adrenal-dependant hyperadrenocorticism do not suppress.

  f. There are a number of methods that owners can use to collect urine; as the cat is using the litter box lift the tail a little and collect using a gravy ladle or similar device or replace litter with small gravel stones of the type used in aquariums or other nonabsorbent litter such as small plastic beads.

2. **Endogenous (basal) ACTH** secretion is elevated in cases of PDH, but suppressed in ADH:

  a. **Protocol**: A blood sample is collected, placed into an EDTA tube, spun immediately, and the plasma transferred into a plastic tube. The plasma is then frozen and shipped frozen to the laboratory.

  b. In cats with PDH, the plasma ACTH concentration is usually above 45 pg/mL (9.9 pmol/L), compared to being low (<10 pg/mL or 2.2 pmol/L) in both normal cats and those with adrenal tumors. Results between 10 and 45 pg/mL (2.2 and 9.9 pmol/L) are considered nondiagnostic.

3. **Abdominal radiographs** may reveal nonspecific changes such as an increased fat deposition, osteopenia, distension of the urinary bladder, dystrophic mineralization, and hepatomegaly. Occasionally the adrenal glands may be identified if they are calcified or markedly enlarged; however, the presence of adrenal mineralization should not be overinterpreted as it occurs in ~30% of normal cats.

4. **Abdominal ultrasonography, CT, or MRI** can all be used to determine the shape and size of the adrenal glands:

  a. **Ultrasonography is a relatively useful method of determining adrenal size** and can aid in the differentiation of ADH from PDH. Unilateral adrenal enlargement is typical of an adrenal tumor whereas bilateral enlargement usually indicates PDH, although it can occasionally result from bilateral adrenal tumors.

  b. **CT and MRI can also be used to image the pituitary gland** as well as the adrenal glands; about **50% of the pituitary tumors are large enough to be visualized using these techniques.**

D. Making a diagnosis of hyperadrenocorticism can be very difficult as the clinical signs are often less dramatic than in dogs and the results of the specific tests are often inconsistent. Therefore, it is usually necessary to use a combination of tests.

V. Differential Diagnoses

See Table 7.1 for the differential diagnoses for skin fragility and for insulin resistant diabetes mellitus (also see Chapter 16).

VI. Treatment

A. There are several options for the treatment of feline hyperadrenocorticism. However, the ideal treatment remains to be determined as there have been few large-scale studies assessing treatment protocols.

B. **Various medical therapies** have been attempted in cats but these have generally given poor results. It has been suggested that medical therapy should perhaps be reserved for presurgical stabilization, rather than long-term control:

  1. While mitotane has been shown to be well tolerated in healthy cats, it has been used to treat very few cats with hyperadrenocorticism. Use of this drug gave poor results in one cat at 25 mg/kg/q 24 h for 25 days, longer courses and/or higher doses have been more effective in a small number of cases.

  2. Treatment with ketoconazole can cause considerable toxicity and has given very mixed results when used in cats with hyperadrenocorticism.

  3. Metyrapone has shown potential positive effects in a small number of cats; however, it can be difficult to obtain.

  4. There is little information available on the use of l-deprenyl for the treatment of feline hyperadrenocorticism.

5. **Trilostane** has given the most promising results of the medical approaches, albeit in a small number of published cases. Trilostane inhibits 3β-17-hydroxysteroid dehydrogenase, and therefore blocks the synthesis of adrenal and gonadal steroid hormones:
   a. It has been used for the treatment of both PDH and ADH in dogs with good results.
   b. In cats with PDH that were treated with trilostane, there was a reduction in their clinical signs and their endocrine tests improved. Although they still required exogenous insulin, they survived for many months on treatment.
   c. Trilostane has also been used to treat a single feline case of bilateral adrenal enlargement with excessive sex hormone production (but no hypercortisolemia), in which it induced moderate clinical improvement.
   d. Trilostane has typically been given at 30 mg/cat orally q 12–24 h (ranging from 10 mg/cat q 24 h to 60 mg/cat q 12 h), long term. Side effects appear to be rare in cats, although trilostane is not recommended in patients with renal insufficiency, and in some dogs, it causes mild lethargy and decreased appetite, and very rarely, is associated with adrenal necrosis leading to hypoadrenocorticism.
   e. It should be used with caution in cats, and close monitoring is essential (repeated serum biochemistry, hematology and assessment of the pituitary–adrenal axis).
6. **Cobalt irradiation** for the treatment of PDH by the ablation of the pituitary tumor has been used in a small number of cats. To date, this technique has given mixed results, although there are reports of some good survival times and resolution of diabetes in a few cases.

C. **Surgical options** for the treatment of hyperadrenocorticism include **adrenalectomy** and **hypophysectomy**:
   1. Historically, the difficulties with medical therapy have meant that **adrenalectomy** has been considered the treatment of choice in cats with hyperadrenocorticism; however, this may be changing with the apparent success of trilostane treatment (see above). Where a single adrenal tumor is present, the removal of the **affected adrenal gland** is recommended. However, if PDH or bilateral adrenal tumors are present **bilateral adrenalectomy** is recommended:
      a. Postoperative complications may be reduced by early diagnosis. However, while surgery can provide successful treatment, the risk of **hemorrhage, fatal perioperative hypoadrenal crisis, cardiac or renal failure, sepsis, or surgical complications** are great and the procedure should only be performed by an experienced surgical team.
      b. A further complication is the diabetic state of the cat and this must also be given consideration. While attempting to treat the cause of the hyperadrenocorticism, exogenous insulin is still necessary to control blood glucose and reduce loss of beta cells from glucose toxicity. Various combinations of short-, intermediate-, or long-acting insulin have been administered for stabilization of the diabetes, but these may be required at relatively high doses. However, since the severity of the insulin resistance can fluctuate, it is recommended that home monitoring be performed to facilitate good glycemic control and increase the probability of diabetic remission. If home monitoring cannot be performed, it is recommended that doses do not exceed 2.2 IU/kg/dose.
      c. Short-term postoperative glucocorticoid administration is needed after unilateral adrenalectomy because the contralateral gland will be temporarily atrophied. However, long-term treatment will be needed after bilateral adrenalectomy and should also include mineralocorticoids.
   2. **Transsphenoidal hypophysectomy** is the treatment of choice in humans with PDH and has been successfully performed in a small number of cats with PDH. However, facilities offering this technique are limited as it requires specialist surgical facilities, the same type of perioperative management as with bilateral adrenalectomy, and poses **many potential complications**.

VII. Prognosis
A. **Without treatment, the prognosis is poor;** most cats die or are euthanized within a month of diagnosis:
   1. Surgical options are not without risk. If successful, surgery for PDH will reduce the signs of hyperadrenocorticism, but carries with it the risk of hypoadrenal crisis. In addition, tumor expansion may eventually lead to neurological signs. If **adrenal tumors are successfully removed, the hyperadrenocorticism should resolve** and the diabetic state may become less insulin resistant or even resolve.

2. Medical management with **trilostane** appears to ameliorate the signs of hyperadrenocorticism but it may not alter the need for exogenous insulin; and diabetic cats are still susceptible to diabetic complications. Irrespective of these complications, the authors have had success treating cats with trilostane with **survival times of approximately 18 months.**

VIII. Prevention

No known prevention.

References and Further Readings

Boag AK, Neiger R, Church DR. Trilostane treatment of bilateral adenal enlargement and excessive sex steroid hormone production in a cat. *J Soc Admin Pharmacol* 2004;45:263–266.

Bruyette DS. Adrenal function testing. *In*: August AR, ed. *Consultations in Feline Internal Medicine*. Philadelphia: W.B. Saunders, 1994.

Cauvin AL, Witt AL, Groves E. The urinary corticoid:creatinine ratio (UCCR) in healthy cats undergoing hospitalization. *JFSM* 2003;5:529–533.

Chapman PS, Kelly DF, Archer J, et al. Adrenal necrosis in a dog receiving trilostane for the treament of hyperadrenocorticism. *J Soc Admin Pharmacol* 2004;45:307–310.

Daley CA, Zerbe CA, Schick RO, et al. Use of metyrapone to treat pituitary-dependent hyperadrenocorticism in a cat with large cutaneous wounds. *JAVMA* 1993;202:956–960.

De Lange MS, Galac S, Trip MR, et al. High urinary corticoid/creatinine ratios in cats with hyperthyroidism. *JVIM* 2004;18:152–155.

Duesburg C, Peterson ME. Adrenal disorders in cats. *Vet Clin North Am Small Anim Pract* 1997;27:321–347.

Duesburg CA, Nelson RW, Feldman EC, et al. Adrenalectomy for the treatment of hyperadrenocorticism in cats: 10 cases (1988–1992). *JAVMA* 1995;207:1066–1070.

Eastwood JM, Elwood CM, Hurley KJ. Trilostane treatment in a dog with functional adrenocortical neoplasia. *J Soc Admin Pharmacol* 2003;44:126–131.

Elliott DA, Feldman EC, Koblik PD, Samii VF, Nelson RW. Prevalence of pituitary tumours among diabetic cats with insulin resistance. *JAVMA* 2000;216:1765–1768.

Feldman EC, Nelson RW. Hyperadrenocorticism in cats (Cushings Syndrome). In: Feldman EC, Nelson RW, eds. *Canine and Feline Endocrinology and Reproduction*, 3rd ed. Philadelphia: WB Saunders, 2004.

Goossens MMC, Meyer HP, Voorhout G, et al. Urinary excretion of glucocorticoids in the diagnosis of hyperadrenocorticism in cats. *Domest Anim Endocrinol* 1995;12:355–362.

Gunn-Moore D. Feline Endocrinopathies. *Vet Clin North Am Small Anim Pract* 2005;35:171–210.

Henry CJ, Clark TP, Young DW, et al. Urine cortisol:creatinine ratios in healthy and sick cats. *JVIM* 1996;10:123–126.

Immink WF, van Toor AJ, Vos JH, et al. Hyperadrenocorticism in four cats. *Vet Q* 1992;15:81–85.

Jones CA, Refsal KR, Steven BJ, et al. Adrenocortical adenocarcinoma in a cat. *JAAHA* 1992;28:59–62.

Kaser-Hotz B, Rohrer CR, Stankeova S, et al. Radiotherapy of pituitary tumours in five cats. *J Small Anim Pract* 2002;43:303–307.

Meij BP, Voorhout G, Rijnberk A. Progress in transsphenoidal hypophysectomy for treatment of pituitary-dependant hyperadrenocorticism in dog and cats. *Mol Cell Endocrinol* 2002;197:89–96.

Meij BP, Voorhout G, Van Den Ingh TS, et al. Transsphenoidal hypophysectomy for treatment of pituitary-dependant hyperadrenocorticism in 7 cats. *Vet Surg* 2001;30:72–86.

Moore LE, Biller DS, Olsen DE. Hyperadenocortiissm treated with metytapone followed by bilateral adrenalectomy. *JAVMA* 2000;217:691–694.

Myers NC, Bruyette DS. Feline adrenocortical diseases: Part II-Hypoadrenocorticism. *Sem Vet Med Surg (Small Anim)* 1994;9:144–147.

Neiger R, Witt AL, Noble A, et al. Trilostane therapy for the treatment of pituitary-dependent hyperadrenocorticism in 5 cats. *JVIM* 2004;18:160–164.

Nelson RW, Feldman EC, Smith MC. Hyperadreenocorticism in cats: Seven cases (1978–1987). *JAVMA* 1988;193:245–250.

Peterson ME, Kemppainen RJ. Dose-response relation between plasma concentrations of corticotropin and cortisol after administration of incremental doses of cosyntropin for corticotropin stimulation testing in cats. *AJVR* 1993;54:300–304.

Peterson ME, Kintzer PP, Foodman MS, Piccolie A, Quimby FW. Adrenal function in the cat: Comparision of the effects of cosyntropin (synthetic ACTH) and corticotrophin gel stimulation. *AJVS* 1984;37:331–333.

Peterson ME, Steele P. Pituitary-dependent hyperadrenocorticism in a cat. *JAVMA* 1986;189:680–683.

Schwedes CS. Mitotane (o, p'-DDD) treatment in ac at with hyperadrenocorticism. *J Soc Admin Pharmacol* 1997;38:520–524.

Skelly BJ, Petrus D, Nicholls PK. Use of trilostane for the treatment of pituitary-dependant hyperadrenocorticism in a cat. *J Soc Admin Pharmacol* 2003;44:269–272.

Smith MC, Feldman EC. Plasma enodgenous ACTH concentrations and plasma cortisol responses to synthetic ACTH and dexamethasone sodium phosphate in healthy cats. *AJVR* 1987;48:1717–1724.

Sparkes AH, Adams DT, Douthwaite JA, Gruffydd-Jones TJ. Assessment of adrenal function in cats: Responses to intravenous synthetic ACTH. *JSAP* 1990;31:2–5.

Valentine RW, Silber A. Feline hyperadrenocorticism: A rare case. *Feline Practice* 1996;24:6–11.

Watson ADJ, Church DR, Emslie DJ, Middleton DJ. Comparative effects of proligestone and megestrol acetate on basal plassma gluscose concentrations and cortisol responses to exogenous adrenocorticotrophic hormone in cats. *Res Vet Sci* 1989;47:374–376.

Watson PJ, Herrtage ME. Hyperadrenocorticism in six cats. *J Soc Admin Pharmacol* 1998;39:175–184.

Widmer WR, Guptill L. Imaging techniques for facilitating diagnosis of hyperadrenocorticism in dogs and cats. *JAVMA* 1995;206(12):355–362.

Willard MD, Nachreiner RF, Howard VC, Fooshee SK. Effect of long-term administration of ketoconazole in cats. *AJVR* 1986;47:2510–2513.

Zerbe CA. Feline hyperadrenocorticism. In: Kirk RW, ed. Current Veterinary Therapy X. Philadelphia: W.B. Saunders, 1989.

Zerbe CA, Refsal KR, Peterson ME, et al. Effect of non-adrenal illnes on adrenal function in the cat. *AJVR* 1987;48:451–454.

Zimmer C, Horauf A, Reusch C. Ultrasonographic examination of the adrenal gland and evaluation of the hypophyseal-adrenal axis in 20 cats. *JSAP* 2000;41:156–160.

CHAPTER 8

Primary Functioning Adrenal Tumors Producing Signs Similar to Hyperadrenocorticism Including Atypical Syndromes in Cats

Nicki Reed and Danièlle Gunn-Moore

Pathogenesis

- Very rare condition.
- Adrenocortical carcinoma producing excessive progesterone.

Classical Signs

- Older cats.
- Clinical signs similar to hyperadrenocorticism: polyuria, polydipsia, skin changes including alopecia and dermal fragility.

Diagnosis

- Identification of an adrenal mass and demonstration of elevated progesterone levels.

Treatment

- Adrenalectomy.
- Medical management with trilostane.

I. Pathogenesis
A. **Excessive hormone production from an adrenocortical neoplasm:**
   1. **Zona glomerulosa** produces mineralocorticoids (aldosterone).
   2. **Zona fasciculata** produces predominantly cortisol, corticosterone, and deoxycorticosterone.
   3. **Zona reticularis** produces predominantly androgens, estrogens, and progesterones.

Clinical Endocrinology of Companion Animals, First Edition. Edited by Jacquie Rand.
© 2013 John Wiley & Sons, Inc. Published 2013 by John Wiley & Sons, Inc.

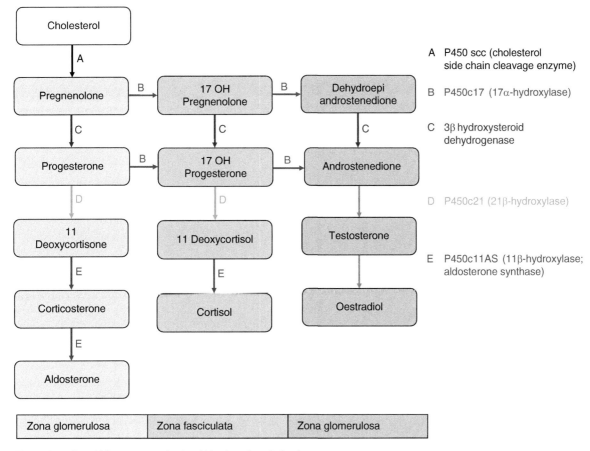

Figure 8.1   Steroid hormone synthesis within the adrenal gland.

B. All steroid hormones are synthesized from cholesterol (see Figure 8.1).
C. Excessive circulating hormone levels may arise as a result of:
    1. Increased production or secretion from **neoplastic cells** of the adrenal cortex due to increased adrenal cortical cell mass.
    2. **Aberrant synthetic pathways** leading to altered steroidogenesis; deficiency of some enzymes may lead to increased levels of precursors not yet reported in cats.
    3. **Increased peripheral conversion** of precursors (not yet reported in cats).
D. **Progesterone particularly may mimic signs of hyperadrenocorticism when present in excess:**
    1. Progesterone can **bind to cortisol binding protein,** displacing cortisol and increasing levels of free but not total cortisol.
    2. Both increased progesterone and increased free cortisol have a negative feedback effect on the hypothalamic–pituitary–adrenal axis, affecting the adrenocorticotropic hormone (ACTH) stimulation test and decreasing total cortisol.
    3. Progesterone can **bind** directly to the **glucocorticoid receptor** in dogs and man (although this has not been shown for cats).
    4. Progesterone may cause **insulin antagonism,** contributing to hyperglycemia and glucosuria.
E. Risk factors for development of adrenocortical neoplasias have not been identified.
F. The condition is very rare, with only six cases reported in the literature. Of these six cases, two had concurrent hyperaldosteronism (see Table 8.1).

Table 8.1 Previously reported cases of hyperadrenocorticism associated with non-cortisol producing adrenal gland tumors.

Signalment	ACTH ST	LDDST	Sex steroids	Diagnosis	Management	Outcome	Reference
Himalayan; 7 yo; MN	Consistent with iatrogenic HAC	Normal, but delayed suppression (0.1 mg/kg)	High basal progesterone, with increase post-ACTH ST	Left adrenal cortical carcinoma Secreting progesterone	Adrenalectomy	Alive 12 months post surgery	Boord and Griffin (1999)
DSH; 7 yo; MN	Consistent with iatrogenic HAC	Normal (0.01 mg/kg)	High basal progesterone and testosterone; minimal increase with ACTH ST	Right adrenal cortical carcinoma Secreting progesterone and testosterone Metastasis in lung	Aminoglutethimide (4 weeks)	Died 3 months post diagnosis	Rossmeisl et al. (2000)
DLH; 9 yo; MN	Consistent with iatrogenic HAC	Normal (0.1 mg/kg)	High basal progesterone	Adrenal cortical carcinoma Secreting progesterone	Aminoglutethimide Adrenalectomy	Survived 1 year post surgery	Feldman and Nelson (2004)
DLH; 12 yo; MN	Consistent with iatrogenic HAC	Normal (0.01 mg/kg)	High basal progesterone, with increase post-ACTH ST	Right adrenal cortical carcinoma Secreting progesterone and aldosterone	Adrenalectomy	Died 3 days post surgery	DeClue et al. (2005)
Russian Blue; 8 yo; MN	Consistent with iatrogenic HAC	Normal	High basal progesterone	Bilateral adrenal cortical carcinomas Secreting progesterone	N/A	N/A	Quante et al. (2009)
DSH; 14 yo; FN	Consistent with iatrogenic HAC	n/d	High basal progesterone, with increase post-ACTH ST	Left adrenal mass Secreting progesterone and aldosterone	Benazepril, aspirin, spironolactone, insulin, and potassium	Euthanized 8 weeks post diagnosis	Briscoe et al. (2009)

DSH—domestic short hair; yo—years old; MN—male neutered; DLH—domestic long hair; FN—female neutered; ACTH ST—adrenocorticotropin stimulation test; HAC—hyperadrenocorticism; LDDST—low-dose dexamethasone suppression test; n/d—not done; N/A—not applicable.

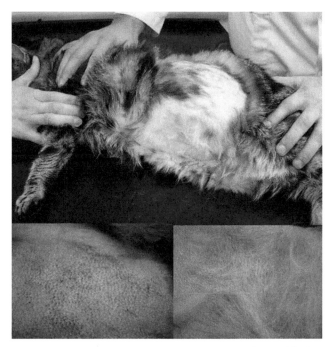

Figure 8.2 Coat changes in a cat with progesterone-secreting adrenal mass—top: bilateral flank alopecia; lower left: comedones; lower right: prominent vessels.

II. Signalment

A. All recorded cases have been **middle-aged to old cats** (range 7–14 years).

B. No breed predisposition has been identified.

C. The majority of reported cases (five of six) have been in neutered male cats.

III. Clinical Signs

A. **Polydipsia and polyuria** are consistent features. This may be due to progesterone causing an increase in free cortisol or due to insulin antagonism.

B. **Polyphagia** is an inconsistent finding, only specifically reported in two cases.

C. **Coat changes** generally consist of bilaterally symmetrical alopecia, often most prominent ventrally. The hair may be easily epilated, and the coat may appear dry or greasy. Comedones, scale, and prominent blood vessels are other skin changes reported in this condition (see Figure 8.2).

D. **Dermal atrophy** is often reported, with skin fragility resulting in spontaneous tearing in two cases.

E. The abdomen may appear pendulous or distended.

F. Behavioral changes, notably aggression, have been reported in one case.

G. Evidence of cardiac disease such as gallop rhythm, cardiac murmur, cardiomegaly, and/or pericardial effusion has been identified in 50% of the cases.

IV. Diagnosis

A. **Routine hematology** may be unremarkable, although microcytosis was reported in one case.

B. **Elevated blood glucose** and fructosamine consistent with concurrent insulin antagonism is often identified.

C. **Hypokalemia** was identified in three of six cases. The presence of hypokalemia should alert the clinician to pursue investigation for concurrent hyperaldosteronism, which was confirmed in two of six cases.

D. Urinalysis may identify **glucosuria**.

E. **ACTH stimulation tests** usually show a minimal increase in cortisol poststimulation, consistent with a pattern of iatrogenic hyperadrenocorticism. Basal cortisol values may also be low due to the suppressive effect of progesterone and increased free cortisol on the hypothalamic–pituitary–adrenal axis.

F. **Low-dose dexamethasone suppression tests (LDDST)** have shown varied response, partly due to the use of different doses of dexamethasone. Due to low basal cortisol values, the degree of suppression may appear minimal; however, values at 4 and 8 h are low, which is consistent with the response expected from a normal cat.

G. **Elevation in basal progesterone** is a consistent feature. Progesterone was measured following ACTH stimulation in four cases and did show an increase; however, a dynamic test is not necessary.

H. Assessment of other adrenocortical steroid hormones may identify abnormal levels of other sex hormones, such as testosterone.

I. **Abdominal ultrasonography** to demonstrate the presence of an adrenal mass. Adrenocortical carcinomas are predominantly unilateral, but a bilateral condition has also been reported.

J. **Histopathology** to confirm the presence of carcinoma; ideally with immunohistochemistry to demonstrate functional production of progesterone.

V. Differential Diagnoses

A. **Hyperadrenocorticism** is the primary differential from the history and clinical signs. A low basal cortisol may increase the suspicion for a progesterone-secreting tumor over a cortisol-secreting tumor, supported by minimal increase in response to ACTH stimulation. Basal progesterone levels should enable differentiation from classical hyperadrenocorticism.

B. **Diabetes mellitus** may be associated with some of the clinical signs (polydipsia, polyuria, polyphagia, abdominal distension, hyperglycemia, and glucosuria), but does not usually present with skin changes and coat changes, if present are usually confined to a poor, seborrheic coat.

C. **Paraneoplastic alopecia**, typically associated with pancreatic neoplasia often has a similar ventral distribution. The skin often has a glistening appearance and does not tend to exhibit fragility; a skin biopsy could differentiate the two conditions.

D. **Feline-acquired skin fragility syndrome** may be iatrogenic in association with administration of glucocorticoids or progestogens, and can also be seen in association with diabetes mellitus or severe liver disease. Idiopathic cases have also been reported.

VI. Treatment

A. **Surgical treatment:**

1. **Adrenalectomy** has the potential to be curative; however, metastatic disease may be present at the time of diagnosis.

2. Complications associated with adrenalectomy include hemorrhage, poor wound healing, thromboembolic disease and postoperative hypoadrenocorticism.

3. Perioperative management with glucocorticoids and mineralocorticoids should be considered due to atrophy of the contralateral adrenal gland.

4. Preoperative medical management should be considered to allow resolution of the skin fragility prior to surgery.

B. **Medical treatment:**

1. **Aminoglutethimide** is an inhibitor of P450scc, the side chain cleavage enzyme responsible for converting cholesterol to pregnenolone (see Figure 8.1). Its use has been reported in two cats, which showed initial clinical improvement with a dose of approximately 6 mg/kg. Side effects reported in humans include nausea, anorexia, and rashes. In one cat treated for 6 weeks resolution of diabetes mellitus and skin thinning was followed by development of gynecomastia. It was thought that the rapid fall in progesterone levels may have stimulated prolactin secretion.

2. **Trilostane** is a competitive inhibitor of 3β-hydroxysteroid dehydrogenase (see Figure 8.1). By blocking the synthetic pathways of progesterone, it could theoretically allow reversal of the clinical signs. Trilostane therapy has been used for treatment of typical hyperadrenocorticism in cats, with some success reported at doses of 30–60 mg/cat/PO q 24 h. However, it has not been used to treat this form of atypical hyperadrenocorticism and its use in a case of excessive estradiol and testosterone production in a cat failed to show an improvement in steroid hormone levels, despite a moderate improvement in clinical signs. While this therapy may control clinical signs, it would not address the underlying carcinoma, but it may be useful for stabilizing patients prior to surgery.

3. Concurrent diabetes mellitus (see Chapter 16) and hyperaldosteronism (see Chapter 12) if present should also be managed appropriately.

VII. Prognosis

A. Surgical management has resulted in variable survival times of 3 days to >1 year post surgery.

B. Medical management has resulted in shorter survival times of 8 weeks to 3 months.

C. **A guarded prognosis** would have to be given due to the insidious onset of the clinical signs, which may lead to a protracted diagnosis with the increased risk of metastatic spread prior to therapy.

VIII. Prevention

A. Due to the rare and spontaneous nature of these tumors, no advice can be given regarding prevention.

References and Further Readings

Boag AK, Neiger R, Church DB. Trilostane treatment of bilateral adrenal enlargement and excessive sex steroid hormone production in a cat. *J Small Anim Pract* 2004;45:263–266.

Boord M, Griffin C. Progesterone secreting adrenal mass in a cat with clinical signs of hyperadrenocorticism. J Am Vet Med Assoc 1999;214:666–669.

Briscoe K, Barra VR, Foster DF, et al. Hyperaldosteronism and hyperprogesteronism in a cat. *J Feline Med Surg* 2009;11:758–762.

DeClue AE, Breshears LA, Pardo ID, et al. Hyperaldosteronism and hyperprogesteronism in a cat with an adrenal cortical carcinoma. *J Vet Intern Med* 2005;19:355–358.

Feldman EC, Nelson RW. Hyperadrenocorticism in cats (Cushing's syndrome) In: Feldman EC, Nelson RW, eds. *Canine and Feline Endocrinology and Reproduction*, 3rd edn. St. Louis, Missouri: Saunders, 2004, pp. 358–393.

Gross TL, Ihrke PJ, Walde EJ, Affolter VK. *Skin Diseases of the Dog and Cat*, 2nd edn. Oxford: Blackwell Science Ltd., 2005.

Quante S, Sieber-Rückstühl N, Wilhelm S, et al. Hyperprogesteronism due to bilateral adrenal carcinomas in a cat with diabetes mellitus. *Schweiz Arch Tierheilkd* 2009;151:437–442.

Rossmeisl JH, Scott-Moncrieff JCR, Siems J, et al. Hyperadrenocorticism and hyperprogesteronemia in a cat with an adreno-cortical adenocarcinoma. *J Am Anim Hosp Assoc* 2000;36:512–517.

CHAPTER 9

Hyperadrenocorticism in Ferrets

Nico J. Schoemaker

Pathogenesis

- Surgical neutering results in elevated gonadotropins.
- Luteinizing hormone (LH) receptors in the adrenal gland become activated.
- Elevated LH results in secretion of androgens and estrogens.

Classical Signs

- No sex predilection.
- Most ferrets are >3 years.
- Symmetrical alopecia.
- Estrous in neutered female ferrets (jills) and increased sexual behavior in neutered male ferrets (hobs).
- Increased skin odor.
- Pruritus.
- Urinary blockage in hobs due to periprostatic or periurethral cysts.

Diagnosis

- Ferret with classical signs.
- Ultrasound assists in locating affected adrenal gland(s).
- Hormone analysis is helpful for monitoring treatment.

Treatment

- Surgery has long been the treatment of choice.
- GnRH agonists, such as deslorelin and previously leuprolide acetate, are very effective in managing the majority of cases.
- Melatonin is reported, but not advised.

I. Pathogenesis

A. Adrenal disease can refer to changes of the adrenal cortex and/or the adrenal medulla. Pathologic changes involving the adrenal medulla are most often the result of a pheochromocytoma (uncommon in ferrets).

Clinical Endocrinology of Companion Animals, First Edition. Edited by Jacquie Rand.
© 2013 John Wiley & Sons, Inc. Published 2013 by John Wiley & Sons, Inc.

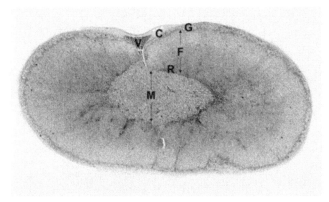

Figure 9.1 Histological section of an adrenal gland of a healthy ferret: M=medulla, R=zona reticularis, F=zona fasciculata, G=zona glomerulosa, C=capsule, V=adrenolumbar vein.

The **most common form of adrenal disease in ferrets is hyperadrenocorticism,** also referred to as adrenocortical disease, in which the adrenal cortex is affected. The adrenal cortex consists of three layers:

1. The zona glomerulosa, which is the outermost layer of the adrenal cortex and produces mineralocorticoids (primarily aldosterone).
2. The zona fasciculata, which consists of an outer and inner part and produces glucocorticoids (cortisol and corticosterone) and androgens.
3. The zona reticularis, the most interior zone, which is extremely variable in its prominence and cellular composition. This zone contains the smallest cells of the adrenal cortex and produces primarily androgens (Figure 9.1).

Thus, in principle, three distinct syndromes may arise in adrenocortical hyperfunction: hyperaldosteronism, hypercortisolism, and hyperandrogenism. In **neutered pet ferrets, hyperandrogenism is the most common form of hyperadrenocorticism,** resulting in **increased plasma concentrations of androstenedione, 17-hydroxyprogesterone, and estradiol.**

B. Three different aetiologies have been suggested for the high occurrence of hyperandrogenism in ferrets. These include (early) neutering of ferrets, housing ferrets indoors, and genetic background:

1. **Neutering**—In recent years, evidence has been gathered that **increased concentrations of gonadotropins,** which occur **after neutering** (due to the loss of negative feedback), stimulate the adrenal cortex, eventually leading to an **adrenocortical neoplasm.** Important research findings in this area indicate that a **significant correlation exists between the age at neutering and the age at onset of hyperandrogenism,** and that luteinizing hormone receptors in the adrenal cortex of ferrets are only functional in the altered adrenal glands and not in healthy adrenal glands. Initially it was believed that neutering at an early age was the main factor responsible for the high occurrence of hyperadrenocorticism in ferrets. The disease is, however, just as common in the Netherlands, where most pet ferrets are neutered between 6 and 12 months of age, compared to the USA, where most pet ferrets are neutered at an age of 6 weeks. Although less common, it should be noted that adrenal disease may also occur in intact ferrets, but is more difficult to diagnose as most clinical signs are difficult to differentiate from the normal hormonally driven physiological changes that occur in healthy intact ferrets.
2. **Housing ferrets indoors**—The hypothesis that ferrets that are kept indoors have a higher chance of developing hyperandrogenism compared to ferrets housed outdoors is consistent with the above-mentioned hypothesis. Ferrets that are kept indoors will generally be exposed to more hours of light per day than ferrets that are housed outdoors, resulting in increased gonadotropin levels. This applies to neutered as well as intact ferrets. The fact that adrenal gland disease is less common in the United Kingdom can be explained by the fact that many ferrets there are still kept outdoors without being neutered.
3. **Genetic background**—In the USA, a specific breeding facility, which provides an estimated 80% of all American ferrets, has been blamed for the high occurrence of hyperandrogenism in American ferrets. This claim, however, does not account for the high prevalence of hyperandrogenism in other parts of the

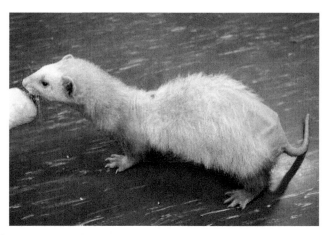

Figure 9.2 Alopecia in a ferret with hyperadrenocorticism.

world (e.g., the Netherlands). Dutch ferrets are not sourced from this facility and therefore do not have the same genetic background. Although the breeding facility cannot be blamed for the high incidence of hyperandrogenism in ferrets, this does not mean that a genetic background for the disease is not possible. In humans, three different hereditary syndromes have been recognized in which multiple endocrine neoplasms are seen (MEN1, MEN2a, and MEN2b). Since insulinomas and adrenal gland tumors are frequently seen simultaneously in ferrets, a condition similar to MEN in humans may exist. At the present time, however, no proof for a genetic predisposition has been found.

C. It has been reported that approximately 85% of ferrets with hyperadrenocorticism have **enlargement of one adrenal gland without atrophy of the contralateral adrenal gland**. In the other 15% of cases, bilateral enlargement is present.

D. The adrenal glands can be histologically classified as (nodular) **hyperplasia, adenoma, and adenocarcinoma**. The histological diagnosis, however, does not provide information on functionality of the tumor nor does it provide any prognostic information. Pituitary tumors have not been found to be associated with adrenal tumors in ferrets.

E. The prevalence of hyperandrogenism in Dutch ferrets during a period of 3 months has been reported to be 0.55% (95%, confidence interval: 0.2–1.1%). There are no reports on what percentage of ferrets eventually develop neoplastic adrenal glands. This may be as high as 75%.

F. A case of LH-dependent hypercortisolism (Cushing's disease) has been diagnosed by the author. The major complaint in this ferret was severe polyuria and polydipsia (PU/PD).

G. A case of primary hyperaldosteronism has also been reported in a ferret.

II. Signalment

Although initial reports suggested that the majority of ferrets with adrenocortical disease were females, a Dutch study could not confirm this sex predilection. In the author's practice in the Netherlands, slightly more male than female ferrets with hyperandrogenism are seen. In the USA, diagnosis of hyperandrogenism in ferrets may occur as early as 2 years of age. In the Netherlands, however, most cases are seen in ferrets older than 3 years of age. This age difference is a reflection of the age at which ferrets are neutered in each country.

III. Clinical Signs

A. **Alopecia**, which is frequently symmetrical, is commonly, but not always seen (Figure 9.2). Sometimes only a thinning of the hair coat is seen. Loss of hair at the base of the tail in the absence of ectoparasites is also suggestive for hyperandrogenism. Alopecia usually begins in spring, which coincides with the start of the breeding season, and may disappear without treatment. The next year, the alopecia commonly recurs after which it usually does not resolve spontaneously at the end of the breeding season.

The skin is usually not affected, although some excoriations may be seen. While hair loss on the tail may be a preliminary presentation of hyperandrogenism, it is also frequently seen in ferrets with seasonal alopecia. It is important to differentiate between these two conditions.

B. A **neutered jill with vulvar swelling** (the most recognizable sign of estrous) which is older than 3 years is likely to have an adrenal tumor.

C. **Recurrence of sexual behavior after neutering** in hobs, but sometimes also in jills, is frequently seen. This is often accompanied by an increased skin odor produced by the sebaceous glands.

D. **Dysuria** and eventually urinary obstruction may be seen in hobs. These clinical signs can be attributed to the presence of periprostatic or periurethral cysts, which are formed under the influence of adrenal androgen secretion. This association is frequently overlooked by practitioners who are not familiar with this disease.

E. **Mammary gland enlargement** is sometimes seen in jills.

F. **Pruritus**—a sign which is commonly associated with an infectious cause for alopecia—is frequently seen in ferrets with hyperandrogenism. No cause for this pruritus has been documented. The author has specifically looked for an association between the pruritus and a (secondary) *Malassezia* infection, but did not find this association.

G. **PU/PD** are reported in ferrets with hyperandrogenism. It is not clear, however, whether adrenal hormone production is responsible for these signs, or if these (elderly) ferrets have concurrent kidney disease. In a minority of cases, a LH-dependent hypercortisolism may be responsible for the PU/PD.

IV. Diagnosis

A. **Clinical signs**—Although many advanced techniques can be used in diagnosing hyperadrenocorticism in ferrets, the recognition of clinical signs related to the production of sex steroids remain the most important.

B. **Abdominal palpation**—Further confirmation can sometimes be obtained by palpating a (tiny) firm mass craniomedial to the cranial pole of the kidney(s), representing the enlarged adrenal gland(s). The right adrenal gland is more difficult to palpate due to the overlying right caudate process of the caudate liver lobe.

C. **Plasma hormone analysis**—Hormones that are commonly elevated include **androstenedione, estradiol, and 17-hydroxyprogesterone.** Blood can be sent to the Clinical Endocrinology Service of the College of Veterinary Medicine, University of Tennessee, for analysis of these hormones. Dehydroepiandrosterone sulfate used to be included in this panel, but is currently no longer incorporated. Elevation of one or more of the abovementioned hormones is considered to be diagnostic for hyperadrenocorticism. However, **plasma concentrations of these hormones in intact female ferrets are identical to those in hyperadrenocorticoid ferrets.** This hormone panel is therefore not considered of aid by the author in differentiating between a ferret with hyperandrogenism and one with an active ovarian remnant. Hormone measurement, however, can be used to monitor treatment and progression of this disease.

Plasma concentrations of ACTH and α-MSH do not change in ferrets with hyperandrogenism and are therefore not helpful for making a diagnosis.

Plasma cortisol concentrations have—just as in dogs—been found to be nondiagnostic as well.

ACTH stimulation tests and dexamethasone suppression tests—as commonly used in dogs with Cushing's syndrome—are not considered diagnostic in ferrets.

D. **Urinary hormone analysis**—An increased urinary corticoid:creatinine ratio (UCCR) can be found in ferrets with adrenocortical disease. The UCCR, however, is considered to be of limited diagnostic value because this ratio is also increased in intact ferrets during the breeding season and in ferrets with an active ovarian remnant. If a large population of ferrets needs to be screened for hyperandrogenism, the UCCR may function as a preliminary screening test.

E. **Abdominal ultrasonography**—Abdominal ultrasonography is **very useful to determine size and location of the affected adrenal glands.** This technique does not provide any information on hormone release. It is therefore possible that only one adrenal gland is enlarged, while both adrenal glands contribute to the androgen release. It is also possible that a ferret has hyperandrogenism without being able to determine which adrenal gland is affected. Abdominal ultrasonography is useful for visualization of an ovarian remnant (an important differential diagnosis). Other abdominal organs, such as the prostate, can also be evaluated.

It may be difficult to distinguish an adrenal gland from an abdominal lymph node. By using specific landmarks, the adrenal glands can be fairly easily detected in nearly 100% of ferrets. The left adrenal gland is located lateral to the aorta, at the level of the origin of the cranial mesenteric and celiac arteries. The right adrenal gland is more difficult to locate. The caudate process of the caudate liver lobe may be used as an acoustic window. When using this window, the three major vessels (aorta, portal vein, and caudal vena cava)

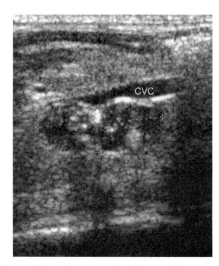

Figure 9.3   Ultrasound image of an enlarged right adrenal gland of a ferret with hyperandrogenism. The gland is located dorsal to the caudal vena cava (CVC). A mineralisation is seen in the center (white arrow).

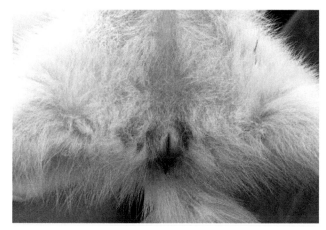

Figure 9.4   Swollen vulva and thinning of the abdominal fur. Swelling can be seen both in a ferret during estrous as well as in a ferret with hyperandrogenism.

in that area are located. The vena cava is the most lateral and dorsal of the three. The portal vein has a much wider diameter compared to the caudal vena cava. The right adrenal gland is attached to the dorsolateral surface of the caudal vena cava, at the level of and/or immediately cranial to the origin of the cranial mesenteric artery (Figure 9.3). The adrenal glands of ferrets with hyperandrogenism may have one or more of the following signs: a significantly **increased thickness**, a **rounded appearance**, a **heterogeneous structure**, an **increased echogenicity,** and sometimes contain signs of mineralization.

V.   Differential Diagnoses

A.   **Hormonal**—The most important differential diagnoses for a jill with signs of hyperandrogenism are a non-ovariectomized animal or one with active remnant ovaries (Figure 9.4). A Sertoli cell tumor in intact hobs and hypothyroidism are also possible, but are considered rare.

B.   **Infectious**—Dermatophytosis and demodicosis may lead to alopecia and pruritus in ferrets. A bacterial dermatitis may also present in a similar way. In all these conditions, skin lesions will be present. These lesions, other than an incidental superficial scratch mark, are not seen in ferrets with hyperandrogenism.

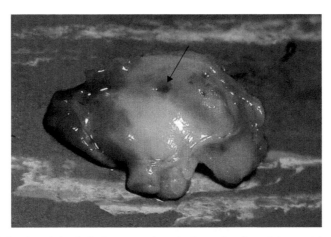

Figure 9.5   Photo of the right adrenal gland of a ferret seen from the internal surface of the caudal vena cava showing vessels entering the adrenal gland (arrow).

C. **Noninfectious**—Severe alopecia and pruritus in a ferret has been seen due to food intolerance. This ferret had identical signs to those seen in a typical ferret with hyperandrogenism. Ultrasonography, hormone analysis, and surgery, however, could not confirm this diagnosis. As soon as the ferret was switched to a different commercial diet, the signs started to disappear and the animal was asymptomatic within a couple of weeks.

VI. Treatment

The optimal treatment for hyperandrogenism in ferrets is a **combination of surgery and placement of an implant containing deslorelin** (a depot GnRH analogue). Many different factors influence the eventual choice of treatment. An owner may decline surgery based on criteria such as the age of the ferret, presence of concurrent disease (cardiomyopathy), risk of surgery when the right or both adrenal glands are involved, and financial limitations.

A. **Surgery**—Surgical removal of the left adrenal gland is relatively easy. The adrenal gland is dissected out of the retroperitoneal fat and the adrenolumbar vein is ligated. The location of the right adrenal gland makes it much more difficult to remove. The close proximity to the liver and the dorsolateral attachment to the caudal vena cava makes a dorsal approach more logical. This is in fact the surgical approach to the adrenal glands in humans. In ferrets, however, an abdominal approach is most commonly used. Since there is a close connection between the right adrenal gland and the caudal vena cava (Figure 9.5), either a part of the adrenal needs to be left attached to the vena cava (Figure 9.6) or part of the wall of the vein has to be removed. Ligation of the caudal vena cava is only possible if this vein is already occluded for a major portion of its diameter and collateral veins have opened up. If this is not the case, there is a risk of hypertension distal to ligation which may lead to acute kidney failure. Different surgical protocols have been proposed for removing bilateral adrenocortical tumors. Many advise to leave part of an adrenal gland behind, while others advise to remove both adrenal glands. It would seem likely that hypoadrenocorticism would occur after removing both glands, but this seems to occur only in a minority of cases. Cryosurgery and injection with alcohol has also been proposed. With cryosurgery, however, it is uncertain how much tumor has actually been destroyed. Alcohol injection in dog testes has been found to be very painful. Since less painful alternatives are present, this technique is not advised by the author.

B. **Hormone treatment:**

1. **GnRH agonist**—The most effective drugs at the present time are the depot GnRH agonists of which **leuprolide acetate** (Lupron Depot, TAP Pharmaceutical Products Inc.) is the most well known. This drug is not registered for use in animals, but for men with prostate cancer. **Deslorelin** is another GnRH analogue. This drug is commercially available in the form of an implant for chemical castration of male dogs in Australia (Suprelorin®, Peptech Animal Health Pty Limited, Australia) and Europe (Suprelorin®,

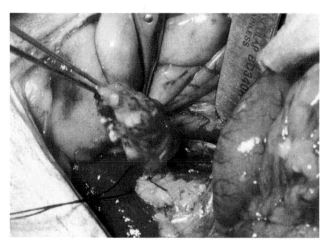

Figure 9.6   Resection of an adrenal tumor from the caudal vena cava of a male ferret with hyperandrogenism. In this case, the tumor could be dissected free from the vena cava.

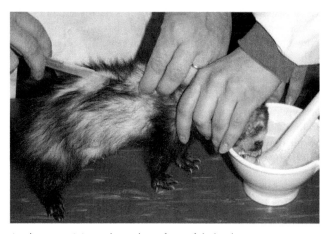

Figure 9.7   Placement of an implant containing a slow release form of deslorelin (GnRH agonist) in a ferret. Distraction with food enables placement of the implant without anesthesia.

Virbac Animal Health, France). Advantages of these implants over leuprolide acetate are: (1) the drug does not need to be reconstituted; (2) it lasts much longer than the depot injections; (3) it is registered for use in animals; and (4) it is cheaper. These implants have been found to be very effective for treating hyperandrogenism in ferrets. As it is now commercially available, it has become the drug of choice (Figure 9.7).

Leuprolide acetate provides a suitable alternative where deslorelin is not available. The Lupron 30-day Depot formulation is given in a dose of 100 μg IM for ferrets <1 kg and 200 μg IM for ferrets over 1 kg. This drug will suppress adrenocortical hormone release for at least 1 month in ferrets and may even last up to 3 months. Some veterinarians use a 3-month formulation (which is exactly three times as expensive), but this drug does not seem to work three times longer than the 30-day formulation.

It may seem strange that a depot GnRH agonist is used in ferrets with hyperadrenocorticism, when the increased release of GnRH and gonadotropins that occur post neutering are responsible for the disease in the first place. To understand the mechanism behind this treatment, it is important to know that pituitary and hypothalamic hormones are released in a pulsatile fashion. Gonadotropins are only released when GnRH is secreted in pulses. The depot GnRH agonist overrides the pulsatile release, thereby blocking the release of gonadotropins. **The administration of a depot GnRH agonist therefore results in an initial single release of gonadotropins, followed by baseline concentrations.** This initial release may exaggerate clinical signs, which may last for up to 2 weeks after placement of the implant.

2. **Flutamide**—Flutamide (10 mg/kg, PO, q 12 h) inhibits androgen uptake and may therefore be beneficial in the first weeks of treating ferrets with a GnRH agonist, when gonadotropins are increased.

3. **Melatonin**—Melatonin has also been proposed as a therapeutic option for hyperadrenocorticoid ferrets. Mink receiving such an implant develop appealing thick furs. This has also been reported in ferrets. Melatonin supposedly suppresses the release of GnRH. In the early 1980s, researchers showed that ferrets, which were kept under 8 h light:16 h darkness (8L:16D), would come into estrus only 7 weeks later than ferrets exposed to long photoperiods (14L:10D). It is therefore debatable if melatonin is indeed capable of suppressing the release of gonadotropins. Clinical improvement, however, is seen in hyperadrenocorticoid ferrets either receiving 0.5 mg melatonin daily PO or an implant containing 5.4 mg melatonin. In the study in which melatonin was given orally, however, hormone concentrations, in general, rose and the tumors continued to grow. This treatment may therefore pose a risk to the ferrets because although their condition continues to progress, the clinical signs are effectively masked and this deterioration will not be evident to an owner. Home medication with melatonin, which can been purchased in drugstores in the USA, may delay the initial presentation of ferrets with hyperadrenocorticism to veterinarians.

4. **Ketoconazole and mitotane**—Ketoconazole and mitotane (o,p'-DDD) are well known drugs for treating hypercortisolism in dogs and humans. These drugs have also been tried in ferrets, but both were not considered very effective and should therefore be considered obsolete.

5. **Trilostane**—Trilostane (Vetoryl®, Arnolds Veterinary Products/Dechra Veterinary Products), a 3β-hydroxysteroid dehydrogenase (3β-HSD) blocker, has become an important drug for treating pituitary-dependent hyperadrenocorticism in dogs. Since 3β-HSD is necessary for the synthesis of androstenedione and 17-hydroxyprogesterone, it is tempting to speculate that this drug would be very effective in treating ferrets with hyperadrenocorticism. In a pilot study, 5 mg Trilostane was given orally once daily to a ferret with hyperadrenocorticism. Within a month, the owner complained that the alopecia and vulva swelling in the ferret increased. Plasma hormone analysis showed a decreased 17-hydroxyprogesterone concentration but increased concentrations of androstenedione, oestradiol, and dehydroepiandrosterone sulfate. These results can be explained by the fact that a decrease of 3β-HSD may lead to an activation of 17,20-lyase and thus the androgen pathway. More research is therefore necessary before this drug can safely be administered to ferrets.

VII. Prognosis
A. **Without treatment:**
1. Ferrets with adrenal pathology may survive for years with this condition. Pruritus, however, may be unbearable for the animal, and some of these animals appear to be more lethargic as well. Rupture of the caudal vena cava may occur if the right adrenal gland invades this vein.
2. Anemia due to prolonged hyperestrogenism is rare in jills with adrenal tumors.
3. Ferrets with urinary blockage need immediate medical intervention (cystocentesis, catheterization, and placement of a prepubic catheter) to combat uremia and/or bladder rupture.
B. **After surgery:**
1. After surgical removal of a unilateral adrenal tumor, the disease commonly recurs due to development of disease in the contralateral adrenal gland. It is therefore advised to administer a deslorelin implant at the time of surgery to prevent further stimulation of the contralateral gland.
C. **After deslorelin treatment:**
1. Approximately 10% of ferrets seem to develop adrenal carcinomas after 1.5–2 years of treatment. More research is necessary to better understand the pathogenesis and incidence of this phenomenon. In the meantime, young ferrets with an adrenal tumor may benefit from surgical removal of the affected adrenal gland in conjunction with hormone therapy to reduce the risk of such complications.
2. In a small proportion of ferrets, adrenal tumors are no longer under control of pituitary LH release and produce their hormones autonomously. In these cases, deslorelin therapy is not effective.

VIII. Prevention

A. Since surgical neutering in ferrets has been implicated as an etiological factor in the development of hyperandrogenism in this species, a search for alternative contraceptive methods has been made. In jills, neutering is necessary to prevent pancytopenia due to elevated estradiol plasma concentrations during a persistent estrous. In hobs, there is no medical need for castration. Males are mainly castrated to (1) prevent reproduction; (2) reduce intraspecies aggression enabling them to be kept in groups; and (3) decrease the intensity of the musky odor produced by the sebaceous glands.

In hobs, deslorelin implants suppress plasma follicle stimulating hormone (FSH) and testosterone concentrations, decrease testis size, and inhibit spermatogenesis. In addition, the musky odor, sexual behavior, as well as aggressive behavior are reduced. The suppressed testosterone concentrations indicate that LH plasma concentrations are also suppressed. In jills, deslorelin implants may induce a temporary estrous, which may last up to 4 weeks. In general, however, this period will last up to 2 weeks.

Deslorelin is therefore considered a suitable alternative for surgical neutering in ferrets. Whether these implants will actually reduce the incidence of hyperandrogenism in ferrets remains uncertain.

References and Further Readings

Desmarchelier M, Lair S, Dunn M, et al. Primary hyperaldosteronism in a domestic ferret with an adrenocortical adenoma. *J Am Vet Med Assoc* 2008;233:1297–1301.

Kuijten AM, Schoemaker NJ, Voorhout G. Ultrasonographic visualization of the adrenal glands of healthy and hyperadrenocorticoid ferrets. *J Am Anim Hosp Assoc* 2007;43:78–84.

Quesenberry KE, Rosenthal KL. Endocrine diseases. In: Quesenberry KE, Carpenter JW, eds. *Ferrets, Rabbits and Rodents; Clinical Medicine and Surgery*, 2nd edn. Philadelphia: Saunders, 2003, pp. 79–90.

Rosenthal KL, Peterson ME. Evaluation of plasma androgen and estrogen concentrations in ferrets with hyperadrenocorticism. *J Am Vet Med Assoc* 1996;209:1097–1102.

Rosenthal KL, Peterson ME, Quesenberry KE, et al. Hyperadrenocorticism associated with adrenocortical tumor or nodular hyperplasia of the adrenal gland in ferrets: 50 cases (1987–1991). *J Am Vet Med Assoc* 1993;203:271–275.

Schoemaker NJ, Kuijten AM, Galac S. Luteinizing hormone-dependent Cushing's syndrome in a pet ferret (*Mustela putorius furo*). *Domestic Animal Endocrinology* 2008;34:278–283.

Schoemaker NJ, Mol JA, Lumeij JT, et al. Plasma concentrations of adrenocorticotrophic hormone and alpha-melanocyte-stimulating hormone in ferrets (*Mustela putorius furo*) with hyperadrenocorticism. *Am J Vet Res* 2002;63:1395–1395.

Schoemaker NJ, Schuurmans M, Moorman H, et al. Correlation between age at neutering and age at onset of hyperadrenocorticism in ferrets. *J Am Vet Med Assoc* 2000;216:195–197.

Schoemaker NJ, Teerds KJ, Mol JA, et al. The role of luteinizing hormone in the pathogenesis of hyperadrenocorticism in neutered ferrets. *Mol Cell Endocrinol* 2002;197:117–125.

Schoemaker NJ, van Deijk R, Muijlaert B, et al. Use of a gonadotropin releasing hormone agonist implant as an alternative for surgical castration in male ferrets (*Mustela putorius furo*). *Theriogenology* 2008;70:161–167.

Schoemaker NJ, Wolfswinkel J, Mol JA, et al. Urinary excretion of glucocorticoids in the diagnosis of hyperadrenocorticism in ferrets. *Domest Anim Endocrinol* 2004;27:13–24.

Vinke CM, van Deijk R, Houx BB, et al. The effects of surgical and chemical castration on intermale aggression, sexual behaviour and play behaviour in the male ferret (*Mustela putorius furo*). *Appl Anim Behav Sci* 2008;115:104–121.

Wagner RA, Bailey EM, Schneider JF, et al. Leuprolide acetate treatment of adrenocortical disease in ferrets. *J Am Vet Med Assoc* 2001;218:1272–1274.

Wagner RA, Piché CA, Jöchle W, et al. Clinical and endocrine responses to treatment with deslorelin acetate implants in ferrets with adrenocortical disease. *Am J Vet Res* 2005;66:910–914.

CHAPTER 10

Hyperadrenocorticism and Primary Functioning Adrenal Tumors in Other Species (Excluding Horses and Ferrets)

Michelle L. Campbell-Ward

Pathogenesis

- Hyperadrenocorticism associated with pituitary dysfunction or adrenal neoplasia has been described in rodents and birds.
- Iatrogenic hyperadrenocorticism may result from the administration of exogenous corticosteroids.

Classical Signs

- Polyuria, polydipsia, polyphagia, and weight loss.
- Bilaterally symmetrical alopecia (rodents).

Diagnosis

- Generally based on history and clinical signs.
- Laboratory confirmation is difficult due to patient size and a lack of validated protocols.
- Definitive diagnosis may only be possible at necropsy.

Treatment

- Scant information is available regarding medical and surgical treatment options for spontaneous hyperadrenocorticism.
- In cases of iatrogenic origin, discontinue exogenous corticosteroid therapy.

Hyperadrenocorticism and functional adrenal tumors in **ferrets and horses** are covered in **Chapters 9 and 11,** respectively. This chapter focuses on these conditions in pet rodents and birds.

Clinical Endocrinology of Companion Animals, First Edition. Edited by Jacquie Rand.
© 2013 John Wiley & Sons, Inc. Published 2013 by John Wiley & Sons, Inc.

I. Pathogenesis
A. **Rodents:**
   1. Hyperadrenocorticism is an uncommon diagnosis in pet gerbils but is seen in **repeatedly bred and aging laboratory gerbils.** The disease is often linked to myocardial necrosis/fibrosis, diabetes, and obesity in this species. Elevated serum triglycerides, enlarged pancreatic islets, thymic involution, adrenal hemorrhage, adrenal lipid depletion, and hepatic lipidosis may also be seen. Some affected animals may have pheochromocytomas.
   2. Adrenocortical adenoma is one of the most common benign neoplasms in the Syrian hamster. Adrenocortical adenocarcinoma and a pituitary chromophobe adenoma have also been reported in **hamsters** and these **neoplasms have been implicated in clinical cases of hyperadrenocorticism.**
   3. There is a single case report describing hyperadrenocorticism in the guinea pig.
B. **Birds:**
   1. Only **limited information** is available regarding spontaneous hyperadrenocorticism in pet birds.
   2. Pituitary adenomas are the most commonly reported neuroendocrine tumors in birds. Pituitary carcinoma and adenocarcinoma have also been reported. These pituitary tumors may be nonfunctional or hypersecrete adrenocorticotropic hormone (ACTH) and be associated with bilateral adrenal hyperplasia. Primary neoplastic diseases of the adrenal gland are also reported in birds and can vary from benign adenomas to malignant adenocarcinomas.
   3. It would appear that adrenocorticotropic hormones and prolactin have a greater effect on blood sugar than insulin in birds. Many suspected diabetic patients seen may in fact be Cushingoid.
   4. Chronic stress may result in adrenal hypertrophy from continual ACTH stimulation.
C. **All:**
   1. **Iatrogenic hyperadrenocorticism** may occur in any species secondary to the **administration of exogenous corticosteroids. Birds** appear to be **more sensitive to the secondary effects of corticosteroids** than mammals.

II. Signalment
D. In gerbils, the disease occurs in higher prevalence in older breeders (both males and females) although a cause and effect relationship has not been established.
E. In hamsters, older males are overrepresented.

III. Clinical Signs
F. **Rodents:**
   1. Bilaterally symmetrical alopecia, often of the flank/thigh area.
   2. Hyperpigmentation.
   3. Skin thinning.
   4. Hepatomegaly.
   5. Polydipsia.
   6. Polyuria.
   7. Polyphagia.
   8. Behavioral changes.
   9. Weight loss.
   10. Bilateral exophthalmos has been reported in a guinea pig.
G. **Birds:**
   1. Polyuria.
   2. Polydipsia.
   3. Weight loss or gain.
   4. Polyphagia.
   5. Feather picking.
   6. Reproductive abnormalities.
   7. Muscular weakness and atrophy.
   8. Intra-abdominal fat accumulation.

IV. Diagnosis
A. **Rodents:**
1. The diagnosis is generally **presumed on the basis of history and clinical signs**.
2. The practicalities of obtaining blood from small patients to run diagnostic tests may prove problematic. Additionally, it is important to consider that both cortisol and corticosterone rise through stress due to handling and restraint and during pregnancy.
3. In hamsters, demonstration of **elevated blood cortisol** (normal range 13.8–27.6 nmol/L [0.5–1.0 µg/dL]) has been described in clinical cases. Alkaline phosphatase may also be elevated (normal range 8–18 IU/L, raised >40 IU/L—secondary to hepatomegaly).
   a. As hamsters secrete both **corticosterone and cortisol**, it has been suggested that both should be measured to assess adrenocortical function accurately.
4. Measurement of **basal salivary cortisol** values and the **ACTH stimulation test** have been validated in **guinea pigs** and proved to be useful in confirming the diagnosis in the single case report in this species.
   a. 20 IU ACTH was administered intramuscularly and saliva samples collected before and 4 h after administration. Saliva samples were analyzed by radioimmunoassay and post-ACTH cortisol levels were markedly elevated in the patient compared to controls.
5. There is one report of urine cortisol:creatinine ratio being used as a screening test for a suspected case in a hamster. A 24 h urine sample was collected for analysis, however, no reference ranges have been established for this test in rodents.
6. Abdominal ultrasonography may reveal enlarged adrenal glands in affected rodents.
B. **Birds:**
1. There are **no reported cases of hyperadrenocorticism in birds with antemortem confirmation of the diagnosis**.
2. In all avian species tested **corticosterone**, not cortisol, is the main corticosteroid produced by the "adult" adrenal gland. So theoretically, confirmation of clinical suspicion of hyperadrenocorticism (Cushing's syndrome) can be attempted by determining the plasma corticosterone level before and after ACTH stimulation. An exaggerated increase in corticosterone after ACTH stimulation is expected in clinical cases; however, it must be remembered that corticosterone concentrations may be affected by the time of day, season, reproductive activity, genetics, and degree of stress. A one-time determination of corticosterone concentration in the blood does not accurately reflect adrenocortical function and is not considered an appropriate diagnostic tool in birds.
3. ACTH stimulation protocols have been established in psittacines, raptors, chickens, and ducks.
   a. A baseline blood sample is collected.
   b. 16–50 units of ACTH are administered intramuscularly.
   c. A second blood sample is collected 1–2 h after ACTH administration.
   d. Quantification of corticosterone in both blood samples requires an assay specific to this hormone, for example, radioimmunoassay.
   e. In general, ACTH causes a peak corticosterone response within 30–60 minutes after injection with a return to baseline levels within 120–240 minutes. Pre- and post-ACTH corticosterone concentrations vary significantly among avian species. In healthy cockatoos, macaws, Amazon parrots, and lorikeets, the mean post-ACTH corticosterone concentrations are 4–14 times the mean baseline concentration. The sensitivity and specificity of the test remains undetermined and further investigation is required in relation to interpretation of test results.
4. Extrapolating from mammalian medicine, a dexamethasone suppression test may also be used to aid the diagnosis of hyperadrenocorticism. There is limited information available regarding its use in pet birds, but some research has been undertaken in relation to the effects of dexamethasone on corticosterone levels in pigeons and chickens.
5. Hemogram "stress" abnormalities may be seen, for example, leukocytosis and heterophilia.
6. It may be valuable to evaluate hepatic function as concurrent hepatopathy is likely (e.g., hepatic lipidosis).
7. Hyperglycemia and glucosuria may be seen.
8. Necropsy, histopathology, and immunohistochemistry may be required for definitive diagnosis.

V. Differential Diagnoses

A. **Gerbils/hamsters:**
   1. Ectoparasites.
   2. Dermatophytosis.
   3. Epitheliotropic lymphoma (hamsters).

B. **Guinea pigs:**
   1. Cystic ovarian disease (see Chapter 47).
   2. Vitamin C deficiency.
   3. Alopecia of pregnancy.
   4. Barbering.
   5. Diabetes mellitus (see Chapter 17).

C. **Birds:**
   1. Diabetes mellitus (see Chapter 17).

VI. Treatment

A. **Rodents:**
   1. In the hamster, there is one report of effective treatment with **metyrapone** 8 mg orally given daily for 1 month. Alopecia resolved within 12 weeks of treatment. However, in another hamster, metyrapone at the same dosage and mitotane (5 mg q 24 h for 30 days) were both ineffective.
   2. In a guinea pig, 2–6 mg **trilostane** per os q 24 h was used successfully. Careful monitoring of basal salivary cortisol concentrations was essential to ensure adequate therapy and reduce potential side effects at higher dose rates (inappetence and weight loss).
   3. Surgical removal of the affected gland via flank laparotomy (if a functional adrenal tumor is diagnosed). Techniques have been described for various species.

B. **Birds:**
   1. Mitotane has been suggested as a therapeutic consideration in birds. However, no reports of medical or surgical treatment of hyperadrenocorticism in birds have been described. This is likely a consequence of the difficulty in achieving an antemortem diagnosis.

C. **Iatrogenic hyperadrenocorticism:**
   1. Discontinue exogenous corticosteroid therapy.

VII. Prognosis

A. There is limited information available regarding prognosis of adrenal dysfunction in these species. Due to the likelihood of concurrent disease and limited therapeutic options, survival times of geriatric patients with pituitary or adrenal neoplasia are likely to be short.

VIII. Prevention

A. There are no known preventative measures for spontaneous hyperadrenocorticism in rodents or birds.

B. Iatrogenic hyperadrenocorticism may be avoided by judicious use of therapeutic corticosteroids in all species. Due to their apparent increased sensitivity, **particular care should be taken when considering glucocorticoid therapy in birds**: the dosage should be lower than in mammals, the duration of the treatment limited, short-acting corticosteroids selected in preference to longer acting formulations, and topical application chosen when possible.

References and Further Readings

Adamcak A, Kaufman A, Quesenberry K. What's your diagnosis: Generalized alopecia in a Syrian hamster. *Lab Anim* 1998;27(6):19–20.

Bauck LB, Orr JP, Lawrence H. Hyperadrenocorticism in three teddy bear hamsters. *Can Vet J* 1984;25(6):247–250.

Brink-Johnsen T, Brink-Johnsen K, Kilham L. Gestational changes in hamster adrenocortical function. *J Steroid Biochem* 1981;14:835–839.

de Matos R. Adrenal steroid metabolism in birds: Anatomy, physiology and clinical considerations. *Vet Clin North Am Exot Anim Pract* 2008;11:35–57.

Lawrie A. Systemic non-infectious disease. In: Harcourt-Brown N, Chitty J, eds. *BSAVA Manual of Psittacine Birds*, 2nd edn. Gloucester: British Small Animal Veterinary Association, 2005, pp. 245–265.

Lumeij JT. Endocrinology. In: Ritchie BW, Harrison GJ, Harrison LR, eds. *Avian Medicine—Principles and Application*. Lake Worth: Wingers, 1994, pp. 582–606.

Martinho F. Suspected case of hyperadrenocorticism in a golden hamster (*Mesocricetus auratus*). *Vet Clin North Am Exot Anim Pract* 2006;9:717–721.

Orr H. Rodents: Neoplastic and endocrine disease. In: Keeble E, Meredith A, eds. *BSAVA Manual of Rodents and Ferrets*. Gloucester: British Small Animal Veterinary Association, 2009, pp. 181–192.

Ottenweller JE, Tapp WN, Burke JN, et al. Plasma cortisol and corticosterone concentrations in the golden hamster (*Mesocricetus auratus*). *Life Sci* 1985;37:1551–1558.

Percy DH, Barthold SW. *Pathology of Laboratory Rodents and Rabbits*, 3rd edn. Ames: Blackwell Publishing, 2007.

Rees Davies R. The small sick psittacid. In: Harcourt-Brown N, Chitty J, eds. *BSAVA Manual of Psittacine Birds*, 2nd edn. Gloucester: British Small Animal Veterinary Association, 2005, pp. 266–279.

Starkey SR, Morrisey JK, Stewart JE, et al. Pituitary-dependent hyperadrenocorticism in a cockatoo. *J Am Vet Med Assoc* 2008;232(3):394–398.

Wesche P. Rodents: Clinical pathology. In: Keeble E, Meredith A, eds. *BSAVA Manual of Rodents and Ferrets*. Gloucester: British Small Animal Veterinary Association, 2009, pp. 42–51.

Westerhof I, Pellicaan CH. Effects of different application routes of glucocorticoids on the pituitary-adrenocortical axis in pigeons (*Columbia livia domestica*). *J Avian Med Surg* 1995;9(3):175–181.

Westerhof I, Van den Brom WE, Mol JA, et al. Sensitivity of the hypothalamic-pituitary-adrenal system of pigeons (*Columbia livia domestica*) to suppression by dexamethasone, cortisol, and prednisolone. *Avian Dis* 1994;38:435–445.

Zeugswetter F, Fenske M, Hassan J, et al. Cushing's syndrome in a guinea pig. *Vet Rec* 2007;160(25):878–880.

CHAPTER 11

Hyperadrenocorticism (Pituitary Pars Intermedia Dysfunction) in Horses

Catherine McGowan

Pathogenesis

- Equine hyperadrenocorticism is almost invariably associated with pituitary dysfunction, a condition referred to as pituitary pars intermedia dysfunction (PPID).
- As the name suggests, it affects the pars intermedia of the pituitary gland not the pars distalis.
- It causes a loss of dopaminergic inhibition of the pituitary pars intermedia resulting in increased pituitary peptide production including α-melanocyte-stimulating hormone (α-MSH), adrenocorticotropic hormone (ACTH), and β-endorphin.
- PPID is a neurodegenerative disease associated with aging, most closely related to human Parkinson's disease.

Classical Signs

- It is a common (20%) problem of horses, ponies, and donkeys 15 years of age and older with no breed or sex predilection.
- A variable combination of clinical signs is seen, the most common of which is hirsutism.
- Other signs include polyuria and polydipsia, hyperhidrosis, muscle catabolism, and weight redistribution resulting in a loss of epaxial musculature and a potbellied appearance.
- Secondary infections and/or delayed wound healing are commonly encountered.
- Laminitis is frequently the most devastating consequence and may necessitate euthanasia.

Diagnosis

- Hirsutism is pathognomonic for PPID but diagnosis should be confirmed in all horses where treatment is initiated in order to have baseline endocrine values for monitoring purposes.
- Basal ACTH concentration or the low-dose dexamethasone stimulation test are most commonly used.
- ACTH or α-MSH response to thyrotropin-releasing hormone or domperidone can also be used.

Clinical Endocrinology of Companion Animals, First Edition. Edited by Jacquie Rand.
© 2013 John Wiley & Sons, Inc. Published 2013 by John Wiley & Sons, Inc.

● Resting blood insulin and glucose concentrations are nonspecific but are recommended for monitoring purposes.

Treatment

● Dopamine agonists—pergolide mesylate is the drug of choice.
● Management of the horse including attention to hooves, teeth, deworming and clipping the hair coat, as well as clinical and endocrinological follow up are critical to the success of treatment.

I. Pathogenesis
A. The pathophysiology of PPID is **different from that of hyperadrenocorticism in other species:**
1. It is **almost invariably associated with pituitary dysfunction,** hence the name pituitary pars intermedia dysfunction (PPID). The condition has also been referred to, sometimes misleadingly, as equine Cushing's disease/syndrome, pituitary/hypophyseal/chromophobe adenoma, pars intermedia adenoma/hyperplasia, diffuse adenomatous hyperplasia of the pituitary, and pituitary-dependent hyperadrenocorticism. The preferred name pituitary pars intermedia dysfunction or PPID will be used throughout this chapter:
   a. Unlike Cushing's disease in dogs and humans, adrenocortical hyperplasia and hypercortisolemia are not consistent findings in horses with PPID.
   b. Only one case of adrenal gland–dependant equine Cushing's syndrome has been reported.
   c. Iatrogenic hyperadrenocorticism has also been reported but is much less common than PPID.
2. As the name suggests, PPID affects the pars intermedia of the pituitary gland:
   a. The pituitary gland (hypophysis) is comprised of two lobes: the anterior lobe (adenohypophysis) and the posterior lobe (neurohypophysis). The anterior lobe is further divided up into three parts; the *pars intermedia, distalis,* and *tuberalis.*
   b. When the pituitary gland is viewed histologically, three distinct areas can be appreciated, the pars nervosa (or neurohypophysis), the pars distalis, and the pars intermedia. The **part of the pituitary gland affected in the horse with PPID is the *pars intermedia*** (Figure 11.1).
   c. The pars intermedia is comprised entirely of the melanotrope cell type that synthesizes and processes a range of proopiomelanocortin (POMC) peptides. The melanotrope processes the parent POMC peptide further than the pars distalis so that the range of peptides produced are different from the pars distalis and include alpha-melanocyte-stimulating hormone (α-MSH), corticotrophin like intermediate peptide (CLIP), beta endorphin, and gamma-lipotropin. While POMC processing is markedly elevated, the relative proportions of peptides released from affected horses appears unchanged when compared with normal horses (Figure 11.2).
   d. Excessive hormone production leads to **hyperplasia** of that part of the pituitary gland which **may or may not then progress to adenoma formation** (Figure 11.3).
3. PPID involves a **loss of dopaminergic inhibition** of the pituitary pars intermedia:
   a. The pars distalis is well vascularized and receives releasing and inhibitory factors from the hypothalamus that control secretion.
   b. The pars intermedia is poorly vascularized and relies on neurotransmitters released from axons from the hypothalamus to control secretion, especially tonic inhibition by dopamine, mediated by dopaminergic D2 receptors on the melanotropes.
   c. The loss of tonic inhibition by dopamine mediated by the D2 receptor is responsible for excess pars intermedia activity and PPID.
4. PPID is a **neurodegenerative disease associated with aging,** most closely related to human Parkinson's disease:
   a. This is a factor that is important to convey to owners of affected horses as older terms such as pituitary adenoma or tumor may imply to owners that this condition is untreatable or that the prognosis is hopeless.

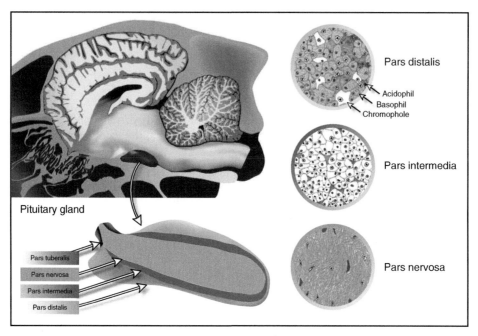

Figure 11.1   Equine pituitary anatomy and histology. (Photo courtesy of Cathy McGowan.)

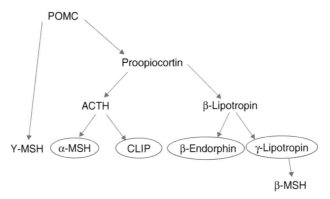

Figure 11.2   Proopiomelanocortin processing by pars intermedia melanotropes. ACTH, adrenocorticotropic hormone; CLIP, corticotrophin like intermediate peptide; MSH, melanocyte-stimulating hormone; POMC, proopiomelanocortin.

b. In studies of pituitary glands, there was a marked reduction in dopamine (to <12% of the control value) in affected horses compared with controls, but no change in serotonin concentrations between horses with PPID and control horses.

c. Immunohistological studies of pituitary glands of horses with PPID have shown that there is a marked reduction (to <20% of the control value) in tyrosine hydroxylase, a marker of functional dopaminergic neurons, and a 50% reduction in the cell bodies of the dopaminergic neurons compared to controls, as in Parkinson's disease.

d. Further, studies have shown an increased oxidative stress marker, 3-nitrotyrosine, and expression of alpha-synuclein in horses with PPID with both of these also found to occur in patients with Parkinson's disease.

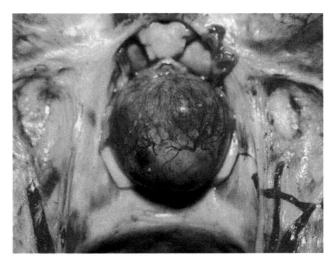

Figure 11.3   Enlarged pituitary gland post mortem in a horse. (Image courtesy of Prof. Derek Knottenbelt.)

Table 11.1   Mean age, clinical signs, and their frequency of occurrence in eight case series of horses with pituitary pars intermedia dysfunction.

Clinical sign	Heinrichs et al. (1990)	Hillyer et al. (1992)	Boujon et al. (1993)	van der Kolk et al. (1993)	Couetil et al. (1996)	Schott et al. (2001)	Donaldson et al. (2002)	McGowan and Neiger (2003)
Total number studied	19	17	5	21	22	77	27	20
Mean age (years)	19	20	18	21	21.5	23	19 (median)	19
Hirsutism	47%	94%	100%	100%	95%	83%	59%	100%
Laminitis	NR	82%	NR	24%	59%	52%	74%	80%
Weight loss or redistribution	NR	88%	60%	38%	50%	47%	33%	65%
Lethargy	NR	82%	20%	NR	41%	36%	19%	95%
Polyuria/polydipsia	26%	76%	NR	NR	32%	34%	7%	55%
Hyperhidrosis	NR	59%	60%	5%	14%	33%	29%	30%
Bulging supraorbital fat	NR	12%	40%	19%	9%	30%	26%	50%
Concurrent infections	21%	66%	40%	19%	36%	NR	30%	35%

NR = not recorded.

II. Signalment
A. PPID is a **common condition**, affecting approximately 20% of horses, ponies, and donkeys 15 years of age and older with **no breed or sex predilection**:
  1. The **average age of diagnosis is 15–20 years** (Table 11.1).
  2. The **main risk factor for development of PPID is increasing age.**

(a)

(b)

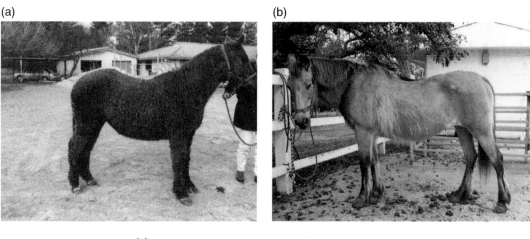

(c)

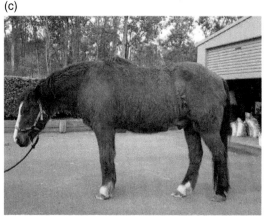

Figure 11.4   Hirsutism is the most common clinical sign in horses with PPID.

　　　3. PPID is very rare in horses < 10 years of age.
B.　Despite earlier clinical case series reporting a seemingly increased proportion of ponies affected, ponies are not considered to be at increased risk. Ponies may appear overrepresented because:
　　　1. People may be more likely to keep ponies for longer than horses due to easier management.
　　　2. Hirsutism is often more noticeable in pony breeds.
III.　Clinical Signs
A.　A **variable combination of clinical signs** may be seen (Table 11.1):
　　　1. The clinical syndrome falls across a spectrum of advancing severity associated with advancing disease.
　　　2. The total number of clinical and historical signs of PPID increases in proportion with increasing plasma concentrations of the pituitary peptides ACTH and α-MSH.
　　　3. A similarly **variable spectrum of pituitary pathology** is described from focal or multifocal hypertrophy or hyperplasia, to diffuse adenomatous hyperplasia, to adenomatous hyperplasia with microadenomas, to adenoma formation.
B.　**Clinical signs** are hallmarked by **hirsutism** (excessive hair growth):
　　　1. An owner-reported **history of delayed shedding or a long hair coat is the most significant historical finding** associated with PPID.
　　　2. Hirsutism is not a normal feature of aging and is **pathognomonic for PPID.**
　　　3. Hirsutism may range from delayed shedding each year, uneven hair coat with patches of alopecia, to a permanent long or even curly hair coat (Figure 11.4).

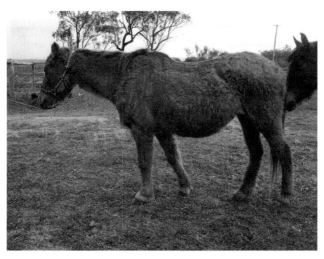

Figure 11.5   Muscle catabolism and weakness, with a potbelly and "sway back" appearance.

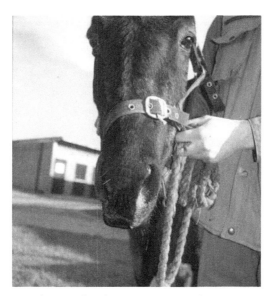

Figure 11.6   Sinusitis in this horse secondary to reduced immunity associated with PPID.

C. Despite the relatively low proportion of ACTH among POMC peptides released from the abnormal pars intermedia, **many of the clinical signs are attributed to hyperadrenocorticism:**

1. These include **polyuria and polydipsia** probably associated with direct effect of cortisol on antidiuretic hormone (ADH) production, although likely to be exacerbated by osmotic diuresis in hyperglycemic horses.

2. **Muscle catabolism** and weight redistribution:

   a. Horses usually appear **underweight, with loss of muscle over their back and a potbellied appearance,** attributed to the catabolic effects of hypercortisolemia (Figure 11.5).

   b. These signs are also associated with atrophy of type II muscle fibers, typical of steroid-induced myopathy as found in other species.

3. **Susceptibility to infections and reduction in healing,** for example, oral ulcerations, skin infections, periodontal disease, and sinusitis (Figure 11.6):

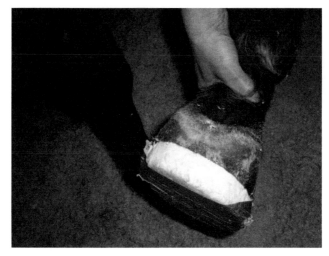

Figure 11.7   Styrofoam pads support this aged mare with PPID with severe (Grade 3) laminitis.

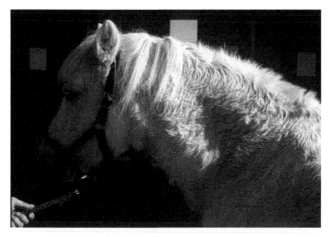

Figure 11.8   Pony demonstrating marked hyperhidrosis.

a. Unexplained periodontal disease, sinusitis, or recurrent infections in the aged horse should alert practitioners to the possibility of PPID.

4. **Recurrent or chronic laminitis,** most likely via the induction of insulin resistance secondary to the prolonged hyperadrenocorticism (Figure 11.7):

a. Laminitis is frequently the most devastating consequence and **may necessitate euthanasia.**

b. Laminitis in an aged horse without evidence of systemic illness or history of a feeding accident should be investigated in every instance for an underlying endocrinopathy (equine metabolic syndrome and/or PPID).

D. **Other clinical signs** may be attributable to other POMC peptides. However, the effects of other peptides secreted from the pars intermedia are not well known; neither are the effects of compression of the pars nervosa or pars distalis which may occur in some horses:

1. **Lethargy** is often attributed to excess β-endorphin activity.

2. **Hyperhidrosis** (excessive sweating) may be associated with catecholamine effects from the adrenal medulla, as a result of hirsutism reducing thermoregulatory capability or even due to the effects of compression of an enlarged pituitary gland onto the thermoregulatory centers (Figure 11.8).

3. Effects from an adenoma or enlarged pituitary on the brain stem are rare, although blindness has been reported:

    a. Anatomically, effects on the optic chiasm would be most likely from an enlarged pituitary gland (Figure 11.3), although further extension from an adenoma would be very unlikely.

    b. Seizures have been rarely reported in horses with PPID but the cause of the seizures has not been demonstrated to be due to the pituitary disease.

E. PPID causes a combination of clinical signs, especially lethargy and wasting, which are often considered indicative of a poor quality of life. However, these clinical signs have been consistently and successfully reversed by medical therapy.

F. **Clinical Pathology:**

    1. **Routine hematology and biochemistry are not useful in the diagnosis of PPID** as horses with PPID have no significant difference from age-matched normal horses:

        a. A stress leukogram, as seen in dogs, is not present.

        b. Aged horses, irrespective of whether they have PPID or not tend to have a relative lymphopenia.

        c. Inflammatory changes, if present, represent concurrent illness rather than the effects of hypercortisolemia.

    2. Routine hematology, serum biochemical analysis, and urinalysis may, however, provide valuable information about concurrent problems in an aged horse.

    3. **Routine hematology and biochemistry are also useful in the assessment and monitoring** of a horse with PPID with respect to **prognosis and response to therapy.**

IV. Diagnosis

A. Diagnosis of PPID is based on **history, clinical signs, and laboratory findings:**

    1. A **variety of diagnostic laboratory tests is available** but one limitation is that a gold standard antemortem test has yet to be identified. A definitive diagnosis may be achieved via postmortem examination in combination with clinical signs but this is of limited value to the practicing clinician.

B. It is important to consider the **reasons for diagnosis**, before deciding on a diagnostic protocol:

    1. **Aims of diagnosis:**

        a. To determine the need for treatment.

        b. To obtain prognostic information.

        c. To obtain baseline information in order to monitor the response to therapy.

        d. To differentiate from insulin resistance or equine metabolic syndrome.

C. **To determine the need for treatment:**

    1. If the reason for diagnosis is to **initiate and potentially monitor therapy**, then the method of diagnosis needs to be **most accurate** as treatment is expensive and lifelong.

    2. There are basically **two types of endocrine tests, basal and dynamic.**

    3. **Basal tests** are those that can be obtained with a **single sample** and are popular with veterinarians and clients due to **simplicity and reduced cost**, especially considering that testing may need to be repeated regularly following diagnosis:

        a. However, the benefits may be partially offset by the **reduction in sensitivity and specificity of diagnosis.**

    4. **Basal plasma ACTH concentration is currently the best option for a basal diagnostic test:**

        a. Sensitivities and specificities of >80% have been reported with a single cutoff value, with increased sensitivities and specificities >90% if seasonally adjusted reference ranges are used instead of a single cutoff value.

        b. **ACTH concentrations will increase in the autumn months,** with horses with PPID potentially having more pronounced increases.

        c. Some laboratories are now able to correct for the seasonal effects on ACTH and can provide altered diagnostic ranges for samples collected during this period.

        d. **Cutoff values** for diagnosis of PPID using basal plasma ACTH concentration will **vary depending on the assay used**, but, for example, for the Immulite® 1000, a value of 6.5 pmol/L (29.7 pg/mL) can be used as a cutoff for non-autumn months (>80% sensitivity and specificity), or 10.3 pmol/L (47 pg/mL) for autumn months (>90% sensitivity and specificity).

Table 11.2   Protocol for the low dose dexamethasone suppression test in horses.

- Collect a baseline serum blood sample followed by injection of 40 μg/kg dexamethasone intramuscularly.
- Collect a second serum sample between 18 and 24 h later and submit both to a laboratory for cortisol analysis. (Heparinized plasma samples can also be taken.)
- Cortisol is reasonably stable so both samples can be submitted as whole blood together, although it is pertinent to chill the samples (in a refrigerator).
- Normal horses show suppression of cortisol concentration of around 70–80% from baseline.
- Following administration of dexamethasone, affected horses have serum cortisol >40 nmol/L (1.45 μg/dL) from a baseline of around 100 nmol/L (3.62 μg/dL) while normal horses have suppression to <20 nmol/L (0.72 μg/dL).
- The "gray zone" in horses that suppress between 20 and 40 nmol/L (0.72 and 1.45 μg/dL) is difficult to interpret. Horses with high baseline values (>150 nmol/L (5.44 μg/dL)) usually have slightly less suppression and values less than 40 nmol/L are considered a normal suppression in this case. However, if in doubt, the test should be repeated or a basal adrenocorticotropic hormone concentration determined to help confirm the result.

e. ACTH is **labile** and the EDTA plasma samples should be separated and chilled within 3 h of collection, frozen within 12 h, and sent frozen to the laboratory. Plasma samples must not be kept in glass tubes as the ACTH is adsorbed onto glass.

f. This can be achieved in practice provided you take a pipette, plastic storage container, and cooler with ice packs with you (many laboratories provide collection packs). Blood can be collected in **an EDTA vacutainer, allowed to separate by gravity, and separated and chilled on ice within an hour.** It is advisable to check with your laboratory for any additional requirements they may have before collecting the sample.

5. **Basal α-MSH** may offer some advantages over basal ACTH as it is **specific to the pars intermedia** and not part of the adrenocortical axis (less affected by stress), but **is well correlated to ACTH in the field setting.**

6. **Dynamic endocrine testing** can provide **much greater diagnostic sensitivity and specificity** over simple measurement of basal hormone levels because they evaluate the integrity of endocrine regulatory feedback loops:

a. **The low-dose dexamethasone suppression test has the highest reported sensitivity and specificity for the diagnosis of PPID.** When samples are collected 20 h apart, the test has been reported to approach 100% sensitivity and specificity (Table 11.2).

b. The aim of the test is to **detect a failure of suppression of cortisol following the administration of dexamethasone** in horses with PPID.

c. The rationale is that the ACTH and resultant adrenal cortisol production from affected horses are not affected by negative feedback. The pars intermedia is not affected by negative feedback, so affected horses fail to show a suppression of cortisol following administration of the exogenous glucocorticoid, dexamethasone.

d. The test is affected by season, with the **potential for false-positive diagnoses during the autumn months.**

e. The dexamethasone suppression test is **not affected by the time of day**; however, frequently it is convenient to perform an overnight test starting the afternoon before.

7. **Other dynamic tests** include the combined dexamethasone suppression/thyrotropin-releasing hormone (TRH) stimulation test and ACTH or α-MSH response to domperidone or TRH. These tests may offer increased diagnostic capability but are **not considered as first choice for field testing.**

8. Risks of dynamic endocrine tests:

a. Some veterinarians and horse owners have raised concern about the possibility of exacerbating laminitis or inducing an attack of laminitis due to administration of dexamethasone.

b. In the author's opinion, there is little doubt that excessive prolonged doses of corticosteroids can cause laminitis, particularly in a predisposed horse. However, the risk of the dexamethasone suppression test is minimal, and the benefits outweigh the risks. The dose given is low, less than half a single therapeutic dose, and given only once.

D. **To obtain prognostic information and to obtain baseline information in order to monitor the response to therapy:**
  1. A horse with unequivocal hirsutism and three or more clinical signs of PPID may not require a diagnostic test to determine the need for treatment. However, prior to commencement of treatment, **baseline and prognostic tests should be obtained.**
  2. **Insulin is the most important prognostic test** and will **correlate with laminitis:**
     a. PPID horses with high insulin (>1305 pmol/L [188 μIU/mL]) are more likely to develop laminitis and not survive 2 years compared to those with low to moderate elevations (<430 pmol/L [62 μIU/mL]).
     b. **Fasting samples** in horses that are managed with defined feeding periods are ideal, with one option being to collect the sample prior to the morning feed after an overnight fast of 6 h or to collect at 12 pm midday after the morning feed has been removed at least 4 h before.
  3. **Blood-glucose concentration is also useful for prognostic purposes:**
     a. Blood glucose concentration is not very sensitive as a diagnostic test as **not all horses with PPID develop hyperglycemia**; however, **those that do have hyperglycemia often have more advanced disease**, possibly with additional disease stress and/or pancreatic exhaustion.
  4. **ACTH concentration** has been correlated with the number of clinical signs of PPID and so **very high values** (except during the autumn) can be considered a **poor prognostic indicator:**
     a. ACTH concentration should decrease on pergolide therapy and can be used to adjust the dose if improvements of ACTH do not occur.

V. Differential Diagnoses
A. In cases where hirsutism is not apparent or laminitis is the primary clinical sign, it is important to differentiate PPID from **Equine metabolic syndrome** (see Chapter 20), both of which are associated with insulin resistance:
  1. Dynamic or basal tests of pituitary peptides or the dexamethasone suppression test will be the best way to differentiate the two syndromes (see above).
B. In the absence of hirsutism, other clinical signs suggestive of PPID may be explained by a number of differential diagnoses:
  1. Polyuria and polydipsia may be caused by neurogenic or nephrogenic diabetes insipidus, psychogenic polydipsia, or hyperglycemia of various origins (pancreatic disease, pheochromocytoma).
  2. Weight loss and muscle wasting may be associated with dental disease, parasitism, or other age-related conditions.

VI. Treatment
A. There are several factors to consider regarding if and when to treat:
  1. **Medical therapy does improve quality of life of affected horses.**
  2. All owners should be informed and given the option of treatment.
  3. **General preventive care and improved husbandry** by owners as an adjunct to medical therapy is **important** including hoof care, regular deworming, clipping, and dental care.
  4. **Attention to diet is also important.** Horses with PPID are aged and potentially in a catabolic state so it is important to provide a balanced diet with **adequate high quality protein and to supplement for trace minerals and vitamins.** Large reductions in caloric intake are not recommended, although **ensuring PPID horses are not overfed** so as to remain/become fat is important.
B. Many veterinarians and owners will wait until clinical laminitis develops; however, this is not advised as this may increase the risk of euthanasia when the first episode occurs.
C. In the past, medical treatment of PPID has fallen into **three basic classes of medication:**
  1. Cortisol inhibitors (trilostane).
  2. Serotonin antagonists (cyproheptadine).
  3. Dopamine agonists (pergolide and bromocriptine).
D. The **current recommendation is to use pergolide mesylate** (Prascend®, Boehringer Ingelheim; [1 mg scored tablets]) as **first-line therapy:**
  1. Medical treatment of PPID has been used for almost 30 years with early reports in textbooks and review articles originally advocating cyproheptadine, pergolide, or bromocriptine predominantly on a theoretical basis from extrapolation from the human literature.

2. However, based on cumulative evidence, pergolide has become the standard of care recognized in the equine internal medicine literature in horses with PPID.

3. Pergolide (Prascend®, Boehringer Ingelheim) has recently been licensed in some EU countries for use in horses.

E. **Dopamine agonists: Pergolide and Bromocriptine:**

   1. The first report of medical treatment of PPID in the scientific literature described a single horse given three dopamine agonists after which the effects of POMC peptides and cortisol were measured.

   2. This landmark study demonstrated the benefit of dopamine agonists:

      a. There was inhibition of all the measured POMC peptides (ACTH, β-endorphin, CLIP, α-MSH, and β-MSH) by dopamine infusion, bromocriptine given subcutaneously or orally, and pergolide given orally.

   3. Practically, **pergolide mesylate was shown to be the most appropriate dopamine agonist** among the three used. In oral capsule form at a dose rate of 5 mg given once was **well tolerated and effective at lowering POMC peptides** for the duration of the measurement period (48 h):

      a. Dopamine infusion was short acting and produced a rebound increase in POMC peptides following cessation of the infusion.

      b. Bromocriptine was poorly absorbed orally, and while therapeutic levels and an appropriate response were attained, the amount given (100 mg) was much larger per body weight than in man and not well tolerated by the horse. In an attempt to overcome this, subcutaneous injections were used, but these caused local swelling and reactions.

   4. Retrospective clinical trial data have shown **pergolide treatment to decrease plasma ACTH concentration and improve clinical signs based on owner reports in as many as 85% of horses with PPID over approximately 2 months of therapy.**

   5. Pergolide therapy has been shown in several publications to be **superior to cyproheptadine therapy** and other studies have shown pergolide treatment to be effective after a failed period of cyproheptadine treatment:

      a. When the effects of pergolide and cyproheptadine were compared in a retrospective study of PPID, only two of seven owners reported clinical improvement after treatment using cyproheptadine while 17 of 20 owners reported that pergolide treatment resulted in clinical improvement.

      b. In another study, pergolide was also shown to be a more effective treatment for PPID than cyproheptadine in terms of clinical response (17/20 favorable outcome for pergolide vs 3/7 for cyproheptadine) and normalizing the results of endocrine tests (7/20 vs 1/7, respectively).

   6. Pergolide has been associated with **few side effects** where horses start at a dose of 0.002 mg/kg. The most frequently reported side effect is that of **mild inappetence or reduced appetite** and the majority of horses respond to a reduction in dose and then a more gradual increase in dose:

      a. Side effects of inappetence and depression were more commonly reported in earlier studies where initial doses were at the high end of the dose range.

   7. The general approach to treatment with pergolide is start at a low dose, increase until clinical signs and endocrine values are well controlled (or signs of intolerance, e.g., inappetence are observed), and then slowly reduce to the lowest effective dose for each horse:

      a. Due to severity and stage of disease and the individual physiological response to therapy, **individual horses may respond differently to treatment.**

      b. **A dose of 0.001–0.002 mg/kg q 24 h,** which represents low dose therapy, is **an appropriate starting dose.**

      c. The dose should be **increased slowly from the starting dose, every 2–4 weeks,** depending on clinical and endocrinological response to **up to 0.01 mg/kg q 24 h.**

      d. Many horses may be able to be maintained on 0.002 mg/kg (low dose), but in the author's opinion, attempting to maintain horses on a lower dose places the horse at risk of treatment failure due to inadequate dose.

F. **Cortisol inhibitors: Trilostane:**

   1. Trilostane is a competitive inhibitor of 3-β-hydroxysteroid dehydrogenase.

   2. In a 2-year prospective study in 20 horses with PPID, trilostane at 1 mg/kg q 24 h PO was demonstrated to be effective in reducing the clinical signs of PPID, and horses showed a reduction in the cortisol response to TRH 30 days after commencing treatment.

3. Trilostane acts peripherally to reduce clinical signs of disease:
   a. It reduces the effects of hyperadrenocorticism by **inhibiting adrenal cortical glucocorticoid production**.
4. **Clinical signs**, for example, laminitis, muscle catabolism and polyuria/polydipsia and secondary infections **can be reduced**.
5. Trilostane can be considered as an **adjunct therapy** for PPID rather than the main treatment (i.e., pergolide).

G. Serotonin antagonists: cyproheptadine:
   1. Cyproheptadine has been advocated for the management of PPID in horses on the basis of the fact that high doses of serotonin may stimulate the release of ACTH from the pars intermedia.
   2. However, in studies in horses, serotonin stimulation had been shown to have no influence on gene expression of POMC in the pars intermedia.
   3. While a marked reduction in dopamine (to <12% of the control value) in PPID affected horses compared with controls has been shown, there was no change in serotonin (5-HT) concentrations between horses with PPID and control horses.
   4. Despite the lack of pathophysiological justification, there have been **some reports of clinical benefit from the use of cyproheptadine** and it has been used more recently as an **adjunct therapy in horses responding poorly to pergolide therapy**. The reported dose is 0.25 mg/kg PO q 24 h for 4–8 weeks, increasing to q 12 h dosing at that time if there is a poor response on the basis of clinical signs and repeat laboratory testing.
   5. However **the majority of data supports a lack of effect of cyproheptadine** and it has been suggested that any improvement noted with cyproheptadine is due to management adjustments (deworming, dental work, and improved nutrition) rather than the effects of the drug itself.
   6. In one study, management adjustments had been performed before the onset of therapy and no effect of cyproheptadine therapy could be detected.

H. **Monitoring:**
   1. Once treatment has been initiated, it is important to **continue to monitor the horse clinically as well and endocrinologically**.
   2. Horses affected with PPID are aged, and as such **more susceptible to diseases associated with aging** including dental disease, lameness, respiratory disorders and skin disorders.
   3. Owners should be encouraged to monitor appetite, hair coat (clip if necessary), water intake and bed wetting when housed, body condition score including estimation of muscle loss as well as fat score, laminitis/lameness, and general demeanor.
   4. Horses with PPID will be more susceptible to secondary infections and **regular clinical examinations and hematological and biochemical profiles** are warranted.
   5. Monitoring will be quite regular initially as the horse starts treatment.
   6. Clinical data as well as **baseline plasma ACTH concentration or dexamethasone suppression test, serum insulin concentration, and blood or urine glucose measurement** can be performed:
      a. The author recommends monthly monitoring initially, with adjustment to the dose of pergolide depending on the response.
      b. Subsequent monitoring can be 3 monthly to 6 monthly, depending on the horse's response.
   7. A suggested treatment and monitoring protocol is outlined in Table 11.3.

VII. Prognosis
A. In general, **milder cases respond extremely well to medical therapy** and **treated horses can return to full function,** many cases able to compete in their respective disciplines.
B. **More severe cases** often respond well too, but very advanced cases or those complicated with secondary or concurrent disease, common in aged horses, may not:
   1. In such cases, it is important to **utilize endocrinological and clinical variables to determine the response to medical therapy** and formulate a prognosis.
   2. The **prognosis is poor if ACTH and insulin remain markedly elevated despite appropriate therapy** at recommended doses.

Table 11.3   Example of a treatment and monitoring protocol for horses with pituitary pars intermedia dysfunction.

This example assumes no concurrent disease and controlled laminitis at the time of treatment. If concurrent disease or uncontrolled laminitis are present, clinical examinations and repeat diagnostic evaluation will necessarily fall within in a shorter time frame.

1. Obtain baseline endocrine and clinical values, for example, basal insulin and glucose, basal adrenocorticotropic hormone (ACTH), and documented clinical examination findings.
2. Owners should be encouraged to monitor appetite, hair coat, water intake and bed wetting when housed, body condition score including estimation of muscle loss as well as fat score, laminitis/lameness, and general demeanor monthly.
3. Calculate the starting dose of pergolide based on 0.002 mg/kg PO q 24 h to the nearest 0.5 mg.

Horse body weight (kg)	Starting daily dose (mg)	Dosage range (μg/kg)
200–350	0.5	1.3–2.5
350–600	1.0	1.7–2.5
601–850	1.5	1.8–2.5

4. After 1 month of once daily treatment, reevaluate baseline endocrine and clinical values as well as owner-reported improvements. You should expect one or more clinical signs to improve and/or the basal ACTH to have returned to normal or close to normal range for that time of year.
5. If clinical and/or endocrine improvements are not noted, increase the dose by 0.001 mg/kg.
6. Reevaluate monthly with increases in the dose by 0.001 mg/kg until clinical signs and endocrinological variables have improved or a maximal dose of 0.01 mg/kg has been reached.
7. If signs of inappetence or depression are observed, reduce the dose by increments of 0.001 mg/kg and investigate for concurrent disease.
8. Once the signs have been successfully controlled, veterinary monitoring can reduce to two to four times per year.
9. Owners should continue to monitor at least monthly and alert their veterinarian if there is deterioration in any clinical sign.
10. If signs are well controlled for >3 months, a slow reduction in the dose by 0.001 mg/kg/month can be attempted, with a minimal dose not less than 0.002 mg/kg.

C.   Horses treated with medical therapy earlier, especially prior to the development of laminitis, have the best outcome.

D.   Long-term therapy has been shown to be safe and evidence of reduced effectiveness of pergolide over the time frames used for horses (2–7 years) has not been observed.

While affected horses tend to be older, they should not be undervalued or overlooked. Trends in horse ownership are changing and aged horses are more frequently presented for veterinary care. They may be highly experienced athletes or valued by their owners as a companion or teacher.

VIII. Prevention

A.   Although there are no specific preventative measures, the importance of early diagnosis and initiation of therapy cannot be overstated.

References and Further Readings

Aleman M, Watson JL, Williams DC, et al. Myopathy in horses with pituitary pars intermedia dysfunction (Cushing's disease). *Neuromuscul Disord* 2006;16(11):737–744.
Beck D. Effective long-term treatment of a suspected pituitary adenoma with bromocriptine mesylate in a pony. *Equine Vet Educ* 1992;4:119–122.

Beech J. Tumors of the pituitary gland (pars intermedia). In: Robinson NE, ed. *Current Therapy in Equine Medicine*. Philadelphia: WB Saunders, 1983, pp. 164–169.

Beech, J. Tumors of the pituitary gland (pars intermedia). In: Robinson NE, ed. *Current Therapy in Equine Medicine 2*. Philadelphia: WB Saunders, 1987, pp. 182–185.

Beech J. Treatment of hypophysial adenomas. *Compendium on Continuing Education for the Practicing Veterinarian* 1994;16:921–923.

Beech J. Diseases of the pituitary gland. In: Colahan PT, Merritt AM, Moore JN, et al., eds. *Equine Medicine and Surgery*, Vol. 2, 5th edn. St Louis: Mosby, 1999, pp. 1951–1967.

Boujon CE, Bestetti GE, Meier HP, et al. Equine pituitary adenoma: A functional and morphological study. *J Comp Pathol* 1993;109(2):163–78.

Cohen ND, Carter GK. Steroid hepatopathy in a horse with glucocorticoid-induced hyperadrenocorticism. *J Am Vet Med Assoc* 1992;200:1682–1684.

Couetil L, Paradis MR, Knoll J. Plasma adrenocorticotropin concentration in healthy horses and in horses with clinical signs of hyperadrenocorticism. *J Vet Int Med* 1996;10(1):1–6.

Donaldson MT, Lamonte BH, Morresey P, et al. Treatment with pergolide or cyproheptadine of pituitary pars intermedia dysfunction (equine Cushing's disease). *J Vet Int Med* 2002;16(6):742–746.

Donaldson MT, McDonnell SM, Schanbacher BJ, et al. Variation in plasma adrenocorticotropic hormone concentration and dexamethasone suppression test results with season, age, and sex in healthy ponies and horses. *J Vet Intern Med* 2005;19(2):217–222.

Dybdal NO, Hargreaves KM, Madigan JE, et al. Diagnostic testing for pituitary pars intermedia dysfunction in horses. *J Am Vet Med Assoc* 1994;204(4):627–632.

Dybdal N, Levy M. Pituitary pars intermedia dysfunction in the horse. Part II: Diagnosis and treatment. In: *Proceedings of the 15th Annual Forum of the American College of Veterinary Internal Medicine*. 1997, pp. 470–472.

Heinrichs M, Baumgärtner W, Capen CC. Immunocytochemical demonstration of proopiomelanocortin-derived peptides in pituitary adenomas of the pars intermedia in horses. *Vet Pathol* 1990;27(6):419–425.

Hillyer MH, Taylor FRG, Mair TS, et al. Diagnosis of hyperadrenocorticism in the horse. *Equine Vet Educ* 1992;4:131–134.

Jørgensen HS. Studies on the neuroendocrine role of serotonin. *Dan Med Bull* 2007;54(4):266–88.

Love S. Equine Cushing's disease. *Br Vet J* 1993;149(2):139–153.

McFarlane D. Advantages and limitations of the equine disease, pituitary pars intermedia dysfunction as a model of spontaneous dopaminergic neurodegenerative disease. *Ageing Res Rev* 2007;6(1):54–63.

McFarlane D, Toribio RE. Pituitary pars intermedia dysfunction (equine Cushing's disease). In: Reed SM, Bayly WM, Sellon DC, eds. *Equine Internal Medicine*, 3rd edn. St Louis: Saunders, 2010, pp. 1262–1270.

McGowan TW. *Aged horse health management and welfare*. PhD Thesis, University of Queensland. 2009.

McGowan CM, Neiger R. Efficacy of trilostane for the treatment of equine Cushing's syndrome. *Equine Vet J* 2003; 35(4):414–418.

McGowan CM, Frost R, Pfeiffer DU, et al. Serum insulin concentration in horses with equine Cushing's syndrome: Prognostic value and response to a cortisol inhibitor. *Equine Vet J* 2004;36(3):295–298.

Miller MA, Pardo ID, Jackson LP, et al. Correlation of pituitary histomorphometry with adrenocorticotrophic hormone response to domperidone administration in the diagnosis of equine pituitary pars intermedia dysfunction. *Vet Pathol* 2008;45(1):26–38.

Millington WR, Dybdal NO, Dawson R, Jr., et al. Equine Cushing's disease: Differential regulation of beta-endorphin processing in tumors of the intermediate pituitary. *Endocrinology* 1988;123(3):1598–1604.

Orth DN, Holscher MA, Wilson MG, et al. Equine Cushing's disease: Plasma immunoreactive proopiolipomelanocortin peptide and cortisol levels basally and in response to diagnostic tests. *Endocrinology* 1982;110(4):1430–1441.

Perkins GA, Lamb S, Erb HN, et al. Plasma adrenocorticotropin (ACTH) concentrations and clinical response in horses treated for equine Cushing's disease with cyproheptadine or pergolide. *Equine Vet J* 2002;34(7):679–685.

Schott HC, Coursen CL, Eberhart SW, et al. The Michigan Cushing's project. In: *Proceedings of the 47th Annual Convention of the American Association of Equine Practitioners*. 2001, pp. 22–24.

Schott HC, 2nd. Pituitary pars intermedia dysfunction: Equine Cushing's disease. *Vet Clin North Am Equine Pract* 2002a;18(2):237–270.

Schott HC, 2nd. Pituitary pars intermedia dysfunction: Equine Cushing's disease. In: Robinson, NE, ed. *Current Therapy in Equine Medicine*, 5th edn. Philadelphia: Saunders, 2002b, pp. 807–811.

Schott HC, 2nd. Pituitary pars intermedia dysfunction: challenges of diagnosis and treatment. In: *52nd Annual Convention of the American Association of Equine Practitioners*. San Antonio, Texas. Ithaca: International Veterinary Information Service (www.ivis.org); Document No. P5308.1206, 2006.

Toribio RE. Pars intermedia dysfunction (equine Cushing's disease). In: Reed SM, Bayly WM, Sellon DC, eds. *Equine Internal Medicine*, 2nd edn. Philadelphia: Saunders, 2004, pp. 1327–1337.

Toribio RE. Adrenal glands. In: Reed SM, Bayly WM, Sellon DC, eds. *Equine Internal Medicine*, 3rd edn. St Louis: Saunders, 2010, pp. 1248–1251.

van der Kolk JH, Ijzer J, Overgaauw PA, et al. Pituitary-independent Cushing's syndrome in a horse. *Equine Vet J* 2001;33(1):110–112.

van der Kolk JH, Kalsbeek HC, van Garderen E, et al. Equine pituitary neoplasia: A clinical report of 21 cases (1990–1992). *Vet Rec* 1993;133(24):594–597.

Wilson MG, Nicholson WE, Holscher MA, et al. Proopiolipomelanocortin peptides in normal pituitary, pituitary tumor, and plasma of normal and Cushing's horses. *Endocrinology* 1982;110(3):941–954.

CHAPTER 12

Primary Hyperaldosteronism

Andrea M. Harvey and Kent R. Refsal

Hyperaldosteronism

Pathogenesis

- Primary hyperaldosteronism is most commonly due to a aldosterone-secreting adrenal neoplasm (adenoma or carcinoma).
- Usually unilateral neoplasia, but can be bilateral.
- Bilateral adrenal hyperplasia has been described but fewer reports to date.

Classical Signs

- Middle-aged to older cats and dogs, no breed or sex predispositions.
- Hypokalemic polymyopathy.
- Hypertensive retinopathy/sudden onset blindness in cats.
- Clinical signs similar to hyperadrenocorticism in dogs if tumor is also secreting glucocorticoids.

Diagnosis

- Elevated plasma aldosterone concentration.
- Exclusion of diseases associated with secondary hyperaldosteronism and/or low/normal plasma renin activity and/or high aldosterone:renin ratio.
- Presence of adrenal mass (in the case of neoplasia).
- Adrenal tumors may secrete excess of multiple corticosteroids; elevated concentrations of other hormones may be documented.

Treatment

- Antihypertensive treatment (amlodipine besylate).
- Potassium supplementation.
- Spironolactone (aldosterone antagonist).
- Adrenalectomy for unilateral adrenal neoplasia is the preferred treatment.

Clinical Endocrinology of Companion Animals, First Edition. Edited by Jacquie Rand.
© 2013 John Wiley & Sons, Inc. Published 2013 by John Wiley & Sons, Inc.

I. Pathogenesis

A. **Hyperaldosteronism results from increased secretion of aldosterone from the adrenal glands** and may be of primary or secondary etiology:

    1. **Primary hyperaldosteronism (PHA)** occurs when there is an inappropriate increase in aldosterone secretion, independent of the renin–angiotensin–aldosterone system (RAAS). It was first reported in 1983 in a cat with an adrenocortical carcinoma. Since 1999, it has been reported in 35 more cats and 9 dogs; PHA is increasingly recognized as a cause of hypokalemia and/or hypertension, especially in cats.

    2. **Secondary hyperaldosteronism** occurs as a response to stimulation of the RAAS and, therefore, may occur as a compensatory response to counteract dehydration, hypotension, reduced renal perfusion (most commonly secondary to renal disease), or sodium deficiency (reduced intake or increased loss).

B. **The RAAS** acts to maintain the volume of extracellular fluid, circulatory pressure, and electrolyte homeostasis:

    1. Active release of renin is stimulated predominantly by decreased renal perfusion, detected by baroreceptors in the afferent arterioles.

    2. In the circulation, renin acts on angiotensinogen, to form angiotensin I, which is then converted to angiotensin II by angiotensin-converting enzyme.

    3. Angiotensin II has potent biological effects, mediating vasoconstriction, promoting renal tubular sodium reabsorption, stimulating aldosterone release from the adrenal cortex, and exerting negative feedback on renin release.

C. **Aldosterone** is synthesized from cholesterol through a series of intermediary metabolites including progesterone, 11-deoxycorticosterone, and corticosterone in the zona glomerulosa of the adrenal cortex. In the kidneys, aldosterone acts on the distal collecting tubules and collecting ducts, promoting sodium reabsorption with concurrent loss of potassium and hydrogen ions.

D. **Stimulation of the RAAS, therefore, results in an increased circulatory pressure via vasoconstriction and sodium retention, with subsequent loss of potassium and hydrogen ions.**

E. **PHA is most commonly caused by adrenal neoplasia:**

    1. **Unilateral adrenocortical adenoma or carcinoma** occurs with approximately equal frequency in cats. Adrenocortical carcinomas appear to predominate in dogs. Metastases from adrenal carcinomas have been reported in both cats and dogs.

    2. **Bilateral adrenal adenomas** have also been recognized in two cats. Another cat was reported to have developed a right adrenal carcinoma 2 years after a left adrenal adenoma was surgically removed.

    3. **Adrenal tumors may produce excesses of multiple corticosteroids:**

        a. **Concurrent hyperaldosteronism and hyperprogesteronism** has been described with adrenal neoplasia in two cats, and one of the authors (AH) has observed a few similar cases. The affected cats also had diabetes mellitus and dermatologic changes, both attributed to progesterone excess.

        b. Elevations of both aldosterone and corticosterone associated with adrenal tumors have been reported in two dogs, where the clinical signs raised initial suspicion for hyperadrenocorticism.

    4. **Concurrent elevations of aldosterone, progesterone, and corticosterone may be more common in cats than previously recognized.** A recent laboratory survey of feline sera submitted for assay of aldosterone identified elevations of progesterone of potential clinical significance in almost half of the samples where baseline aldosterone exceeded 3000 pmol/L.

    5. **A pathologic mineralocorticoid excess can occur even when there are low concentrations of aldosterone.** Case reports of people and one dog have identified adrenal tumors where mineralocorticoid steroidogenesis did not advance beyond production of **11-deoxycorticosterone**. This intermediate metabolite of steroidogenesis exerts mineralocorticoid bioactivity and, thus, signs identical to PHA when produced in excess.

F. **Nontumorous hyperaldosteronism (idiopathic adrenal hyperplasia)** has been described in a series of 11 cats and in 1 dog:

    1. Affected animals have clinical signs consistent with mineralocorticoid excess despite normal or mildly elevated baseline concentrations of aldosterone.

    2. Hyperplasia of the zona glomerulosa was the lesion described when the opportunity for histopathologic examination was made available.

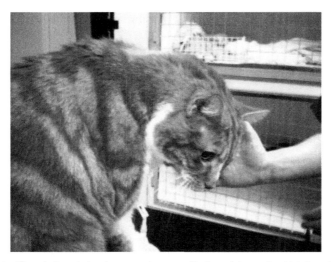

Figure 12.1 The cat was significantly hypokalemic—note the ventroflexion of the neck which is a classic presentation of hypokalemic polymyopathy. The cat was unable to lift his head. (Photo courtesy of Dr Séverine Tasker of The Feline Centre, Langford Veterinary Services, University of Bristol.)

II. Signalment

A. **Middle-aged to older cats and dogs:**
   1. Reported ages of onset range from 5 to 20 years, with an average of 11 years for cases of adrenal neoplasia.
   2. Age of onset for cases of adrenal hyperplasia appears similar, with ages ranging from 11 to 18 years in the reported feline cases. An 8-year-old Yorkshire terrier is the single dog reported with this condition.
B. **No breed predispositions noted:**
   1. Most reported cases have been domestic shorthair cats, with one each of domestic longhair, Siamese, Burmese, and Burmilla being diagnosed with adrenal neoplasia.
   2. Adrenal tumors causing hyperaldosteronism have been reported in a German shorthaired pointer, Doberman pinscher, beagle, and mixed breed dogs.
C. **No sex predisposition exists;** almost all reported cases have been neutered, with roughly equal proportions of female and male for both cats and dogs.

III. Clinical Signs

A. The major clinical signs are similar, whether PHA results from adrenal adenoma, carcinoma, or hyperplasia.
B. **Most commonly,** the major initial presenting signs relate directly to **increased aldosterone concentrations** and can be divided broadly into **two main groups:**
   1. **Hypokalemic polymyopathy:**
      a. **Most common presentation for adrenal neoplasia** cases. Cervical ventroflexion is most frequently reported (Figure 12.1), but hind limb weakness and ataxia, or, less commonly, limb stiffness, dysphagia, and collapse may also be seen. Clinical signs associated with myopathy may be mild and episodic or severe and acute in onset.
      b. Hypokalemic polymyopathy is a less common major presenting sign for adrenal hyperplasia cases (3 of 11 reported feline cases).
   2. **Retinopathy associated with hypertension in cats:**
      a. Intraocular hemorrhage or acute onset blindness resulting from retinal detachment (Figure 12.2a, b) due to hypertension is less commonly the main presenting sign in cases of adrenal neoplasia (2 of 36 reported cats). However, subclinical hypertension is common in cats and has been reported in dogs with aldosterone-secreting adrenal neoplasia.
      b. Hypertensive retinopathy appears to be a **more common major presenting sign in cases of adrenal hyperplasia** (7 of 11 reported cats). Overall, hypertension appears to be more severe in this group of cats; systolic blood pressure was above 185 mm Hg in all 11 reported cases and was > 200 mm Hg in 6/11 cats.

(a)   (b)

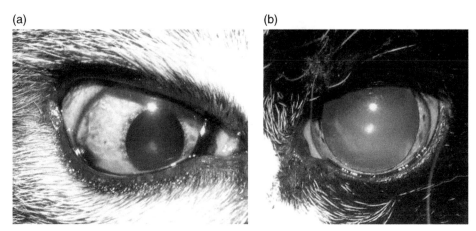

Figure 12.2   (a) Iridal hemorrhage in a cat with systemic hypertension. (b) Retinal detachment in a cat with systemic hypertension. The cat presented with sudden onset blindness. Note that the retinal blood vessels are clearly visible, a typical appearance with retinal detachment. (Photos courtesy of Tim Knott, Rowe Veterinary Group, UK.)

C. **Clinical signs related to glucocorticoid/progestin excess:**
   1. **Hyperadrenocorticism in dogs**—In addition to signs of muscle weakness, dogs with hyperaldosteronism will often display polyuria, polydipsia, and a potbellied appearance. The attending clinician may initially suspect hyperadrenocorticism.
   2. **Hyperprogesteronism in cats:**
      a. There are two detailed case reports of cats with aldosterone-secreting adrenal tumors that have had concurrent hyperprogesteronism, and the authors have also encountered a few cats with concurrent hyperaldosteronism and hyperprogesteronism that presented similarly to the reported cases.
      b. **Signs of hyperprogesteronism usually predominate,** resulting in very similar clinical signs to those encountered with hypercortisolemia, namely **secondary diabetes mellitus, polyuria, polydipsia, polyphagia, poor coat condition, seborrhea, thin fragile skin, and a potbellied appearance** (Figure 12.3a, b). Elevated serum progesterone concentrations may contribute to muscle weakness, which may be attributed initially to hypokalemic polymyopathy. Clinical signs of hypertension also may be present.
D. **Less common clinical signs:**
   1. **Other possible clinical signs associated with hypertension** may include neurological signs such as seizures, ataxia, and behavioral changes as a result of central nervous edema, hemorrhage, or ischemia.
   2. **Polyuria and polydipsia** in 15% of cats with aldosterone-secreting adrenal neoplasia.
   3. **Polyphagia** in 10% of cats with aldosterone-secreting adrenal neoplasia. Adrenocortical cortisol secretion was normal, but other hormones were not assessed. Therefore, whether the polyphagia is due to the hyperaldosteronemia or to an excess of a different hormone is unknown.
E. **Clinical signs related to renal disease:**
   1. In the cats with nontumorous hyperaldosteronism (i.e., adrenal hyperplasia), laboratory evidence of progressive renal disease is common.
   2. Three of 11 cats underwent necropsy confirming bilateral adrenal hyperplasia along with **histopathological renal changes consisting of hyaline arteriolar sclerosis, glomerular sclerosis, tubular atrophy, and interstitial fibrosis.** Such changes are classically recognized in humans with bilateral adrenal hyperplasia, suggesting the renal disease is a consequence of hyperaldosteronism. Clinical signs related to progressive renal disease may, therefore, develop in cats with adrenal hyperplasia.
F. **Clinical signs related to concomitant illness:**
   1. **Cats with PHA can be older, so concurrent disease may be present** which may divert attention from the possibility of hyperaldosteronism, for example, concomitant chronic kidney disease or hyperthyroidism may be assumed wrongly to be the sole cause of hypokalemia and/or hypertension.

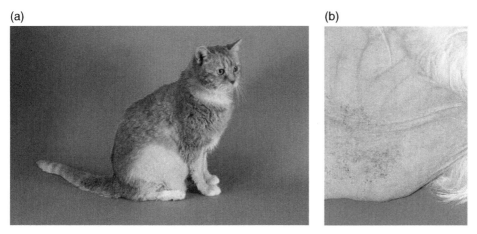

Figure 12.3   Both cats were diagnosed with concurrent hyperaldosteronism and hyperprogesteronism due to unilateral adrenal carcinomas. (a) This cat's initial presenting problems were progressive symmetrical alopecia, seborrhea oleosa, and abdominal distension. With time, diabetes mellitus, polyphagia, failure of hair regrowth, and hind limb weakness developed. (b) Note the very thin skin and prominent cutaneous blood vessels commonly seen in cases of hyperprogesteronism. (Photos courtesy of Langford Veterinary Services, Bristol, UK.)

2. The presence of left ventricular hypertrophy, systolic heart murmur, tachycardia, gallop rhythm, or dysrhythmias strongly suggest the presence of cardiomyopathy which may be secondary to hypertension and/or concurrent disease such as hyperthyroidism. Cardiac disease associated solely with PHA has not been described in cats but may be possible due to cardiac effects of aldosterone. If a patient in congestive heart failure has an elevated plasma aldosterone concentration, however, secondary hyperaldosteronism should be the primary consideration.

3. Multiple endocrine neoplasia type 1 has been reported in one cat with an aldosterone-producing adenoma and concurrent insulinoma and functional parathyroid adenoma.

IV. Diagnosis—Laboratory Assessment and Diagnostic Imaging
A. **Hematological and biochemical features:**
   1. No specific hematological abnormalities have been identified for PHA.
   2. On serum biochemistry, **hypokalemia** is most often present; **however, the degree is variable:**
      a. Hypokalemia, especially in cats, is identified for many other reasons and other causes should be excluded first.
      b. Persistence of hypokalemia despite supplementation with potassium is a common factor that prompts suspicion of hyperaldosteronism.
      c. **Most reported cases of PHA due to adrenal neoplasia were moderately to severely hypokalemic;** however, this could, in part, reflect the fact that persistent hypokalemia may be considered a prerequisite before hyperaldosteronism is considered as a differential diagnosis.
      d. In the described cases of **adrenal hyperplasia, hypokalemia was much less common and usually only mild.**
      e. The presence of only mild hypokalemia or **normokalemia does not, therefore, exclude the possibility of PHA.** It should be considered as a differential diagnosis for hypertension even in the absence of hypokalemia.
      f. **Serum sodium concentrations usually are normal.** Hypernatremia has been reported only in three cats with PHA and, in all cases, was mild. The lack of significant hypernatremia may be explained by concurrent volume expansion secondary to sodium retention.
      f. **Creatine kinase usually is elevated in cats with polymyopathy,** with the degree of elevation also highly variable.

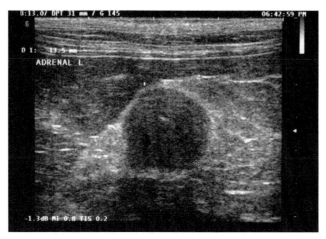

Figure 12.4   Ultrasound image illustrating the typical hypoechoic appearance of an adrenal mass of the right adrenal gland. (The left adrenal gland is also visible.) The histopathology was consistent with an adrenal adenoma. A unilateral adrenalectomy was successful in managing the case. (Image Langford Veterinary Services, Bristol, UK.)

    f. **Metabolic alkalosis is often present,** likely related to aldosterone-mediated excretion of hydrogen ions.

    g. **Blood urea nitrogen and serum creatinine concentrations may be elevated** at the time of diagnosis, and progression of renal disease may be the cause of death in some cases:

        1) The presence of azotemia may hinder the diagnosis of PHA in some cases, because the presence of hypokalemia and/or hypertension may be considered a consequence of primary renal disease.

        2) **Progressive renal disease is likely to occur as a sequela of uncontrolled PHA** (particularly due to adrenal hyperplasia) with renal damage occurring because of a combination of elevated intraglomerular capillary pressure, inflammation, and fibrosis, which are a direct effect of angiotensin II and chronic hypokalemia. Until there is routine access to a plasma renin activity assay or clinical validation of a mineralocorticoid suppression test in veterinary medicine, **differentiation of primary renal disease (with or without secondary hyperaldosteronism), from PHA with secondary renal disease, will pose a diagnostic challenge** for clinicians.

B. **Diagnostic imaging:**

  1. **Radiography:**

    a. **Adrenal masses are rarely visible radiographically,** but if the mass is large enough to be seen on radiographs, it is more likely to be an adrenocortical carcinoma than an adenoma. Presence of adrenal calcification is not necessarily significant as up to approximately 33% of normal older cats can have adrenal calcification.

    b. Pulmonary metastases can occur, albeit infrequently; therefore, thoracic radiographs to screen for metastases should be performed prior to consideration of surgery.

  2. **Ultrasonography:**

    a. **Currently ultrasonography is the best described imaging modality for detecting adrenal masses in dogs and cats.**

    b. In all reported feline cases of PHA in which adrenal ultrasonography has been performed, **unilateral adrenal enlargement with evidence of an adrenal mass** has been identified, ranging from 10 to 46 mm in diameter in cats and larger in dogs (Figure 12.4).

    c. The contralateral adrenal gland may appear normal in appearance or may be unidentifiable. It is **vital that the contralateral gland be assessed,** because bilateral adrenal neoplasia has also been reported.

    d. Ultrasonography should also attempt to identify the **presence and extent of invasion of the caudal vena cava** by the tumor or related thrombus and the presence of metastases to other organs. A close association of the tumor with the caudal vena cava usually is evident.

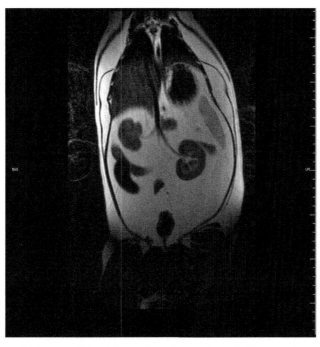

Figure 12.5　T_2-weighted sagittal MRI scan of the abdomen from the cat shown in Figure 12.4, demonstrating the significantly enlarged right adrenal gland in comparison to the left. Note the slight compression but no evidence of invasion into the caudal vena cava. (Image Langford Veterinary Services, Bristol, UK.)

    e. With **adrenal hyperplasia, subtle abnormalities** such as an increase in adrenal echogenicity or areas of calcification and thickening and/or rounding of one pole of one or both adrenal glands may be present. However, **in some cases, there are no visible changes.**

  3. Advanced imaging:

    a. Other imaging modalities, including magnetic resonance imaging (MRI), computed tomography (CT), and saphenous venography, have been reported in a small number of cases in an attempt to establish the extent of the adrenal mass before undertaking surgery (Figure 12.5).

    b. Due to the small number of cases of aldosterone-secreting tumors in which these modalities have been utilized, their benefit for affected patients is unclear. However, as such studies are useful for preoperative planning for other types of adrenal tumors, their performance should be considered in cases of hyperaldosteronism as well.

C. Endocrine assays:

  1. Plasma Aldosterone Concentration (aldosterone):

    a. **Confirming the diagnosis relies mainly on demonstration of an elevated aldosterone concentration.**

    b. The assay is widely available at commercial endocrine laboratories and requirements for collection and handling of serum or plasma are routine. There is no evidence of diagnostic benefit in performing an ACTH stimulation test for aldosterone measurement.

    c. **Aldosterone has been elevated in all reported cases of feline PHA associated with adrenal neoplasia.** Mineralocorticoid excess has been reported in a dog with an adrenocortical carcinoma due to a hormone other than aldosterone, that is, 11-deoxycorticosterone.

    d. There is wide variation in aldosterone concentration in normal animals and those with secondary hyperaldosteronism. Therefore, results must be assessed relative to clinical signs. Demonstration of **elevated aldosterone concentration alone does not distinguish between primary and secondary hyperaldosteronism.**

    e. Histopathological confirmation of the neoplasm together with resolution of clinical signs and normalization of aldosterone postoperatively assist in confirming the diagnosis in adrenal neoplasia cases.

f. In cases of early PHA, and particularly in bilateral adrenal hyperplasia cases, aldosterone **can be within the upper end of reference range at initial presentation.**

g. **Ideally, aldosterone should be interpreted together with plasma renin activity,** which would be expected to be elevated in cases of secondary hyperaldosteronism and low or normal in cases of PHA.

2. Plasma renin activity:

a. **Reliably distinguishing primary from secondary hyperaldosteronism requires assessment of activity of the renin–angiotensin system,** which is most commonly done by measuring plasma renin activity.

b. **Measuring plasma renin activity is problematic.** The assay is not widely commercially available for veterinary application. Plasma samples must be processed quickly and kept frozen until assay to avoid falsely decreased results. **Falsely elevated plasma renin activity** results can occur from the use of **some drugs** (e.g., angiotensin-converting enzyme inhibitors and β-blockers). Dietary salt intake also may influence plasma renin activity.

c. Plasma renin activity in cats with PHA due to adrenal neoplasia have been low or normal, so normal renin activity does not exclude the possibility of hyperaldosteronism caused by an adrenal tumor.

3. Aldosterone:renin activity ratio:

a. The aldosterone:renin activity ratio is the most reliable screening test for PHA in human medicine, with a high ratio being indicative of the diagnosis.

b. Use of the ratio has assisted in the diagnosis of the 11 reported cases of nontumorous PHA. The cats had high-normal to increased aldosterone and low-normal or decreased plasma renin activity at presentation. Elevation of the aldosterone:renin activity ratio was the evidence for inappropriate excess of aldosterone secretion.

c. **Nontumorous PHA is more difficult to diagnose without assessment of plasma renin activity** and aldosterone:renin activity ratio. Potential causes of **secondary hyperaldosteronism** should be excluded with appropriate testing including investigation for **renal, liver, and cardiac disease.** However, given that nontumorous PHA can cause progressive renal disease, distinguishing between PHA and secondary hyperaldosteronism in an azotemic patient is problematic without assessing plasma renin activity.

4. Mineralocorticoid function tests:

a. In human medicine, **mineralocorticoid function tests** are used as confirmatory tests for PHA, as false positive results can arise using the aldosterone:renin activity ratio alone.

b. **Mineralocorticoid function tests** assess the response to treatments designed to suppress the RAAS (e.g., oral sodium loading, saline infusion, fludrocortisone administration with sodium supplementation, and the captopril challenge test).

5. Mineralocorticoid function tests are being investigated for use in cats:

a. Preliminary studies showed that administration of enalapril for 5 days or increased dietary sodium intake did not suppress production of aldosterone in healthy cats.

b. Administration of fludrocortisone acetate (0.05 mg/kg) for 4 days decreased the urinary aldosterone:creatinine ratio in healthy cats.

6. Measurement of other steroid hormones:

a. Assessment of progesterone, corticosterone, and cortisol responses to ACTH stimulation and dexamethasone suppression testing may be warranted if clinical signs raise concern for glucocorticoid excess.

b. In case reports to date, cats with hyperaldosteronism and hyperprogesteronism and a dog with increased corticosterone related to an adrenocortical tumor have had normal to low baseline concentrations of cortisol with subnormal responses to ACTH-stimulation.

c. Assays for aldosterone, cortisol, or progesterone are readily available at veterinary diagnostic laboratories. Assays for corticosterone or 11-deoxycorticosterone may have to be arranged in specialty laboratories that perform steroid assays for characterization of congenital adrenal hyperplasia in humans.

7. **Due to the current difficulty in measuring plasma renin activity and lack of a defined mineralocorticoid suppression test in cats, two different diagnostic algorithms are suggested.** Both are based initially on identification of appropriate clinical signs and documentation of an elevated aldosterone, and then one is further based on the ideal situation where aldosterone:renin activity ratio and/or **mineralocorticoid function tests** are available (Figure 12.6a); the other is an alternative algorithm which can be used when

there is a lack of available aldosterone:renin activity ratio and/or **mineralocorticoid function tests** (Figure 12.6b).

V. Differential Diagnoses
A. **Hypokalemia:**
  1. **Reduced intake** (e.g., anorexia, IV fluids containing inadequate potassium).
  2. **Increased loss:**
    a. Gastrointestinal loss (e.g., vomiting and diarrhea).
    b. Urinary loss (e.g., renal disease, diuresis, diabetic ketoacidosis and PHA).
  3. **Intracellular translocation** (e.g., metabolic alkalosis, hyperthyroidism, insulin therapy, and Burmese hypokalemic polymyopathy).
B. **Hypertension:**
  1. Renal disease.
  2. Hyperthyroidism.
  3. PHA.
  4. Pheochromocytoma.
  5. Other diseases that are associated with hypertension in humans and may be associated with hypertension in cats but have not yet been identified as a cause of feline hypertension include obesity, diabetes mellitus, and hyperadrenocorticism.

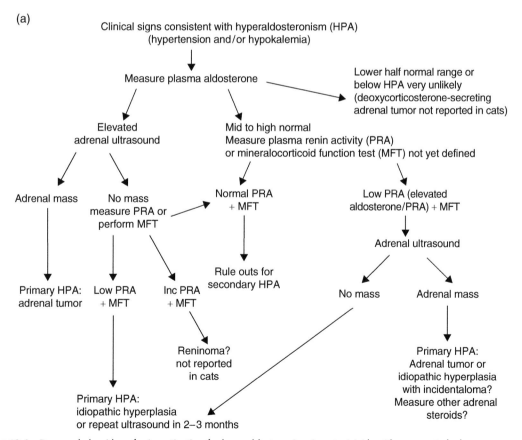

Figure 12.6 Proposed algorithms for investigation for hyperaldosteronism in cats. (a) Algorithm suggested when measurement of plasma renin activity/mineralocorticoid function tests available.

(b)

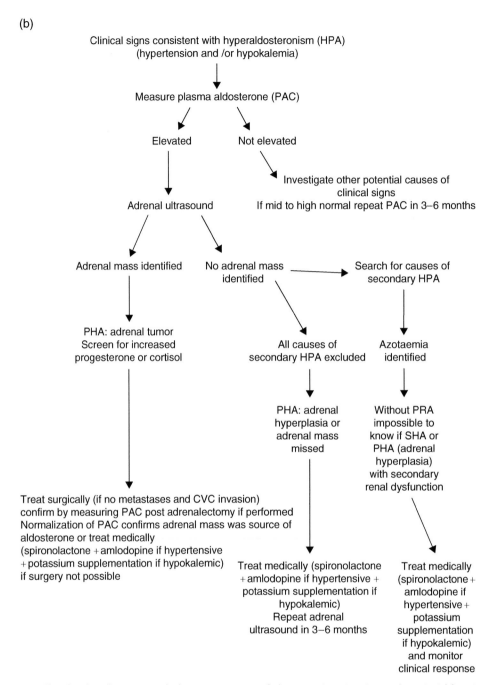

Clinical signs consistent with hyperaldosteronism (HPA)
(hypertension and /or hypokalemia)

Measure plasma aldosterone (PAC)

Elevated   Not elevated

Investigate other potential causes of
clinical signs
If mid to high normal repeat PAC in 3–6 months

Adrenal ultrasound

Adrenal mass identified   No adrenal mass   Search for causes of
                                 identified   secondary HPA

PHA: adrenal tumor
Screen for increased   All causes of   Azotaemia
progesterone or cortisol   secondary HPA excluded   identified

                                PHA: adrenal   Without PRA
                                hyperplasia or   impossible to
                                adrenal mass   know if SHA or
                                missed   PHA (adrenal
                                                       hyperplasia)
                                                       with secondary
                                                       renal dysfunction

Treat surgically (if no metastases and CVC invasion)
confirm by measuring PAC post adrenalectomy if performed
Normalization of PAC confirms adrenal mass was source of
aldosterone or treat medically
(spironolactone + amlodopine if hypertensive
+ potassium supplementation if hypokalemic)   Treat medically (spironolactone   Treat medically
if surgery not possible   + amlodopine if hypertensive +   (spironolactone +
                                                   potassium supplementation if   amlodopine if
                                                   hypokalemic)   hypertensive +
                                                   Repeat adrenal   potassium
                                                   ultrasound in 3–6 months   supplementation
                                                                                        if hypokalemic)
                                                                                        and monitor
                                                                                        clinical response

Figure 12.6 (cont'd)   (b) Algorithm suggested when measurement of plasma renin activity/mineralocorticoid function tests not available. (Reproduced from Refsal KR, Harvey AM. *Consultations in Feline Internal Medicine*, Chapter 24, Volume 6. St Louis, MO: Saunders Elsevier, Figure 24.9 A and B, 2010, p. 262. With permission.)

C. **Adrenal mass:**
1. Functional neoplasm (adenoma or carcinoma):
   a. Adrenal cortex: may secrete aldosterone, progesterone, cortisol, corticosterone, testosterone, or other corticosteroids.
   b. Adrenal medulla: may secrete epinephrine/norepinephrine.
2. Nonfunctional neoplasm (e.g., incidentaloma and metastatic neoplasm).
3. Benign mass, for example, hematoma and abscess.

D. **The most important differential diagnoses for both hypertension and hypokalemia occurring together are renal disease and PHA. As progressive renal disease can occur as a consequence of PHA, all patients with significant hypertension and/or hypokalemia should be assessed for the possibility of PHA.**

VI. Treatment

A. **Medical management:**
1. Initial treatment of PHA is directed at **controlling hypokalemia and/or hypertension.**
2. **Treatment of hypokalemia:**
   a. Potassium supplementation has been effective using potassium gluconate at doses of 2–6 mEq PO q 12 h in cats.
   b. In three dogs (30–45 kg body weight) with mineralocorticoid excess related to adrenocortical neoplasia, the daily amount of oral potassium supplementation ranged from 8 to 60 mEq.
   c. Intravenous potassium chloride-supplemented fluids may be required in more severely hypokalemic cases.
3. **Treatment of hypertension:**
   a. **Amlodipine besylate** (0.625–1.25 mg/cat PO q 24 h) is the initial treatment of choice for hypertension due to hyperaldosteronemia in cats. Most hypertensive cats become normotensive with amlodipine treatment, but higher doses sometimes are required. Hypertension can become refractory to treatment.
   b. The best therapy in affected dogs is unknown.
4. **Antagonism of aldosterone:**
   a. **Spironolactone**, a competitive aldosterone receptor antagonist, is also recommended (2–4 mg/kg PO q 24 h for cats or dogs), assisting in the control of both hypokalemia and hypertension.
   b. Severe facial dermatitis in Maine coon cats was reported as a potential side effect of spironolactone.
5. Treatment of concurrent excess of other steroids:
   a. Effective medical management has not yet been described in cats. Use of aminoglutethimide has been reported for preoperative stabilization in one cat but was of questionable benefit. One author (AH) has used trilostane in one cat, but it was not successful in suppressing progesterone concentrations. However, trilostane remains the best therapeutic option and further data are needed.
   b. Administration of mitotane achieved suppression of aldosterone, cortisol, and corticosterone in a dog with an adrenal mass, but the onset of dermatologic and neurologic signs resulted in euthanasia by day 129 after diagnosis.
   c. Current experience with medical management of adrenal tumors that secrete excesses of other corticosteroids in addition to aldosterone is very limited. General principles regarding use and monitoring of multiple therapeutic agents would be the same for cats and dogs. A course of such medical management could also be employed to improve the condition of the animal in preparation for adrenalectomy.

B. **Surgical management:**
1. **Unilateral adrenalectomy** is a potentially curative treatment for unilateral adrenal masses and is the preferred therapy; however, it is a high risk procedure and should be performed only by a skilled surgeon where intensive care facilities are available:
   a. **High perioperative mortality;** approximately 33% (5/15 cats) of reported cats died intraoperatively or postoperatively, most commonly as a result of severe, acute hemorrhage from the caudal vena cava. **However, it should be noted that experience so far is limited, with surgery performed in a small number of cats.**

b. Patients should be stabilized medically prior to surgery and meticulous preoperative planning is required. A successful laparoscopic adrenalectomy has been described in a cat (Smith et al. 2012).

c. Complications of postoperative adrenal insufficiency have not been associated with excision of aldosterone-secreting tumors in cats; however, patients should be monitored for this. Postoperative hyperkalemia, requiring transient administration of fludrocortisone, has been occasionally encountered.

d. Cats or dogs with concurrent hyperprogesteronism or hypercortisolemia pose additional surgical risks, including wound dehiscence, sepsis, and thromboembolic disease and can have postoperative glucocorticoid deficiency.

VII. Prognosis

A. **Adrenal neoplasia:**

1. **The prognosis does not appear to be worse for cats with nonmetastatic carcinomas compared to those with adenomas.**

2. Medical management alone has been associated with nonmetastatic survival times of 7 months to 984 days, in four of five treated cats. The survival time in one cat receiving medical treatment alone was limited to 50 days, attributed to owner noncompliance. Cause of death is most commonly chronic kidney disease, thromboembolic disease, or refractory hypertension.

3. **Adrenalectomy** is associated with a good prognosis if the patient survives the immediate peri- and postoperative periods. Ten of fifteen adrenalectomized cats survived the postoperative period with 8 surviving at least a year; two cats were alive 3.5 and 5 years postoperatively. One of the authors (AH) has experienced successful management of concurrent hyperaldosteronism and hyperprogesteronism with adrenalectomy; however, follow-up times are currently still short.

B. **Nontumorous PHA.** There is a lack of available long-term follow-up data. Most cases would be expected to eventually succumb to renal disease but may be well managed medically with amlodipine and spironolactone for some time.

VIII. Prevention

No known prevention.

Hyperaldosteronism in Other Species

A. There is a single case report of PHA as a result of an adrenocortical adenoma in a 6-year-old neutered female domestic **ferret.**

B. **High concentrations of sex hormones** were also present.

C. Clinical signs began with lethargy, alopecia, and pruritus and progressed to include dyspnea and weakness. Hypertension and severe hypokalemia were noted, and an abdominal mass was palpated.

D. Hypertension and hypokalemia were effectively managed medically, as discussed for cats; however, continued dyspnea necessitated euthanasia 2 months postdiagnosis.

E. Concurrent cardiac disease causing pulmonary edema was identified at postmortem examination.

References and Further Readings

Ash RA, Harvey AM, Tasker S. Primary hyperaldosteronism in the cat: A series of 13 cases. *J Feline Med Surg* 2005;7:173.
Behrend EN, Weigand CM, Whitley EM, et al. Corticosterone- and aldosterone-secreting adrenocortical tumor in a dog. *J Am Vet Med Assoc* 2005;226:1662.
Breitschwerdt EB, Meuten DJ, Greenfield CL, Anson LW, Cook CS, Fulghum RE. Idiopathic hyperaldosteronism in a dog. *J Am Vet Med Assoc* 1985;187(8):841–845.
Briscoe K, Barrs VR, Foster DF, Beatty JA. Hyperaldosteronism and hyperprogesteronism in a cat. *J Feline Med Surg* 2009;11(9):758–762.
De Clue AE, Breshears LA, Pardo ID, et al. Hyperaldosteronism and hyperprogesteronism in a cat with an adrenal cortical carcinoma. *J Vet Intern Med* 2005;19:355.
Desmarchelier M, Lair S, Dunn M, Langlois I. Primary hyperaldosteronism in a domestic ferret with an adrenocortical adenoma. *J Am Vet Med Assoc* 2008;233(8):1297–1301.

Djajadiningrat-Laanen SC, Galac S, Cammelbeek SE, van Laar KJ, Boer P, Kooistra HS. Urinary aldosterone to creatinine ratios in cats before and after suppression with salt or fludrocortisone acetate. *J Vet Int Med* 2008;22(6):1283–1288.

Javadi S, Djajadiningrat-Laanen SC, Kooistra HS, et al. Primary hyperaldosteronism, a mediator of progressive renal disease in cats. *Domest Anim Endocrinol* 2005;28:85.

MacDonald KA, Kittelson MD, Kass PH. Effect of spironolactone on diastolic function and left ventricular mass in Maine coon cats with familial hypertrophic cardiomyopathy. *J Vet Int Med* 2008;22(2):335–341.

Machida T, Uchida E, Matsuda K, et al. Aldosterone-, corticosterone- and cortisol-secreting adrenocortical carcinoma in a dog: Case report. *J Vet Intern Med Sci* 2008;70:317.

MacKay AD, Holt PE, Sparkes AH. Successful surgical treatment of a cat with primary aldosteronism. *J Feline Med Surg* 1999;1:117.

Moore LE, Biller DS, Smith TA. Use of abdominal ultrasonography in the diagnosis of primary hyperaldosteronism in a cat. *J Am Vet Med Assoc* 2000;217:213.

Refsal KR, Harvey AM. Primary hyperaldosteronism. In: August JR, ed. *Consultations in Feline Internal Medicine*, Chapter 24. St Louis, MO: Saunders Elsevier, 2010, pp. 254–267.

Reine NJ, Hohenhaus AE, Peterson ME, et al. Deoxycorticosterone-secreting adrenocortical carcinoma in a dog. *J Vet Intern Med* 1999;13:386.

Rijnberk A, Kooistra HS, van Vonderen IK, Mol JA, Voorhout G, van Sluijs FJ, IJzer J, van den Ingh TS, Boer P, Boer WH. Aldosteronoma in a dog with polyuria as the leading symptom. *Domest Anim Endocrinol* 2001;20(3):227–240.

Shiel R, Mooney C. Diagnosis and management of primary hyperaldosteronism in cats. *In Pract* 2007;29:194.

Smith RR, Mayhew PD, Berent AC. Laparoscopic adrenalectomy for management of a functional adrenal tumor in a cat. *J Am Vet Med Assoc* 2012;241(3):368–372.

CHAPTER 13

Pheochromocytoma in Dogs

Claudia E. Reusch

Pathogenesis

- Catecholamine-producing tumor mostly from adrenal medulla, in rare cases from extra-adrenal chromaffin tissue.
- Slow growing, but potentially malignant.
- Clinical signs result from catecholamine excess or size/invasiveness of tumor.
- Catecholamine secretion from the tumor is highly unpredictable.

Classical Signs

- Highly variable, occur several times per day or reoccurrence after days, weeks, or months.
- Weakness and episodic collapse most frequent signs.
- Hypertension only in approximately 50% of dogs.

Diagnosis

- Very challenging due to vague clinical signs.
- Clinical diagnosis usually made on a combination of clinical suspicion, detection of an adrenal mass by ultrasonography, and, if available, increased urinary normetanephrine:creatinine ratio.
- Definitive diagnosis by histopathology.

Treatment

- Adrenalectomy.
- Preoperative medical management with phenoxybenzamine.

I. Pathogenesis

A. The **cells of the adrenal medulla are called pheochromocytes** or chromaffin cells. They can be regarded as modified postganglionic sympathetic neurons lacking axons. Innervation is by preganglionic fibers of the sympathetic nervous system which induce the release of catecholamines into the bloodstream. Some

Clinical Endocrinology of Companion Animals, First Edition. Edited by Jacquie Rand.
© 2013 John Wiley & Sons, Inc. Published 2013 by John Wiley & Sons, Inc.

extra-adrenal chromaffin tissue is also present adjacent to the aorta, in the carotid bodies, or viscera and within sympathetic ganglia.

B. Pheochromocytomas are **rare catecholamine-producing neuroendocrine tumors** which arise from the adrenal medulla in the vast majority of cases. **Occasionally, tumors derive from extra-adrenal chromaffin tissue and are referred to as paragangliomas:**

    1. **Pheochromocytomas are potentially malignant in dogs. Local invasion into the adjacent vessels and other tissues is seen in more than 50% of dogs** (based on necropsy results at the time of death); sites of metastasis are regional lymph nodes, spleen, liver, kidney, pancreas, lung, heart, bone, and CNS. In the case of a large tumor, **extraluminal compression of blood vessels is possible.**

    2. The tumors are **usually slow growing. Size is extremely variable** and ranges between a few millimeters to more than 10 cm in diameter at the time of diagnosis.

    3. **Most tumors are unilateral,** but in approximately 5–10% of cases both adrenal glands are affected. They **may coexist with cortisol-producing adrenocortical tumors, ACTH-producing pituitary tumors, or other endocrine tumors.**

    4. **Clinical signs are the result of catecholamine excess and/or rarely from the space-occupying or invasive nature of the tumor.**

C. Catecholamines are synthesized from the amino acid tyrosine and include dopamine, norepinephrine (noradrenaline) and epinephrine (adrenaline). They are stored within chromaffin cells until release. Plasma half-life of catecholamines is very short (1–3 min). They are metabolized into the inactive compounds normetanephrine and metanephrine (Figure 13.1):

    1. Catecholamines bind to α- and β-adrenergic receptors (respectively to their subtypes α_1, α_2, β_1, β_2, and β_3) and **induce "fright, fight, and flight" reactions.** Most importantly, they **increase heart rate and contractility, blood pressure, respiration rate;** relax the gastrointestinal tract and urinary bladder musculature; **and increase blood glucose, free fatty acids, and alertness (Table 13.1).**

    2. **In healthy dogs, the content of the adrenal medulla is approximately 30% norepinephrine and 70% epinephrine.** Both are stored within chromaffin cells and are secreted in response to exercise, danger, surgery, hypovolemia, hypotension and hypoglycemia, as well as many other stress-associated stimuli.

    3. **In dogs with pheochromocytoma, the proportion of the hormones may be different from that of normal dogs.** According to preliminary studies, the tumors may secrete more norepinephrine than epinephrine. **Hormone secretion may be constant or sporadic and is highly unpredictable.** The mechanism responsible for the release of catecholamines from a tumor is not well understood.

II. Signalment

A. The disease may occur at any age; however, it is **most commonly seen in older dogs (≥8 years).**

B. There is no apparent sex and breed predisposition.

III. Clinical Signs

A. The clinical presentation is **highly variable.**

B. Signs **may be apparent several times per day or may only reoccur after days, weeks, or months.** Severity of the disease ranges from dramatic and life threatening to very mild. **Some pheochromocytomas are hormonally silent.**

C. Due to their mostly paroxysmal appearance, **clinical signs are usually not evident at the time of physical examination.**

D. There does not seem to be a correlation between severity of clinical signs and tumor size.

E. **Clinical signs may be categorized as** (Table 13.2):

    1. **Nonspecific:** anorexia, weight loss, lethargy.

    2. **Related to the cardiorespiratory system and/or hypertension:** tachypnea, panting, tachycardia, cardiac arrhythmias (mainly tachyarrhythmias), collapse, pale mucous membranes, nasal, gingival, or ocular hemorrhage, and acute blindness due to retinal detachment.

    3. **Related to the neuromuscular system:** weakness, anxiety, pacing, muscle tremors, seizures.

    4. **Miscellaneous:** polyuria/polydipsia, vomiting, diarrhea, painful abdomen.

    5. **Related to large, malignant tumors:** abdominal distension, ascites, and hind-limb edema. Intraabdominal or retroperitoneal hemorrhage due to tumor rupture is also possible, but occurs rarely.

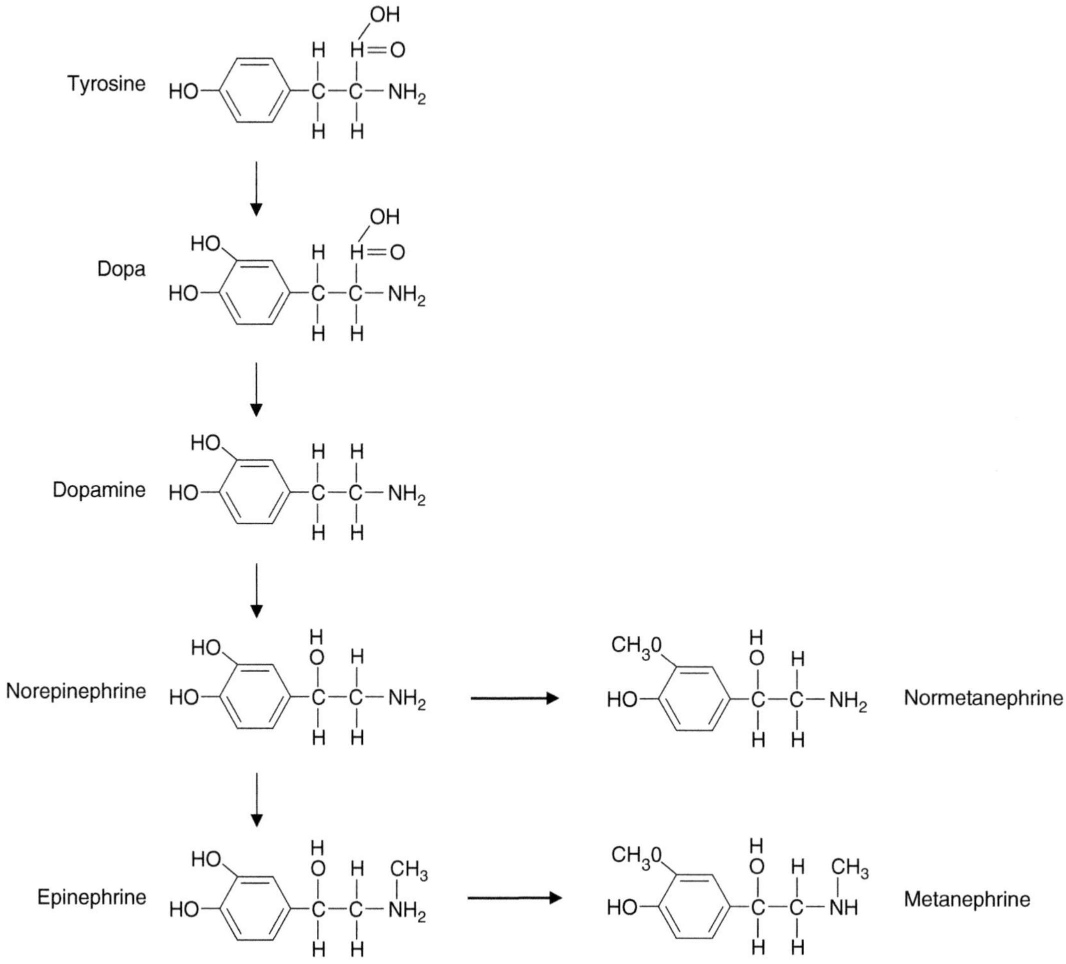

Figure 13.1 Biosynthesis and metabolism of catecholamines (simplified).

Table 13.1 Responses of selected tissues to catecholamines.

Organ/tissue	Receptor type	Effect
Cardiovascular system	β_1	Increase in heart rate, increase in contractility
	α_2	Vasoconstriction
	β_2	Vasodilation in skeletal muscle arterioles, coronary arteries, and all veins
Bronchial muscles	β_2	Relaxation
Gastrointestinal tract	α, β	Decrease in motility
Pancreatic islets	α	Decrease in insulin and glucagon secretion
	β	Increase in insulin and glucagon secretion
Liver	α, β	Increase in glycogenolysis and gluconeogenesis
Adipose tissue	β	Increase in lipolysis
Urinary bladder	α	Increase in sphincter tone
	β	Relaxation of M. detrusor

Table 13.2   Clinical signs in dogs with pheochromocytoma.

Categories	Clinical signs
Unspecific	Anorexia, weight loss, lethargy
Related to cardiorespiratory system and/or hypertension	Tachypnea, panting, tachycardia, arrhythmias, collapse,* pale mucus membranes, nasal-, gingival-, ocular hemorrhage, acute blindness
Related to neuromuscular system	Weakness,* anxiety, pacing, muscle tremor, seizures
Miscellaneous	PU/PD, vomiting, diarrhea, painful abdomen
Related to large, malignant tumor	Abdominal distension, ascites, hind-limb edema, intra-abdominal or retroperitoneal hemorrhage

* Most frequent signs.

F. The **most common signs are weakness and episodic collapse.**
G. **Other signs may be seen in metastatic disease, depending on the organ involved.** Ataxia and paresis have been described in dogs with metastasis in the vertebral canal.
H. Similar neurological signs (e.g., pain, ataxia, paresis, paralysis) may be seen if a paraganglioma metastasizes to the spinal cord.

IV. Diagnosis
A. Since clinical signs are vague, **diagnosis of pheochromocytoma is challenging.** Additional difficulties may arise from the fact that the frequency of concurrent disease is high (approximately 50%) and may affect diagnostic test results. **Clinical diagnosis usually is a combination of clinical suspicion, detection of an adrenal mass by ultrasonography, and, if available, demonstration of an increased urinary normetanephrine: creatinine ratio. Definitive diagnosis is by histopathology.**
B. Clinical pathology:
    1. There are **no consistent abnormalities** on complete blood count, serum biochemistry, and urinalysis.
    2. **Various findings are possible, none of which would raise specific suspicion of pheochromocytoma:** mild nonregenerative anemia, stress leukogram, mild thrombocytopenia or thrombocytosis, increased serum alkaline phosphatase or alanine aminotransferase activity, azotemia, hypoalbuminemia, mild hyperglycemia, hypercholesterolemia, proteinuria, hypoisosthenuria, or isosthenuria. **Laboratory results may also be completely normal.**
C. Blood pressure measurement (Table 13.3):
    1. **Hypertension is one of the hallmarks** of the disease. However, hypertension is **not pathognomonic** for pheochromocytoma and is also frequently found in hyperadrenocorticism, which is one of the most important differential diagnoses.
    2. Due to the episodic secretion of catecholamines, hypertension is only **present in approximately 50% of dogs at the time of examination. With repetitive measurements on consecutive days, hypertension may be picked up in a higher percentage of dogs.**
    3. Hypertension **varies from mild to severe.** "Typical" systolic measurements are between 200 and 240 mm Hg, the maximum systolic blood pressure reported so far is 325 mm Hg.
D. Diagnostic imaging:
    1. Radiography:
        a. **Abdominal radiographs are of limited value** for the workup of dogs with pheochromocytoma. Detection of a soft tissue mass in the area of the adrenal glands may be possible with large masses or masses which are calcified; the latter, however, is rare with pheochromocytomas.
        b. **Thoracic radiographs** are helpful to search for pulmonary metastasis.
    2. **Abdominal ultrasonography:**
        a. Ultrasonography has **major advantages over radiography** for adrenal imaging: higher resolution to visualize small masses, potential to detect retroperitoneal effusion and tumoral invasion into

Table 13.3   Blood pressure in dogs with pheochromocytoma.

No. of dogs with pheochromocytoma revealing hypertension (total no. of dogs with blood pressure measurements)	Measuring technique	Definition of systolic hypertension (mmHg)	Range of systolic blood pressure (mmHg)	Reference
1 (1)	Indirect, oscillometric Indirect, Doppler	Not given	200–240 200–240	Williams and Hackner (2001)
0 (1)	Indirect, Doppler	Not given	110	Whittemore et al. (2001)
1 (1)	Indirect, Doppler	Not given	240	Brown et al. (2007)
6 (7)	Indirect, Doppler	>160	164–325	Gilson et al. (1994)
10 (23)	Indirect, oscillometric	>160	135–214	Barthez et al. (1997)
3 (5)	Indirect, Doppler	>160	55–270	Kook et al. (in press)

surrounding vessels and tissues, and assessment of other abdominal organs for distant metastasis. Sensitivity is higher than radiography, but is not 100%.

b. The adrenal glands are **usually evaluated with a 7.5 MHz transducer**. There are a number of techniques for locating the adrenal glands with the patient either in dorsal or lateral recumbency. We prefer to image the left adrenal with the patient in dorsal recumbency and the right adrenal with the patient in left lateral recumbency.

c. Often pheochromocytoma is only considered as a diagnosis after an adrenal mass has been detected by ultrasonography.

d. Masses have a **wide range in size** (a few millimeters to more than 10 cm in diameter).

e. **Small masses can be embedded within the parenchyma so that the shape of the adrenal gland appears normal.** Detection requires high resolution of the ultrasound equipment and good operator skills. With larger masses, normal shape is lost.

f. **Masses may be hypoechoic, isoechoic, or hyperechoic to the adjacent renal cortex or have mixed echogenicity.** They may also contain anechoic, non-far-enhancing areas which represent foci of necrosis and hemorrhage (Figure 13.2).

g. **Mineralization is rare** in pheochromocytomas, in contrast to cortisol-producing masses.

h. **No pattern of echogenicity or architecture is specific for pheochromocytomas**, other adrenal masses, for example, cortisol-producing tumors, look similar.

i. **Invasion into surrounding vessels (most often into the caudal vena cava) with tumor thrombosis may be detectable**; color flow Doppler methodology may be helpful.

j. Tumors are **usually unilateral**, with the contralateral adrenal gland being of normal shape and size.

k. However, **exceptions occur**, such as bilateral pheochromocytomas, coexistence with other tumor types (e.g., cortisol-producing adrenal tumor) or with pituitary-dependent hyperadrenocorticism, rendering interpretation of ultrasonographic findings difficult.

3. **CT and MRI:**

a. Both modalities are **more sensitive than ultrasonography** for identifying adrenal masses and, in particular, characterizing the extent of local invasion. They may, therefore, be superior for determining if the mass is surgically resectable.

b. They also **do not allow a definitive diagnosis**, that is, discrimination between pheochromocytoma and other adrenal masses.

c. CT and MRI **require general anesthesia and the use of contrast media which may carry the risk of a hypertensive crisis and cardiac arrhythmias.**

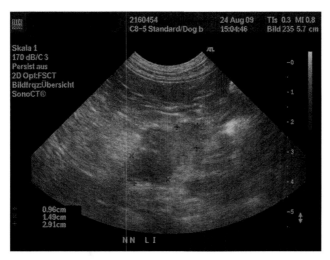

Figure 13.2   Ultrasonographic image of a pheochromocytoma in the left adrenal gland of an 11-year-old Cairn terrier. The shape of the mass is highly irregular with mixed echogenicity, size (longest dimensions) is approximately 2.9×1.5 cm. (Courtesy of the Unit of Diagnostic Imaging, Vetsuisse Faculty Zurich, Switzerland.)

4. Scintigraphy and positron emission tomography:
   a. Scintigraphy with ^{123}I-labeled metaiodobenzylguanidine (^{123}I-MIBG) and positron emission tomography with *p*- [^{18}F]fluorobenzylguanidine (p-[18 F]PFBG) take advantage of the fact that the radiopharmaceuticals have similar uptake mechanisms as norepinephrine and accumulate in the adrenal medulla.
   b. They may be more specific for the diagnosis of pheochromocytoma than the other imaging modalities and may aid in differentiating adrenal masses.
   c. However, sensitivity may be lower. The use of the techniques has so far only been described in a very small number of dogs.
   d. Scintigraphy may also be useful to detect bone metastasis at an earlier stage of the disease than radiography.
5. Fine needle aspiration and biopsy:
   a. **Nearly no information is available** on fine needle aspirate or biopsy of pheochromocytoma in dogs.
   b. **Potential risks associated with the aspiration/biopsy procedure itself are hemorrhage, arrhythmias, and hypertensive crisis.**
   c. Additionally, small samples may not always allow differentiation between cortical and medullary tumors nor between benign and malignant tumors.
6. Hormonal testing:
   a. **In humans**, diagnosis of pheochromocytoma is mainly based on biochemical detection of excessive amounts of catecholamines (epinephrine, norepinephrine) and their metabolites (metanephrine, normetanephrine) in urine collected over 24 h. Measurement of plasma metanephrines is a more recently available test:
      1. Both tests (urine and plasma) have **high sensitivity and specificity.**
      2. **False-negative results** may occur in patients with mild disease or with intermittent catecholamine secretion.
      3. **False-positive results** are possible with various diseases and drugs, for example, phenoxybenzamine, calcium channel blockers, metoclopramide, glucocorticoids, and β-blockers.
   b. **In dogs**, urinary catecholamine and metanephrine concentrations have only recently been evaluated:
      1. Dogs with pheochromocytoma have **significantly higher urinary ratios of epinephrine, norepinephrine, and normetanephrine:creatinine than healthy dogs.** The least overlap is seen with regard to the urinary normetanephrine:creatinine ratio (Figure 13.3).

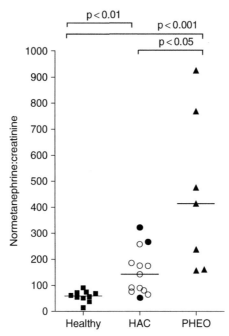

Figure 13.3 Urinary normetanephrine:creatinine ratios in healthy dogs (n=10), dogs with hyperadrenocorticism (HAC, *n*=13), and dogs with pheochromocytoma (PHEO, *n*=7). In the group of dogs with HAC open circles represent dogs with pituitary-dependent hyperadrenocorticism, closed circles dogs with cortisol-producing adrenal tumors.

2. When the ratios were compared between dogs with pheochromocytoma and dogs with hyperadrenocorticism (as one of the main differential diagnoses), only the urinary normetanephrine:creatinine ratio was significantly higher in dogs with pheochromocytoma (Figure 13.3).

3. A cutoff value of urinary normetanephrine:creatinine ratio of four times normal is associated with pheochromocytoma. However, lower values do not exclude the disease and repetitive testing may therefore be required.

4. Sample collection and urine processing have specific requirements such as need for sample acidification, protection from light, and cooled or frozen storage. Close collaboration with the laboratory is, therefore, necessary.

V. Differential Diagnoses

A. Since clinical signs are often vague and nonspecific and usually associated with more common diseases, pheochromocytoma is often not considered as a differential diagnosis.

B. **Depending on the clinical presentation, diseases of various organ systems have to be considered:**

1. Cardiovascular.
2. Respiratory.
3. Neuromuscular.
4. Metabolic/endocrine.

C. Due to the routine use of abdominal ultrasonography, the finding of an adrenal mass has become frequent. **Differential diagnoses for adrenal masses are:**

1. Hypersecretory tumors:
   a. Cortisol-producing (most frequent).
   b. Cortisol-precursor-producing, for example, 17-α-hydroxy-progesterone.
   c. Pheochromocytoma.
   d. Aldosteronoma (very rare in dogs).
2. Nonfunctional masses:
   a. Myelolipoma.
   b. Cyst.

      c. Abscess.
      d. Hematoma.
      e. Metastasis.

VI. Treatment

A. **Adrenalectomy is the treatment of choice** and should be performed as soon as possible:

  1. **Preoperative medical management:**

    a. Medical therapy with the noncompetitive α-adrenergic blocker **phenoxybenzamine should be started immediately after diagnosis and given for at least 1–2 weeks before surgery.**

    b. Phenoxybenzamine decreases perioperative mortality in dogs undergoing adrenalectomy for pheochromocytoma. Although the exact mechanism is unknown, the beneficial effects may be due to phenoxybenzamine's ability to block the effects of excessive adrenergic stimulation, that is, reverses vasoconstriction and hypovolemia.

    c. **Optimal dose of phenoxybenzamine has not been studied** in dogs. Currently, we start with 0.25 mg/kg BID and increase gradually every few days until a dosage of 1–2 mg/kg BID is reached. **Careful monitoring is required since some dogs may develop hypotension;** in those cases, the dosage of phenoxybenzamine should be decreased.

  2. **Anesthesia and surgery:**

    a. Surgical removal of a pheochromocytoma is a **high risk procedure and is technically demanding.** Therefore, it should only be done by a team of experienced surgeons and anesthetists in a facility in which intensive postoperative care is guaranteed.

    b. **Monitoring by EKG and systemic blood pressure measurement should be done during surgery and for 1–2 days thereafter.**

    c. **Potential life-threatening complications are common, in particular during induction of anesthesia and manipulation of the tumor.** They include severe tachycardia and various other types of cardiac arrhythmias, hypertension, hypotension, and hemorrhage. Those complications **may also occur postoperatively.**

B. **Medical management:**

  1. In some dogs, **adrenalectomy may not be an option** due to tumor size, extensive invasion into surrounding tissue, distant metastasis, serious concurrent disease, or owner constraints.

  2. Medical management may also be an option in dogs with recurrence of pheochromocytoma after surgery or in which tumor resection was incomplete.

  3. Treatment of choice is phenoxybenzamine. The aim is to control the effects of excessive catecholamine secretion; the drug does not have an effect on tumor growth or metastasis.

  4. Starting dosage of phenoxybenzamine is 0.25 mg/kg BID which is gradually increased until clinical signs are controlled, hypotension occurs, or a maximum dosage of 1 mg/kg BID is reached.

VII. Prognosis

A. Prognosis **depends on many factors** such as general condition of the patient, size and invasiveness of the tumor, experience of the surgeon and anesthetist, quality of postoperative care, and occurrence of perioperative complications.

B. In dogs that survive the perioperative period, survival for several years is possible.

C. Very little data are available for dogs which are only treated medically. Survival for more than a year has been seen in some cases.

VIII. Prevention

No known prevention.

References and Further Readings

Barthez PY, Marks SL, Woo J, et al. Pheochromocytoma in dogs: 61 cases (1984–1995). *J Vet Intern Med* 1997;11:272–278.
Berry CR, DeGrado TR, Nutter F, et al. Imaging of pheochromocytoma in 2 dogs using *p*-[^{18}F]Fluorobenzylguanidine. *Vet Radiol Ultrasound* 2002;43:183–186.

Berry CR, Wright KN, Breitschwerdt EB, et al. Use of [123]Iodine metaiodobenzylguanidine scintigraphy for the diagnosis of a pheochromocytoma in a dog. *Vet Radiol Ultrasound* 1993;34:52–55.

Besso JG, Penninck DG, Gliatto JM. Retrospective ultrasonographic evaluation of adrenal lesions in 26 dogs. *Vet Radiol Ultrasound* 1997;38:448–455.

Bouayad H, Feeeney DA, Caywood DD. Pheochromocytoma in dogs: 13 cases (1980–1985). *J Am Vet Med Assoc* 1987;191:1610–1615.

Brown S, Atkins C, Bagley R, et al. Guidelines for the identification, evaluation, and management of systemic hypertension in dogs and cats. *Journal of Veterinary Internal Medicine* 2007;21:542–558.

Gilson SD, Withrow SJ, Wheeler SL, et al. Pheochromocytoma in 50 dogs. *J Vet Intern Med* 1994;8:228–232.

Herrera MA, Mehl ML, Kass PH, et al. Predictive factors and the effect of phenoxybenzamine on outcome in dogs undergoing adrenalectomy for pheochromocytoma. *J Vet Intern Med* 2008;22:1333–1339.

Kook PH, Boretti FS, Hersberger M, et al. Urinary catecholamine and metanephrine to creatinine ratios in healthy dogs at home and in a hospital environment and in 2 dogs with pheochromocytoma. *J Vet Intern Med* 2007;21:388–393.

Kook PH, Grest P, Quante S, et al. Urinary catecholamine and metanephrine to creatinine ratios in 7 dogs with pheochromocytoma. *Vet Rec* 2010;166:169–174.

Platt SR, Sheppard BJ, Graham J, et al. Pheochromocytoma in the vertebral canal of two dogs. *J Am Anim Hosp Assoc* 1998;34:365–371.

Rizzo SA, Newman SJ, Hecht S, et al. Malignant mediastinal extra-adrenal paraganglioma with spinal cord invasion in a dog. *J Vet Diagn Invest* 2008;20:372–375.

Rosenstein DS. Diagnostic imaging in canine pheochromocytoma. *Vet Radiol Ultrasound* 2000;41:499–506.

Santamarina G, Espino L, Vila M, et al. Aortic thromboembolism and retroperitoneal hemorrhage associated with a pheochromocytoma in a dog. *J Vet Intern Med* 2003;17:917–922.

Von Dehn BJ, Nelson RW, Feldman EC, et al. Pheochromocytoma and hyperadrenocorticism in dogs: Six cases (1982–1992). *J Am Vet Med Assoc* 1995;207:322–324.

Whittemore JC, Preston CA, Kyles AE, et al. Nontraumatic rupture of an adrenal gland tumor causing intra-abdominal or retroperitoneal hemorrhage in four dogs. *J Am Vet Med Assoc* 2001;219:329–333.

Williams JE, Hackner SG. Pheochromocytoma presenting as acute retroperitoneal hemorrhage in a dog. *J Vet Emerg Crit Care* 2001;11:221–227.

CHAPTER 14

Pheochromocytoma in Cats

Danièlle Gunn-Moore and Kerry Simpson

Pathogenesis

- Functional tumor of the adrenal medullary chromaffin cells.

Classical Signs

- Highly variable; polyuria, polydipsia, aggression, agitation, hyphema, inappetence, lethargy, intermittent vomiting, tachypnea, and seizures.

Diagnosis

- Demonstration of a mass and increased catecholamines or their serum metabolites.

Treatment and Prognosis

- Surgical resection with or without therapy for hypertension and treatment of concurrent neoplasia.
- Outcome is highly variable.

I. Pathogenesis

A. The **adrenal medulla** contains **chromaffin cells** which are derived from the neuroectoderm and are able to **synthesize, store,** and secrete the catecholamines **epinephrine (adrenaline)** and **norepinephrine (noradrenaline):**
  1. In addition to the chromaffin cells within the adrenal medulla, there are occasional extra-adrenal chromaffin cells within and about the sympathetic ganglia.
B. **Pheochromocytoma are tumors of neuroectodermal origin that arise from the chromaffin cells within the adrenal medulla.** Occasionally, tumors of chromaffin cells may occur at distant locations; these **extra-adrenal pheochromocytomas are termed paragangliomas. Both pheochromocytomas and paragangliomas are rare in the cat.**
C. The chromaffin cells within the adrenal medulla are capable of amine precursor uptake and decarboxylation. Synthesis of epinephrine and norepinephrine commences with the hydroxylation of tyrosine by tyrosine hydroxylase, to form dihydroxyphenylalanine (DOPA), which is in turn converted to dopamine (Figure 14.1).

Clinical Endocrinology of Companion Animals, First Edition. Edited by Jacquie Rand.
© 2013 John Wiley & Sons, Inc. Published 2013 by John Wiley & Sons, Inc.

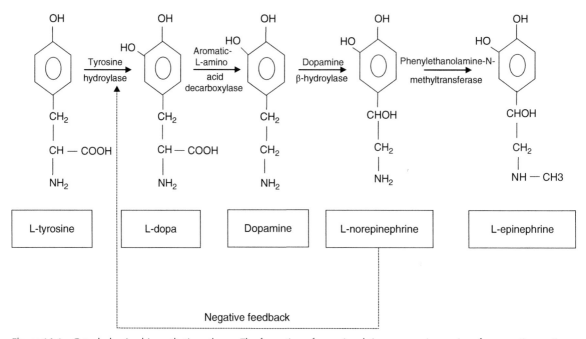

Figure 14.1 Catecholamine biosynthetic pathway: The formation of norepinephrine occurs via a series of enzymatic reactions. (Adapted from **Landsburg L, Young JB.** Catecholamines and the adrenal medulla. In: Bondy PK, Rosenburg LE, eds. Metabolic Control and Disease, 8th edn. Philadelphia, PA: WB Saunders, 1980, pp. 1621–1693.)

Once formed dopamine is transported into intracellular vesicles within the chromaffin cell, where the enzyme dopamine β-hydroxylase converts it to noradrenaline. The formed noradrenaline can then undergo methylation to form adrenaline, which accounts for 60% of the adrenal catecholamine output in the cat:

1. A rise in the noradrenaline level has a negative feedback on the enzyme tyrosine hydroxylase (the rate limiting step in the formation of the catecholamines) (Figure 14.1).

D. **In pheochromocytoma, this negative feedback is lost,** and increased catecholamine synthesis can occur. **Pheochromocytoma typically release norepinephrine.** However, some produce both epinephrine and norepinephrine, and occasionally cases produce epinephrine alone:

1. In humans, the secretion of dopamine or other peptides have been reported, including vasoactive intestinal peptide, somatostatin, calcitonin, corticotrophin-releasing hormone, adrenocorticotrophic hormone (ACTH), atrial natriuretic peptide, α-melanocyte-stimulating hormone, parathyroid-related peptide, and opioid peptides.

E. In the normal adrenal gland, catecholamine release is mediated by neural impulses. Since pheochromocytomas are not innervated, catecholamine release is thought to occur by diffusion of storage granules:

1. However, this process is poorly understood, with **unpredictable release of catecholamines** in response to physiological stressors such as hypotension, hypoxia, hypoglycemia, fear, and stress.

2. It is also recognized that catecholamines may be released in response to physical manipulation of the tumor and **in response to a variety of drugs** including metoclopramide and histamine.

3. While most tumors produce paroxysms of hormone release, some produce hormones constantly.

F. The variety of substances produced by these tumors, coupled with the (often) paroxysmal nature of secretion, makes pheochromocytoma hard to diagnose.

II. Signalment

A. To date, the authors are only aware of nine cases of pheochromocytoma, and one paraganglioma diagnosed in cats. All cases have occurred in domestic short-haired cats; six in males and three in females. A wide variety of ages have been reported, ranging from **7 to 18 years.**

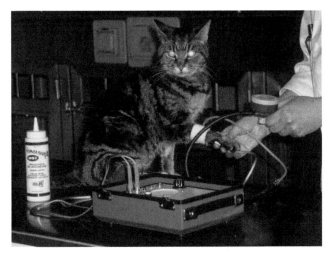

Figure 14.2 Assessment of blood pressure should be a routine part of the physical examination of any cat suspected of having an adrenal gland disorder.

III. Clinical Signs

A. The **clinical signs associated with pheochromocytoma can result from the presence of the mass, excretion of excessive amounts of catecholamines, and/or the presence of other neoplasms.** Many of the clinical signs are vague:

   1. The paroxysmal nature of hormone excretion means that clinical signs may be present intermittently. The frequency and length of these paroxysms has not been documented in cats, however, in people they can occur as frequently as several times per day, or as infrequently as several times per month, and may last from 1 min to several hours.

B. In the cat, reported clinical signs include polyuria, polydipsia, aggression, agitation, hyphema, inappetence, lethargy, intermittent vomiting, tachypnea, and seizures.

C. In the majority of cats, **physical examination has been reported to be relatively normal**; however, documented abnormalities include a **heart murmur** (two cases), palpable **abdominal mass** (three cases), potbellied appearance (one case, with concurrent hyperadrenocorticism), and poorly kept hair coat (two cases).

IV. Diagnosis

A. Investigations should include assessment of **blood pressure** (Figure 14.2); which has been elevated in at least two cases.

B. **Routine laboratory evaluation is generally unremarkable** or demonstrates nonspecific alterations such as azotemia, increased ALT, decreased potassium, hypercarbia, and increased triglycerides and creatine kinase.

C. **Urinalysis** is typically unremarkable, although several authors have reported a specific gravity below 1.030.

D. Abdominal **radiography** has detected an abdominal mass in one case and is reported to be useful in the identification of masses in 30–56% of canine cases. However, the presence of adrenal mineralization should not be overinterpreted as it occurs in ~30% of normal cats. Thoracic radiography should be performed as this may reveal cardiomegaly, metastasis, or concurrent neoplasms.

E. **Abdominal ultrasonography** has been used to detect tumors in many of the feline cases. This can also be used to detect metastasis or concurrent disease and in assessment for neoplastic invasion of the kidney or vena cava:

   1. In cats, tumors of the adrenal gland have ranged from 0.76 cm to 2.2 cm (normal short axis measurement for the adrenal gland being reported as 0.29–0.53 cm). The single paraganglioma was a 3 × 4 cm mass.

F. **CT** and **MRI** have been employed in other species for the detection of pheochromocytoma and for assessment of disease progression.

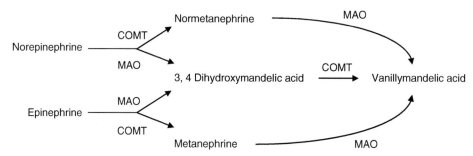

Figure 14.3 Catabolic pathways for the breakdown of catecholamines. Unchanged catecholamines and their metabolites are excreted primarily in the urine. MAO, monoamine oxidase; COMT, catechol-o-methyl transferase. (Modified from **Levine RJ**, **Landsberg L.** In: Bondy PK, Rosenburg LE, eds. Duncan's Diseases of Metabolism, 7th edn. Philadelphia, PA: WM Saunders, 1974, p. 1196.)

G. In people nuclear **scintigraphy** techniques, using either iodine metaiodobenzylguanidine (I-MIBG) or somatostatin (octreotide) have proven useful in the detection of pheochromocytoma and for staging the disease.

H. In order to demonstrate that an adrenal mass is functional and producing catecholamines, chemical confirmation should be performed. This can be achieved by **assessing the urinary excretion of unconjugated catecholamines and/or their metabolites** (Figure 14.3):

1. Ideally, this involves a 24-h urine collection, performed while the patient is at rest. The urine should be acidified to achieve pH <3 and refrigerated.
2. Alternatively, spot urine samples can be assessed, and results expressed per unit of creatinine; however, the sporadic nature of catecholamine secretion from these tumors makes this technique less than ideal.
3. Unfortunately, the logistics of sample collection, storage and lack of normal data for cats, make these techniques problematic.

I. **Plasma levels of norepinephrine, epinephrine, and dopamine can be assessed**, although there is wide variation within normal animals, and high levels can be invoked by stress or excitement. Assessment in dogs has suggested that plasma levels of norepinephrine >1500 pg/mL and epinephrine >300 pg/mL are consistent with a diagnosis of pheochromocytoma.

J. Alternatively, in order **to diagnose a pheochromocytoma, an α_2-agonist can be administered.** This decreases neurologically mediated release of catecholamines from normal adrenal glands, which does not occur with pheochromocytoma:

1. In people, blood pressure and serum catecholamine levels are assessed at baseline and 3 h post administration of **clonidine** (0.3 mg/70 kg). Blood pressure should decrease after clonidine administration, but in people with pheochromocytoma, the serum catecholamine levels remain >500 pg/mL and decrease by <50%.

K. Other protocols which are described in the human literature involve the administration of **phentolamine** (a rapidly acting α_2-antagonist) while monitoring for a decrease in blood pressure. However, this test yields many false-positive results in people and is associated with life-threatening hypotension and shock.

L. Alternatively, drugs such as **histamine, tyramine, metoclopramide, and glucagon can be administered to stimulate catecholamine secretion.** Again this is generally not recommended as these tests also yield a high number of false positive results and can mediate a hypertensive crisis in patients with pheochromocytoma.

M. **To date, neuroendocrine tests have only been performed in two reported feline cases:**

1. In the first, plasma adrenaline concentration was twice that of an age-matched control cat and reduced to a subnormal level postsurgical removal of the mass.
2. More recently, plasma normetanephrine and metanephrine levels were assessed in a cat with pheochromocytoma and compared to normal cats and sick cats with nonadrenal illness. While the metanephrine levels were not significantly different between the groups, normetanephrine levels were significantly higher in the cat with pheochromocytoma, suggesting that in some cases, assessment of these metabolites may be useful in cats.

Table 14.1   Main differential diagnoses for adrenal masses and hypertension in the cat.

	Differential diagnosis
Adrenal mass	Hyperadrenocorticism
	Hyperaldosteronism (Conn's syndrome)
	Phaeochromocytoma
	Nonsecretory tumors
Hypertension	Chronic renal failure
	Hyperthyroidism
	Hyperaldosteronism
	Hyperadrenocorticism
	Acromegaly
	Phaeochromocytoma

V.   Differential Diagnosis
See Table 14.1.

VI.   Treatment
A.   **Surgical removal** of the mass remains the treatment of choice for pheochromocytoma. However, prior to surgery the cat should be stabilized:

1.   In humans, an α-adrenergic antagonist such as **phenoxybenzamine** is administered for 2–4 weeks prior to surgery to decrease the effects of chronic vasoconstriction and therefore result in fewer hypertensive crisis in the perioperative period.

2.   Alternative therapies used in people include **prazosin hydrochloride**, the calcium channel blocker, nifedipine, and ACE inhibitors.

3.   In the face of acute perioperative hypertensive crises, intravenous phentolamine or sodium nitroprusside can be administered.

4.   If cardiac tachyarrhythmias are present, it is recommended that a β-blocker is used. However, drugs with β2 activity should only be used with preexisting α-adrenergic blockade in order to avoid exacerbating hypertension. Propranolol (0.4–1.2 mg/kg PO q 8–12 h) has been recommended for use in the cat. The short-acting β-blocker, esmolol (200–500 µg/kg IV over 1 min, then 25–200 µg/kg/min IV constant rate infusion) can be used to treat intraoperative arrhythmias.

5.   During the operative period, the blood pressure should be closely monitored. Of the cases reported in cats; five underwent exploratory laparotomy, one of these cases died after removal of the tumor, and another was euthanized following the development of thromboembolic complications postoperatively. The remaining three demonstrated dramatic decreases in blood pressure upon removal of the neoplasm. In all three cases, the hypotension was successfully managed by either the administration of dopamine or by increasing the rate of administration of fluid therapy. One of these cases went on to develop chronic hypertension, a phenomenon that has been reported occasionally in people after successful removal of pheochromocytoma, but is poorly understood.

VII.   Prognosis
A.   The prognosis for cats with pheochromocytoma appears **highly variable**. Of the reported cases, only five underwent exploratory laparotomy and surgery, with two further cases being euthanized for concurrent disease (lymphoma and pyelonephritis), and pulmonary metastases reported in a further case. Of those cats undergoing surgery, two were euthanized in the perioperative period and three survived surgery, with follow-up being reported at 3 weeks, 18 months, and 36 months:

1.   **In people and dogs, pheochromocytoma are recognized in association with concurrent neoplasms;** 50–54% of dogs are reported as having concurrent tumors.

2.   A similar correlation may exist in cats. Of the reported cases, one cat had a concurrent adrenocortical adenoma (this was successfully removed at the same surgery as the pheochromocytoma, and the cat

was reported to be alive 36 months post surgery), one cat had concurrent apocrine gland adenocarcinoma (this cat died of thromboembolic complications in the postoperative period); a further case was identified with concurrent bronchoalveolar carcinoma, which was removed at a successive surgery (the cat remaining alive and well, despite persistent hypertension, at 18 months post diagnosis), and one case was euthanized because concurrent lymphoma. In the light of these findings, care should be taken to assess any cats with pheochromocytoma for concurrent neoplasms.

VIII. Prevention
No known prevention.

References and Further Readings

Barthez PY, Marks SL, Woo J. Pheochromocytoma in dogs: 61 cases (1984–1995). *JVIM* 1997;11:272–278.

Calsyn JDR, Green RA, Davis GJ, Reilly CM. Adrenal pheochromocytoma with contralateral adrenocortical adenoma in a cat. *JAAHA* 2010;46:36–42.

Carpenter JL, Andrews LK, Holzworth J. Tumors and tumorlike lesions. *In*: Holzworth J, ed. *Diseases of the Cat: Medicine and Surgery*. Philadelphia, PA: W.B. Saunders, 1987.

Chun R, Jakovljevic S, Morrison WB, Denicola DB, Cornell KK. Apocrine gland adenocarcinoma and pheochromocytoma in a cat. *JAAHA* 1997;33:33–36.

Duesburg C, Peterson ME. Adrenal disorders in cats. *Vet Clin North Am Small Anim Pract* 1997;27:321–347.

Henry CJ, Brewer WG, Montgomery RD, Groth AH, Cartee RE. Clinical vignette: Adrenal pheochromocytoma. *JVIM* 1993;7:199–201.

Kemppainen RJ, Behrend E. Adrenal physiology. *Vet Clin North Am Small Anim Pract* 1997;27:173–186.

Maher ER. Pheochromocytoma in the dog and cat: Diagnosis and management. *Semin Vet Med Surg (Small Anim)* 1994;9:158–166.

Maher ER, Mcneil EA. Pheochromocytoma in dogs and cats. *Vet Clin North Am Small Anim Pract* 1997;27:359–380.

McMillan F. Functional pancreatic islet cell tumor in a cat. *JAAHA* 1985;21:741–746.

Myers NC, Bruyette DS. Feline adrenocortical diseases: Part II—Hypoadrenocorticism. *Semin Vet Med Surg (Small Anim)* 1994;9:144–147.

Patnaik AK, Erlandson RA, Lieberman PH, Welches CD, Marretta SM. Extra-adrenal pheochromocytoma (paraganglioma) in a cat. *JAVMA* 1990;197:104–106.

Wimpole JA, Adagra C, Billson M, Pillai DN, Foster D. Plasma metanephrines in healthy cats, cats with non-adrenal disease and a cat with phaeochromocytoma. *JFMS* 2010;12(16):435–440.

Zimmer C, Horauf A, Reusch C. Ultrasonographic examination of the adrenal gland and evaluation of the hypophyseal-adrenal axis in 20 cats. *JSAP* 2000;41:156–160.

CHAPTER 15

Canine Diabetes Mellitus

Linda Fleeman and Jacquie Rand

Pathogenesis

- Diabetes mellitus is caused by absolute or relative insulin deficiency.
- In populations in which female dogs are routinely neutered, the majority of cases have type 1 diabetes mellitus caused by immune destruction of pancreatic β cells.
- In approximately 30%, diabetes is due to extensive pancreatic damage from chronic pancreatitis.
- In intact bitches, a form analogous to human gestational diabetes can occur during diestrus or pregnancy.
- Canine diabetes also occurs in association with corticosteroid therapy, hyperadrenocorticism, or progesterone-induced acromegaly.

Classical Signs

- Most diabetic dogs are over 5 years of age with the highest prevalence occurring between 8 and 12 years of age.
- Intact females are at increased risk, especially if they are also overweight.
- Typical signs are polydipsia, polyuria, lethargy, weight loss, polyphagia, poor hair coat, and reduced immunity.

Diagnosis

- Hyperglycemia (blood glucose concentration >200 mg/dL [>11 mmol/L]) with glucosuria and consistent clinical signs.

Treatment

- The two primary goals of therapy for diabetic dogs are:
  1. Resolution of all clinical signs.
  2. Avoidance of insulin-induced hypoglycemia.
- An additional goal is diabetic remission for those dogs with reversible causes of insulin resistance such as diestrus, pregnancy, or progesterone-induced acromegaly.
- Lifelong exogenous insulin therapy is usually required unless there is prompt diabetic remission.

Clinical Endocrinology of Companion Animals, First Edition. Edited by Jacquie Rand.
© 2013 John Wiley & Sons, Inc. Published 2013 by John Wiley & Sons, Inc.

- It is important to feed consistent meals at fixed times so the postprandial period matches periods of maximal insulin activity.
- Successful management requires lifelong monitoring and reappraisal of the treatment regimen.
- Serial blood glucose concentration curves should be combined with additional indicators of glycemic control, such as changes in water intake, body weight, and urine glucose concentrations when appraising insulin dose.
- If chronic pancreatitis is present, it is important to manage the consequences and risk factors of this condition.

I. Pathogenesis

A. In dogs, multiple underlying pathological processes result in diabetes and the most common are type 1, other specific types of diabetes, and diestrual.

B. **In populations in which female dogs are routinely neutered, at least 50% of diabetic dogs have type 1 diabetes** based on histological and autoantibody evidence of immune destruction of β cells:
   1. Clinical and epidemiological factors in dogs closely match those of human patients with the human latent autoimmune diabetes of adults (LADA) form of type 1 diabetes.
   2. **Type 1 diabetes is** due to **absolute insulin deficiency** caused by **immune destruction of pancreatic β cells.**
   3. Evidence is mounting for a **genetic basis** for canine diabetes mellitus.
   4. The association with the **major histocompatibility complex** alleles on the dog leukocyte antigen gene strongly suggests that the immune response has a role in pathogenesis.
   5. **Multiple environmental factors likely initiate β-cell autoimmunity:**
      a. Once begun, β-cell destruction proceeds by common pathogenic pathways.
      b. A seasonality to the diagnosis of canine diabetes, with the **incidence peaking in winter**, suggests that environmental influences might have a role in disease progression just prior to diagnosis.

C. **Diestrual or gestational diabetes:**
   1. Results from a **relative insulin deficiency** associated with **insulin resistance.**
   2. Diabetes diagnosed in a bitch during either **pregnancy or diestrus** is comparable to human gestational diabetes.
   3. The periodic influence of diestrus-associated insulin resistance likely contributes to the **increased risk of intact female dogs** for developing diabetes.
   4. **Hormonal influences** during diestrus and pregnancy:
      a. **Progesterone** stimulates the mammary glands to produce **growth hormone.**
      b. Both hormones induce insulin resistance.
      c. In some cases, excess growth hormone production causes clinical signs of acromegaly (see Chapter 40).
   5. The risk of diabetes is increased in intact bitches if they are **also overweight**, probably due to an **additive effect of diestrus- and obesity-associated insulin resistance.**
   6. **Swedish Elkhounds have higher insulin levels during diestrus** than other breeds, and they have an increased risk for developing diabetes.

D. **Other specific types of diabetes:**
   1. **Diabetes caused by chronic pancreatitis** is the result of an **absolute insulin deficiency** due to extensive **inflammatory destruction of pancreatic tissue:**
      a. Pancreatitis is responsible for the development of diabetes mellitus in **approximately 30% of diabetic dogs** and, thus, is the **most common "other specific type" of diabetes in dogs.**
      b. Progressive destruction of **both endocrine and exocrine tissue** will result in loss of insulin-secreting β cells, glucagon-secreting α cells, and exocrine acinar cells:
         1) **Glucagon** has an important role in the **counter-regulatory response to hypoglycemia** and is therefore crucial in protecting diabetic dogs from the life-threatening consequences of insulin overdose.
         2) **Impaired glucagon counter-regulatory response** to insulin-induced hypoglycemia in diabetic dogs has been associated with episodes of **clinical hypoglycemia.**

c. Diabetic dogs with chronic pancreatitis can also develop **exocrine pancreatic insufficiency (EPI)**.

d. Although no evidence exists that type 2 diabetes occurs in dogs or that obesity-associated insulin resistance has a key role in the pathogenesis of canine diabetes; there is evidence that **obesity is a risk factor for canine pancreatitis.** Insulin resistance associated with obesity will also exacerbate other causes of insulin resistance if present, and magnify the adverse effect on glycemic control of loss of β-cell function from any other cause.

e. Environmental factors such as **feeding high fat diets resulting in lipemia and disturbances in lipid metabolism** have been implicated as potential etiological factors in dogs with obesity-associated pancreatitis and likely play a role in the development of pancreatitis in diabetic dogs.

2. **Diabetes associated with diseases that cause insulin resistance:**

a. Canine diabetes mellitus secondary to **glucocorticoid therapy, hyperadrenocorticism, or acromegaly** are less common "other specific types of diabetes."

b. As most dogs do not develop diabetes with chronic glucocorticoid therapy or spontaneous hyperadrenocorticism, progression to overt diabetes might require preexistent, underlying reduced β-cell mass or function, for example, from immunological processes or chronic pancreatitis.

E. Insulin deficiency results in the classical signs of diabetes mellitus: **polyuria, polydipsia, weight loss, an increased appetite, and lethargy:**

1. Polyuria is the result of **osmotic diuresis** caused by persistent glucosuria. The patient compensates by increasing water intake to prevent dehydration.

2. Weight loss and lethargy occur because insulin deficiency results in **decreased ability to metabolize the nutrients absorbed from the gastrointestinal tract as well as urinary loss of glucose and amino acids.** Diabetic dogs partially compensate by increasing food intake.

II. Signalment

A. **Most diabetic dogs are over 5 years** of age with the highest prevalence occurring between **8 and 12 years of age.**

B. **Intact females** are at increased risk, especially if they are also overweight.

C. Although **mixed breed dogs are more commonly affected,** some pure breeds are overrepresented.

D. **Breed predisposition** for developing diabetes **varies with geographic region:**

1. In the USA, breeds at increased risk for developing diabetes include Miniature Schnauzer, Bichon Frise, Miniature poodle, and Samoyed.

2. In the UK, Samoyeds, Tibetan terriers, Cairn terriers, Miniature Schnauzers, Yorkshire terriers, Border terriers, and Labrador retrievers are overrepresented.

3. In Sweden, the most commonly affected breeds are Australian terrier, Samoyed, Swedish Elkhound, and Swedish Lapphund.

III. Clinical Signs

A. **Uncomplicated diabetes mellitus:**

1. Diabetic dogs classically present with **polyuria, polydipsia, weight loss, an increased appetite, and lethargy.**

2. The onset of these classic clinical signs is typically **insidious,** ranging from **weeks to months in duration,** and may initially be unnoticed or considered insignificant by the owner.

B. **Sick diabetic dogs:**

1. The importance of the compensatory role of polydipsia and polyphagia in the pathophysiology of diabetes mellitus becomes apparent when they do not occur. **Any concurrent illness in diabetic dogs that causes inappetence or anorexia and vomiting is rapidly complicated by dehydration, depression, and ketosis.**

2. The **majority of diabetic dogs that present with diabetic ketoacidosis have at least one concurrent disease,** with **acute pancreatitis being the most common diagnosis.**

3. When present, **chronic pancreatitis** is likely the result of recurrent episodes of subclinical or clinical acute pancreatitis.

a. It can be associated with **minimal clinical signs** in some dogs.

b. Other dogs have **recurrent episodes of clinical acute pancreatitis of variable severity.**

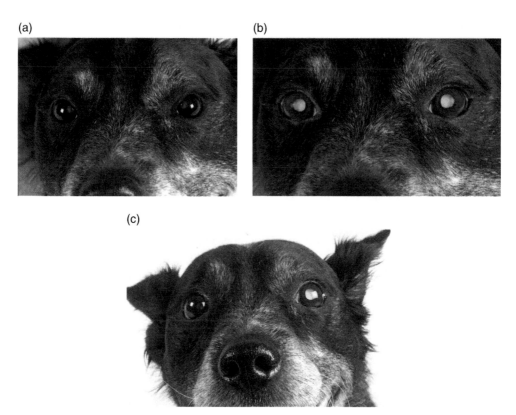

Figure 15.1 Development of diabetic cataracts in a dog. (a) An 11-year-old crossbred dog photographed shortly after diagnosis of diabetes mellitus. (b) The same dog 3 months later. Diabetic cataracts had developed rapidly and the owners reported sudden vision loss. (c) The same dog following phacoemulsification surgery to remove the cataract from the right eye. (From Fleeman LM, Rand JS. Long-term management of the diabetic dog. *Waltham Focus* 2000;10:16.)

4. **Concurrent exocrine pancreatic insufficiency (EPI):**
   a. Is usually characterized by **continued weight loss despite high calorie intake and good glycemic control.**
   b. Affected dogs often will produce **feces three or more times per day** which may or may not be normal in appearance.
C. **Diabetic cataracts:**
   1. Cataract formation is the **most common,** and one of the most important, **long-term complications** associated with diabetes in dogs (Figure 15.1).
   2. They are **irreversible and can progress quite rapidly.**
   3. Approximately **30% of diabetic dogs already have reduced vision at initial presentation.**
   4. Cataracts will develop **within 5–6 months of diagnosis in the majority** of diabetic dogs and, by 16 months, approximately 80% have significant cataract formation.
   5. **Mild or subclinical uveitis** is present in most dogs with diabetic cataracts:
      a. It is evidenced by perilimbal hyperemia and reduced intraocular pressure.
      b. If lens-induced uveitis is not treated, it can progress and cause **permanent ocular damage.**
   6. The **risk of cataract development** seems to be **unrelated to the level of hyperglycemia,** but **increase with age.**
IV. Diagnosis
A. Diagnosis of diabetes mellitus is based on the presence of **hyperglycemia** (fasting blood glucose concentration >200 mg/dL [>11 mmol/L]) **and glucosuria with compatible clinical signs.**
B. Increased serum **liver enzyme activities and concentrations of cholesterol and triglycerides** are commonly noted in newly diagnosed diabetic dogs. In most cases, they return to within the reference range with successful diabetic management.

C. **Bacterial cystitis:**
1. Should be screened for in all cases when diabetes is first documented.
2. Diagnosis requires **microbial urine culture** because results of a routine urinalysis and sediment exam in diabetics can be misleading.
3. It is commonly present in diabetic dogs and sometimes is not associated with obvious clinical signs.
D. The diagnosis of **concurrent pancreatitis** can be difficult because all available diagnostic tests have limitations:
1. The most sensitive test is measurement of canine **serum pancreatic lipase immunoreactivity (cPLI).**
2. The most specific test is **ultrasonography performed by a skilled operator.**
3. **Low serum trypsin-like immunoreactivity (TLI)** may identify concurrent **EPI:**
    a. Measurement of TLI to diagnose EPI is most useful when severe insufficiency exists.
    b. The TLI concentration can be transiently increased when there is concurrent EPI and active pancreatic inflammation.
    c. Thus, diagnosis of EPI may be missed if the inflammation increases the TLI concentration to within the normal range.
4. For diabetic dogs suspected to have concurrent EPI but not confirmed by TLI concentration, a **therapeutic trial with oral pancreatic enzyme supplementation** might assist with diagnosis.
E. In dogs with poorly controlled diabetes:
1. **Diagnosis of other concurrent conditions such as hyperadrenocorticism or hypothyroidism can be challenging.**
2. Glycemia and the clinical signs of diabetes should be as well controlled as possible before performing tests such as the low-dose dexamethasone suppression test, the ACTH stimulation test, or free T4 assay which can be affected by diabetes and lead to false diagnoses of hyperadrenocorticism and hypothyroidism.

V. Differential Diagnoses
A. Differential diagnoses for **polydipsia and polyuria** in dogs:
1. Includes **chronic renal failure, hypercalcemia, hyperadrenocorticism, hypoadrenocorticism, and pyelonephritis** as well as less commonly encountered problems such as hepatic insufficiency, hyperthyroidism, central diabetes insipidus, and psychogenic polydipsia (see Chapter 42).
2. An important differential diagnosis for polydipsia and polyuria in **intact bitches** is **pyometra.**
3. **Glucosuria without hyperglycemia** (blood glucose concentration <180 mg/dL [<10 mmol/L]) occurs with **renal glycosuria:**
    a. Primary renal glycosuria is a hereditary disease in **Basenjis and Norwegian Elkhounds.**
    b. Acquired renal glycosuria is usually caused by **toxic damage to the proximal renal tubules.**
B. Differential diagnoses for **weight loss with a normal or increased appetite** in dogs include **gastrointestinal malassimilation disorders and EPI,** cachexia associated with conditions such as **malignant neoplasia and cardiac failure,** and endocrinopathies such as **hyperthyroidism.**
C. Differential diagnoses for polyphagia include **hyperadrenocorticism,** drug therapy with **corticosteroids or phenobarbital, gastrointestinal malassimilation disorders, EPI, and primary polyphagia,** that is, neurological disease.

VI. Treatment
A. **Treatment of diabetes in sick dogs:**
1. Diabetes mellitus with or without ketoacidosis presents an additional treatment challenge in **dogs that are sick and require hospitalization.**
2. The majority of diabetic dogs that present with diabetic ketoacidosis have at least one concurrent disease, with **acute pancreatitis being the most common:**
    a. With appropriate therapy, dogs with both acute pancreatitis and diabetic ketoacidosis appear to have a **similar chance of survival** as those with diabetic ketoacidosis alone, although they typically **require hospitalization for a longer period.**
    b. Management of acute pancreatitis is primarily directed at the various clinical sequelae.
    c. The goal of treatment is to support the patient until there is spontaneous recovery.

3. Diabetic dogs with **anorexia** have a **high risk of hypokalemia:**
   a. **Intravenous fluids should be supplemented** with 30–40 mEq/L (30–40 mmol/L) of potassium (KCl or a 50:50 combination of KCl and KPO$_4$) **from the outset.**
   b. Potassium depletion:
      1) Results from decreased intake due to anorexia and increased loss due to vomiting and diuresis.
      2) Fluid therapy causes dilution of circulating potassium levels and promotes further renal loss.
      3) Insulin therapy and correction of acidosis causes potassium to move from the extracellular space into cells.
   c. In critically ill patients, **adjustment of the amount of potassium supplementation should ideally be based on results of serum potassium concentration monitoring.**
4. If the patient was previously diagnosed with diabetes and is on maintenance insulin, **longer-acting insulin preparations such as lente or neutral protamine Hagedorn (NPH) insulin should be discontinued and replaced with short-acting insulin until the animal is recovered and eating well:**
   a. Suitable short-acting preparations include **regular insulin** (e.g., Actrapid, Novo Nordisk), **lispro insulin** (Humalog, Eli Lilly) or insulin aspart (NovoRapid, NovoLog [in USA]; Novo Nordisk).
   b. Administration protocols involving either **constant rate intravenous infusion** or **intermittent intramuscular/subcutaneous injections** are effective:
      1) **Constant rate intravenous infusion protocols are often simpler and less labor intensive** for management of prolonged anorexia in diabetic dogs.
      2) The main constraint is that a **separate fluid administration line and infusion pump is required** in addition to those used for supportive fluid therapy.
   c. An **initial insulin infusion rate of 50 mU/kg/h** is recommended:
      1) This rate is easily achieved by administering a 50 mU/mL solution (**25 U insulin in 500 mL saline) at 1 mL/kg/h.**
      2) All flow rates and doses should be **based on estimated ideal body weight** and not actual body weight.
      3) Aim for a decrease in blood glucose concentration of approximately 50 mg/dL/h (3 mmol/L/h).
   d. **When the patient's blood glucose concentration reaches 180–270 mg/dL (10–15 mmol/L):**
      1) The initial rate should be **halved** to 25 mU/kg/h (0.5 mL/kg/h of this solution).
      2) At the same time, the **maintenance fluids should be changed to contain 2.5% dextrose** and 30–40 mEq/L (30–40 mmol/L) potassium.
   e. The insulin infusion rate is **adjusted up or down** to maintain blood glucose concentration at **145–270 mg/dL (8–15 mmol/L).**
   f. **If the dog's illness is associated with substantial insulin resistance:**
      1) An insulin infusion flow rate of up to 150 mU/kg/h (**3 mL/kg/h** of the solution described above) may be required to maintain blood glucose concentration at 145–270 mg/dL (8–15 mmol/L).
      2) As the dog recovers and insulin resistance resolves, the **insulin infusion flow rate will need to be decreased.**
   g. **If there is not substantial insulin resistance,** a reliable means of achieving a fairly stable blood glucose concentration in an anorexic diabetic dog is to balance intravenous infusion of insulin at 25 mU/kg/h (**0.5 mL/kg/h** of the solution described above) with a maintenance infusion of 2.5% dextrose in 0.45% saline with 30–40 mEq/L (30–40 mmol/L) potassium at **6 mL/kg/h.**
   h. **When a previously anorexic diabetic dog begins to eat,** the intravenous insulin flow rate usually needs to be increased to manage postprandial glycemia.
5. **Once the diabetic dog has recovered** and has a normal appetite:
   a. Therapy with short-acting insulin can be discontinued.
   b. A maintenance protocol using a longer-acting insulin preparation administered every 12 h can be introduced or resumed.
   c. **Intravenous insulin infusion should continue until immediately prior to subcutaneous administration of longer-acting insulin.**
6. Intermittent intramuscular/subcutaneous injections are also effective and in some settings are simpler for clinical staff to administer and less expensive for the client:

a. Low doses of regular or lispro insulin can be used.

b. **An initial dose of 0.25 U/kg** is injected intramuscularly after intravenous fluid therapy has commenced with Lactated Ringer's solution with 30–40 mEq/L (30–40 mmol/L) potassium. For dogs weighing < 10 kg, a starting dose of 2 U/dog is appropriate.

c. **Intramuscular insulin doses are repeated every hour at 0.1 U/kg**, or 1 U for dogs weighing < 10 kg, until a blood glucose concentration of 145–270 mg/dL (8–15 mmol/L) is achieved. Aim for a decrease in glucose concentration of approximately 50 mg/dL/h (3 mmol/L/h).

d. When a blood glucose concentration of 145–270 mg/dL (8–15 mmol/L) has been achieved, the **maintenance fluids should be changed to contain 2.5% dextrose** and 30–40 mEq/L (30–40 mmol/L) potassium. Insulin therapy is then continued at **0.1–0.4 U/kg subcutaneously every 4–6 h** as required to maintain a blood glucose concentration of 145–270 mg/dL (8–15 mmol/L). Monitoring blood glucose concentration at least every 2 h is recommended at this stage.

B. **Management of diabetic dogs requiring elective general anesthesia:**
1. **Half the usual dose of insulin should be administered in the morning when food is withheld.**
2. Whenever possible, **general anesthesia should be scheduled early in the day** so, if the procedure allows, the patient can be recovered and discharged to the home environment before the next insulin injection and meal are due.
3. **Intravenous administration of an insulin constant rate infusion is recommended** while the dog is hospitalized with the goal of maintaining blood glucose concentration at **110–270 mg/dL (6–15 mmol/L):**
   a. Blood glucose concentration should be **monitored every 1–2 h** and intravenous fluids continued until discharge.
   b. **If the blood glucose concentration is 110–270 mg/dL (6–15 mmol/L),** intravenous infusion of insulin (solution of 25 U insulin in 500 mL saline) at 25 mU/kg/h (0.5 mL/kg/h) with a maintenance infusion of 2.5% dextrose in 0.45% saline with 20–40 mEq/L (20–40 mmol/L) potassium at 6 mL/kg/h is recommended.
   c. **If the blood glucose concentration is >270 mg/dL (>15 mmol/L),** intravenous infusion of insulin at 25 mU/kg/h (0.5 mL/kg/h of the solution described above) with a maintenance infusion of lactated Ringer's solution with 20–40 mEq/L (20–40 mmol/L) potassium is recommended.
   d. **If the blood glucose concentration is <110 mg/dL (<6 mmol/L),** a maintenance infusion of 2.5% dextrose in 0.45% saline with 20–40 mEq/L (20–40 mmol/L) potassium at 6 mL/kg/h is recommended and **insulin infusion should be withheld** until the blood glucose concentration is >110 mg/dL (>6 mmol/L).

C. **Choosing a blood glucose meter:**
1. **A wide range of portable blood glucose meters are available:**
   a. Most are sufficiently accurate and precise to be useful for monitoring blood glucose concentration in diabetic dogs.
   b. **Meters designed for use by humans often give lower results** than the laboratory reference method.
2. The **AlphaTRAK blood glucose meter** (Abbott Animal Health):
   a. Is designed specifically for veterinary patients.
   b. Gives **precise and more accurate blood glucose measurements for dogs** than blood glucose meters designed for human samples.
   c. It requires only 0.3 μL of blood and, therefore, is suitable for **home monitoring** of blood glucose concentration as well as for **hospital use.**
   d. The AlphaTRAK meter provides results above the laboratory reference method more often than most human blood glucose meters and **can potentially miss hypoglycemia in insulin-treated patients.**
3. **If there is ever any doubt about the accuracy of a blood glucose concentration measurement, the best approach is to repeat the measurement** using the same meter or a laboratory reference method.

D. **Options for monitoring blood glucose concentration in hospitalized dogs:**
1. **Continuous monitoring of subcutaneous or interstitial glucose concentration:**
   a. Provides **several advantages** for diabetic dogs compared with traditional methods of serial blood glucose monitoring, with the major one being that **glucose measurements are obtained every 3–5 min** allowing clinicians to base treatment decisions on much more detailed glycemic data.
   b. The **Guardian® REAL-Time Continuous Glucose Monitoring System (CGMS) (Medtronic)** provides glucose results **in real time** and uses wireless technology:

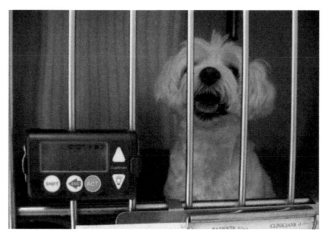

Figure 15.2 The Guardian® REAL-Time Continuous Glucose Monitoring System (CGMS) (Medtronic) provides glucose concentration results in real time using wireless technology, so the monitor does not need to be attached to the patient. The monitor provides data when it is within 2.0 yd (1.8 m) of the sensor and thus works well when attached to the front of the patient's kennel door.

1) The **monitor does not need to be attached to the patient** (Figure 15.2).

2) **Strong correlation exists between interstitial and blood glucose concentrations** in diabetic dogs with a delay of 5–12 min.

3) Importantly, the CGMS system **can facilitate detection of brief periods of hypoglycemia** (Figure 15.3).

4) **Limitations** of the system include a **2–3 h set up period** before glucose readings are obtained and the requirement for 2–3 **blood samples to be collected every 24 h during monitoring for calibration**. It is preferable to avoid calibrating the CGMS when blood glucose is changing rapidly.

5) **The most reliable location for placement of the CGMS sensor is the dorsal neck** (Figure 15.4)

6) The CGMS provides **clinically accurate glucose concentrations in ketoacidotic dogs**, although the device may not function as well in severely dehydrated patients.

7) **The CGMS does *not* provide reliable data in dogs during general anesthesia.**

c. Other continuous interstitial glucose monitors, such as the **GlucoDay (Menarini Diagnostics)** and **other Medtronic CGMS**:

1) Do not provide results in real time and so glycemic data are not available until the device is disconnected from the dog.

2) They are, therefore, **less useful for monitoring sick diabetic dogs in which ongoing treatment decisions are based on current blood glucose measurements**.

3) They are more appropriately used in the hospital or home environment for monitoring glycemia in stable patients.

d. As with all methods of monitoring glycemia, it is not advisable to rely on continuous interstitial glucose monitors as the sole monitoring tool.

e. If there is doubt about the accuracy of interstitial glucose results, the best approach is to immediately obtain a blood glucose measurement.

2. **Venous blood can be obtained by direct venipuncture, from an indwelling peripheral or central intravenous catheter or by lancing the marginal vein of the lateral pinna:**

a. Application of topical **local anesthetic cream** to the site prior to venipuncture and use of a **very small gauge needle** will improve patient comfort and cause minimal damage to the vein.

b. Blood collection from indwelling peripheral and central intravenous catheters is very well tolerated:

1) **Catheters** in diabetic dogs should be **flushed with heparinized saline (1 U/mL)** following blood collection to protect against thrombus formation and catheter occlusion.

c. Small venous blood samples can be readily obtained from the **marginal vein of the lateral pinna** of dogs:

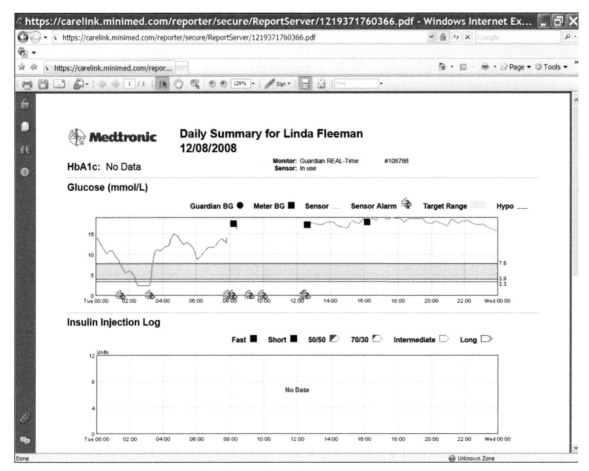

Medtronic

Daily Summary for Linda Fleeman
12/08/2008

Monitor: Guardian REAL-Time   #108788
Sensor: In use

HbA1c: No Data

Glucose (mmol/L)

Guardian BG ●   Meter BG ■   Sensor ___   Sensor Alarm ✤   Target Range   Hypo ___

Insulin Injection Log

Fast ■   Short ■   50/50 ▨   70/30 ▢   Intermediate ▢   Long ▷

No Data

Figure 15.3 Graphical output from a Guardian® REAL-Time Continuous Glucose Monitoring System (CGMS) manufactured by the diabetes division of Medtronic, Inc. attached to a diabetic dog with a history of poor diabetic control. Note the precipitous decrease in interstitial glucose concentration from midnight until approximately 3 a.m., followed by a brief 20-min period of hypoglycemia, and then very rapid rebound to hyperglycemia within 10 min. The dog showed no clinical signs of hypoglycemia and remained asleep during this period. The data were interpreted as evidence of Somogyi phenomenon and a recommendation was made to decrease the insulin dose. *The Guardian® REAL-Time Continuous Glucose Monitoring System is not approved by U.S. FDA for use in any animals.*

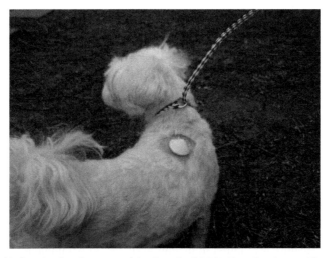

Figure 15.4 The most reliable location for placement of the Guardian® REAL-Time Continuous Glucose Monitoring System (CGMS) sensor in diabetic dogs is the dorsal neck.

(a) (b) (c)

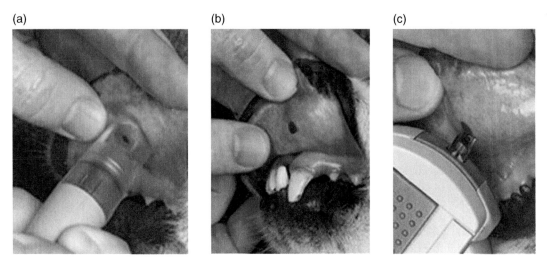

Figure 15.5 Measurement of capillary blood glucose concentration from the buccal mucosa. (a) The upper lip adjacent to the canine tooth is turned up to expose the buccal mucosa and saliva is wiped away with a swab. (b) The vacuum-lancing device is applied to the buccal mucosa at the level of the canine tooth. (c) The vacuum-lancing device is removed when an adequate amount of blood is present on the mucosal surface. The test tip of the glucose meter is applied to the blood drop and the sample is drawn into the test strip.

    1) The area should first be warmed with a damp cloth, warmed moist cotton ball, or heat pack.

    2) Second, **petroleum jelly is applied to the area and the vein nicked with a lancing device.** The petroleum jelly causes the blood drop to bead on the surface and prevents spreading of the sample into the surrounding fur.

    3) Occasionally, **gentle massage** around the nick site is required to generate a sufficient drop.

    4) The technique can be performed with minimal physical restraint and is usually well tolerated.

3. **Measurement of capillary blood glucose concentration in diabetic dogs is an alternative to the techniques using venous blood:**

    a. Similar to the marginal pinnal vein method, major advantages of capillary blood glucose measurement are that it can **reliably be performed with minimal restraint and in patients with difficult venous access.**

    b. Sites suitable for collection of capillary blood samples in dogs include:

        1) **The buccal mucosa.**

        2) **The medial aspect of the pinna.**

        3) **The main paw pad.**

        4) **The carpal pad.**

        5) **An elbow callus.**

        6) **Skin that has been clipped of hair, for example, the base of the tail.**

    c. **Collection of capillary blood from the buccal mucosa** employs a technique similar to that used for assessment of buccal mucosal bleeding time:

        1) The upper lip adjacent to the canine tooth is everted to expose the buccal mucosa and saliva is wiped away.

        2) **A standard or a vacuum-lancing device** such as the CareLance (i-SENS) **is applied to the mucosa at the level of the canine tooth** and the device is triggered.

        3) **If a standard lancing device is used,** the device is removed once it has been triggered and the upper lip is held away from the sampling site until the blood drop has reached sufficient size.

        4) **If a vacuum-lancing device is used,** the piston is slowly released and a vacuum forms within the end cup, causing the mucosal surface to bulge and the blood drop to enlarge.

        5) A glucose meter that can operate with sample sizes $<5\,\mu L$, such as the AlphaTRAK meter (Abbott Animal Health), is required to maximize success in obtaining a glucose measurement; the volume of blood obtained can be a limiting factor for meters requiring larger volumes (Figure 15.5).

d. For **collection of capillary blood from skin sites:**
   1) The lancing device is placed on the site and triggered.
   2) If a standard lancing device is used, the area surrounding the site can be gently massaged to encourage enlargement of the blood drop.
   3) If a vacuum-lancing device is used, the vacuum action causes the blood drop to enlarge.
   4) When the medial pinna is sampled, a folded gauze swab is held against the lateral pinna to provide support as the device is triggered. It is important that **digital pressure against the folded swab is not excessive** because this may occlude blood flow to the site of sampling and prevent enlargement of the blood drop.
E. Goals of long-term management:
   1. The **two primary goals of therapy** for diabetic dogs are:
      a. **Resolution of clinical signs.**
      b. **Avoidance of insulin-induced hypoglycemia.**
   2. An **additional goal is diabetic remission:**
      a. Remission is possible for dogs with diabetes due to severe insulin resistance if they have sufficient residual β-cell function.
      b. Remission **requires** both reduction of hyperglycemia by **treating with insulin** plus **prompt elimination of insulin resistance.**
      c. Remission is **most likely in animals with diestrus or gestational diabetes** and in those that develop diabetes while receiving medication known to cause insulin resistance, such as **glucocorticoids.**
   3. **Resolution of all clinical signs is best achieved using a regimen of fixed daily insulin doses and feeding consistent meals:**
      a. **Lethargy tends to resolve rapidly** and dogs become more active and responsive soon after initiation of insulin therapy.
      b. **Weight loss** is usually arrested before optimal glycemic control is achieved.
      c. Complete resolution of **polyuria and polydipsia** will not occur until the **blood glucose concentration is below the renal threshold (approximately 200 mg/dL [11 mmol/L]) most of the time.**
      d. In the majority of diabetic dogs, the process of **cataract** formation has unfortunately already been initiated before control of hyperglycemia is achieved.
   4. **Avoidance of insulin-induced hypoglycemia:**
      a. Is **very important** as the condition can result in irreversible **brain damage or death.**
      b. A **conservative approach to insulin dosing, twice daily insulin administration, and complementary nutritional strategies** greatly reduce the risk.
F. Choosing the right insulin preparation for long-term management:
   1. **A large variety of human insulin preparations are available as well as veterinary preparations registered specifically for use in dogs and cats** (Table 15.1):
      a. Although limited veterinary information exists on most of the recently released human products, all are potentially efficacious for treatment of diabetic dogs.
      b. Good glycemic control can be achieved with most insulin preparations.
      c. Some preparations are easier to use, because they have a more predictable effect between dogs and in the same dog on different days.
      d. Generally, **the longer the duration of action of insulin, the greater the variability in response between dogs receiving the same dose.**
   2. Lente insulin:
      a. The only preparation available is **Vetsulin** (in the USA) or **Caninsulin** (elsewhere in the world) made by MSD Animal Health, a **40 U/mL porcine insulin zinc suspension specifically registered for veterinary use.**
      b. There is **good evidence that this insulin product is effective for the treatment of diabetes in dogs.**
      c. It has an **intermediate duration** of action.
      d. It is a combination of **30% short-acting semilente and 70% longer-acting ultralente insulins;** the combination results in a relatively **predictable and rapid peak effect.**
      e. The median duration of action is 14 h:

Table 15.1   Currently available insulin products.*

Type of insulin	Concentration (U/mL)	Brand name(s)	Manufacturer	Size of multiuse vials (mL)	Injection pen availability
Veterinary insulin preparations					
Insulin zinc suspension (lente)	40	Vetsulin;* Caninsulin	MSD Animal Health	2.5 and 10; 2.7 mL cartridges	VetPen in 2 sizes: 0.5–8U (0.5 U increments) and 1–6 U (1 U increments)
Protamine zinc insulin (PZI)	40	ProZinc	Boehringer Ingelheim	10	None
Traditionally available human insulin preparations					
Regular insulin	100 (and 500**)	Humulin R	Eli Lilly	3 and 10	None
Regular insulin	100	ActRapid	Novo Nordisk	10	NovoPens including Junior/Demi[a]
Isophane (NPH) insulin	100	Humulin N	Eli Lilly	10	HumaPen Luxura incl. HD;[a] Humulin N Pen[b]
Isophane (NPH) insulin	100	Protaphane	Novo Nordisk	10	NovoPens incl. Junior/Demi;[a] InnoLet;[a] NovoLet[b]
50% regular and 50% isophane (NPH)	100	Mixtard 50/50	Novo Nordisk	None	NovoPens including Junior/Demi;[a] InnoLet[a]
30% regular and 70% isophane (NPH)	100	Mixtard 30/70	Novo Nordisk	None	NovoPens including Junior/Demi;[a] InnoLet[a]
30% regular and 70% isophane (NPH)	100	Humulin 70/30	Eli Lilly	10	HumaPen Luxura incl. HD;[a] Humulin 70/30 Pen[b]
New human insulin preparations					
Insulin lispro	100	Humalog	Eli Lilly	3 and 10	Humapen Luxura including HD;[a] Autopen;[a] KwikPen[b]
Insulin aspart	100	NovoLog; NovoRapid	Novo Nordisk	10	NovoPens including Junior/Demi;[a] FlexPen[b]
Insulin glulisine	100	Apidra	Sanofi Aventis	10	OptiClik;[a] SolarStar[b]
50% lispro and 50% lispro protamine	100	Humalog Mix 50/50	Eli Lilly	10	HumaPen Luxura including HD;[a] KwikPen[b]
30% aspart and 70% aspart protamine	100	NovoLog Mix 70/30; NovoMix 30	Novo Nordisk	10	NovoPens including Junior/Demi;[a] FlexPen[b]
25% lispro and 75% lispro protamine	100	Humalog Mix 75/25	Eli Lilly	10	HumaPen Luxura including HD;[a] KwikPen[b]
Insulin glargine	100	Lantus	Sanofi Aventis	10	Autopen;[a] SolarStar[b]
Insulin detemir	100	Levemir	Novo Nordisk	10	NovoPens including Junior/Demi;[a] FlexPen[b]

*Availability and brand names of commercial insulin products and injection devices change over time and vary between countries. Availability of Vetsulin in the USA has recently been affected.

**500 U/mL included to alert reader to its existence, but no indication for its use exists in small animals.

[a] Insulin injection pen that uses 3 mL cartridge refills. All deliver 1 U dose increments, except for the NovoPen Junior/Demi and the HumaPen Luxura HD which deliver 0.5 U increments.

[b] Prefilled disposable 3 mL insulin injection pen. All deliver 1 U dose increments, except for the NovoLet which delivers 2 U dose increments.

      1) Significant **lowering of blood glucose concentration occurs in the majority (90%) of dogs for 12 h or more.**

      2) Thus, it is suited to a **twice daily dosing regimen in diabetic dogs and a meal can be fed at the time of the insulin injection.**

  f. The **40 U/mL veterinary preparation** is **advantageous for small dogs,** which might require a total insulin dose of only 1 or 2 U:

      1) It is recommended that VetPen insulin dosing pens are used to ensure accuracy and precision of dosing.

      2) If syringes are to be used, dosing is simpler and more accurate if specific U-40 syringes are prescribed with this product.

  g. Availability of Vetsulin in the USA has recently been affected; however, supply of Caninsulin elsewhere is not affected and has been reliable for many years.

3. **Isophane/NPH insulin:**

  a. Examples are Humulin N (Eli Lilly) and Protaphane (Novo Nordisk).

  b. Has an intermediate duration of action and is **effective** for the treatment of diabetes in dogs **when administered twice daily.**

  c. **Postprandial hyperglycemia can occur in some well-regulated diabetic dogs when meals with high insoluble fiber content are fed at the same time** as NPH insulin injection.

  d. Thus, the ideal time for feeding such meals might be 1–2 h after the insulin injection, which may not be convenient for many owners.

4. **Premixed combinations of 30% regular and 70% isophane (NPH) insulin:**

  a. Humulin 70/30 (Eli Lilly) and Mixtard 30/70 (Novo Nordisk) are still available in most countries.

  b. They are 100 U/mL premixed combinations of 30% short-acting and 70% intermediate-acting insulin.

  c. They have a **similar action to lente insulin in most dogs, although in others, duration is shorter. They are suited to a twice-daily dosing regimen in diabetic dogs where the meals are fed at the same time as the insulin injections.**

5. **Recombinant human protamine zinc insulin:**

  a. The release of ProZinc (Boehringer Ingelheim) provides a veterinary product to fill the gap in the market created by the discontinuation of PZI-VET.

  b. It is **not generally recommended as a first choice therapy** for diabetic dogs as it has a less predictable action with a slower onset than lente insulin or the 70% or 100% NPH preparations.

6. **Premixed combinations of short-acting lispro or aspart insulin with longer-acting protamine insulin:**

  a. Humalog Mix 75/25 (Eli Lilly) is marketed for human diabetics as an improved product that can be used twice-daily, a replacement for Humulin 70/30. It is a mix of 75% insulin lispro protamine suspension and 25% insulin lispro injection (rDNA origin).

  b. NovoLog 70/30 (Novo Nordisk) is a similar product with **70% insulin aspart protamine and 30% insulin aspart.**

  c. In humans, compared with Humulin 70/30, Humalog Mix 75/25 and NovoLog 70/30 have a more rapid and predictable onset of glucose-lowering activity, with greater reduction in postprandial glycemia when administered with a meal, and appear to have a similar duration of action to lente (Vetsulin/Caninsulin) in many dogs. Because of the rapid onset of action, initial dosing should be conservative (0.25 U/kg lean body weight).

  d. Currently **no information has been published on the use of these new premixed combinations for the management of diabetes in dogs:**

      1) Research in diabetic dogs is warranted as the product(s) might prove reliable and efficacious when administered twice-daily at the same times as meals.

      2) Based on data in humans, it appears the risk of hypoglycemia might be greatest in the first 2 h after injection in dogs, so it will likely be crucial that meals are always consumed at the time of injection.

7. **Insulin glargine and insulin detemir:**

  a. Products are Lantus (Sanofi Aventis) and Levemir (Novo Nordisk).

  b. They are **long-acting synthetic insulin analogues:**

      1) Developed for human diabetics to provide continuous basal insulin concentrations that inhibit hepatic glucose production.

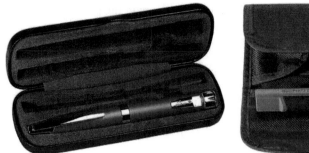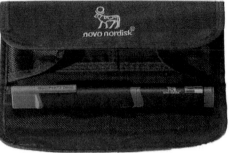

Figure 15.6 The HumaPen Luxura HD pen (Eli Lilly) and the NovoPen Junior (USA)/Demi (elsewhere) pens (Novo Nordisk) deliver accurate and precise insulin doses in 0.5 U increments.

2) The therapeutic aim is to mimic the physiological pattern of basal insulin secretion of healthy subjects.

3) In humans, the **basal insulin levels** provided by these products are supplemented at meal times by administration of short-acting insulin preparations that act during the postprandial period.

c. Preliminary investigation of the treatment of diabetic dogs with **glargine insulin** indicated that the **success rate might be lower** than with lente insulin.

d. **Levemir insulin is more potent** than insulin preparations traditionally used in diabetic dogs:

1) Thus, its **usefulness in small dogs is limited.**

2) A small study that evaluated the management of diabetic dogs using **detemir with daily dosage adjustments based on daily blood glucose concentration testing** suggested that such a protocol **might be a useful option** for dogs inadequately controlled with other insulin preparations.

e. Until there is further evaluation of their efficacy for the treatment of diabetes in dogs, **insulin glargine or detemir are not recommended as a first choice of insulin therapy.**

G. Insulin dosing pens:

1. Insulin dosing pens are **designed to be used by people with no formal medical training:**

a. The goal is to make the task of **measuring and administering insulin doses easier, less painful, and more accurate and precise.**

b. They can provide the same benefit for diabetic animals and their owners.

2. **Insulin dosing pens are much more accurate and precise than insulin syringes:**

a. For example, when administering a dose of 1U of a 100 U/mL insulin preparation, the mean dose delivered using the Autopen (Owen Mumford) is 0.93 U (range: 0.63–1.20 U) and for the SolarSTAR pen (Sanofi Aventis) is 1.02 U (range: 0.60–1.40 U).

b. In comparison, for pediatric nurses administering a dose of 1 U using 0.3 mL or 0.5 mL insulin syringes, the mean±SD dose was 1.64±0.38 (range: 0.65–2.80 U).

c. Importantly, it can be seen that **most syringe-measured low doses exceed the intended dose.**

3. **HumaPen Luxura HD pen (Eli Lilly) and the NovoPen Junior (USA)/Demi (other countries) pens (Novo Nordisk):**

a. They are specifically designed for use in babies and children and **deliver accurate and precise insulin doses in 0.5 U increments** (Figure 15.6).

b. As these pens can be used with the 3 mL cartridges of all the intermediate-acting 70% and 100% NPH insulin preparations, they are particularly suitable for use in diabetic dogs.

4. **Storage:**

a. Before insulin cartridges are opened, they should be stored in the refrigerator.

b. However **once opened and in use, most pens should *not* be refrigerated but instead kept at room temperature,** that is, <30 °C (<86 °F) away from direct heat and light.

5. Using a pen:

a. **Before each use, insulin dosing pens typically need to be primed** with 2 U until a stream of insulin appears, which can seem wasteful to those not familiar with the protocol.

b. During injection, the **needle must be left in the skin for several seconds** while the injection button is held down.

c. When the needle is removed after injection, it is normal for a drop of insulin to be visible on the tip of the needle.

H. **Avoiding insulin-induced hypoglycemia and dosing errors:**

1. A prudent approach for the majority of diabetic dogs is to adopt a **twice-daily insulin-dosing regimen** at the outset.

2. High doses of insulin and episodes of hypoglycemia are more common in diabetic dogs that receive insulin only once daily.

3. **Insulin dosing pens are recommended** because they are associated with fewer dosing errors and more accurate dosing.

4. **If it is not possible to administer an insulin injection on time, the best approach is to skip that injection and resume insulin administration at the next scheduled time:**

    a. Missing a single injection will have negligible consequences. However, regularly missing insulin injections will likely result in poor control and may precipitate diabetic ketoacidosis.

    b. In contrast, late administration of insulin can lead to overlap of insulin action (and therefore overdose) if the following insulin injection is administered on time.

    c. The usual meal can be fed whenever an insulin injection is missed.

5. Insulin overdose:

    a. Overdose may occur when there is good glycemic control resulting in **lower blood glucose levels at the time of insulin administration** (for example, less than 180–215 mg/dL or 10–12 mmol/L). Appropriate dose adjustment based on knowledge of how the dog typically responds, and careful home monitoring is advised to achieve excellent glycemic control while avoiding hypoglycemia.

    b. Diabetic dogs with good glycemic control should, therefore, be closely monitored.

6. A variety of management and medical factors **increase the risk of insulin overdose**, including:

    a. **Incomplete mixing of insulin suspensions.**

    b. **Administration of insulin at irregular intervals.**

    c. **Inappetence.**

    d. **Excessive exercise.**

    e. **Improved insulin sensitivity** associated with the end of diestrus, discontinuation of drugs that induce resistance, or treatment of concurrent disease such as hyperadrenocorticism.

7. **When a diabetic dog does not eat or eats less than one quarter of the accompanying meal:**

    a. **Half the usual insulin dose should be administered** because the risk of hypoglycemia is increased if insulin is administered when the dog does not eat.

    b. Inappetence or anorexia might signify the presence of concurrent disease.

    c. Therefore, owners should **seek prompt veterinary advice whenever a diabetic dog shows unexpected inappetence or anorexia.**

8. Care must be taken when dispensing insulin syringes to owners to ensure that there is no confusion regarding dosing:

    a. For example, the graduations on many 1 mL insulin syringes are equal to 2 U, while graduations on most 0.3 mL and 0.5 mL insulin syringes are 1 U.

    b. In addition, graduations on syringes designed for use with 100 U/mL insulin represent a different volume from graduations on syringes designed for use with 40 U/mL insulin.

9. Care must also be taken when dispensing insulin dosing pens:

    a. Only insulin dosing pens designed for the specific insulin preparation will deliver accurate doses. **If a cartridge of another brand of insulin is inserted, the pen might appear to function normally but typically much smaller insulin doses are delivered.**

    b. The instructions for use of the insulin dosing pen must always be followed exactly.

I. **What to do if clinical hypoglycemia occurs:**

1. If **mild signs of hypoglycemia** develop, the owner should **feed a meal of the dog's usual food:**

    a. **Hand-feeding** might be necessary to encourage the dog to eat.

    b. If the dog is unwilling or unable to eat:

1) **Syrup containing a high glucose concentration** can be administered orally.

2) Suitable syrups are marketed for use by human diabetics and should be kept in reserve by all owners of diabetic dogs.

3) When the dog recovers, a meal of the dog's usual food should be fed immediately.

c. The owner should then **contact their veterinarian before the next insulin injection is due,** at which point dosage reduction is usually recommended.

2. If **profound hypoglycemia** occurs or mild hypoglycemia does not respond to the above treatment:

a. Oral glucose can always be tried first if safe for the owner and dog, for example, if the dog is conscious and not having a seizure.

b. If oral glucose is not successful, the hypoglycemia should be managed initially with an intravenous **bolus of 50% dextrose at a dosage of 1 mL/kg (0.5 g/kg)** administered slowly.

c. **The bolus should be followed with an intravenous constant rate infusion** of 2.5% dextrose in 0.45% saline at 6 mL/kg/h until the blood glucose is >180 mg/dL (>10 mmol/L).

d. The dog's usual food can be fed as frequent small meals.

e. **Insulin should be withheld until the blood glucose is >180 mg/dL (>10 mmol/L),** which may sometimes take several days.

J. Nutritional management:

1. **Feeding consistent meals at fixed times each day is crucial to successful management of diabetes in dogs:**

a. **Commercial dog foods usually result in postprandial elevation of blood glucose concentration from 1 to 6 h** following consumption.

b. **Meals should be timed so that maximal exogenous insulin activity occurs during the postprandial period:**

1) Thus, dogs **should be fed within 1 h** of administration of lente or NPH insulin.

2) In some dogs receiving NPH insulin, postprandial hyperglycemia is reduced by feeding the meal 1–2 h after the insulin injection, and this has been reported to improve glycemic control in dogs fed diets with high insoluble fiber content.

3) When a **twice-daily insulin dosing regimen** is used, a feasible compromise is to **feed the dog just before or immediately following each insulin injection.**

c. The majority of diabetic dogs will readily consume meals twice-daily if the meals are **highly palatable; each meal should contain half the dog's daily caloric requirement.**

d. Dogs are more likely to readily accept a diet that has a **formulation similar to the diet they were consuming before diagnosis of diabetes.** A practical approach is to obtain a **diet history** at the time of diagnosis and then **negotiate an agreement with the owner on a set meal** that will be fed every 12 h.

e. In the majority of cases, the most appropriate meal comprises a **complete and balanced commercial dog food formulated for adult maintenance with <10% of the calories from treats or other foods.**

f. For **finicky eaters,** the meal should be fed at the time of insulin administration and remain available until the expected end of the period of maximal exogenous insulin activity.

g. If **treats** are fed, they should be consumed **during the expected period of maximal exogenous insulin activity.** All treats containing high sugar or fat should be avoided.

2. **Particular care should be taken to ensure a consistent source and content of dietary carbohydrate:**

a. The major determinant of the postprandial glycemic response in dogs is the total carbohydrate content of the meal.

b. As many of the clinical signs of diabetes mellitus are attributable to hyperglycemia, it is rational to limit the glycemic load following each meal.

c. Therefore, a **moderately carbohydrate-restricted diet (e.g., carbohydrate <30% ME) is recommended.**

3. **Clinical benefit for diabetic dogs of feeding a high-fiber diet compared to a typical adult maintenance diet with moderate-fiber** content (30–40 g/1000 kcal) **has not been clearly demonstrated:**

a. Based on the evidence of a recent randomized clinical trial, **routine recommendation of high-fiber, moderate-carbohydrate, moderate-fat diets is not indicated** for diabetic dogs managed with lente insulin.

b. Importantly, **the traditionally recommended high-fiber, moderate-fat diet caused significant weight loss,** and thus is **not suitable for diabetic dogs with thin body condition.**

c. For diabetic dogs managed with NPH insulin, some evidence exists that the **traditionally recommended high-fiber diet can actually cause greater postprandial hyperglycemia than other diets.**

d. In addition, increased dietary fiber content in excess of that routinely recommended for healthy dogs might be associated with other **unwanted side effects, such as inappetence, diarrhea, and flatulence.**

4. **Dietary fat restriction** (e.g., fat <30% ME) should be considered for diabetic dogs with concurrent chronic pancreatitis or persistent hypertriglyceridemia:

a. **Hypertriglyceridemia has been proposed as a possible inciting cause of canine pancreatitis.**

b. Pancreatitis is commonly seen in diabetic dogs, indicating that the diabetic state might also be a risk factor for pancreatitis.

c. However, **dogs with diabetes secondary to chronic pancreatitis likely also have substantial loss of exocrine pancreatic function and will be at increased risk for loss of body weight** when fed a restricted fat diet.

d. **A more targeted approach is to only recommend dietary fat restriction for diabetic dogs if there is persistent hypertriglyceridemia once good glycemic control has been established.**

e. Clinical response to the diet should be evaluated by monitoring body weight and serum triglyceride concentration.

5. The optimal level of dietary protein for diabetic dogs has not been determined:

a. It is rational that recommendations would be no different than for nondiabetic dogs.

b. **As both carbohydrate and fat are usually restricted in diabetic dogs, dietary protein will often provide a substantial source of calories** (e.g., protein >30% ME).

K. **Monitoring clinical signs and response to therapy at home:**

1. **Establishing a practical routine for the dog's owner:**

a. Many owners of diabetic dogs welcome the opportunity to monitor their pet's response to therapy, although compliance can be very variable.

b. **Compliance is markedly improved if a close rapport between the owner and the clinician managing the case exists as well as appropriate individualization of the dog's therapeutic and monitoring regimen.**

c. The clinician must invest time to **educate the owner about canine diabetes and its management** as well as to provide **support and guidance while the owner becomes accustomed to the treatment and monitoring procedures and establishes a practical routine.**

2. The primary aim of therapy in diabetic dogs is to achieve resolution of clinical signs:

a. **Thus, it is important to regularly monitor signs such as the volume of water drunk and body weight.**

b. **If the dog drinks >60 mL/kg/day or is lethargic or losing weight, adjustment of the insulin dose is probably required.**

3. **Owners of diabetic dogs should be encouraged to keep detailed records of their dog's progress** (Figure 15.7):

a. **Appetite, general demeanor, and behavior** should be recorded daily.

b. **Insulin dose and meal composition and amount consumed** should be recorded twice daily.

c. **Water intake over 24 h** should be measured at least once weekly:

1) **If more than one pet drinks from the same bowl, it is still useful to measure the volume drunk by all the animals.**

2) The diabetic dog typically is the reason for most of the variation in water consumed in multi-pet households.

d. **Urine glucose and ketones** should be measured at least once weekly:

1) **Persistent negative glucosuria might indicate an increased risk of hypoglycemia.**

2) Ketonuria usually indicates illness or very poor diabetic control.

e. **Body weight** should ideally be recorded once weekly, preferably always using the same scale.

4. **In addition to appraisal of the owner's insulin dosing technique, compliance of both the owner and the patient with the feeding recommendations must be routinely evaluated to ensure appropriate timing and consistency of the meals.** An approach that is often successful following each reappraisal is to recommend the "dose" of food along with the dose of insulin to educate the owner of the importance of carefully weighing or measuring the food in the same manner that they carefully prepare the dose of insulin.

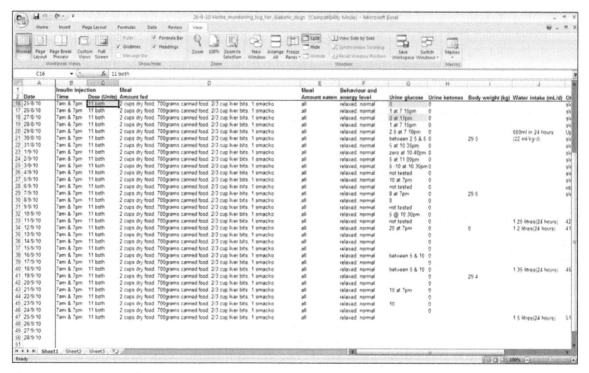

Figure 15.7   An example of a spreadsheet that can be used by an owner of a diabetic dog to record their pet's clinical progress.

L. **Measurement of long-term glycemia: fructosamine and glycosylated hemoglobin:**
1. Measurement of **fructosamine or glycosylated hemoglobin** is an additional method for assessing glycemic control.
2. Fructosamine and glycosylated hemoglobin concentrations provide **approximate measures of average blood glucose concentration over the preceding 2–4 weeks and 3–4 months**, respectively, and thus are indicators of longer-term diabetic control.
3. Measurement of either is **most useful when there is little available information about recent clinical signs** or when results of serial blood glucose measurements do not match with the reported clinical signs.
4. Monitoring the trends in serial measurements of fructosamine or glycosylated hemoglobin in an individual diabetic dog allows evaluation of glycemic response to management changes.
5. **A major limitation with these measures is that they represent average glycemia and give no information about the degree of fluctuation around that average:**
    a. Therefore, they **do not indicate the risk of hypoglycemia** on the current insulin regimen.
    b. It is recommended that an **additional monitoring tool, such as a serial blood glucose curve, be used to determine how to adjust insulin therapy.**
M. **Monitoring glucose concentrations at home:**
1. Some owners are able to perform **home serial blood glucose concentration curves:**
    a. **Single, sporadic measurements provide little useful clinical information** for monitoring glycemic control, with the exception of measurements taken when there are signs suggesting hypoglycemia or vague clinical signs of unknown origin. **Serial blood glucose concentration curves** that follow a similar protocol to those obtained in hospital provide the most accurate information for adjustment of insulin dose.
    b. As with blood glucose curves obtained in a hospital, **results must be related to the dog's clinical signs.**
    c. A practical approach is to **use knowledge of the dog's clinical signs to guide the timing of home-generated blood glucose curves.** For example, if there is marked variability in 24 hour water intake, owners can be advised to **perform a glucose curve during a period when the dog is not drinking much water and/or there is no glucosuria.** This approach would increase the chance of detecting hypoglycemia.

d. **Home-generated serial blood glucose curves are as reliable as hospital-generated curves**, and may provide better information in dogs affected by stress of hospital visits.

e. Home-generated serial blood glucose curves also demonstrate the same considerable **day-to-day variability** in glucose concentrations as hospital-generated curves, particularly in dogs that are not yet well controlled.

f. The **major advantages** of home-monitoring are:

    1) Measurements can be easily obtained at any time and can be repeated if equivocal results are obtained.

    2) Cost is minimal compared with a veterinary visit.

    3) The effect of hospitalization on appetite and stress hyperglycemia are avoided.

    4) Blood glucose can be promptly measured if there are signs suggestive of hypoglycemia.

g. Samples can be obtained either from the **marginal vein of the lateral pinna, by collection of capillary blood, or by direct venipuncture**, as described previously.

h. For successful integration in the pet's diabetic management, it is important that clinic staff take the time to educate the owner on use of the meter and allow the owner to practice obtaining samples from their pet to identify the best sites for that dog-owner combination:

    1) Once an owner is familiar with the technique, they usually need **practice with the dog at home** before they develop sufficient skill to generate a serial blood glucose curve.

    2) **Micromanagement with frequent adjustment of insulin dose should be avoided.**

    3) Owners who choose home monitoring often need to be advised against overzealous blood glucose measurement and interpreting the results themselves.

2. **Continuous interstitial glucose concentration monitoring systems can also be used** in the home environment and have **similar advantages and limitations** as when used on hospitalized patients:

a. **Continuous glucose monitoring systems that give results in real time** (e.g., the Guardian® REAL-Time CGMS, Medtronic) and systems that **provide data at the end of the monitoring period** (e.g., GlucoDay (Menarini Diagnostics) can both be used at home.

b. **Important advantages** of continuous monitoring systems over intermittent blood glucose measurement are that they **facilitate detection of brief periods of hypoglycemia** and **provide information overnight**.

c. **One limitation** is that the systems must be **calibrated with blood glucose concentration two to three times every 24 h**, so that there is still a requirement for blood sampling during monitoring.

d. Cost is another limitation, particularly the ongoing cost of the glucose sensors.

N. Hospital-generated **serial blood glucose concentration curves**:

1. **Serial blood glucose concentration curves are most useful in cases where the clinical history is inadequate and home glucose monitoring is not being performed.** However, it is important to recognize that, if used alone, they can be an unreliable clinical tool for evaluation of insulin dose in individual diabetic dogs because of high **day-to-day variability** in results and the impracticality of performing multi-day consecutive curves:

a. **Additional indicators of glycemic control**, such as changes in water intake, appetite, body weight, and urine glucose concentrations, should always be considered when appraising insulin dose.

b. The large day-to-day variability of the curves and the serious sequelae that might result from insulin overdose justify the need for a **conservative approach to dosage recommendation**. For example, when blood glucose measurements and assessment of clinical signs indicate that there is very good glycemic control, dosage increases should typically be limited to increments of 0.5 or 1.0 U of insulin.

2. One of the **principal reasons** for performing a serial blood glucose curve in a diabetic dog is to **evaluate whether the insulin dose can be increased without risk of inducing hypoglycemia**:

a. The risk of hypoglycemia is particularly important whenever recommending **insulin doses >1 U/kg**.

b. Although assessment of clinical signs is valuable for identifying dogs with poor glycemic control, it is often not effective for identifying dogs at risk of clinical hypoglycemia.

3. The **standard protocol** for generating a serial blood glucose curve in a veterinary clinic is:

a. **Admit the dog into the clinic before administration of the morning insulin injection.**

b. Obtain a baseline blood glucose reading.

Table 15.2   Guidelines for evaluation of serial blood glucose concentration curves in diabetic dogs.

If the nadir is <55 mg/dL (3 mmol/L), or the dog has shown clinical signs of hypoglycemia	Decrease the 12 hourly insulin dose by 50%
If the nadir is 55–90 mg/dL (3–5 mmol/L), or if either pre-insulin blood glucose value is <180 mg/dL (10 mmol/L)	Decrease the 12 hourly insulin dose by 20% (rounded down to nearest unit of insulin)
If the final pre-insulin blood glucose is <90 mg/dL (5 mmol/L)	Withhold insulin overnight and feed the dog as usual. Decrease the 12 hourly insulin dose by 20% (rounded down to the nearest unit of insulin) the following morning. If the pre-insulin blood glucose is <55 mg/dL (3 mmol/L), decrease the 12 hourly insulin dose by 50%.
If the nadir is 90–145 mg/dL (5–8 mmol/L) and both pre-insulin blood glucose values are >180 mg/dL (10 mmol/L)	The dog likely has optimal clinical control and does not require an insulin dosage adjustment.
If the nadir is >145 mg/dL (8 mmol/L), and the pre-insulin blood glucose values are >180 mg/dL (10 mmol/L)	Increase the 12 hourly insulin dose by 20% (rounded down to nearest unit of insulin).
If very high blood glucose measurements are recorded in an insulin-treated diabetic dog, e.g., values in excess of 550 mg/dL (30 mmol/L)	The possibility of insulin resistance should be considered if insulin dose is >1 U/kg.

The findings of a serial blood glucose curve should always be related to the history, physical examination findings, and changes in body weight before a final decision is made regarding insulin dose. If a diabetic dog is not lethargic, has a stable body weight, has no ketonuria, is drinking <60 mL/kg/day, and glycemic control is very good, but an increase or decrease in insulin dosage is suggested by the serial blood glucose curve, then insulin dosage adjustments of no more than 1 U are advised, regardless of the dose the dog is receiving.

   c. The **usual insulin dose and meal is then given.**
   d. **Blood glucose measurements are obtained every 2 h until the next insulin injection is due.**
4. Having the owner administer the morning insulin injection provides an opportunity **to review injection technique and correct any problems.**
5. If the dog refuses to eat, subsequent blood glucose values are likely to be lower than if the dog eats normally:
   a. In this situation, **it is probably best to cancel the serial blood glucose curve** on that day and reschedule.
   b. The protocol can be modified on the next occasion to allow **the owner to take the dog home or to a less stressful environment after the baseline blood glucose reading is obtained and the usual meal fed there.**
   c. The dog should be returned to the hospital before the next blood glucose reading is due.
   d. **Alternatively, the morning pre-insulin blood glucose reading can be omitted** from the serial blood glucose curve and the dog brought to the hospital after the morning insulin injection and meal have been given at home.
6. Guidelines for evaluation of serial blood glucose curves in diabetic dogs are primarily based on the **nadir,** or lowest blood glucose reading obtained, and the two **pre-insulin blood glucose values** (Table 15.2):
   a. The first pre-insulin blood glucose value is the reading obtained before the morning insulin injection:
      1) The **pre-insulin blood glucose values provide an indication of the likely blood glucose level when the dog is due for an insulin injection at home.**
      2) Appropriate adjustment of dose using dosing guidelines (Table 15.2) is important to avoid hypoglycemia as the effects of the previous insulin injection might overlap with the next insulin dose and produce an additive effect.
   b. The second pre-insulin blood glucose is the sample taken before the next insulin injection is due, usually 12 h after the first.
   c. The **nadir** (lowest) concentration, together with consideration of pre-insulin blood glucose concentration, provides an indication of the **maximal insulin dose that can be used to avoid hypoglycemia:**

      1) **The nadir can occur at any point in the blood glucose curve,** including just prior to an insulin injection.

      2) The time to nadir influences dose recommendations but can vary considerably, even in the same dog over consecutive visits.

7. **Severe episodes of hypoglycemia following insulin overdose can result in compensatory hyperglycemia, also termed the Somogyi phenomenon:**

    a. The hyperglycemia sometimes **persists for several days.**

    b. Serial blood glucose assessment performed shortly after an episode of clinical hypoglycemia may result in a curve similar to that obtained following insulin underdosing.

8. **If there is ever any doubt about the interpretation of a serial blood glucose curve, it is always safest to err on the side of caution and decrease the dog's insulin dose.**

9. Home measurement of blood glucose concentrations at the time of vague or suggestive signs of hypoglycemia is valuable in differentiating subsequent compensatory hyperglycemia from other causes of hyperglycemia.

O. **Insulin resistance:**

1. The majority of uncomplicated diabetic dogs are stabilized on an insulin dose of approximately 0.5 U/kg and few require doses >1.0 U/kg.

2. **Insulin resistance should be suspected at insulin doses exceeding 1.5 U/kg.**

3. Errors in insulin handling or administration should be differentiated from insulin resistance and occasionally can mimic insulin resistance.

4. The **major differential diagnoses for insulin resistance are:**

    a. Concurrent disease or drug therapy.

    b. Compensatory hyperglycemia secondary to insulin overdose (Somogyi phenomenon).

5. **Errors in insulin handling or administration:**

    a. **Insulin can become inactivated** if exposed to temperatures >30°C (>86°F) or light for prolonged periods or if shaken vigorously:

      1) Most insulin suspensions must be **gently mixed prior to administration** or doses might vary greatly. It is recommended that Vetsulin (USA)/Caninsulin (elsewhere) be well mixed prior to dosing to ensure accuracy.

      2) **An expedient method of ruling out the possibility of inactivated insulin** when investigating apparent insulin resistance is to change to a new vial of insulin.

    b. **Administration issues:**

      1) A wide range of insulin syringes are available and **inadvertently changing to a different type of syringe** can lead to dosing errors.

      2) Dosing errors are less frequent with insulin dosing pens than with needles and syringes.

      3) However, insulin-**dosing pens must be primed prior to administration of each dose to ensure there is no air in the system.**

      4) It is also important to **check that the dosing dial has returned to the "zero" position after each dose.**

      5) Although experienced owners of diabetic dogs rarely report difficulty with administration of insulin to their pet, it is important to **review their injection technique for errors** whenever insulin resistance is investigated.

6. Concurrent disease or drug therapy causing insulin resistance:

    a. May be suspected based on **history and physical examination findings** and can be further investigated by performing **hematology, serum biochemistry, urinalysis, and microbial culture and sensitivity of the urine.**

    b. **Almost any concurrent disease can cause insulin resistance** that affects diabetic control.

    c. **Hyperadrenocorticism and hypothyroidism** are two important causes of insulin resistance in diabetic dogs, and they can present a diagnostic challenge in a diabetic dog.

    d. **Systemic and topical corticosteroids** are the drugs most commonly associated with insulin resistance.

    e. **Obesity** causes insulin resistance.

    f. Other causes of insulin resistance can include **liver disease, dental infections, neoplasia, organ failure, and hyperlipidemia.**

g. Anti-insulin antibodies occur in some insulin treated dogs but their clinical significance is unclear, and they are only very occasionally suspected as a cause of insulin resistance. In humans, they more often prolong the duration of insulin action than result in insulin resistance.

h. Insulin resistance and poor glycemic control lasting several days is often associated with episodes of active pancreatitis in dogs with underlying chronic pancreatitis. Dogs may be inappetent and/or have vomiting associated with the episodes:

i. Once a cause of insulin resistance has resolved or is removed, insulin sensitivity can be expected to improve and there will be increased risk of hypoglycemia unless the insulin dose is decreased.

7. Compensatory hyperglycemia secondary to insulin overdose (Somogyi phenomenon) is one of the most common causes of insulin resistance in diabetic dogs:

a. There is typically a **period of good glycemic control** that is followed by deteriorating glycemic control despite increasing insulin doses:

1) The period of good glycemic control may be very brief.

2) It is sometimes missed, **especially if dose adjustment is based only on results of serial blood glucose concentration curves without careful consideration of the dog's clinical signs.**

b. In **insulin**-treated diabetic people, hypoglycemic events occur more frequently during the night than during the day:

1) The same may be true for dogs.

2) **Therefore, insulin-induced hypoglycemia may be missed with only day time monitoring. Continuous subcutaneous glucose monitors are a useful diagnostic aid for detecting night time hypoglycemia** (Figure 15.3).

c. Compensatory hyperglycemia often persists for several days following insulin-induced hypoglycemia.

d. For diabetic dogs receiving insulin doses >1.5 U/kg where administration/dosing errors and concurrent disease/drugs have been ruled out, **it is recommended that the insulin dose be decreased to 0.5 U/kg and the response to the change monitored:**

1) If insulin resistance was due to compensatory hyperglycemia secondary to insulin overdose, **there is typically marked clinical improvement within 1–2 weeks.**

2) If there is another cause of insulin resistance, **clinical signs typically become much worse within 24 h; the previous insulin dose can be resumed** and the investigation for another cause continued.

P. **Excessively short- or long-duration of insulin action may result in poor glycemic control** with ensuing hyperglycemia and/or hypoglycemia:

1. Excessively short- or long-duration of insulin action may be suspected based on results of serial blood glucose testing.

2. **Serial blood glucose curves vary from day-to-day along with apparent duration of action.**

3. Excessively short duration of insulin action:

a. The diagnosis must be **supported by compatible clinical signs such as polydipsia;** in some dogs polydipsia repeatedly occurs for only a few hours before an insulin injection is due.

b. Must be **differentiated from compensatory hyperglycemia secondary to insulin-induced hypoglycemia.**

c. Can be associated with **insulin resistance and investigation for concurrent disease** is indicated.

d. If short duration is confirmed and insulin overdose and concurrent disease ruled out, **the same insulin preparation may be administered every 8 h or a different insulin preparation with an expected longer duration may be trialed.**

4. **Long duration of insulin action as a cause of hyper- and/or hypoglycemia:**

a. Usually responds to a decrease in the **12 hourly insulin dose.**

b. It is not usually necessary to decrease the frequency of insulin administration.

Q. **Management of concurrent chronic pancreatitis:**

1. Chronic pancreatitis in diabetic animals can have **important clinical implications:**

a. In addition to the **possibility of episodes of acute pancreatitis,** progressive destruction of both endocrine and exocrine tissue will result in loss of insulin-secreting β cells, glucagon-secreting α cells, and exocrine acinar cells:

  1) Therefore, **the glucagon counter-regulatory response to hypoglycemia might be reduced.**

  2) Avoidance of insulin overdose is one of the primary goals of treatment of diabetic animals and is especially important in patients suspected to have chronic pancreatitis.

 b. Loss of body weight and condition despite polyphagia are presenting signs for both diabetes mellitus and EPI:

  1) If weight loss continues despite adequate glycemic control, the possibility of concurrent EPI should be considered.

  2) Evaluation of frequency of defecation (more than twice a day) **and fecal consistency** (may or may not be normal) **can assist with diagnosis.**

  3) Serum TLI concentration should be measured and/or a therapeutic trial with pancreatic enzyme supplementation performed (Figure 15.8).

  4) The goal is to **identify EPI early in the clinical course** so pancreatic enzyme supplementation can be started before excessive body condition is lost.

2. Reducing the risk of pancreatitis in diabetic dogs:

 a. Hypertriglyceridemia has been proposed as a possible inciting cause of canine pancreatitis:

  1) Increased serum triglyceride concentrations are commonly seen in diabetic dogs.

  2) Thus, the diabetic state might also be a risk factor for pancreatitis.

 b. Restriction of dietary fat is an important part of the management of hypertriglyceridemia in dogs and is recommended for diabetic dogs **when hypertriglyceridemia cannot be corrected by exogenous insulin therapy:**

  1) Fasting serum triglyceride concentrations can be monitored to identify persistent hypertriglyceridemia and to assess the response to feeding a fat-restricted diet (Figure 15.9).

  2) Dietary fat restriction (i.e., <30% ME) should be recommended **for all diabetic dogs with fasting serum triglyceride concentration** >500 mg/dL (>5.5 mmol/L).

  3) For diabetic dogs with good glycemic control, dietary fat restriction to <30% ME is recommended if fasting serum triglyceride concentration is >400 mg/dL (>4.4 mmol/L.)

  4) Fasting triglyceride levels are expected to decrease in response to dietary fat restriction.

  5) Therefore, if fasting serum triglyceride concentration is >400 mg/dL (>4.4 mmol/L) when the dog is being fed a diet with <30% ME fat, further restriction of dietary fat to <20% ME is recommended.

 c. An alternative or adjunct to monitoring fasting serum triglyceride concentrations is to **monitor postprandial concentrations:**

  1) Fasting triglyceride concentration might not accurately predict the postprandial peak concentration in dogs, which could be an important limitation when monitoring response to dietary fat restriction.

  2) As serial postprandial blood sampling is routine in diabetic dogs when assessing glycemia, it is convenient to also evaluate triglycerides at the same time:

   a) Point-of-care meters such as the CardioChek PA test system can be used.

   b) Peak blood triglyceride concentration will most likely occur 2–6 h after a typical meal formulated for adult maintenance, so **blood triglyceride concentrations should be measured at 2, 4, and 6 h after a meal.**

VII. Prognosis

A. **Well-controlled diabetic dogs have a similar chance of survival to that of non-diabetic dogs of the same age and gender,** although **death is still more frequent during the first 6 months of therapy.**

B. The **case-fatality rate** of diabetic dogs seen at referral veterinary hospitals in North America has **decreased from 37% to 5% over the past 30 years:**

 1. In a review of diabetic dogs 27 years ago, 50% were alive 2 months after initial diagnosis and went on to be successfully managed, often for periods of several years.

 2. Major improvements in the level of care and therapy available for diabetic dogs have been achieved since then, and the survival rate is now much higher.

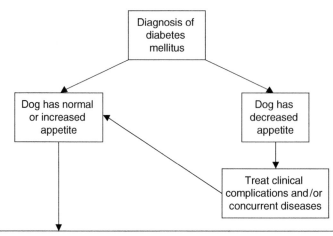
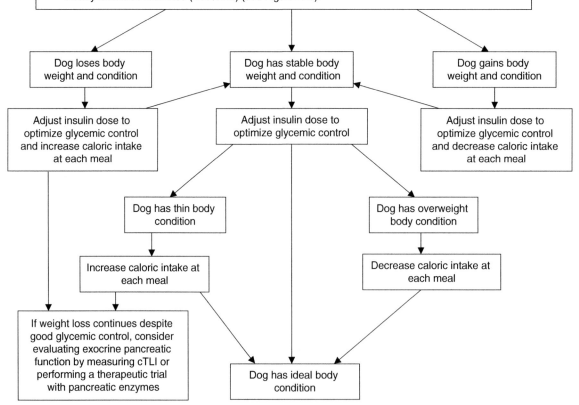

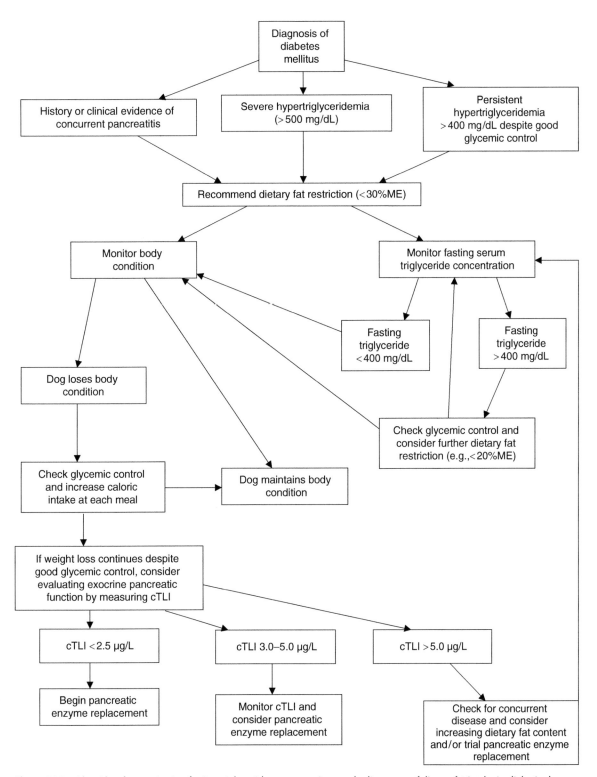

Figure 15.9   Algorithm for monitoring fasting triglyceride concentrations and adjustment of dietary fat intake in diabetic dogs.

VIII. Prevention

A.   Type 1 diabetes mellitus in dogs is likely caused by multiple interacting genetic and environmental influences and there is no information on prevention of this form of diabetes.

B.   Diestrus and gestational diabetes can be prevented by neutering of female dogs. For entire bitches, the risk of developing diabetes might be decreased by maintenance of lean body condition.

C.   There is little available information on prevention of chronic pancreatitis leading to diabetes in dogs. It is possible that maintenance of lean body condition and early treatment of hyperlipidemia might decrease the incidence or progression of chronic pancreatitis in dogs.

References and Further Readings

Alejandro R, Feldman E, Shienvold FL, et al. Advances in canine diabetes mellitus research: Etiopathology and results of islet transplantation. *J Am Vet Med Assoc* 1988;193:1050–1055.

Briggs CE, Nelson RW, Feldman EC, et al. Reliability of history and physical examination findings for assessing control of glycemia in dogs with diabetes mellitus: 53 cases (1995–1998). *J Am Vet Med Assoc* 2000;217:48–53.

Casella M, Wess G, Reusch CE. Measurement of capillary blood glucose concentration by pet owners: A new tool in the management of diabetes mellitus. *J Am Anim Hosp Assoc* 2002;38:239–245.

Catchpole B, Ristic JM, Fleeman LM, et al. Canine diabetes mellitus: Can we learn new tricks from old dogs? *Diabetologia* 2005;48:1948–1956.

Davison LJ, Herrtage ME, Catchpole B. Study of 253 dogs in the United Kingdom with diabetes mellitus. *Vet Record* 2005;156:467–471.

Davison LJ, Slater LA, Herrtage ME, et al. Evaluation of a continuous glucose monitoring system in diabetic dogs. *J Small Anim Practice* 2003;44;435–442.

Davison LJ, Weenink SM, Christie MR, et al. Autoantibodies to GAD65 and IA-2 in canine diabetes mellitus. *Vet Immunol Immunopathol* 2008;126(1–2):83–90.

Fall T, Hedhammar A, Wallberg A, et al. Remission of diestrus diabetes in Elkhounds is predicted by glucose concentrations at diagnosis and by time to surgery from onset of clinical signs (Abstract). In: *ECVIM-CA Congress*, abstract 95, Toulouse, France. 2010, p. 259.

Fall T, Johansson KS, Juberget A, et al. Gestational diabetes mellitus in 13 dogs. *J Vet Intern Med* 2008:22(6):1296–1300.

Feldman EC, Nelson RW (eds). Canine diabetes mellitus. In: *Canine and Feline Endocrinology and Reproduction.* St Louis: Elsevier, 2004, pp. 486–538.

Fleeman LM, Rand JS. Management of canine diabetes. *Vet Clin North Am Small Anim Pract* 2001:31:855–880.

Fleeman LM, Rand JS. Evaluation of day-to-day variability of serial blood glucose curves in diabetic dogs. *J Am Vet Med Assoc* 2003;222(3):317–321.

Fleeman LM, Rand JS. Diabetes mellitus: Nutritional strategies. In: Pibot P, Biourge V, Elliott D, eds. *Encyclopedia of Canin Canine Nutrition.* Paris, France: Aniwa Publishing, 2006, pp. 192–215.

Fleeman LM, Rand JS, Markwell PJ. Lack of advantage of high-fibre, moderate-carbohydrate diets in dogs with stabilised diabetes. *J Small Anim Practice* 2009;50: 604–614.

Fleeman LM, Rand JS, Morton JM. Pharmacokinetics and pharmacodynamics of porcine insulin zinc suspension in eight diabetic dogs. *Vet Rec* 2009;164:232–237.

Ford SL, Rand JS, Ghormley TM, et al. Evaluation of detemir insulin in diabetic dogs managed with home blood glucose monitoring (Abstract). In: *ACVIM Forum*, Anaheim, CA, USA, 2010, pp. 442.

Fracassi F, Boretti F, Sieber-Ruckstuhl N, et al. Use of insulin glargine in dogs with diabetes mellitus (Abstract). In: *ECVIM-CA Congress Proceedings*, abstract 99. Toulouse, France, 2010, p. 260.

Guptill L, Glickman L, Glickman N. Time trends and risk factors for diabetes mellitus in dogs: Analysis of Veterinary Medical Data Base records (1970–1999). *Vet J* 2003;165;240–247.

Hess RS, Saunders M, van Winkle TJ. et al. Concurrent disorders in dogs with diabetes mellitus: 221 cases (1993–1998). *J Am Vet Med Assoc* 2000:217(8):1166–1173.

Rand JS, Fleeman LM, Farrow HA, et al. Canine and feline diabetes mellitus: Nature or nurture? *J Nutr* 2004:134:2072S–2080S.

Reineke EL, Fletcher DJ, King LG, et al. Accuracy of a continuous glucose monitoring system in dogs and cats with diabetic ketoacidosis. *J Vet Emerg Crit Care* 2010;20(3):303–312.

Thoresen SI, Lorenzen FH. Treatment of diabetes mellitus in dogs using isophane insulin penfills and the use of serum fructosamine assays to diagnose and monitor the disease. *Acta Vet Scand* 1997;38(2):137–146.

Wiedmeyer CE, Johnson PJ, Cohn LA, et al. Evaluation of a continuous glucose monitoring system for use in dogs, cats, and horses. *J Am Vet Med Assoc* 2003:223:987–992.

CHAPTER 16

Feline Diabetes Mellitus

Jacquie Rand

Pathogenesis

- Hyperglycemia occurs as a result of a relative or absolute deficiency of insulin.
- Most cases are presumed to have type 2 diabetes.
- Other specific types of diabetes occur secondary to acromegaly, hyperadrenocorticism, and pancreatitis and account for a minority of cases in general practice.

Classical Signs

- Most cats are >8 years of age, with a peak onset of 10–13 years of age.
- Moderate to marked polyuria/polydipsia, usually of 2–12 weeks duration prior to diagnosis.
- Weight loss, polyphagia, or inappetence.
- More often overweight, but may be normal weight or underweight.

Diagnosis

- Persistent hyperglycemia with glycosuria.

Treatment

- Long-acting insulin, low-carbohydrate diet, and normalization of body condition.

Prognosis

- Excellent with appropriate therapy if type 2 diabetes; with comorbidities such as pancreatitis or acromegaly, prognosis is good to guarded depending on therapeutic options available.

I. Pathogenesis

A. Most diabetic cats appear to have **type 2 diabetes mellitus**, previously called adult-onset diabetes or noninsulin-dependent diabetes:

   1. **Type 2 diabetes is characterized** by decreased insulin secretion, insulin resistance, and amyloid deposition in the pancreatic islets:

Clinical Endocrinology of Companion Animals, First Edition. Edited by Jacquie Rand.
© 2013 John Wiley & Sons, Inc. Published 2013 by John Wiley & Sons, Inc.

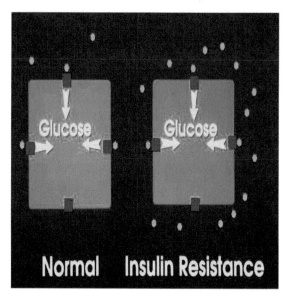

Figure 16.1   Insulin resistance requires more insulin (stars) to be secreted to achieve the same glucose uptake (arrows) into cells (large rectangles) via insulin receptors (small squares) to maintain blood glucose concentrations in the normal range compared with when insulin sensitivity is normal. (With permission from Rand JS.)

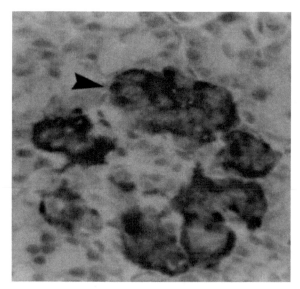

Figure 16.2   Normal pancreatic islet with surrounding exocrine tissue. Beta cells are stained in the islet to show the hormone amylin. (From Rand JS, Martin GJ. Management of feline diabetes mellitus. *Endocrinology* 2001:31(5):881–913. With permission. The Veterinary Clinics of North America Small Animal Practice, Elsevier.)

a. When there is insulin resistance (Figure 16.1), more insulin is required to maintain blood glucose concentrations in the normal range compared with when insulin sensitivity is normal. Prolonged demand for increased insulin secretion from the beta cells to overcome insulin resistance eventually leads to beta cell failure.

b. Deposition of amyloid in pancreatic islets is a characteristic finding in diabetic cats and contributes to beta cell loss (Figures 16.2 and 16.3). The amyloid is a precipitate of the hormone amylin which is cosecreted with insulin from beta cells.

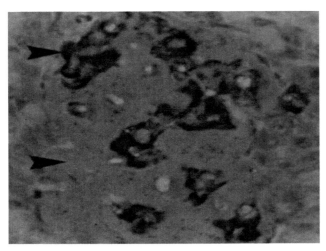

Figure 16.3   Pancreatic islet from a diabetic cat showing extensive amyloid deposition damaging beta cells and reducing insulin secretion. (From Rand JS, Martin GJ. Management of feline diabetes mellitus. *Endocrinology* 2001:31(5):881–913. With permission. The Veterinary Clinics of North America Small Animal Practice, Elsevier.)

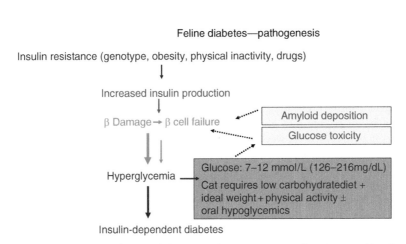

Figure 16.4   Mechanism for development of type 2 diabetes. Insulin resistance stimulates increased insulin secretion to maintain blood glucose in the normal range. With time, chronic hypersecretion of insulin damages the beta cells and blood glucose concentration starts to increase. If this mild increase in blood glucose is detected as being persistent and not attributed to stress, with appropriate management, glucose will normalize. To facilitate the compromised beta cells to secrete sufficient insulin to maintain euglycemia, body condition should be kept lean, a low-carbohydrate diet fed, and physical activity encouraged to increase insulin sensitivity. If this mild hyperglycemia is not detected, persistent low-grade hyperglycemia will further suppress beta cell function through the phenomena of glucose toxicity. Blood glucose will continue to rise, exacerbating glucose toxicity and diabetes ensues, which in most cats is initially insulin dependent. (From Marshall and Rand, 2009. With permission.)

B. **Risk factors for diabetes include** old age, male gender, obesity, physical inactivity, confinement indoors, breed (Burmese in Australia, New Zealand and the UK; Maine coon, domestic longhair, Russian blue, and Siamese in the USA), and repeated or long-acting steroid or megestrol acetate administration. Many of these risk factors cause insulin resistance and increase the demand on beta cells to produce insulin (Figure 16.4).
C. Prevalence of diabetes in cats in North America, the UK, and Australia is approximately 1:81 to 1:250 cats depending on the population studied; prevalence in Burmese cats in Australasia is approximately 1 in 50 cats, with 1 in 10 cats that are 8 years of age or older affected.

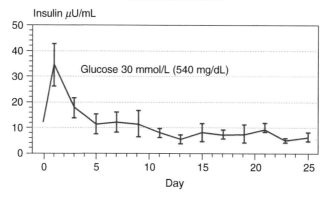

Figure 16.5   Insulin secretion measured in healthy cats over 25 days after an IV glucose infusion was begun at day 0. Persistently high blood glucose concentrations in the range typically seen in newly diagnosed diabetic cats (e.g., 540 mg/dL; 30 mmol/L) causes rapid suppression of insulin secretion from beta cells even in healthy cats, to levels seen in newly diagnosed diabetic cats. This phenomena is called glucose toxicity. Eventually, it leads to beta cell damage and loss of beta cells. (With permission from Rand JS.)

D. At diagnosis, **endogenous insulin secretion is usually very low**:
  1. This is probably because of the combined effects of:
     a. Impaired insulin secretion associated with the beta cell defect causing type 2 diabetes.
     b. Amyloid deposition in the islets which is toxic to beta cells.
     c. Suppression of insulin secretion by glucose toxicity (Figure 16.5).
E. **Glucose toxicity is defined as suppression of insulin secretion by persistently (>24-h duration) high blood glucose.** Good glycemic control is essential to reverse glucose toxicity:
  1. Suppression of insulin secretion by glucose toxicity is **initially functional and reversible,** later it results in structural changes in beta cells. **Over weeks and months, changes become irreversible,** and beta cells are lost.
F. Some cats have **other specific types of diabetes.** Their diabetes results from **another disease process causing decreased insulin secretion or impaired insulin action (insulin resistance).** In primary accession practice in Western countries, other specific types of diabetes account for approximately 5–10% of cases, whereas in referral practice they are more common and account for 20% or more of cases:
  1. **Growth hormone–producing tumors (acromegaly)** appear to be the most common other specific type of diabetes and are **underdiagnosed. Referral institutions** in the UK and USA report acromegaly in approximately **25–30% of diabetic cats;** the high incidence likely reflects the populations studied.
  2. **Pancreatic neoplasia** is a significant cause of diabetes in referred populations of diabetic cats in North America, accounting for as many as 9–18% of feline diabetics necropsied at referral institutions.
  3. **Histological** evidence of **pancreatitis** is commonly associated with feline diabetes (50% of diabetic cats have pancreatitis lesions at necropsy):
     a. In most cats, pancreatitis is not severe enough to cause diabetes alone, but probably contributes to some loss of beta cells.
     b. A small number of cats appear to have diabetes as a result of end-stage pancreatitis.
  4. **Hyperadrenocorticism is an infrequent** specific type of diabetes associated with insulin resistance, but is more common in the cases seen in referral practice.
  5. **Hyperthyroidism** results in glucose intolerance and insulin hypersecretion, which may be the result of insulin resistance in the liver since insulin sensitivity of peripheral tissues seems unaltered. Glucose intolerance and insulin hypersecretion deteriorates in some cats following treatment of hyperthyroidism, which might be the result of weight gain and resultant obesity. In prediabetic cats, the superimposed glucose intolerance of hyperthyroidism could precipitate overt diabetes.
G. **Chronic kidney disease is relatively common** in diabetic cats, firstly because most are **aged,** and secondly, there is increasing evidence that suggests that **diabetic nephropathy** is also a feature of the disease in cats, as

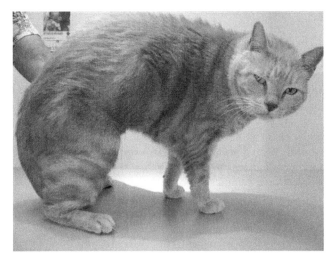

Figure 16.6 A plantigrade stance and/or muscle weakness is observed in a significant proportion of newly diagnosed diabetic cats. Presence of a plantigrade stance is negatively associated with the probability of remission, likely because it indicates long-standing hyperglycemia. (Photo from R. Marshall. With permission.)

is in humans. In a study of 55 diabetic cats, the proportion of persistently azotemic cats increased with age, with the highest frequency (31%) in the ≥10 to <15 years age group, but a surprising 18% of cats had persistent azotemia in the 5 to <10 year age group. Compared to similarly aged sick cats, diabetic cats are statistically more likely to have evidence of microalbuminemia and proteinuria, and histopathologic lesions consistent with diabetic nephropathy have been reported in diabetic cats.

II. Signalment
A. Cats are typically ≥8 years of age and with a peak age of onset of 10–13 years of age.
B. Diabetic cats are more often male than female (2:1 ratio), except for Burmese cats.
C. Body condition is more often overweight (40%) than normal (35%) or underweight (25%).
D. Burmese cats are overrepresented in the UK, Australia, and New Zealand; in the USA, Maine coon, domestic longhair, Russian blue, and Siamese cats are overrepresented.

III. Clinical Signs
A. Earliest signs are **polyuria and polydipsia** (80% of cats), and nocturia and urinary incontinence may be reported.
B. **Weight loss (70%) occurs and is accompanied by increased appetite.** However, polyphagia is only reported by a minority of owners (<20%) at the time of diagnosis.
C. At initial diagnosis, some cats have **decreased appetite** (50%) and are depressed and others are **polyphagic.**
D. **Lethargy or depression** (50%) may be present. Other cats are alert at presentation.
E. **Muscle wasting** (50%) and **weakness** are often present and may be evidenced as reluctance or inability to jump.
F. **Dehydration** (50%) is common in cats that are lethargic and inappetent.
G. **Vomiting** occurs in one-third of cats, but is usually infrequent.
H. **Hepatomegaly** (20%) from hepatic lipidosis and occasionally jaundice may be present.
I. **Rear limb weakness or plantigrade posture** (hocks touching the ground) is present in approximately 50% of diabetic cats secondary to diabetic neuropathy. Weakness is more common than plantigrade posture (Figure 16.6).
J. Acetone odor, which has a similar odor to nail polish remover or acetone, may be evident on the breath, and occurs on average 5 days before ketonuria is detected.
K. Poor unkempt (50%) scurfy hair coat may be evident.

IV. Diagnosis

A. In most cats, a single **blood glucose concentration measurement of >20 mmol/L (360 mg/dL) is diagnostic** of diabetes. However, some sick or very stressed cats occasionally have glucose concentrations >20 mmol/L (360 mg/dL).

B. If **blood glucose is 12–20 mmol/L (216–360 mg/dL), persistent hyperglycemia** must be demonstrated to differentiate diabetes mellitus from acute stress-induced hyperglycemia. Retest cats 4–6 h later and if still hyperglycemic, retest the next day to confirm persistent hyperglycemia. The **presence of typical clinical signs** (polyuria, polydipsia, and polyphagia with weight loss) with **glycosuria** and demonstration of either **increased plasma fructosamine, glycated hemoglobin, beta-hydroxybutyrate,** or **ketonuria** are also useful for differentiating diabetes from stress-induced hyperglycemia.

C. Plasma **fructosamine >400 μmol/L** is indicative of diabetes mellitus. However, some diabetic cats have a normal fructosamine concentration and, occasionally, nondiabetic sick cats have mildly increased fructosamine concentrations. Fructosamine increases above the reference range (400 μmol/L) within 7–10 days of marked hyperglycemia (e.g., 30 mmol/L; 540 mg/dL) and takes 3 weeks to plateau:

    1. One study showed that fructosamine concentration was only intermittently above the upper limit of the reference range in cats with persistent hyperglycemia of 17 mmol/L (mg/dL) for 6 weeks.

    2. Measurement of fructosamine is most useful in situations where the clinical history is poor. However, assessing urine for glucose and ketones and hospitalizing the cat and repeating blood glucose measurements later may be simpler, quicker, and more informative for obtaining a diagnosis. Retest blood glucose 4–6 h later, and if still hyperglycemic and ketonuria is absent, retest the next day to confirm persistent hyperglycemia. The presence of ketonuria and hyperglycemia has close to a 100% specificity for diabetes mellitus.

D. **Glycosylated hemoglobin** (HbA1c) has been used for both diagnosis and monitoring of diabetic cats, but is less commonly used than fructosamine. It reflects blood glucose concentration over the previous 6–8 weeks. Some veterinary laboratories provide routine analysis and there are also point-of-care meters available. There is considerable variation in the literature on the reference range in cats, depending on the assay used. As with fructosamine, there is some overlap in values between normal and diabetic cats, especially those with more acute onset of signs or with less severe hyperglycemia.

E. **Persistent hyperglycemia** longer than 24 h is associated with diabetes mellitus in nearly all cats. Demonstration of **persistent hyperglycemia** (≥10 mmol/L; 180 mg/dL) **unassociated with acute stress or concomitant serious illness is diagnostic.** Diabetic cats with blood glucose below the renal threshold (14–16 mmol/L; 250–290 mg/dL) will have no or minimal signs of diabetes:

    1. Occasionally, **transient hyperglycemia** longer than 24 h duration occurs **with serious illness** and resolves within a few days. These cats likely have underlying impaired glucose tolerance:

        a. Illness-associated hyperglycemia rarely results in blood glucose concentrations >19 mmol/L (342 mg/dL).

    2. If **persistent (≥24h) hyperglycemia** (>12 mmol/L; 216 mg/dL) is present in a **sick cat,** begin treatment with appropriate doses of insulin, even if it is not clear if the hyperglycemia is illness associated.

    3. **Hyperglycemia longer than 24 h suppresses insulin secretion, and therefore should be managed promptly.**

F. Plasma **beta-hydroxybutyrate >1 mmol/L (10 mg/dL)** is indicative of diabetes mellitus. However, some diabetic cats have normal plasma beta-hydroxybutyrate:

    a. A **urine dipstick** may be used with **serum or heparinized plasma to detect ketonemia.** A positive test indicates ketonemia. It detects mainly oxaloacetate rather than beta-hydroxybutyrate, the predominant ketone in cats.

    b. **Ketonemia** detected by laboratory measurement of **beta-hydroxybutyrate** occurs within about **2 weeks of marked hyperglycemia.**

    c. **Ketonuria detectable with a urine dipstick** occurs approximately **5 days** after plasma beta-hydroxybutyrate exceeds the renal threshold and is measurable in urine.

V. Differential Diagnoses

A. **Stress hyperglycemia results from struggling or illness. Beware of misdiagnosis** in cats with stress hyperglycemia from illness or struggling, which also have concomitant disease that produces similar signs to diabetes mellitus, for example, renal failure or hyperthyroidism:

1. **Stress hyperglycemia associated with struggling can increase blood glucose** by as much as **10 mmol/L (180 mg/dL)** and result in transient hyperglycemia. However, blood glucose concentration is generally <10 mmol/L (180 mg/dL) within 4–6 h if the cat is hospitalized and further struggling does not occur.
2. **Stress hyperglycemia associated with illness** may persist for several days and exceed 20 mmol/L (360 mg/dL). If blood glucose remains elevated in a sick cat for 12–24 h, treat the cat with appropriate doses of insulin and closely monitor blood glucose.

B. **Hyperthyroidism** may produce similar signs of weight loss, polyphagia, and polyuria/polydipsia in an old cat. Generally the polydipsia in hyperthyroidism is less pronounced. Elevated thyroxine concentration is diagnostic, but in sick cats with hyperthyroidism, thyroxine concentration may be high end of the normal range.

VI. Treatment

A. **General principles:**
1. **The primary goal of therapy** in a newly diagnosed cat is to achieve euglycemia with **remission of insulin therapy** (called diabetic remission).
2. Cats in which remission is not possible, the primary **goals** are to **resolve the clinical signs of diabetes** and to **avoid** life-threatening **clinical hypoglycemia.**

B. **Diabetic remission:**
1. **Achieving noninsulin dependence or diabetic remission** improves the health and quality of life for the cat, decreases the cost and inconvenience for the owner, and should be the **main goal determining choice of therapy** in newly diagnosed diabetic cats.
2. Depending on the treatment implemented, 20–90% of newly diagnosed diabetic cats will undergo remission of their diabetes in 1–4 months (mean 2 months), if good glycemic control is achieved.
3. **Early control of hyperglycemia** is a **critical** factor in achieving **diabetic remission**. Cats started on an intensive protocol of glycemic control within 6 months of diagnosis were significantly more likely to achieve diabetic remission (84% remission rate) than those intensively controlled later than 6 months (34% remission, $p = 0.0002$).
4. Excellent glycemic control facilitates diabetic remission by enabling beta cells to recover from glucose toxicity. Excellent glycemic control is aided by use of **long-acting insulin, especially glargine and detemir** administered twice daily, and a low-carbohydrate diet, together with careful **monitoring of blood glucose concentration** and appropriate dose adjustments:
   a. **Remission rates of approximately 90%** or more can be achieved in **newly diagnosed diabetic cats** treated with **glargine or detemir,** provided blood glucose is monitored closely (at least once a week) and the insulin dose adjusted to achieve excellent glycemic control.
5. Remission is more **common in diabetic cats recently treated with insulin-antagonistic drugs,** such as megestrol acetate or long-acting steroids, and cats without signs of diabetic neuropathy.
6. Other factors associated with remission are mean blood glucose <16 mmol/L (290 mg/dL) within 3 weeks of initiation of treatment and older age of cat. Cats less likely to achieve remission had increased cholesterol, evidence of plantigrade stance, and required a higher maximum dose of insulin to gain glycemic control (median dose was 50% higher 0. 66 vs 0.43 U/kg)

C. **Oral hypoglycemic agents:**
1. Oral hypoglycemic agents work by stimulating insulin secretion and/or improving insulin sensitivity or decreasing glucose absorption.
2. **For initial management,** cats with clinical signs of diabetes should be **treated with insulin. Better glycemic control will be achieved using insulin** rather than oral hypoglycemic agents or diet alone:
   a. **Insulin is more potent in decreasing blood glucose;** this enables beta cells to overcome the effects of glucose toxicity.
3. Approximately **5–30% of cats have adequate clinical control using oral hypoglycemic drugs** which stimulate insulin secretion. The sulphonylurea, glipizide, is the most widely used oral hypoglycemic drug for cats. However, **remission rates are significantly lower** (18%) using oral hypoglycemic agents than with insulin (>80%) in newly diagnosed diabetic cats.
4. Oral hypoglycemic drugs are most useful as sole treatment when:
   a. Beta cells are not markedly suppressed by glucose toxicity (e.g., blood glucose is <14 mmol/L [<250 mg/dL]).

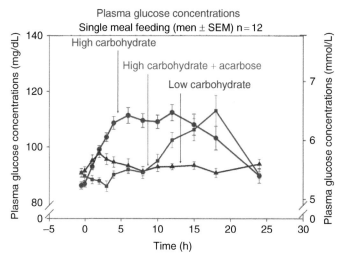

Figure 16.7 Blood glucose concentrations measured over 24 h in healthy cats after eating a meal of a high-carbohydrate (50% ME) or low-carbohydrate (6% ME) diet. Note that blood glucose concentrations after eating a high-carbohydrate diet remain elevated for 20 h after eating and are significantly higher than after eating a low-carbohydrate diet. Some cats fed with the high-carbohydrate diet were administered acarbose at 25 mg/kg orally at the time of feeding. Acarbose decreases blood glucose concentrations for 8 h after eating and must be dosed twice daily, even if the cat eats only once a day. Feeding a low-carbohydrate diet is as effective as acarbose. Acarbose is useful in diabetic cats with advanced renal failure that require a low-protein (high-carbohydrate) diet to decrease azotemia. (With permission from Rand JS, unpublished data.)

    b. The owner refuses to give insulin injections. However, this decision markedly reduces the probability of remission. A better option is to hospitalize the cat and intensively treat with insulin for 3–4 weeks with the aim of inducing remission.
  5. Acarbose decreases glucose absorption from the gastrointestinal tract and can be used as an adjunct to insulin therapy. However, the same effect on blood glucose concentration can be achieved by feeding a low-carbohydrate diet (Figure 16.7):
    a. Acarbose is indicated in cats with **advanced renal failure** that require a restricted protein diet which is consequently high in carbohydrate. Acarbose must be administered orally twice daily and is of most benefit in cats eating most of their food at the time of acarbose administration rather than *ad libitum* eating.
D. Choice of insulin:
  1. The **insulin chosen will influence the probability of remission**; because remission has substantial health benefits for the cat, and cost and lifestyle benefits for the owner, choice of insulin should be governed by maximizing remission in newly diagnosed diabetic cats.
  2. Based on one study in **newly diagnosed diabetic cats, glargine was associated with the highest remission rates (>90%)** followed **by beef/pork PZI (40%)** and **porcine lente (30%)** insulin. **Recombinant PZI and beef/pork PZI have been shown to have similar efficacy** in cats.
  3. Detemir is reported to have similar remission rates to glargine in cats.
  4. Based on remission rates in newly diagnosed diabetic cats, glargine and detemir are first choice insulins in cats and PZI is a second choice insulin. Lente insulin is a third choice insulin, and NPH is not recommended. Ultralente is unavailable in most countries.
  5. However, in many European countries, there is a legal requirement to first use an insulin licensed for veterinary use. Use of these insulins reduces the probability of remission. **It is recommended that if remission is not achieved within 4–6 weeks of therapy with a veterinary-use insulin, detemir or glargine should be used in newly diagnosed diabetic cats.**
  6. Glargine (Lantus, Aventis) or **detemir (Levemir, Novo Nordisk) are the insulins of choice in diabetic cats.** They have a longer duration of action resulting in significantly higher remission rates in newly diagnosed diabetic cats. They are also associated with lower rates of clinical hypoglycemia:
    a. Glargine and detemir should be administered twice daily to have the highest probability of remission.

7. **Lente and NPH (Isophane) insulins** have **too short a duration of action** to be recommended as a first choice insulin in diabetic cats. Remission rates are significantly lower (30%) in newly diagnosed diabetic cats than with glargine and detemir (>90% remission rates in newly diagnosed diabetic cats). However, clinical control is often good, and signs of diabetes resolve in the majority of cats:
   a. Lente and NPH must be given at least twice daily in all cats, and many cats would have better glycemic control with treatment three to four times daily.
   b. For approximately 2–4 h twice a day, there is minimal exogenous insulin action when using these insulins. This means that most diabetic cats have episodes of marked hyperglycemia >16 mmol/L (>288 mg/dL) twice daily, which exacerbates glucose toxicity, and makes diabetic remission less likely than when using longer acting insulins.
8. **Because** of the small doses used in cats, 40 U/mL insulin is preferable to 100 U/mL insulin. However, expected duration of action is more important than concentration. All human-use insulin is 100 U/mL in Western countries. Using 0.3-mL insulin syringes is advantageous when using 100 U/mL insulin. Small doses (<1U) can also be dispensed by calculating the number of drops/U for a given needle size and discarding the appropriate number of drops prior to administering the desired dose. Hold the syringe vertically with the needle pointing down to count drops/U, and to discard drops prior to administering required dose.
9. Beef or pork insulins have a longer duration of action than human insulin. Most insulin licensed for veterinary use was pork or beef/pork mixes, but many are no longer available. At the time of writing, veterinary-use insulins are recombinant PZI (PZIVet; Boehringer Ingelheim Vetmedica) and porcine lente (Caninsulin/Vetsulin; Intervet/Schering Plough). Recombinant human-use insulin is either identical in amino acid sequence to human insulin or has substitutions to alter duration of action. The new insulin analogues developed for use in people have very prolonged action, and therefore **species of origin is no longer a consideration in choice of insulin** in cats.
10. **Eating does not need to be coordinated with insulin administration**, because the postprandial increase in blood glucose is very prolonged in cats. The postprandial period depends on the amount eaten and the carbohydrate content of the food. For example, for diets with high carbohydrate content (>40% ME; metabolizable energy), the postprandial increase is 12–14 h if fed twice daily and 15–24 h for once daily (Figure 16.7).
11. **Feed a low-carbohydrate diet** (<15% of energy from carbohydrate) because it lowers blood glucose, reduces insulin requirement, and increases the probability of remission (Figure 16.7):
   a. It is very important to continue to feed a low-carbohydrate diet once the cat is in remission, to continue to minimize the demand on beta cells to secrete insulin.
12. **Underweight and normal bodyweight** cats need a high-quality, calorie-dense feline diet that is palatable. Feed a low-carbohydrate diet (<15% of energy) and adjust amount fed to maintain ideal body condition:
   a. **A diet** with **12% of energy from carbohydrate (ME)** resulted in significantly higher remission rates (68%) in diabetic cats than a diet with 26% energy from carbohydrate (42% remission). Typical premium dry cat foods have 30–40% energy from carbohydrate and supermarket brands have typically 40–50%. For comparison, prescription weight loss feline diets are typically around 20% to <30% and diabetic diets are 6–24%.
   b. Because **chronic kidney disease** is not uncommon in diabetic cats (persistent azotemia was present in 17% of diabetic cats 5–10 year age, and 31% diabetic cats >10 years of age), dietary selection should consider phosphate content. Nonprescription diets with very low carbohydrate that are predominantly meat or fish based have high phosphate content and should not be fed to diabetic or prediabetic cats with evidence of chronic kidney disease.
13. **Obese cats** should have their energy intake restricted to reduce body weight by 1–2% per week. Use a **low-carbohydrate diet (<15% ME)** formulated for management of diabetes and obesity; diets designed for weight loss have increased concentrations of essential nutrients. Canned diets appear to improve satiety in some cats compared to dry food. **Obesity decreases insulin sensitivity by 50%,** and puts greater demand on beta cells to secrete insulin, and **therefore should be managed as a priority**, even if the cat achieves remission without substantial weight loss.

14. **Hypoglycemia kills cats:**

    a. Teach owners to recognize signs (abnormal fear, hiding, **dazed drunken look, dilated pupils, wobbliness, weakness, head or body tremors, twitching, seizures, or coma**). Signs may occur with little warning in cats that have apparently excellent clinical control of their diabetes.

    b. In cats with mild signs, feed the cat immediately, preferably with a palatable, high-carbohydrate food, for example, a maintenance dry cat food for adult cats. Signs often resolve within 1–2 h.

    c. For cats with marked signs, the owner should immediately start treatment with honey or a glucose syrup designed for human diabetic patients, given per os. If the cat is having seizures, rub honey or syrup into the gums, or give per rectum using the lubricated insulin syringe (provided the needle can be removed), and seek veterinary attention immediately.

    d. Cats with **severe signs require intravenous (IV) glucose or glucagon**:

       1. Give 50% dextrose at 0.5–1.0 mL/kg IV.

       2. If IV access is not possible, 50% dextrose (0.5–1.0 mL/kg) or corn syrup (0.25–0.5 mL/kg) administered per os or rubbed on the gums may be effective, but glucagon 0.25–1.0 mg intramuscularly (IM) is superior. Glucagon must be followed by IV dextrose once seizures have stopped to maintain blood glucose.

    e. **Reevaluate the cat**; usually the insulin dose needs to be decreased by 50–70%. Some cats will no longer require insulin, because their diabetes is in remission:

       1. It is important to **check if the cat is being inadvertently overdosed**. This can occur when different syringes have been dispensed with a different volume per gradation than was previously used. For example, for many brands of syringes, the **gradations on a 1-mL (100 U/mL) syringe represent 2 U, whereas on a 0.5-mL syringe they represent 1 U**. If owners are switched to 1-mL syringes, the dose may be inadvertently doubled if the same number of graduations are used to dose the insulin. Similarly, a switch from syringes designed for U100 insulin to those for U40 insulin may result in an inadvertent 2.5 times increase in dose.

    f. As in humans, glargine and detemir use appears to be less frequently associated with clinical hypoglycemic episodes, although biochemical hypoglycemia is common in cats on protocols designed to rigorously control blood glucose concentrations.

15. **For treatment of "sick" and ketoacidotic diabetic cats see Chapter 19, Ketoacidosis.**

16. Treatment of "healthy" diabetic cats:

    a. If the cat is not very depressed or dehydrated, start **glargine or detemir subcutaneously**. The same starting dose is suitable for PZI and lente insulin (Tables 16.1 and 16.2):

       1. Use an initial dose of **0.25 U/kg ideal body weight q 12 h, if blood glucose is between 12 and 19 mmol/L (220–350 mg/dL)**.

       2. Use an initial dose of **0.5 U/kg ideal body weight q 12 h, if blood glucose is 20 mmol/L (360 mg/dL) or more**.

       3. Alternatively, start with 1 U/cat and increase sequentially as required.

17. Response to treatment can be evaluated in a number of ways, and no individual modality should be used as the sole parameter for adjusting therapy.

18. A combination of measurement of blood glucose concentrations together with owner assessment of clinical signs, and changes in body weight, water intake, and urine glucose are the best indicators of glycemic control.

19. **Measurement of blood glucose concentration** is the **cornerstone of effective monitoring** and adjustment of insulin dose and is **essential** if a cat is to have the **best chance of diabetic remission**.

20. **Glycemic control should also be monitored** using **clinical parameters (water intake, urine glucose concentration, and body weight)**.

21. **Water drunk** is a better indicator of mean blood glucose and level of clinical control than is fructosamine concentration:

    a. Water drunk of ≤10 mL/kg/24 h on canned food or ≤60 mL/kg/24 h on dry food indicates excellent glycemic control.

    b. **Water drunk** should be measured at home on at least 2 consecutive days to provide a more accurate estimate. Ideally, an owner should keep a daily diary of water drunk if blood glucose con-

Table 16.1   Dosing protocol for cats on long-acting insulin (glargine, detemir, and PZI) and glucose monitoring every weeks for 4–6 weeks and then every 2 weeks until stable or in remission.

Parameter used for dosage adjustment	Change in dose
Use an initial dose 0.5 U/kg of ideal body weight BID if blood glucose is ≥360 mg/dL (≥20 mmol/L) and 0.25 U/kg BID if glucose <360 mg/dL (<20 mmol/L)	
If preinsulin blood glucose concentration >216 mg/dL (>12 mmol/L) *and/or* If nadir blood glucose concentration >180 mg/dL (>10 mmol/L)	Increase by 0.25–1 U per injection Use water drunk and urine glucose as a guide to dose change
If preinsulin blood glucose concentration 180<216 mg/dL (10–12 mmol/L) *and/or* If nadir blood glucose concentration is 90–160 mg/dL (5–9 mmol/L)	Same dose
If nadir glucose concentration is 65–72 mg/dL (3.5–4 mmol/L)	Water drunk, urine glucose, and next preinsulin glucose concentration to determine if insulin dose is decreased or maintained
If preinsulin blood glucose concentration <180 mg/dL (10 mmol/L) *and/or* If nadir blood glucose concentration is <65 mg/dL (<3.5 mmol/L)	Reduce by 0.5–1 U per injection *or* if total dose is 0.5–1 U SID or less, stop insulin and check for diabetic remission
If clinical signs of hypoglycemia are observed	Reduce by 50%
In fractious cats where blood glucose measurement is not possible, use water drunk and urine glucose to adjust dose. However, glycemic control will likely be inferior, and remission delayed or not obtained	
If water intake is <20 mL/kg on wet food or <60 mL/kg on dry food	Same dose
If water intake is >20 mL/kg/24 h on wet food or >60 mL/kg/24 h on dry food	Increase dose by 0.5–1 U per injection
If urine glucose is ≥2+(scale 0–4 +)	Increase dose by 0.5–1 U per injection
If urine glucose is negative	Reduce dose every 2 weeks by 0.5–1 U per injection. Check for diabetic remission if dose is 0.5–1 U SID

Parameters for changing insulin dosage when using **long-acting insulin** in diabetic cats being assessed with serial blood glucose measurement every 3–4 h over 12 h every 5–7 days. Blood glucose concentrations are adjusted for using a glucose meter calibrated for feline blood.

centration is not being intensively monitored on a daily basis (three or more measurements daily). Water drunk provides useful additional information if measured on 2 consecutive days prior to measurement of a hospital generated blood glucose curve.

c. Measurement of water drunk is a valuable tool for **fractious cats,** where it is difficult to obtain a blood glucose measurement that is not affected by stress:

1. In these cats, combining water drunk with urine glucose measurements can lead to successful management. However, lack of blood glucose measurements limits how tightly blood glucose concentration can be controlled and therefore decreases the probability of diabetic remission.

22. **Monitoring urine glucose is very useful.** This can be accomplished using poorly absorbent litter material such as silicon beads or shredded paper which allows collection of urine for testing with a

Table 16.2 Dosing protocol for cats on intermediate-acting insulin (lente and NPH).

Blood Glucose Variable	Recommendation
Use an initial dose 0.5 U/kg of lean body weight BID if blood glucose is ≥360 mg/dL (≥20 mmol/L) and 0.25 U/Kg BID if glucose <360 mg/dL (<20 mmol/L); do not increase in first week, but decrease if necessary	
If preinsulin blood glucose concentration is <210 mg/dL (<12 mmol/L)	Withhold insulin and check for diabetic remission
If preinsulin blood glucose concentration is 211–250 mg/dL (13–16 mmol/L)	Total dose should be no more than 1 U/cat bid
If nadir blood glucose concentration is <54 mg/dL (<3 mmol/L)	Dose should be reduced by 50%
If nadir blood glucose concentration is 54–90 mg/dL (3–5 mmol/L)	Dose should be reduced by 1 U per injection if poor control of clinical signs of diabetes; dose should remain the same if exemplary control of clinical signs
If nadir blood glucose concentration is 91–180 mg/dL (6–9 mmol/L)	Dose should remain the same
If nadir blood glucose concentration is >180 mg/dL (>10 mmol/L)	Dose should be increased by 1 U per injection
If nadir blood glucose concentration occurs within 3 h of insulin administration or blood glucose returns to baseline within 8 h	Change to long-acting insulin
If the nadir blood glucose concentration occurs at 8 h or later	Once daily administration may be used, although twice daily administration at a reduced dose is preferred

Source: Adapted from: Rand JS, Marshall R. Diabetes mellitus in cats. *Vet Clin North Am Small Anim Pract* 2005;35(1):211.
Parameters for changing insulin dose and frequency based on blood glucose measurements when using **intermediate-acting insulin. Insulin dose adjustments are based on monitoring blood glucose concentration every 2 weeks with serial measurements every 2 h until 2–4 h after nadir.**

dipstick. Alternatively, a litter box glucose detector system such as Glucotest (Nestlé Purina) can be added to the box filler and reacts to urine with a color change to indicate glucosuria. Some owners are able to train the cat to tolerate a dipstick applied to the urine stream during urination. Alternatively, some of the urine-soaked litter can be mixed with water and tested with a dipstick after straining through a cloth.

a. **Weekly urine glucose monitoring** is helpful for **detecting diabetic remission**, especially in cats treated with lente, NPH, or ultralente insulin. Cats with negative urine glucose should have blood glucose concentration evaluated for evidence of remission.

b. With the long duration of action of glargine, there should be minimal periods when blood glucose is >14 mmol/L (240 mg/dL), and hence stable cats should almost always be 0 or 1+ for urine glucose. A value 2+ or greater likely indicates that an increase in dose is required. Urine glucose concentration is less useful for detecting remission in glargine-treated cats, but in contrast to lente-treated cats, it is useful for increasing the insulin dose, especially in fractious cats where blood glucose measurements cannot be obtained without considerable stress (Figure 16.8).

c. Because cats treated with lente, NPH, or ultralente insulin usually have hyperglycemia within 6–10 h after insulin administration, which persists until the next dose, it is not recommended to use urine glucose measurements to increase the dose of these insulins.

23. Monitoring **fructosamine or glycated hemoglobin** concentration can be a useful indicator of glycemic control in cats susceptible to stress hyperglycemia and/or if the owner is unable to measure water intake. Fructosamine concentrations >500–550 μmol/L (normal <400 μmol/L) or glycated hemoglobin >3% to 4% (normal <2.6%) are consistent with poor glycemic control.

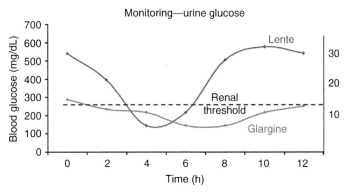

Figure 16.8 Typical blood glucose curve following administration of lente or glargine in diabetic cats. A negative urine glucose concentration is useful for indicating remission in lente- or NPH-treated cats; for approximately 4 h before each insulin injection, there is no exogenous insulin action. Therefore, if there is no glycosuria, it implies significant beta cell function. Basing dose increases on urine glucose when using lente or NPH insulin can result in severe clinical hypoglycemia; nadir glucose concentration may be in the normal range but substantial glycosuria is still present because of the short duration of insulin action. In contrast, because glargine and detemir have a long duration of action with a carryover effect when administered twice daily, urine glucose is often negative in well-controlled cats and is not a specific indicator of remission. However, when blood glucose measurements are problematic, for example, fractious cats, urine glucose concentration can be used to increase the dose. (From Marshall and Rand, 2006. With permission.)

E. **Measurement of blood glucose concentration:**
  1. The distribution of glucose between red blood cells and plasma is different in human beings and cats. As a result, whole blood meters calibrated for human blood consistently read lower than the actual value measured in feline plasma. For some meters, this translates to a value which on average is 1–2 mmol/L (18–36 mg/dL) lower than the actual serum or plasma blood glucose concentration, which translates to 20–40% less for values in the normal or hypoglycemic range.
  2. If using a glucometer internally **calibrated for feline use** (e.g., AlphaTRAK, Abbott Laboratories) or a serum chemistry analyzer, use the published or laboratory reference range for cats, (e.g. **3.6–7.5 mmol/L; 65–135 mg/dL**). If using a **whole blood meter calibrated for human blood,** aim for a target blood glucose concentration of 2.8–5.6 mmol/L (50–100 mg/dL), and if using a plasma-equivalent meter calibrated for human blood, aim for a target blood glucose intermediate between these two ranges. Note that plasma-equivalent test strips can be purchased for meters which previously displayed glucose values for whole blood and will then display plasma-equivalent values.
F. **Monitoring blood glucose concentration:**
  1. The **protocol for serial blood glucose evaluation** comprises administration of the cat's usual meal and insulin dose in the morning and 12 h later at night:
      a. Blood glucose is measured with a portable glucose meter every 2 h (intermediate-acting insulin) or every 3–4 h (long-acting insulin), beginning immediately prior to the morning insulin injection and meal, and continuing until the nadir (lowest glucose concentration) is clearly evident (intermediate-acting insulin) or until the next insulin injection (long-acting insulin).
  2. Results of serial blood glucose concentration testing determine whether the insulin dose should be increased, left unchanged, or decreased, or the type of insulin should be changed.
  3. Dosage changes can be made based on a number of different blood glucose parameters, and optimally should include more than one parameter. **Preinsulin glucose concentration, nadir (lowest) glucose concentration, and mean glucose concentration are most often used.** Nadir glucose concentration is the most important parameter to indicate increases and decreases in dose. When it is in the low end of the normal range, no further dose increases can be made:
      a. Time to nadir and the time to return to baseline glucose concentration are used as indicators for changing insulin type, if the current insulin appears to have too short a duration of action.
G. **Home monitoring** (Figures 16.9–16.11):

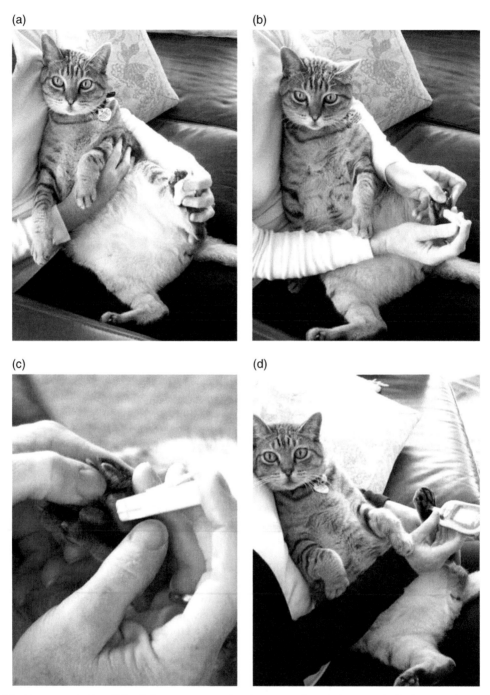

Figure 16.9   Home monitoring of blood glucose concentrations have a number of advantages including more frequent blood glucose measurements on which to base insulin dose increases. Glucose concentration is less likely to be affected by stress or inappetence. Reduced cost and greater convenience for the owner are also factors. (a) Foot pad is warmed to facilitate blood flow using a moist cotton wool ball warmed in microwave or with hot water; (b, c) using lancet to obtain blood sample; and (d) measuring glucose in blood sample with portable glucometer. (Photos from W. Milledge. With permission.)

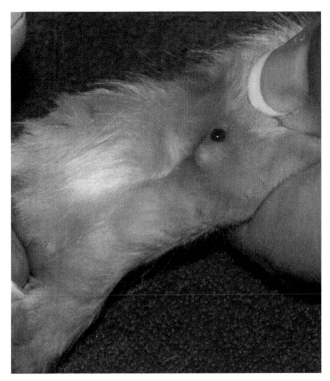

Figure 16.10   A bleb of blood from the pisiform pad being obtained with a lancing device designed for home monitoring. (Photo from S. Ford. With permission.)

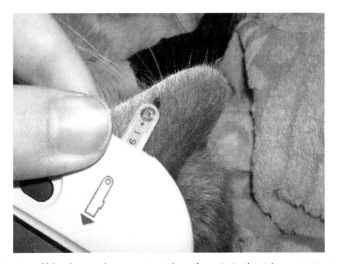

Figure 16.11   Home monitoring of blood using the ear veins. (Photo from S. Ford. With permission.)

1.   Home monitoring provides a number of advantages including **decreasing stress** to the cat. **Stress can lead to spuriously high glucose concentrations** if the cat struggles during examination or blood collection. Home monitoring also **decreases the cost and inconvenience to the owner,** and typically is performed more often than blood glucose measurements by the attending veterinarian, so it provides **increased information** to make blood glucose adjustments.

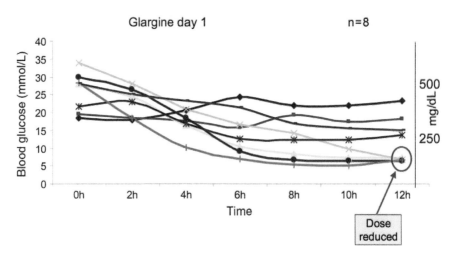

Figure 16.12 Day 1 blood glucose concentrations measured over 12 h in newly diagnosed diabetic cats treated with glargine at 0.5 U/kg if blood glucose ≥20 mmol/L (360 mg/dL). Note range of differing responses. (From Marshall and Rand. With permission.)

2. Typically the measurements taken are **preinsulin glucose concentration**, and then **every 2 h until a nadir** is evident (intermediate-acting insulin) or **every 3–6 h** until the next insulin injection (long-acting insulin).

3. If possible, a blood glucose measurement before bedtime provides additional information.

4. A dosing protocol has been developed (Table 16.3) and successfully used by committed owners prepared to measure blood glucose concentration at least three times daily. Remission rates of 84% were achieved in previously treated cats swapped to the protocol within 6 months of diagnosis.

5. Owners using the protocol need to liaise closely with their veterinarian; initially appointments should be made **weekly for review of the owner's log book** of blood glucose concentrations, insulin dose and clinical signs, and for physical assessment of the cat, including body condition:

    a. The owner must also know how to recognize signs of hypoglycemia and be able to take appropriate action.

6. **Adjusting insulin dose using glargine, detemir, and PZI** (Table 16.1):

    a. If using **glargine, detemir, or PZI, adjust the dose based on nadir** (lowest) glucose and **preinsulin glucose concentration** (concentration immediately before next insulin injection).

    b. In general, increase the dose by ½–1 U/cat q 12 h every **5–7 days** to achieve a nadir glucose concentration of 5–7.5 mmol/L (90–135 mg/dL) (Figures 16.12–16.15). Once clinical signs have resolved and the blood glucose is relatively controlled, a nadir in the normal blood glucose range can be achieved. This is 3.6–7.5 mmol/L (65–135 mg/dL) measured with a meter calibrated for feline blood or 2.8–5.6 mmol/L (50–100 mg/dL) measured with a whole blood meter calibrated for human blood, and intermediate between these two ranges, if measured with a plasma-equivalent meter calibrated for human blood.

7. **Adjusting insulin dose using lente insulin (or NPH or ultralente insulin)** (Table 16.2):

    a. In some countries, insulin registered for veterinary use must be used initially in treating diabetic cats. In those countries, porcine lente insulin (Caninsulin or Vetsulin; Schering-Plough Intervet) is the usually the most available product.

    b. When using **lente, NPH, or ultralente insulin, adjust dose based on nadir (lowest) glucose concentration** and **clinical signs**.

    c. **Do not use preinsulin blood glucose concentration to increase the dose**, only to decrease the dose. There is little appreciable insulin action after 8–10 h, so for most cats on these insulins, the preinsulin glucose concentration cannot be decreased by increasing insulin dose. In general, aim for a glucose

Table 16.3   Dosing protocol for cats on long-acting insulin (glargine and detemir) and home glucose monitoring a minimum of three times per day.

Parameter used for dosage adjustment	Change in dose
Phase 1: Initial dose and first 3 days on glargine or detemir	
Begin with 0.25 IU/kg of ideal weight BID OR If the cat received another insulin previously, increase or reduce the starting dose taking this information into account. Glargine has a lower potency than lente insulin and PZI in most cats	
Cats with a history of developing ketones that remain >17 mmol/L (300 mg/dL) after 24–48 h	Increase by 0.5 IU per injection
If blood glucose is <3.6 mmol/L (<65 mg/dL)	Reduce dose by 0.25–0.5 IU per injection depending on if cat on low or high (>3 U/cat) dose of insulin
Phase 2: Increasing the dose	
If nadir blood glucose concentration >17 mmol/L (>300 mg/dL)	Increase every 3 days by 0.5 IU per injection
If nadir blood glucose concentration 11–17 mmol/L (200–300 mg/dL)	Increase every 3 days by 0.25–0.5 IU per injection depending on if cat on low or high (>3 U/cat) dose of insulin
If nadir blood glucose concentration <11 mmol/L (200 mg/dL) but peak is >11 mmol/L (200 mg/dL)	Increase every 5–7 days by 0.25–0.5 IU per injection depending on if cat on low or high dose of insulin
If blood glucose is <3.6 mmol/L (< 65 mg/dL)	Reduce dose by 0.25–0.5 IU per injection depending on if cat on low or high dose of insulin
If blood glucose at the time of the next insulin injection 3.6–7.5 mmol/L (65–135 mg/dL)	Initially test which of the alternate methods is best suited to the individual cat: a. Feed cat and reduce the dose by 0.25–0.5 IU per injection depending on if cat on low or high dose of insulin b. Feed the cat, wait 1–2 h, and when the glucose concentration increases to >7.5 mmol/L (135 mg/dL) give the normal dose. If the glucose concentration does not increase within 1–2 h, reduce the dose by 0.25 IU or 0.5 IU per injection (as above) c. Split the dose: feed cat, and give most of dose immediately and then give the remainder 1–2 h later, when the glucose concentration has increased to >7.5 mmol/L (135 mg/dL) If all these methods lead to increased blood glucose concentrations, give the full dose if preinsulin blood glucose concentration is 3.6–7.5 mmol/L (65–135 mg/dL) and observe closely for signs of hypoglycemia. In general, for most cats, the best results in phase 2 occur when insulin dose is as consistent as possible, giving the full normal dose at the regular injection time
Phase 3: Holding the dose. Aim to keep blood glucose concentration within 3.5–11 mmol/L (65–200 mg/dL) throughout the day.	
If blood glucose is <3.6 mmol/L (<65 mg/dL)	Reduce dose by 0.25–0.5 IU per injection depending on if cat on low or high dose of insulin

(Continued)

Table 16.3 (*Continued*)

Parameter used for dosage adjustment	Change in dose
If nadir or peak blood glucose concentration >11 mmol/L (> 200 mg/dL)	Increase dose by 0.25–0.5 IU per injection depending on if cat on low or high dose of insulin and the degree of hyperglycemia
Phase 4: Reducing the dose. Phase out insulin slowly by 0.25–0.5 U depending on dose.	
When the cat regularly (every day for at least one week) has its lowest blood glucose concentration in the normal range of a healthy cat and stays under 7.5 mmol/L (135 mg/dL) overall	Reduce dose by 0.25–0.5 IU per injection depending on if cat on low or high dose of insulin
If the nadir glucose concentration is between 3 and 3.5 mmol/L (54 and 63 mg/dL) at least three times on separate days	Reduce dose by 0.25–0.5 IU per injection depending on if cat on low or high dose of insulin
If the cat drops below 3 mmol/L (54 mg/dL) once	Reduce dose immediately by 0.25–0.5 IU per injection depending on if cat on low or high dose of insulin
If peak blood glucose concentration >11 mmol/L (>200 mg/dL)	Immediately increase insulin dose to last effective dose
Phase 5: Remission. Euglycemia for a minimum of 14 days without insulin.	

Criteria for changing insulin dosage when using the long-acting insulin glargine (Lantus), detemir (Levemir) or PZI (ProZinc), together with **home monitoring of blood glucose concentrations** in a protocol aimed at achieving intensive blood glucose control. Blood glucose should be measured at **least three times daily** with a glucometer. This has not been tested with veterinarian-measured blood glucose curves once every week or 2 weeks, and Table 16.1 is recommended if intensive home monitoring is not being performed.

NB. The blood glucose values have been adjusted for use with a portable glucose meter **calibrated for feline blood** (e.g., AlphaTRAK, Abbott Laboratories, CA, USA), where the normal blood glucose range is 3.6–7.5 mmol/L (65–135 mg/dL).* If using a **whole blood meter calibrated for human blood**, aim for a target blood glucose concentration of 2.8–5.6 mmol/L (50–100 mg/dL), and if using a plasma-equivalent meter calibrated for human blood, aim for a target blood glucose intermediate between these two ranges. Note that plasma-equivalent test strips can be purchased for meters which previously displayed glucose values for whole blood.

If using a meter calibrated for use with human blood which displays values for whole blood, these meters may measure 30–40% lower in the low end of the range than glucose concentrations measured using a serum chemistry analyser or a plasma-equivalent meter calibrated for feline use. **Meters calibrated for feline blood may read higher or lower than the actual value, in contrast to consistently low readings for meters validated for human blood**.

Dose increases are per injection per cat.

Source: Adapted from **Roomp PK, Rand JS**. Intensive blood glucose control is safe and effective in diabetic cats using home monitoring and treatment with glargine. *J Feline Med Surg* 2009;11(8):668–682.

* Reeve-Johnson, M, Rand JS, Vankan D et al Reference values for casual blood glucose in healthy, aged cats measured from ear or pad sample using a portable glucose meter *JVIM* 2012;26:755.

nadir of 7–9 mmol/L (126–162 mg/dL) in the first 1–2 months. Later a nadir of 3.6-7.5 mmol/L (65–135 mg/dL) can be achieved in cats that are well controlled.

d. Rebound hyperglycemia may be a consequence of aiming for a low nadir too early in the stabilization process, especially if using lente, ultralente, or NPH insulin or mixes. It also leads to an apparent decrease in duration of action.

8. **Diabetic remission** usually occurs in the first 4 months of therapy, and occurs most often in the 4–6 weeks of treatment in newly diagnosed cats appropriately managed on glargine or detemir and a low-carbohydrate diet. Impending remission is suggested by a **negative urine glucose measurement,** and a preinsulin blood glucose concentration of <12 mmol/L (216 mg/dL). Decrease insulin dose gradually to 0.5–1 U/cat q 12 h or even q 24 h. If urine glucose is still negative and preinsulin blood glucose is still low on a minimal dose of insulin, stop insulin and monitor blood glucose for 12–24 h. If blood glucose remains low, send the cat home on a low-carbohydrate diet and reevaluate in 1 week:

a. **To maximize the probability of remission, insulin dose should be slowly reduced.** Premature cessation of insulin therapy leading to hyperglycemia may delay remission for weeks or months.

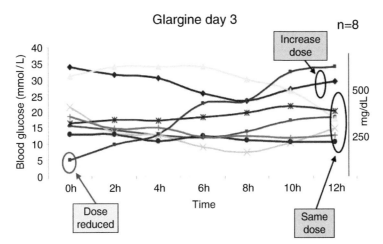

Figure 16.13   Day 3 blood glucose concentrations measured over 12 h in newly diagnosed diabetic cats treated with glargine. Note range of differing responses. (From Marshall and Rand. With permission.)

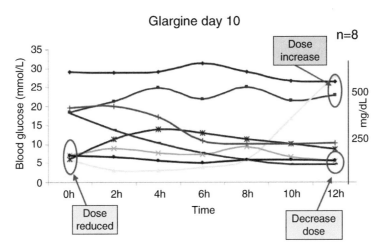

Figure 16.14   Day 10 blood glucose concentrations measured over 12 h in newly diagnosed diabetic cats treated with glargine. Note range of differing responses. (From Marshall and Rand. With permission.)

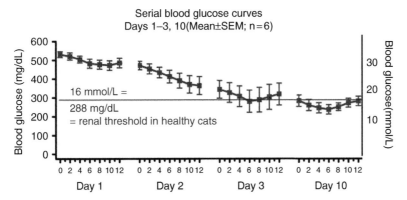

Figure 16.15   Mean blood glucose concentrations measured over 12 h in newly diagnosed diabetic cats on days 1, 3, and 10 after initiation of treatment with glargine at an initial dose of 0.5 U/kg (blood glucose ≥20 mmol/L; 360 mg/dL). Note how rapidly mean blood glucose decreases over time. (From Marshall and Rand. With permission.)

9. Approximately **25–40% of cats in remission relapse** and need to restart treatment with insulin:
  a. Attention to achieving a lean body weight, feeding a low-carbohydrate diet (<15% metabolizable energy (ME) from carbohydrate), and avoiding corticosteroid administration will help to prevent relapse.
  b. Owners should closely monitor blood glucose concentration in remission cats on a weekly basis. If a non-fasted glucose concentration is consistently 10 mmol/L (180 mg/dL) or higher (or fasted >7.5 mmol/L; 135 mg/dL), therapy aimed at achieving euglycemia should be reinstituted. Early institution of insulin therapy facilitates glycemic control being achieved with low doses of insulin, for example, 0.5–1 U q 12–24 h.
  c. If blood glucose is not being monitored at home, the owner should closely monitor water intake and urine glucose. If these increase, insulin therapy should be immediately reinstituted (after confirming increased water consumption is associated with hyperglycemia and not other causes such as chronic kidney disease).
      1) **Of relapsing cats, approximately 25% will achieve a second remission if insulin therapy is promptly reinstituted.**
H. **Poorly controlled cats on high doses of insulin:**
  1. **Cats on insulin doses of >1.5–2 U/kg that are not well controlled should be assessed to determine the cause of the apparent insulin resistance.**
  2. **Problem cats** have **persistent clinical signs** including polydipsia (water drunk >100 mL/kg/24 h), low body condition score, polyphagia, lethargy, and a poor hair coat; an **insulin dose** higher than normal **(1.5–2 or more IU/kg/injection)**; and either a **nadir glucose >10 mmol/L (180 mg/dL)** or **hypoglycemia.**
  3. The **most common problems** resulting in poor control are **excessive dose** when **intermediate-acting insulin** is used, **too short duration of insulin** action, **inadequate insulin action**, and **acromegaly** (resulting in marked insulin resistance and inadequate insulin action).
  4. If inadequate insulin action, first **rule out insulin storage or mixing** (lente) problems by replacing with a new bottle of insulin:
    a. Watch the owner give the insulin to ascertain if **administration technique** is correct and that **air bubbles** in the insulin syringe are not reducing insulin dose (common in elderly owners with failing eyesight).
    b. Check **calibration of the glucose meter** if home monitoring is being used.
    c. Check that a **change in type of insulin syringe** has not lead to an inadvertent change in insulin dose because of differences in volume that each graduation represents on different syringes (0.5- and 1-mL [100-U/mL] syringes and 40-U/mL syringes).
  5. **Poor absorption** can be differentiated from insulin resistance as a cause of inadequate insulin action by giving regular or glargine insulin (0.5 U/kg lean body weight or 2 U/cat) IM and assessing response.
  6. Check **duration of action** and if glucose lowering effect lasts <8–10 h, change to a long-acting insulin such as detemir or glargine:
    a. In many cats treated with the intermediate-acting insulin such as **lente and NPH** (isophane), these **potent insulins rapidly lower blood glucose.**
    b. This **stimulates counter-regulatory responses, even when blood glucose concentration is not in the hypoglycemic range.**
    c. The resulting counter-regulatory response **increases blood glucose concentration** and causes an **apparent short duration** of insulin action and **insulin resistance.**
    d. Because the **glucose lowering effect of lente and NPH in cats is <8–10 h,** most diabetic cats have blood glucose concentrations of 20–24 mmol/L (360–430 mg/dL) at the time of the next insulin dose. Use of a potent insulin with short duration of action such as lente, predisposes cats to premature counter-regulation before glucose concentration reaches the hypoglycemic range, because of the rapid decrease in blood glucose concentration from a high preinjection concentration.
    e. The result is that in some cats, lente and NPH insulins may only lower blood glucose for 2–3 h. This inherent short duration of action of lente, NPH, and ultralente insulins, coupled with the counter-regulation response can result in **insulin dosage being wrongly increased, predisposing to hypoglycemia, rebound hyperglycemia, and insulin resistance.**

7. When **using lente, NPH or ultralente, some cats are mistakenly labeled problem cats** when the clinical signs are well controlled, but **blood glucose measurements are less than ideal:**

   a. This usually occurs when there are **unrealistic goals for glycemic control using intermediate-acting insulin** and lack of understanding that for 2–4 h twice daily, cats treated with these insulins have negligible blood glucose lowering effect from the insulin:

   1) **If the glucose nadir is below 10 mmol/L (182 mg/dL)** after each insulin injection, **peak action occurs >3 h** after administration, and hypoglycemia is not occurring, glycemic control is usually adequate. These cats usually have good clinical control (stable body weight, good coat condition, active, alert, water drunk <100 mL/kg/24 h) but **glycemic control is often inadequate to achieve remission.**

   b. Swapping to a longer acting insulin such as glargine and detemir will usually improve glycemic control and improve the probability of remission.

8. If there is **minimal response to insulin and dose is >1.5–2 U/kg** after at least 3–4 weeks of therapy, obtain a **minimum data base** of CBC, biochemistry, and urinalysis and include feline pancreatic lipase immunoreactivity (**fPLi**), **thyroxine**, and **urine culture** to rule out underlying causes for poor control.

9. Identification and resolution of **chronic infection** can result in improved glycemic control. If significant **dental disease** is present, a full dental including removal of infected tooth roots should be performed, because in some cats diabetic control improves once chronic infection is eliminated.

10. **Acromegaly** is increasingly being recognized as a cause of **insulin resistance and poor glycemic control** in diabetic cats. In some cats, it results in extreme insulin resistance requiring very high insulin doses (e.g., >5–20 U/cat q 12 h) to control blood glucose. Measurement of **insulin-like growth factor (IGF-1)** and **imaging of the brain** are recommended for diagnosis (see Chapter 41).

11. **Hyperadrenocorticism** (see Chapter 7) is a less common cause of poor control.

VII. Prognosis

A. Prognosis is relatively good in insulin-dependent cats, considering average age at diagnosis is 10–13 years. Prognosis is greatly improved if remission is achieved.

VIII. Prevention

A. **Obesity, physical inactivity**, and repeated **long-acting steroid or megestrol acetate** administration are preventable risk factors for type 2 diabetes.

B. Individuals **predisposed to type 2 diabetes** should not become obese, and would likely benefit from a low-carbohydrate diet:

   1. Individuals predisposed to type 2 diabetes through **low insulin sensitivity** (as evidenced by increased fasting glucose to insulin concentration ratio) include obese cats, aged cats of **Burmese breed** (European type) and/or cats being administered **corticosteroids**.

   2. Individuals predisposed to type 2 diabetes through **reduced beta cell function** include cats with evidence of **impaired glucose tolerance** (blood glucose >7.3 mmol/L or 132 mg/dL at 2 h after 0.5 g/kg glucose or 3 h after 1 g/kg glucose IV) or **impaired fasting glucose concentrations** (persistent fasting glucose concentrations 7.6–10 mmol/L; 135–180 mg/dL).

References and Further Readings

Crenshaw KL, Peterson ME. Pretreatment clinical and laboratory evaluation of cats with diabetes mellitus: 104 cases (1992–1994). *J Am Vet Med Assoc* 1996;209(5):943–949.

Link K, Rand J. Changes in blood glucose concentration are associated with relatively rapid changes in circulating fructosamine concentrations in cats. *J Feline Med Surg* 2008;10:583–592.

Marshall R, Rand J, Morton J. Insulin glargine has a long duration of effect following administration either once daily or twice daily in divided doses in healthy cats. *J Feline Med Surg* 2008;10:488–494.

Marshall R, Rand J, Morton J. Glargine and protamine zinc insulin have a longer duration of action and result in lower mean daily glucose concentrations than lente insulin in healthy cats. *J Vet Pharmacol Ther* 2008;31:205–212.

Roomp K, Rand JS. Intensive blood glucose control is safe and effective in diabetic cats using home monitoring and treatment with glargine. *J Feline Med Surg* 2009;11(8):668–682.

Marshall RD, Rand JS, et al. Treatment of newly-diagnosed diabetic cats with glargine insulin improves glycemic control and results in higher probability of remission than protamine zinc and lente insulins. *J Feline Med Surg* 2009;11(8):683–691.

Nelson WN. Diabetes mellitus. In: Ettinger SJ, ed. *Textbook of Veterinary Internal Medicine*, 5th edn. Philadelphia: Saunders, 2000, pp. 1438–1460.

Norman EJ, Mooney CT. Diagnosis and management of diabetes mellitus in five cats with somatotrophic abnormalities. *J Feline Med Surg* 2000;2(4):183–190.

Rand JS. Use of long-acting insulin in the treatment of diabetes mellitus. In: August JR, ed. *Consultations in Feline Internal Medicine*, London: Elsevier Saunders, 2009, vol. 6, pp. 286–296.

Rijnberk A. Acromegaly. In: Ettinger SJ, ed. *Textbook of Veterinary Internal Medicine*, 5th edn. Philadelphia: Saunders, 2000, pp. 1370–1379.

Updated protocols for monitoring are available on: www.uq.edu.au/ccah.

CHAPTER 17

Diabetes Mellitus in Other Species

Michelle L. Campbell-Ward and Jacquie Rand

Diabetes Mellitus in Horses

Pathogenesis

- Diabetes mellitus is defined as persistent hyperglycemia and glucosuria from either absolute or relative hypoinsulinemia; insulin resistance is often an underlying factor.
- Diabetes is an uncommon condition in horses.
- Insulin resistance is commonly associated with metabolic syndrome or pituitary pars intermedia dysfunction in this species.

Classical Signs

- Depression, polyuria, polydipsia, rough hair coat, and weight loss.

Diagnosis

- Demonstration of persistent hyperglycemia.

Treatment

- Underlying conditions, if identified, must be addressed.
- Limited clinical data is available on the use of insulin, glyburide, and metformin.

I. Pathogenesis

A. Diabetes mellitus is defined as **persistent hyperglycemia and glucosuria from either absolute or relative hypoinsulinemia**:

    1. **Chronic insulin resistance** is believed to be a **contributing factor in most horses**.

    2. **Horses are less susceptible than humans and cats** to beta cell failure and **overt diabetes** as a result of chronic insulin resistance.

Clinical Endocrinology of Companion Animals, First Edition. Edited by Jacquie Rand.
© 2013 John Wiley & Sons, Inc. Published 2013 by John Wiley & Sons, Inc.

3. Most cases of insulin resistance in horses are associated with pituitary pars intermedia dysfunction (see Chapter 11), metabolic syndrome (obesity-associated) (see Chapter 20) or hyperlipemia.

4. Diabetes mellitus is associated with disturbances in the secretion of, and sensitivity to, hormones such as insulin, glucagon, catecholamines, growth hormone, and glucocorticoids.

B. **Type 1 diabetes mellitus** is a term used to describe diabetes due to immune-mediated destruction of pancreatic beta cells resulting in low insulin concentrations and hyperglycemia. There are no well documented cases of type 1 diabetes in horses reported in the literature.

C. **Type 2 diabetes mellitus** describes a form of diabetes which occurs secondary to chronic peripheral insulin resistance associated with **genotype and obesity** and results in **absolute or relative beta cell failure**. In the initial stages, it is associated with increased insulin concentrations:

1. **Overt type 2 diabetes** is rarely detected clinically in horses. However, **impaired glucose tolerance and impaired fasting glucose**, stages between normal and diabetic, are relatively common in horses.

2. **Impaired glucose tolerance** refers to delayed return to baseline glucose concentrations after an intravenous glucose challenge, and **impaired fasting glucose** refers to fasting glucose concentrations above the upper limit of the normal range but below those considered diabetic. Although the cut point for diabetes in horses has not yet been defined, glucose concentrations in the range of **7–10 mmol/L or 126–180 mg/dL** are consistent with impaired fasting glucose.

3. The **metabolic syndrome** represents a metabolic state between normal and overt diabetes and in horses and ponies is **more common than diabetes mellitus**. It is associated with **impaired glucose tolerance, insulin resistance, obesity**, and often **laminitis**. It may progress to overt type 2 diabetes mellitus in unmanaged cases. See Chapter 20 for a detailed discussion of impaired glucose tolerance.

D. **Other specific types of diabetes** resulting from beta cell destruction or insulin resistance are **uncommon** in horses. **Pituitary pars intermedia dysfunction** is relatively common in aged horses and is associated with increased production of **adrenocorticotropic hormone (ACTH)** resulting in **insulin resistance**; however, it **rarely progresses to overt diabetes**. Other less common causes of diabetes in horses are **pancreatitis from parasite migration, chronic pancreatitis**, and **ovarian tumors**. **Gestational diabetes** has also been reported with **pregnancy**.

II. Signalment

A. **No specific sex or breed** predispositions have been identified, although horses at risk of developing equine metabolic syndrome or pituitary pars intermedia dysfunction are likely to be overrepresented, including **obese and aged horses and ponies**.

III. Clinical Signs

A. Depression.

B. Polyuria.

C. Polydipsia (water intake >80 L/day).

D. Polyphagia.

E. Progressive weight loss.

F. Rough hair coat.

G. Ketone odor.

IV. Diagnosis

A. Diagnosis is based on **serial measurement of serum glucose to demonstrate persistent hyperglycemia >11.1 mmol/L; 200 mg/dL**:

1. **Persistent hyperglycemia with hypoinsulinemia** is consistent with **advanced beta cell failure** and **insulin-dependent diabetes mellitus**, which may or may not be associated with underlying insulin resistance; **persistent hyperglycemia with hyperinsulinemia** indicates the presence of **insulin resistance and less advanced beta cell failure**.

B. Glucosuria, ketonemia, and ketonuria may also be present.

C. Horses with diabetes mellitus should be investigated to determine the underlying cause, for example, **pituitary pars intermedia dysfunction** or as a **consequence of inadequately managed metabolic syndrome**; various test protocols are available (see Chapters 11 and 20).

V. Differential Diagnoses

A. Older horses that present with signs such as lethargy, **polyuria, polydipsia,** and **weight loss** should be screened for **pituitary pars intermedia dysfunction,** as this a more frequent cause of these clinical signs than diabetes mellitus; in such cases, polyuria/polydipsia is probably the result of a direct effect of cortisol on antidiuretic hormone (ADH) production (unless overt diabetes has developed secondary to chronic insulin resistance).

B. Factors that induce **temporary hyperglycemia** should be excluded, for example:
1. High carbohydrate diets.
2. Stress.
3. Exercise.
4. Glucocorticoid treatment.
5. Sedation with xylazine and ketamine.

C. Horses with pheochromocytomas may be hyperglycemic.

VI. Treatment

A. **Depends on the underlying cause and severity of the hyperglycemia:**
1. If impaired glucose tolerance or impaired fasting glucose are the result of inadequately managed metabolic syndrome or pituitary pars intermedia dysfunction, management is as described for these conditions in Chapters 11 and 20.
2. **If overt diabetes mellitus with glucosuria is diagnosed regardless of cause, treatment with insulin is indicated to protect beta cells from glucose toxicity and further loss.** This has been attempted in a number of cases with variable results:
   a. **Concurrent management of underlying conditions such as obesity or pituitary pars intermedia dysfunction** to **reduce insulin resistance** should be a **high priority** because if beta cells are protected, overt diabetes is potentially reversible.
   b. Recommended doses for **insulin** are 0.05–0.1 IU/kg/intravenously q 8–12 h for regular **insulin** and 0.5–4.0 IU/kg/intramuscularly q 12 h for **protamine zinc insulin.**
   c. During treatment, glucose concentrations must be monitored and adjustments to insulin dosing made accordingly. Always start with a low dose.
   d. Insulin administration can lead to hypoglycemic shock and as such a dextrose solution should be available at the initiation of therapy and when adjustments are being made.
3. The role of **supportive treatment** cannot be overemphasized.
4. In one case of pancreatic beta cell failure, treatment with glyburide (0.02 mg/kg) and metformin (1.9 mg/kg) lowered interstitial fluid glucose concentrations to normal ranges.

VII. Prognosis

A. Given the relatively few documented cases of diabetes mellitus in horses, **limited information** regarding prognosis is available.

B. The **frequent association with other significant endocrine diseases** suggests that the **prognosis should be considered guarded** for horses with overt diabetes (hyperglycemia sufficient to cause glucosuria), unless an underlying cause is identified and successfully managed, and hyperglycemia controlled prior to advanced beta cell failure.

C. **Impaired glucose tolerance and impaired fasting glucose** are considered **prediabetic** but can be **reversed** if the underlying cause such as obesity or pituitary pars intermedia dysfunction is managed successfully.

VIII. Prevention

A. There are no specific preventative measures, although **early recognition and provision of appropriate therapy** for cases of **equine metabolic syndrome and pituitary pars intermedia dysfunction** may prevent diabetes mellitus from developing.

Diabetes Mellitus in Ferrets, Rabbits, and Rodents

Pathogenesis

- Spontaneous diabetes mellitus is a very uncommon condition in ferrets, rabbits, and rodents (except degus); the pathogenesis is poorly understood.
- Extrapolation from the development of diabetic models in biomedical research suggests that genetic and dietary factors may be implicated depending on the species.
- Iatrogenic diabetes mellitus in ferrets may occur secondary to surgical insulinoma debulking.

Classical Signs

- Lethargy, weight loss, polyuria or dysuria, polydipsia, altered appetite, and cataracts (rodents).

Diagnosis

- Demonstration of persistent hyperglycemia and glucosuria in an animal with suggestive clinical signs.

Treatment

- For spontaneous diabetes mellitus in ferrets, protocols developed for feline patients are considered appropriate.
- Iatrogenic postsurgical diabetes mellitus in ferrets may resolve without treatment.
- In rabbits and rodents, treatment tends to focus on dietary management and supportive care.

I. Pathogenesis
A. **Ferrets:**
   1. **Spontaneous diabetes mellitus is a very uncommon condition** in ferrets and not well documented in the veterinary literature. In theory, it may be caused by a lack of insulin, insulin resistance or a glucagonoma but the precise **pathogenesis is not completely understood.**
   2. Most cases of diabetes mellitus in this species occur **iatrogenically following aggressive pancreatectomy to debulk insulinomas** (see Chapter 23).
B. **Rabbits/rodents:**
   1. As a general rule, diabetes mellitus is a very rare diagnosis in pet rodents and rabbits. While many laboratory strains have been developed as models for diabetes research with the disease induced experimentally by a variety of mechanisms, the **incidence of spontaneous disease in the pet population appears to be very low** and cases are limited to individual and often anecdotal case reports in species such as rats, gerbils, guinea pigs, and chinchillas.
   2. The one exception appears to be in **degus. Diabetes mellitus is a commonly reported disease in this species** and appears to occur spontaneously when they are fed an **inappropriate diet** (including fruits and pelleted feeds **high in starch**) and become **obese.** The condition is thought to be noninsulin dependent (type 2 diabetes) and may be associated with islet amyloidosis. Viral involvement has also been implicated. Similar to dogs, degus have high aldose reductase activity in the lens. This enzyme converts glucose via an alternative glucose reduction pathway to sorbitol. Sorbitol increases the osmotic pressure and water influx in the lens, and if glucose concentrations are chronically increased, this results in **cataract formation.**
   3. **Genetically linked** spontaneous diabetes mellitus is reported in some lines of **Chinese hamsters.** The disease in this species arises due to degranulation of beta cells and a primary deficiency in insulin synthesis.

II. Signalment
A. No known age or sex predilections have been recognized for spontaneous diabetes mellitus in these species.
B. Certain strains of laboratory rabbits and rodents have been bred specifically as models for diabetes research in the biomedical field; however, these are rarely seen in companion animal clinical practice.

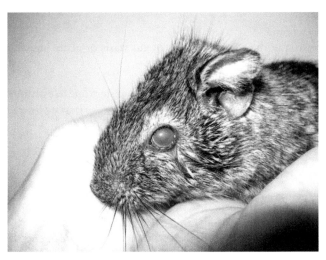

Figure 17.1   Early cataract formation in a diabetic degu. The ocular pathology in this animal resolved following treatment and dietary correction. (Courtesy of Georgina Viktoria Papp and Matyas Liptovszky.)

C. Any ferret that has undergone aggressive surgical excision of an **insulinoma** is considered at risk of developing iatrogenic diabetes mellitus.

III. Clinical Signs
A. **Lethargy/depression.**
B. **Weight loss** or obesity.
C. **Polyphagia** or anorexia/inappetence.
D. **Polydipsia.**
E. **Polyuria** or dysuria.
F. Rapidly forming, bilateral cataracts (especially in guinea pigs and degus) which occur as the hyperglycemia overwhelms the normal metabolic pathways in the lens (Figure 17.1).
G. Infertility (guinea pig sows).

IV. Diagnosis
A. **Ferrets:**
  1. A **persistent blood glucose concentration > 22.2 mmol/L (400 mg/dL) and glucosuria** in a ferret with **consistent clinical signs** is considered diagnostic.
  2. Low blood insulin concentrations and normal to high blood glucagon concentrations may be seen. A **normal or high insulin concentration** accompanied by persistent hyperglycemia may represent **insulin resistance** or the presence of a **glucagonoma.**
  3. Concurrent **ketonuria** may be present in severe cases.
  4. A complete blood count, serum biochemistry panel, survey radiography, and/or ultrasonography are recommended to rule out concurrent disease. Arteriosclerosis and hepatic lipidosis, for example, have been reported in diabetic ferrets.
B. **Rabbits/rodents:**
  1. The diagnosis is made on the basis of serial blood and urine sampling. **Persistent glucosuria, ketonuria, and marked hyperglycemia are highly suggestive of diabetes mellitus** but note that mild glucosuria is not considered a significant finding. The ability to diagnose this disease can be problematic due to difficulties in obtaining repeated blood samples as a result of small patient size. Results may be confounded by the fact that these species often develop a **stress hyperglycemia during handling.**
  2. In guinea pigs, a **glucose tolerance test** has been described.
A baseline blood sample is collected and oral glucose is administered (2 g/kg body weight) following an 18-h fast. Glucose concentrations in guinea pigs with normal glucose tolerance return to baseline by 3 h.

V. Differential Diagnoses

A. **Handling/stress hyperglycemia.**

B. **Hyperglycemia** can be seen in the terminal stages of **gut stasis** or **acute intestinal obstruction in rabbits and rodents.**

C. **Hyperthermia** can be associated with hyperglycemia.

D. Insulin metabolism and blood glucose levels may vary in hamsters due to **estivation and hibernation cycles.**

E. Primary cystitis.

F. Renal disease.

G. Pregnancy toxemia/ketosis.

H. Hepatic lipidosis.

VI. Treatment

A. **Ferrets:**

   1. The **aim of treatment is to try to normalize the blood glucose concentration without the development of hypoglycemia.** Few ferret-specific protocols have been described. As obligate carnivores with a similar glucose metabolism to that of cats, **following the recommendations for feline patients** (see Chapter 16) is considered appropriate.

   2. Treatment is often not required if diabetes has developed as a **postoperative** complication following insulinoma debulking; the condition is often **transient** and the glycemic status normalizes within 1–2 weeks after surgery.

   3. **Insulin therapy is generally indicated if the blood glucose concentration is consistently >16.7 mmol/L (300 mg/dL).** Reported empirical starting insulin doses in ferrets include:

      a. **Neutral protamine Hagedorn** (NPH, isophane insulin), 0.1–1.0 IU/ferret sc q 12 h.

      b. Although ultralente (1 IU/ferret q 24 h) has been reported as efficacious, it is no longer available in most countries.

      c. Glargine is the insulin of choice in cats and would likely be of use in ferrets at a low dose (e.g., initial dose of 0.5 U/ferret and titrate as needed; note glargine cannot be diluted).

      d. Detemir (Levemir, Novo Nordisk) is reported to be efficacious in cats and can be diluted using the manufacturer-supplied Insulin Diluting Medium (Novo Nordisk). Although there are no reports of its use in ferrets, based on its use in dogs and cats, and its ability to be diluted, detemir is potentially a useful insulin for this species. In dogs and cats, the average dose is lower than for other insulins, and a starting dose of ¼ that of other insulins would be recommended (e.g., 0.1–0.2 U/kg q 12–24 h) and titrate upwards. Small doses (<1 U) can be dispensed by calculating the number of drops/U for a given needle size and discarding the appropriate number of drops prior to administering the desired dose. Hold the syringe vertically with the needle pointing down to count drops/U and to discard drops.

      e. After beginning insulin, the dose is gradually increased until the patient is no longer hyperglycemic or ketonuric.

   4. **Insulin therapy should be started in hospital for close monitoring and the ferret discharged only once the blood glucose is stabilized between 6.9 and 11.1 mmol/L (125 and 200 mg/dL).**

   5. **Urine should be monitored closely** by the owner for the presence of glucose and ketones. Realistically, the goal is to have a trace urine glucose reading and negative ketones.

   6. Offering a **low-carbohydrate, high-protein diet** is recommended as an adjunctive measure.

B. **Rabbits/rodents:**

   1. **Dietary modification** to lower fat content (or replace animal fat with vegetable fat), limit starch and fruit intake, and ensure a high protein and high fiber ration is provided.

   2. **Gradual weight reduction in obese patients** is encouraged through calorie restriction, although any weight loss must be slow to avoid inducing hepatic lipidosis.

   3. **Supportive care:**

      a. House on deep absorbent bedding and change daily.

      b. Wet food to increase fluid intake.

      c. Train the owner to give subcutaneous fluids.

      d. Monitor food intake and weight closely.

      e. Reduce stress by ensuring animals have appropriate companionship (e.g., house in pairs) and provide sufficient refuges/hide areas.

4. Medication may be considered if hyperglycemia cannot be controlled by dietary management and supportive care. As in other species, initial doses should be conservatively low and adjusted according to blood and/or urine monitoring. Established protocols do not exist and the literature provides only scant information as a guide:

   a. **Insulin**; the following initial suggested doses have been reported anecdotally:
      1) **NPH insulin**—1 IU q 12 h for a guinea pig; 2 IU q 12 h for a hamster.
      2) **Porcine lente insulin** (Caninsulin; Vetsulin)—1–2 IU/kg subcutaneously q 12 h for a rat; 2 IU q 24 h for a chinchilla.
   b. **Sorbinil**, an aldose reductase inhibitor, has been used in treating and **preventing diabetic neuropathy and cataract** formation in degus.
   c. **Glipizide** has been reported for the treatment of type 2 noninsulin-dependent diabetes mellitus in a guinea pig.

VII. Prognosis
A.   **Guarded to poor in cases of spontaneous diabetes mellitus** as blood glucose concentrations appear to be difficult to regulate in these species.
B.   **Good** in relation to diabetes secondary to **insulinoma** resection.
C.   Spontaneous remission has been reported in guinea pigs.

VIII. Prevention
A.   No specific preventative measures have been identified in relation to spontaneous diabetes mellitus in ferrets.
B.   Given the apparent link between diabetes and obesity and inappropriate dietary management in rodents, the most sensible preventative action for the life of the animal is ensuring **good quality species-appropriate nutrition**, taking care to **avoid overfeeding**.
C.   In colony situations where genetically induced diabetes mellitus is suspected, affected animals should not be allowed to breed.

Diabetes Mellitus in Pet Birds and Reptiles

Pathogenesis

- The existence of true diabetes mellitus in birds and reptiles is debatable and the pathogenesis of disease in suspect cases is unclear.

Classical Signs

- Polyuria and polydipsia.

Diagnosis

- Persistent hyperglycemia with accompanying clinical signs following exclusion of other causes of hyperglycemia.

Treatment

- Can be challenging.
- Supportive care ± medical therapy (e.g., insulin or glipizide).

I. Pathogenesis
A.   **The existence of true diabetes mellitus in birds and reptiles is debatable and the pathogenesis of disease in suspect cases is unclear.** The importance of insulin in birds is not well understood but it is known to be released in response to a wide range of stimuli, not just glucose. Some birds (e.g., ducks) and reptiles (e.g., lizards) have been shown to have high alpha cell predominance in the pancreas and elevated levels of glucagon are thought to play a significant role in the maintenance of blood glucose levels. As such, **glucagon excess** has been proposed as a cause of avian diabetes rather than hypoinsulinemia.

B. In **reptiles**, diabetes may develop secondary to the loss of pancreatic islet cell function due to **severe inflammatory** disease or **trauma**.

C. A **functional pancreatic glucagonoma** has been described in a rhinoceros **iguana** leading to hyperglycemia.

II. Signalment

A. Avian diabetes is most commonly reported in **budgerigars, cockatiels**, and **some larger parrots**; especially those with a history of **obesity and poor nutrition**.

B. Of all the reptile groups, the disease appears to be most often diagnosed in **chelonians**.

III. Clinical Signs

A. **Polyuria** (which may be reported by clients of birds as diarrhea).

B. **Polydipsia**.

C. Weight loss.

D. Polyphagia.

E. Dehydration.

F. Weakness, depression, anorexia, and/or regurgitation especially if concurrent disease is present.

IV. Diagnosis

A. **Birds:**

1. The **normal range for plasma glucose in pet birds is significantly higher than that observed in mammals** with ranges from 10.0 to 27.8 mmol/L (180–500 mg/dL), depending on species. **Values > 44.4 mmol/L (>800 mg/dL) are considered diagnostic for diabetes mellitus.**

2. **Ketonuria and glucosuria** support the diagnosis. When collecting urine for analysis, it is important not to contaminate the sample with feces or uric acid crystals to ensure an accurate result.

3. A **glucose tolerance test** has been described in which 2 g glucose/kg is administered orally to a fasting bird and blood glucose is measured at 0, 10, and 90 min. However, rigorous guidelines on interpretation of results in pet birds do not exist.

B. **Reptiles:**

1. **Persistent hyperglycemia (>11.1–16.65 mmol/L; 200–300 mg/dL)** with or without concurrent glucosuria is consistent with a diagnosis of diabetes mellitus.

2. Blood insulin levels may be useful but normal values have not been established.

C. Collection of a full history, a complete blood count, biochemistry profile, survey radiographs, viral screening, and fecal analysis as appropriate to the case should be undertaken to **rule out other causes of the clinical signs and hyperglycemia.**

V. Differential Diagnoses

A. **Birds:**

1. Transient **stress hyperglycemia**.
2. Hepatic or renal disease.
3. Gastrointestinal disease.
4. Pancreatic neoplasia.
5. Herpes, pox, or polyomavirus resulting in pancreatic pathology.
6. Toxicity or septicemia.
7. Treatment with certain drugs, for example, medroxyprogesterone, aminoglycosides, sulfonamides, tetracyclines, and cephalosporins.
8. Fecal or uric acid contamination of a urine sample.
9. Hyperadrenocorticism (see Chapter 10).
10. Steroid administration.
11. Glucagonoma.

B. **Reptiles:**

1. **Hyperglycemia in reptiles is more often related to metabolic conditions, other systemic diseases and environmental and physiologic variables than true diabetes mellitus.** Some of these include:
   a. Stress.
   b. A recent meal (**hyperglycemia may be seen for several days after a meal**).

    c. Season—temperate species may have higher blood glucose levels at certain times of year, for example, during the breeding season or at emergence from hibernation.

    d. Glucose levels vary with body and liver condition.

    e. Pancreatitis.

    f. Renal failure.

    g. Glucagonoma.

VI. Treatment

A. **General:**

    1. **All attempts to rule out underlying disease and environmental or physiological influences should be made** before the use of insulin or other glucose-regulating drugs is considered.

    2. On the basis of a thorough clinical evaluation, **supportive care** including fluid therapy, alimentation, supplemental vitamins, liver support, and other appropriate chemotherapeutics should be initiated.

    3. **Treatment of any underlying or concurrent condition** must be attempted if the disease is to be adequately controlled.

B. **Glucose-regulating medication in birds:**

    1. Treatment for suspected avian diabetic patients is not always easy or successful. Many patients are small, owner compliance can be poor, and therapeutic protocols have not been well established. In addition, insulin resistance can occur and there may be concomitant pancreatic insufficiency and atrophy. The goal of therapy should be to **eliminate the clinical signs,** rather than provide strict glycemic control.

    2. Some birds appear to respond well to insulin therapy but in others the response can be erratic and vary with the species and individual. The peak and duration of effect of commercially available products is unknown in birds.

    3. All birds undergoing insulin therapy should be hospitalized at the initiation of treatment. The initial **recommended starting dose is 0.1–0.2 IU/kg regular insulin. Serial blood glucose monitoring is recommended**—with samples collected before insulin and every 2–3 h after dosing for up to 24 h. The use of urine reagent strips can be valuable in very small birds where repeat blood sampling is problematic.

    4. Once stable, longer-acting insulin (**neutral Hagedorn or protamine zinc insulin**) may be used. Doses vary significantly and should be titrated. The reported range is **0.067 IU/kg to 3.3 IU/kg intramuscularly q 12–48 h.**

    5. In small patients, regular or NPH insulin may be diluted for accurate dosing. If product-specific diluents supplied by the manufacturer are used, these products appear to remain stable for 30 days once diluted if refrigerated. If non-specific diluents are used (for example, sterile saline or water for injection) the dilution should be made up immediately prior to administration.

    6. **At-home monitoring usually relies on urine testing** (ideally twice daily) but note that **samples can be difficult to obtain if the bird is not polyuric.** To avoid inducing life-threatening hypoglycemia, it is preferable to **maintain the bird at trace/low levels of glucosuria.** Owners should be warned of the signs of hypoglycemia (extreme lethargy, weakness, and seizures).

    7. Recheck visits should be arranged 1 week after initial discharge and thereafter as dictated by alterations in clinical condition. In well-stabilized birds, rechecks may be as infrequent as every 6 months.

    8. Some clinicians report that bovine and porcine protamine-zinc insulin (Caninsulin, Vetsulin) produces the best long-term control of clinical signs whereas human recombinant insulin produces little or no response.

    9. **Oral glipizide 0.5–1.0 mg/kg q 12 h** has been used with varied success.

C. **Glucose-regulating medication in reptiles:**

    1. Little information is available regarding the specific treatment of diabetes in reptiles.

    2. Research indicates that compared with mammals and birds, **reptiles respond very slowly to the administration of mammalian insulin.** For example, insulin given intracelomically may take 24–48 h to be effective, so dosage reevaluations should only be made after several days.

    3. Insulin, glipizide, and somatostatin have been used with limited success in an Asian water dragon.

    4. Starting anecdotal doses for insulin therapy are:

a. Lizards: 5–10 IU/kg q 24–48 h.
b. Snakes and chelonians: 1–5 IU/kg q 24–48 h.

VII. Prognosis
A. No information is available regarding the prognosis of this condition in birds.
B. For reptiles, the prognosis is poor; all documented cases of **persistent hyperglycemia in reptiles** in the literature have failed to survive.

VIII. Prevention
A. No specific preventative measures have been identified for these groups.

References and Further Readings

Chen S. **Pancreatic endocrinopathies in ferrets.** *Vet Clin North Am Exot Anim Pract* 2008;11:107–123.
Datiles MB, Fukui H. **Cataract prevention in diabetic** *Octodon degus* with Pfizer's sorbinil. *Curr Eye Res* 1989;8:233–237.
Durham AE, Rendle DI, Newton JE. The effect of metformin on measurements of insulin sensitivity and beta cell response in 18 horses and ponies with insulin resistance. *Equine Vet J* 2008;40:493–500.
Eiler H, Frank N, Andrews FM, et al. Physiologic assessment of blood glucose homeostasis via combined intravenous glucose and insulin testing in horses. *American J Vet Res* 2005;66:1598–1604.
Harcourt-Brown F. *Textbook of Rabbit Medicine.* Edinburgh: Butterworth Heinemann, 2002.
Hoefer H, Latney L. Rodents: Urogenital and reproductive system disorders. In: Keeble E, Meredith A, eds. *BSAVA Manual of Rodents and Ferrets.* Gloucester: British Small Animal Veterinary Association, 2009, pp. 150–160.
Hudelson KS, Hudelson PM. Endocrine considerations. In: Harrison GJ, Lightfoot TL, eds. *Clinical Avian Medicine*, Vol. 2. Florida: Spix Publishing, 2006, pp. 541–557.
Johnson PJ, Scotty NC, Wiedmeyer C, et al. Diabetes mellitus in a domesticated Spanish mustang. *J Am Vet Med Assoc* 2005;226(542):584–588.
Keeble E. Rodents: Biology and husbandry. In: Keeble E, Meredith A, eds. *BSAVA Manual of Rodents and Ferrets.* Gloucester: British Small Animal Veterinary Association, 2009, pp. 1–17.
Lawrie A. Systemic non-infectious disease. In: Harcourt-Brown N, Chitty J, eds. *BSAVA Manual of Psittacine Birds*, 2nd edn. Gloucester: British Small Animal Veterinary Association, 2005, pp. 245–265.
McArthur S, McLellan L, Brown S. Gastrointestinal system. In: Girling SJ, Raiti P, eds. *BSAVA Manual of Reptiles*, 2nd edn. Gloucester: British Small Animal Veterinary Association, 2004, pp. 210–229.
Montiani-Ferreira F. Rodents: Ophthalmology. In: Keeble E, Meredith A, eds. *BSAVA Manual of Rodents and Ferrets.* Gloucester: British Small Animal Veterinary Association, 2009, pp. 169–180.
Murphy JC, Crowell TP, Hewes KM, et al. Spontaneous lesions in the degu. In: Montali RJ, Migaki G, eds. *The Comparative Pathology of Zoo Animals.* Washington DC: Smithsonian Institution Press, 1980, pp. 437–444.
Orr H. Rodents: Neoplastic and endocrine disease. In: Keeble E, Meredith A, eds. *BSAVA Manual of Rodents and Ferrets.* Gloucester: British Small Animal Veterinary Association, 2009, pp. 181–192.
Pilny AA. The avian pancreas in health and disease. *Vet Clin North Am Exot Anim Pract* 2008;11:25–34.
Pratt SE, Geor RJ, McCutcheon LJ. Repeatability of 2 methods for assessment of insulin sensitivity and glucose dynamics in horses. *J Vet Intern Med* 2005; 19:883–888.
Quesenberry KE, Rosenthal KL. Endocrine diseases. In: Quesenberry KE, Carpenter JW, eds. *Ferrets, Rabbit and Rodents— Clinical Medicine and Surgery*, 2nd edn. St Louis: Saunders Elsevier, 2004, pp. 79–90.
Schott HC, II. Polyuria and polydipsia. In: Reed SM, Bayly WM, Sellon DC, eds. *Equine Internal Medicine*, 3rd edn. St Louis: Saunders Elsevier, 2010, pp. 1214–1218.
Stahl SJ. Hyperglycemia in reptiles. In: Mader DR, ed. *Reptile Medicine and Surgery*, 2nd edn. St Louis: Saunders Elsevier, 2006, pp. 822–830.
Toribio RE. Endocrine pancreas. In: Reed SM, Bayly WM, Sellon DC, eds. *Equine Internal Medicine*, 3rd edn. St Louis: Saunders Elsevier, 2010, pp. 1260–1262.

CHAPTER 18

Canine Diabetic Emergencies

Rebecka S. Hess

Pathogenesis

- Diabetic ketoacidosis (DKA) is a severe form of complicated diabetes mellitus (DM) which requires emergency care.
- Acidosis and electrolyte abnormalities can be life threatening.
- The hyperosmolar hyperglycemic state (HHS) is a rare complication of canine DM which also requires emergency care.
- The hyperosmolarity of the HHS is associated with hypernatremia, but it is not associated with hyperglycemia.

Diagnosis

- In diabetic dogs, a venous pH of < 7.35 and a blood beta-hydroxybutyrate concentration > 2.0 mmol/L or presence of ketones in the urine confirm a diagnosis of DKA.
- A serum osmolality >310 mOsm/L has been used to define hyperosmolarity with severe cases having osmolality >330 mOsm/L).

Treatment

- Fluid therapy and correction of electrolyte abnormalities are the two most important components of therapy for DKA.
- Following 6 h of fluid therapy and electrolyte supplementation for DKA, hyperglycemia is corrected by administration of a rapidly acting insulin.
- Presence of concurrent disease increases the risk for DKA or HHS and must be addressed as part of the diagnostic and therapeutic plan.
- Bicarbonate therapy is usually not needed to treat DKA, and its use is controversial.
- Treatment of HHS is similar to treatment of DKA, except that special attention must be given to slow correction of hypernatremia with 0.9% saline so that the serum sodium concentration decreases no more than 0.5 mEq/L/h.

Clinical Endocrinology of Companion Animals, First Edition. Edited by Jacquie Rand.
© 2013 John Wiley & Sons, Inc. Published 2013 by John Wiley & Sons, Inc.

Prognosis

- About 70% of dogs treated for DKA are discharged from the hospital after a median of 6 days of hospitalization.
- The degree of base deficit is associated with outcome in dogs with DKA.
- Dogs that have concurrent hyperadrenocorticism are less likely to be discharged from the hospital.
- The prognosis for HHS is considered guarded to poor.

I. Pathogenesis

A. **Diabetic ketoacidosis (DKA) is a severe form of complicated diabetes mellitus (DM)** which requires emergency care. Ketones are synthesized from fatty acids as a substitute form of energy, because glucose does not enter cells. Excess keto-acids results in acidosis and severe electrolyte abnormalities, which can be life threatening:

1. **Ketone bodies** are synthesized as an alternative source of energy, when intracellular glucose concentration cannot meet metabolic demands:

   a. Ketone bodies are synthesized from **acetyl-CoA,** which is a product of mitochondrial β-oxidation of fatty acids:

      1) The ATP-dependent oxidation of fatty acids is associated with breakdown of two carbon fragments at a time and results in **formation of acetyl-CoA.**

      2) In nondiabetics, acetyl-CoA and pyruvate enter the citric acid cycle to form ATP. However, in diabetics, glucose does not enter cells in adequate amounts and pyruvate production by glycolysis is decreased. The activity of the citric acid cycle is, therefore, diminished, resulting in **decreased acetyl-CoA utilization.**

      3) The overproduction and underutilization of acetyl-CoA leads to its **accumulation.**

   b. Synthesis of acetyl-CoA is also facilitated by **decreased insulin and increased glucagon concentrations:**

      1) The anabolic effects of insulin include storage of fatty acids in adipose tissue.

      2) Similarly, the catabolic effects of glucagon include lipolysis.

      3) The resultant decreased fatty acid uptake into adipose tissue and increased lipolysis result in elevated acetyl-CoA concentration.

   c. **Acetyl-CoA is the precursor used for ketone body synthesis.**

   d. The three ketone bodies synthesized from acetyl-CoA include **beta-hydroxybutyrate, acetoacetate, and acetone.** Acetoacetate and beta-hydroxybutyrate are anions of moderately strong acids; therefore, their **accumulation results in ketotic acidosis.** Metabolic acidosis may be worsened by vomiting, dehydration, and renal hypoperfusion.

2. **Metabolic acidosis and the electrolyte abnormalities** which ensue are **important determinants in the outcome** of dogs with DKA.

3. It was previously believed that dogs that develop DKA have zero or undetectable **endogenous insulin concentration:**

   a. However, in a study that included seven dogs with DKA, five of them had **detectable endogenous serum insulin concentrations.**

   b. The same study found that two of seven dogs with DKA had **endogenous serum insulin concentration within the normal range.**

   c. Therefore, it is possible that **other factors,** such as **elevated glucagon concentration, contribute** to development of DKA. Glucagon concentration may be elevated due to **concurrent disease.**

B. In contrast to DKA, which is the most common complication of canine DM, the **hyperosmolar hyperglycemic state (HHS)** is a **rare** complication:

1. Traditionally, DKA and HHS have been thought of as two extremes of diabetic complications with DKA characterized mainly by ketosis and acidosis, and **HHS characterized by severe hyperglycemia and dehydration:**

   a. In human beings, DKA was believed to develop acutely, over a 24-h period in young patients with type I DM, whereas **HHS was thought to develop over a 10-day period in older patients with type II DM.**

b. However, more recently, it has become apparent that some **aspects of DKA and HHS can develop simultaneously in an individual.**

c. A mixed state of HHS and DKA is detected in about 30% of humans examined for a diabetic emergency. Additionally, HHS has been well documented in young patients, including pediatric patients with types I or II DM.

2. Therefore, **strict guidelines for clearly differentiating HHS from DKA may not always be clinically important.**

3. The American Diabetes Association has recommended that the terms hyperosmolar nonketotic diabetes or hyperosmolar coma be replaced with the term HHS to illustrate that some degree of ketosis and acidosis may be present in these patients and that varying degrees of mental alterations may be noted.

II. Signalment

A. The **median age of dogs with DKA is 8 years** (range, 8 months to 16 years).

B. Specific **breed or sex** has not been shown to increase the risk of DKA in dogs.

C. Because **HHS is rare**, data are limited but signalment of affected dogs **appears to be similar to those observed in dogs with DKA.**

III. Clinical Signs

A. Clinical signs and physical examination findings in dogs with DKA may be attributed to chronic untreated DM, presence of concurrent disease, or the acute onset of ketoacidosis:

1. The **most common clinical signs** of dogs with DKA are polyuria and polydipsia, lethargy, inappetence or anorexia, vomiting, and weight loss.

2. **Common abnormalities** noted on **physical examination** of dogs with DKA are subjectively overweight or underweight body condition, dehydration, cranial organomegaly, abdominal pain, cardiac murmur, mental dullness, dermatologic abnormalities, dyspnea, coughing or abnormal lung sounds, and cataracts. Some of the findings may be due to concurrent disease and not DKA itself.

B. **Concurrent disease** has been confirmed in approximately **70% of dogs with DKA:**

1. The most common concurrent diseases noted in dogs with DKA are acute pancreatitis, bacterial urinary tract infection, and hyperadrenocorticism.

2. It is possible that presence of concurrent disease results in elevated glucagon concentration and increased risk of DKA.

C. Because **HHS is rare**, data are limited, but **clinical signs appear to be similar to those observed in dogs with DKA.**

IV. Diagnosis

A. In diabetic dogs, a venous pH of < 7.35 and a blood beta-hydroxybutyrate concentration >2.0 mmol/L or presence of ketones in the urine confirm a **diagnosis of DKA.**

B. A thorough diagnostic evaluation is warranted because **most dogs with DKA have a concurrent disorder.** Successful management of the patient depends on the clinician's ability to diagnose and treat the concurrent disorder.

C. **Clinicopathologic abnormalities** are helpful in establishing a diagnosis of DKA and pursuing diagnosis of a concurrent disorder:

1. **Complete blood count:** Approximately 50% of dogs with DKA have a **nonregenerative anemia** (which is not associated with hypophosphatemia), **left-shifted neutrophilia,** or **thrombocytosis.**

2. **Chemistry screen:**

a. **Persistent hyperglycemia** is apparent in all dogs diagnosed with DKA, unless they are insulin treated.

b. **Alkaline phosphatase activity is elevated** in almost all dogs with DKA.

c. **Alanine aminotransferase activity, aspartate aminotransferase activity, or cholesterol** concentration are increased in about half of the dogs with DKA.

d. **Electrolyte abnormalities are common.**

3. **Hypokalemia** and hyperkalemia:

a. Most dogs at initial diagnosis have normo- or hypokalemia although some are hyperkalemic. However, total body potassium is reduced.

b. **Hyperkalemia** may develop as excess positively charged hydrogen ions shift from the extracellular fluid into cells. Positively charged potassium ions then shift out of cells to compensate for the electric shift.

c. Hyperglycemia and hypoinsulinemia contribute to a shift of potassium to the extracellular fluid.

d. Thus, **initially, an animal with DKA may appear to have hyper- or normokalemia.**

e. However, **with rehydration**, potassium ions are lost from the extracellular fluid and **true hypokalemia becomes apparent.**

f. Hypokalemia may be exacerbated by binding of potassium to keto-acids, vomiting, and anorexia.

g. Insulin therapy may worsen hypokalemia as insulin shifts potassium into cells.

h. The **most important clinical significance of hypokalemia in DKA is profound muscle weakness** which may result in respiratory paralysis in extreme cases.

4. **Hypophosphatemia:**

   a. Most dogs are normo- or hypophosphatemic at diagnosis, but some have hyperphosphatemia. Total body phosphorus is reduced.

   b. Hyperphosphatemia develops when phosphate shifts from the intracellular space to the extracellular as a result of hyperglycemia, acidosis, and hypoinsulinemia.

   c. Osmotic diuresis or fluid therapy along with insulin therapy causes extracellular phosphate depletion leading to whole body phosphate depletion.

   d. Hypophosphatemia related to DKA has been **associated with seizures in one dog**.

   e. Severe hypophosphatemia can lead to **hemolysis**; however, anemia can occur in dogs with DKA in the absence of hypophosphatemia as well.

5. In contrast to humans, dogs with DKA **usually do not have low ionized magnesium (iMg^{2+} concentration)** at the time of initial examination. In 78 dogs with uncomplicated DM, 32 dogs with DKA, and 22 control dogs, plasma iMg^{2+} concentration at the time of initial examination was significantly higher in dogs with DKA compared to dogs with uncomplicated DM and control dogs.

6. **Hyponatremia, hypochloremia, and decreased ionized calcium concentration** have also been documented in about 50% of dogs with DKA.

7. **Blood gas analysis:** Venous pH is <7.35 in all dogs with DKA. Lactate concentration is elevated in approximately 33% of dogs with DKA and is not correlated with degree of acidosis.

8. **Urinalysis:**

   a. It is usually indicative of **glucosuria**.

   b. Proteinuria may also be apparent.

   c. **Ketonuria may not be detected** because the nitroprusside reagent in the urine dipstick reacts with acetoacetate and acetone but not with beta-hydroxybutyrate, the dominant ketone body in DKA. **Measurement of serum beta-hydroxybutyrate is more sensitive than measurement of urine ketones.**

   d. The number of white blood cells (WBC) per high power field is usually 5 or less despite the fact that **20% of dogs with DKA have aerobic bacterial growth on urine culture** of a sample obtained by cystocentesis. Lack of pyuria is likely due to immunosuppression of diabetics and decreased ability to mobilize WBC to the site of infection.

9. **Aerobic urine culture is warranted in all dogs with DKA** because urinary tract infections are common, and a **urine sediment may not be an effective screening test** for an infection in these dogs.

D. **Additional testing** such as adrenal or thyroid axis testing, pancreatic lipase immunoreactivity measurement, liver function tests, or liver biopsy will depend on the need to evaluate dogs for **specific concurrent disorders**, depending on their clinical signs and physical examination and clinicopathologic abnormalities.

E. **Imaging modalities** including abdominal radiographs or ultrasound or thoracic radiographs may also be needed in order to evaluate concurrent disorders.

F. **Diagnostic criteria for HHS**:

1. As defined for humans by the American Diabetes Association:

   a. Criteria include a blood glucose concentration >600 mg/dL (33 mmol/L), venous pH >7.30, serum bicarbonate >15 mEq/L, a small or no detectable amount of urine or serum ketone concentration, effective serum osmolality >320 mOsm/kg, and altered mental status.

   b. **Effective osmolality**, which does not depend on blood urea nitrogen, can be calculated using different formulas including the following: Effective $P_{osm} \approx 2 \times$ plasma $[Na^+] + [glucose\ mg/dL]/18$

2. In diabetic dogs, a **diagnosis of HHS** is based on documenting hyperosmolarity in a diabetic:

a. **However,** data regarding the definition of hyperosomlality in diabetic dogs is lacking.

b. In **one** study of 14 diabetic dogs, **normal osmolality (measured or effective) was defined as <310 mOsm/L and marked hyperosmolarity was defined as >330 mOsm/L.**

c. **Although** unproven, hyperosmolarity is unlikely to be clinically significant unless effective serum osmolality is >320 mOsm/kg.

d. **Effective osmolality in diabetic dogs is correlated to Na,** but not to glucose concentration, which has a minor impact.

3. A **search for** a **concurrent disease** is important in HHS.

V. Differential Diagnoses

A. Differential diagnoses for **ketosis** include DKA, acute pancreatitis, starvation, low carbohydrate diet, persistent hypoglycemia, persistent fever, or pregnancy.

B. Differential diagnoses for **metabolic acidosis** include DKA, renal failure, lactic acidosis, toxin exposure, severe tissue destruction, severe diarrhea, or chronic vomiting.

C. In nondiabetics, stress **hyperglycemia,** postprandial hyperglycemia, or hyperglycemia secondary to hyperadrenocorticism, acromegaly, pheochromocytoma, pancreatitis, and other conditions, is usually mild in comparison to the hyperglycemia that develops in DKA.

D. Additional **causes of hyperosmolarity** or hypernatremia in diabetic dogs may include excessive gastrointestinal or renal fluid loss, or rarely, concurrent diabetes insipidus, inadequate water intake, primary hyperaldosteronism, salt poisoning, or iatrogenic hyperosmolar intravenous (IV) fluid administration.

VI. Treatment

A. **Administration and careful monitoring of IV fluid therapy** is the most important component of treatment for DKA:

1. No controlled veterinary studies exist that allow for a sound recommendation as to which commercially available isotonic crystalloid solution is best to use.

2. The American Diabetes Association advocates the use of **0.9% saline** for treatment of DKA because of its relatively high sodium concentration. Since most published literature advocates the use of 0.9% saline (albeit in humans), it is also recommended here for use in dogs.

3. Regardless of which fluid type is used, the dog **must be monitored carefully,** in particular in regard to hydration, mental status, and electrolyte concentrations:

a. **Sodium imbalances should not be corrected at a rate that exceeds 0.5 mmol/L/h.**

b. The rate of fluid administration depends on the percent dehydration of each dog, presence of other conditions (such as heart disease), and ongoing losses (e.g., due to vomiting and diarrhea in acute pancreatitis). However, dogs with DKA are generally very dehydrated and, therefore, the rate of fluid administration is usually high.

c. Fluid therapy **may contribute to a decrease in blood glucose concentration** by improving renal perfusion and decreasing the concentration of counter-regulatory hormones, most importantly glucagon.

d. Fluid therapy also **contributes to resolution of the acidosis.**

B. **Correction and monitoring of electrolyte abnormalities is the second most important component of therapy for DKA.** Electrolyte supplementation **must be monitored frequently,** as adjustment of supplementation rates may be required:

1. A dog that appears hyperkalemic at the time of initial examination may become hypokalemic shortly after fluid therapy has begun. **Hypokalemia** can be treated by administering potassium as an IV continuous rate infusion (CRI) at a rate that should not exceed 0.5 mEq/kg/h (Table 18.1).

2. **When phosphate concentration is <1.5 mg/dL (0.5 mmol/L),** hypophosphatemia is corrected with a CRI of potassium phosphate (the solution contains 4.4 mEq/mL of potassium and 3 mmol/mL (93 mg/mL) of phosphate at a rate of 0.03 mmol/kg/h phosphate IV. Administration of potassium must be taken into account when giving potassium phosphate for correction of hypophosphatemia.

3. A **magnesium sulfate solution** (containing 4 mEq/mL) given IV as a CRI of 1 mEq/kg/24 h has been used successfully for **correction of hypomagnesemia:**

a. **Toxicity of erroneously administered IV magnesium has been reported** in one dog with acute renal disease. Signs of magnesium toxicity included vomiting, weakness, generalized flaccid muscle tone, mental dullness, bradycardia, respiratory depression, and hypotension.

Table 18.1 Potassium supplementation in hypokalemic dogs.*

Serum potassium concentration (mmol/L)	Potassium (mEq) added to 250-mL fluid bag
1.6–2	20
2.1–2.5	15
2.6–3.0	10
3.1–3.5	7

*Not to exceed 0.5 mEq/kg/h.

Table 18.2 Administration of IV insulin in dogs with diabetic ketoacidosis.*

Blood glucose concentration (mg/dL and mmol/L)	Fluid composition	Rate of administration (mL/h)
>250 mg/dL (14 mmol/L)	0.9% NaCl	10
200–250 mg/dL (11–14 mmol/L)	0.45% NaCl + 2.5% dextrose	7
150–200 mg/dL (8–11 mmol/L)	0.45% NaCl + 2.5% dextrose	5
100–150 mg/dL (5.5–8 mmol/L)	0.45% NaCl + 5% dextrose	5
<100 mg/dL (5.5 mmol/L)	0.45% NaCl + 5% dextrose	Stop fluid administration

*2.2 U/kg of regular crystalline insulin added to 250 mL of 0.9% NaCl solution.

b. Care must be taken to **administer IV magnesium only to patients that have documented decreased iMg concentration.**

c. Most dogs with DKA have increased iMg concentration at admission, and, therefore, they do not require IV magnesium supplementation at that time.

4. **Hyponatremia** can be corrected by administering a solution of 0.9% saline.

C. **Correction of hyperglycemia** in DKA is performed by administering a **rapidly acting insulin.** Insulin treatment is **started after 6 h of fluid therapy.** At the moment, **regular insulin** is most commonly used and recommended (Humulin R®, Novolin R®) (Table 18.2):

1. **Regular insulin is administered as an IV CRI or intramuscularly (IM).**
2. When **IV regular insulin is administered as a CRI,** blood glucose is measured every 2 h.
3. When **regular insulin is administered IM,** it is given every hour, and blood glucose is measured every hour:
    a. The initial dose of IM therapy is 0.2 U/kg regular insulin IM, followed by 0.1 U/kg regular insulin IM 1 h later.
    b. Treatment with IM regular insulin is continued with doses of 0.05 U/kg/h, 0.1 U/kg/h, or 0.2 U/kg/h if blood glucose drops by more than 75 mg/dL/h (4 mmol/L), between 50–75 mg/dL/h (3–4 mmol/L), or by <50 mg/dL/h (3 mmol/L), respectively.
4. Several new rapidly acting insulin products have been introduced to the market and are being used successfully in management of humans with DKA. The use of one such insulin, Lispro, is safe and effective in dogs with DKA.
5. A dog **can be transitioned to intermediate- or long-acting insulin,** given subcutaneously, when it is eating full meals reliably:

    a. When the dog reaches a stage in which its appetite is predictable and good, administration of the short-acting insulin is discontinued several hours before the expected administration of the intermediate- or long-acting insulin.

    b. Moderate hyperglycemia should be present when the subcutaneous insulin is administered.

D. **Acidosis in DKA patients** is usually corrected with IV fluid administration and insulin therapy alone. The use of **bicarbonate treatment** for correction of acidosis in humans with DKA **is controversial:**

    1. The American Diabetes Association recommends **bicarbonate supplementation only in DKA patients in which arterial pH remains <7.0 after 1 h of fluid therapy.**

    2. **Possible risks associated with bicarbonate treatment** in humans with DKA include exacerbation of hypokalemia, increased hepatic ketone production, paradoxical cerebrospinal fluid acidosis, cerebral edema, and worsening intracellular acidosis due to increased carbon dioxide production.

    3. **If the American Diabetes Association guidelines were to be applied to dogs, bicarbonate treatment would not be indicated in most dogs with DKA,** because the majority have a venous pH >7.0.

    4. A recent retrospective study of 127 dogs with DKA reported that both the **degree of acidosis and IV sodium bicarbonate therapy were associated with poor outcome.** It is not known if bicarbonate therapy in itself or the severe degree of acidosis that prompted such therapy was the cause of the poor outcome.

    5. Should the clinician deem **bicarbonate therapy** necessary, despite the risks associated with such therapy, a possible bicarbonate treatment protocol may be to administer sodium bicarbonate at **1/2 to 1/3 of [0.3 × body weight × negative base excess]** over a 20-min interval, every 1 h, while monitoring venous pH every hour:

      a. However, it is important to note that **no studies exist to support the above or any other specific bicarbonate treatment** protocol in dogs with DKA.

      b. The American Diabetes Association recommends treating **DKA patients** that maintain a pH of <7.0 after 1 h of fluid therapy with **2 mEq/kg sodium bicarbonate added to 0.9% saline in a solution that does not exceed 155 mEq/L of sodium, over 1 h.** The pH of these patients is monitored every 1 h and treatment is repeated until pH is 7.0 or greater.

E. Presence of concurrent disease is believed to contribute to development of DKA. Therefore, identification of the specific concurrent disease that each dog has and providing the **appropriate treatment directed at alleviating the concurrent disease is indicated.** It is possible that treatment of concurrent disease decreases glucagon secretion and contributes to improved diabetic regulation and resolution of DKA.

F. **Treatment of HHS is similar to treatment of DKA** in that dehydration, hyperglycemia, electrolyte abnormalities, and concurrent disease must be addressed:

    1. However, in treatment of HHS, it is **crucial to lower serum sodium concentration slowly,** in order to decrease the risk of fluid shifting from the extracellular compartment to the brain.

    2. During the hyperosmolar state, **idiogenic osmoles** are formed in the brain, in order to protect the brain from fluid loss. However, once formed, these idiogenic osmoles are cleared slowly, and a rapid decrease in serum osmolality due to rapid lowering of blood sodium concentration could lead to a fluid shift into the brain, and brain edema.

    3. **Therefore, it is crucial that serum sodium concentration be corrected at a rate of <0.5 mEq/L/h:**

      a. **0.9% saline** is the safest fluid, as it is likely to decrease sodium concentration slowly.

      b. However, **careful monitoring of electrolytes is indicated, as in DKA,** to ensure that correction of electrolyte concentrations is appropriate.

VII. Prognosis and Prevention

A. **Most dogs (70%) treated for DKA survive** to be discharged from the hospital. **Median hospitalization time** for dogs with DKA is **6 days:**

    1. At least 7% of dogs develop **recurring episodes** of DKA.

    2. Dogs with coexisting **hyperadrenocorticism** are less likely to be discharged from the hospital.

    3. The degree of **base deficit** is associated with outcome.

B. It is possible that early intervention and prevention of disease concurrent with DM may decrease the incidence of DKA. Since **most dogs with DKA are newly diagnosed diabetics,** it is also possible that early intervention and insulin therapy may prevent complications such as DKA.

C. **Mortality in humans with HHS is high,** and is higher than that reported in humans with DKA:
  1. Mortality in humans with HHS ranges from 15–50% but is difficult to determine due to presence of concurrent disease in many of the patients.
  2. Although the **prognosis is also believed to be guarded to poor in dogs with HHS,** specific numbers or large studies supporting this belief are lacking.

References and Further Readings

American Diabetes Association. Hyperglycemic crises in adult patients with diabetes mellitus. Diabetes Care 2006;29:2739–2748.

Duarte R, Simoes DMN, Franchini ML, et al. Accuracy of serum beta-hydroxybutyrate measurements for the diagnosis of diabetic ketoacidosis in 116 dogs. *JVIM* 2002;16:411–417.

Durocher LL, Hinchcliff KW, DiBartola SP, et al. Acid-base and hormonal abnormalities in dogs with naturally occurring diabetes mellitus. *JAVMA* 2008;232:1310–1320.

Feldman EC, Nelson RW. Diabetic ketoacidosis. In: Feldman EC, Nelson RW, eds. *Canine and Feline Endocrinology and Reproduction.* Philadelphia: W.B. Saunders, 2004.

Fincham SC, Drobatz KJ, Gillespie TN, et al. Evaluation of plasma-ionized magnesium concentration in 122 dogs with diabetes mellitus: A retrospective study. *JVIM* 2004;18:612–617.

Ganong WF. *Review of Medical Physiology*, 18th edn. Stamford: Appleton & Lange, 1997.

Hume DZ, Drobatz KJ, Hess RS. Outcome of dogs with diabetic ketoacidosis: 127 dogs (1993–2003). *JVIM* 2006;20;547–555.

Kitabchi AE, Nyenwe EA. Hyperglycemic crises in diabetes mellitus: Diabetic ketoacidosis and hyperglycemic hyperosmolar state. *Endocrinol Metab Clin North Am* 2006;35:725–751.

Nugent BW. **Hyperosmolar hyperglycemic state.** *Emerg Med Clin North Am* **2005;23:629–648.**

Parsons SE, Drobatz KJ, Lamb SV, et al. Endogenous serum insulin concentration in dogs with diabetic ketoacidosis. *J Vet Emerg Crit* 2002;12:147–152.

Schaer M. Diabetic ketoacidosis and hyperglycemic hyperosmolar syndrome. In: Ettinger SJ, Feldman EC, eds. *Textbook of Veterinary Internal Medicine*, 7th edn. Philadelphia: W.B. Saunders, 2010.

Schermerhorn T, Barr SC. Relationships between glucose, sodium and effective osmolality in diabetic dogs and cats. *JVECC* 2006;16(1):19–24.

Sears KW, Drobatz KJ, Hess RS. Use of lispro insulin for treatment of dogs with diabetic ketoacidosis. *JVIM* 2009;23:696(#40a).

Willard MD, Zerbe CA, Schall WD, et al. Severe hypophosphatemia associated with diabetes mellitus in six dogs and one cat. *JAVMA* 1987;190:1007–1010.

CHAPTER 19

Feline Diabetic Ketoacidosis

Jacquie Rand

Pathogenesis

- Diabetic ketoacidosis is caused by severe insulin deficiency.

Classical Signs

- In its mild form, cats with diabetic ketoacidosis (DKA) appear as typical diabetics.
- In the severe form, cats can present moribund or severely depressed and have marked dehydration.
- Preceding history of polydipsia, polyuria, and weight loss.
- Ketone odor on the breath.

Diagnosis

- Marked hyperglycemia, ketonemia, ketonuria, and acidosis.

Treatment

- Fluid expansion, provision of NaCl-containing fluids, and insulin administration to rapidly correct acidosis.
- Severe form constitutes a medical emergency.

I. Pathogenesis

A. **The extent of insulin deficiency** in diabetic ketoacidosis and the severity of electrolyte and acid-base derangements, as well as the presence of **other comorbidities** directly impact the severity of disease. Signs range from those typical of diabetes to a severe medical emergency requiring immediate intervention:

1. **Severe insulin insufficiency** leads to a **rapid breakdown of fat**, releasing fatty acids into the circulation which are then abnormally oxidized by the insulin-starved liver to ketones, rather than the healthy hepatic metabolism of free fatty acids to triglycerides.

Clinical Endocrinology of Companion Animals, First Edition. Edited by Jacquie Rand.

2. **Free fatty acids** are oxidized to **acetoacetate** which is converted to **beta-hydroxybutyrate or acetone** which can be used as an alternate to glucose as an energy source (see Chapter 18, *Canine diabetic emergencies*, for more details of biochemistry).

3. Insulin insufficiency reduces intracellular glucose concentrations to a level that is insufficient for normal metabolism, resulting in some tissues utilizing increased circulating ketones instead of glucose as their main energy source.

4. If uncomplicated by precipitating conditions, **ketonemia and ketoacidosis can occur approximately 12 and 16 days**, respectively, after glucose-stimulated insulin concentrations are suppressed to fasting levels. **Ketoacidosis** can occur as early as 4 days after ketonemia is first detected.

5. Marked **suppression of insulin secretion** occurs on average **4 days after blood glucose concentrations reach 30 mmol/L (540 mg/dL)**.

6. Increased concentrations of counter-regulatory hormones (e.g., cortisol, glucagon, catecholamines, and growth hormone) may also be involved.

7. Although ketoacidosis can occur purely as a result of marked insulin deficiency, in many cats DKA appears to be associated with precipitating factors such as infection and pancreatitis, especially necrotizing pancreatitis.

8. The ketonemic state causes **central nervous system depression** and ketones act on the **chemoreceptor trigger zone** to produce **nausea, vomiting, and anorexia**. In the kidney, ketones promote osmotic water loss in the urine.

9. **Dehydration** results from inadequate fluid intake in the face of accelerated water loss secondary to glucosuria and ketonuria. The subsequent drop in blood volume reduces tissue perfusion and compounds the acidosis through lactic acid production.

10. In severe cases of DKA, cats have marked dehydration and **extensive loss of electrolytes including sodium, potassium, magnesium, and phosphate**. Some of these plasma deficiencies are **compounded by the intracellular redistribution** of electrolytes occurring **after insulin therapy**.

11. Due to the extreme electrolyte and fluid imbalance, cats with severe DKA can readily develop renal failure. Hyperviscosity, thromboembolism, and severe metabolic acidosis may also be present. All of these conditions are potentially fatal, and a significant number of cats die from the severe form of diabetic ketoacidosis.

12. Clinically and biochemically, cats with DKA and/or hyperosmolar hyperglycemia can be classified into four different categories, which will determine treatment and prognosis:

    a. Cats with minimal depression or dehydration but ketones and acidosis are detected biochemically along with hyperglycemia. These cats are generally managed as "**healthy**" diabetic cats.

    b. Marked depression and dehydration are present along with severe electrolyte abnormalities in the absence of other life-threatening conditions. These cats respond rapidly to appropriate fluid, electrolyte, and insulin therapy and are generally eating and able to be managed on subcutaneous (SC) insulin within 1–2 days.

    c. Severe ketoacidosis compounded by other life-threatening conditions, typically acute necrotizing pancreatitis, sepsis, and/or acute renal failure. Typically these cats require longer than 1–2 days of appropriate therapy before they are eating and can be managed with SC insulin. Of cats dying with ketoacidosis, acute necrotizing pancreatitis was a frequent cause of death.

    d. **Hyperosmolar hyperglycemic state** (formally called nonketotic hyperosmolar diabetes) is a **rare diabetic emergency**. These cats have extreme hyperglycemia (>33 mmo/l. [600 mg/dl], hyperosmolality (>350 mOsm/L), severe dehydration, and severe depression. In the classical criteria for nonketotic hyperosmolar diabetes, ketosis and acidosis are absent, but the American Diabetes Association recommends the use of the term hyperosmolar hyperglycemic state in recognition that approximately 30% of human patients have a mixed condition with some ketosis and acidosis.

B. **Risk factors** for developing diabetic ketoacidosis include:

    1. Undiagnosed diabetes mellitus.

    2. Inadequate insulin dose or dosing frequency or missed insulin dose(s).

    3. Intercurrent illnesses such as sepsis or acute necrotizing pancreatitis.

II. Signalment

A. Signalment is that for diabetic cats, that is, typically cats **>8 years of age**, with most cats between 10–14 years of age.

B. **Risk factors for diabetes** and hence DKA include **senior age, male gender, obesity, Burmese breed of European blood lines, and physical inactivity.** In USA, Maine coon, domestic longhair, Russian blue, and Siamese are overrepresented.

III. Clinical Signs

A. Cats with clinical signs associated with DKA are **moderately to severely dehydrated,** having lost 7–12% of body water on initial presentation.

B. Cats with **severe diabetic ketoacidosis** often present **recumbent with marked dehydration, hypovolemia, metabolic acidosis, and shock.**

C. **Ketone odor,** which has a similar smell to nail varnish remover or acetone, may be evident on the breath.

D. Typically there is a **history of polydipsia and polyuria for weeks to months** and several weeks of prior **weight loss.** However, in some cats, owners do not report polyuria and polydipsia. Lack of owner awareness of the initial classical signs of diabetes puts cats at significant risk of developing DKA.

E. Cats with **mild diabetic ketoacidosis** display typical **diabetic clinical signs** and may have the same preceding history as cats with a more serious form of the disease, but can appear bright and alert on presentation.

F. Severe forms of the disease constitute a potentially fatal medical emergency that needs immediate attention to correct dehydration, electrolyte disturbances, and acidosis.

IV. Diagnosis

A. Most cats have **marked hyperglycemia** (usually >24 mmol/L [436 mg/dL]; range 16 to >35 mmol/L [290 to >630 mg/dL]), **glucosuria, ketonemia** (beta-hydroxybutyrate >0.5 mmol/L; average 4–5 mmol/L), **ketonuria and acidosis** (pH <7.3; TCO_2 i.e. serum bicarbonate <12 mmol/L [12 mEq/L]) (average 8 mmol/L [8 mEq/L]):

    1. The predominant ketone in plasma and urine in cats is **beta-hydroxybutyrate,** but urinary dipsticks detect mainly acetoacetate. However, cats presenting with clinical signs of DKA are typically ketonuric.

    2. Using a cut point of 1.5 mmol/L for urinary ketones, the sensitivity and specificity of urine dipsticks for detecting DKA in cats were reported to be 82% and 95%, respectively; when used with a cut point of 4 mmol/L in plasma, sensitivity/specificity were 100% and 88% for detecting DKA.

    3. Addition of hydrogen peroxide to urine does not improve the sensitivity of urine dipsticks to detect urinary ketones.

    4. Dipsticks and portable meters for measuring beta-hydroxybutyrate are available and are more sensitive for detecting ketosis in cats.

    5. Urine ketones produce a positive dipstick test result approximately 5 days after beta-hydroxybutyrate is detectable in the urine and up to 11 days after beta-hydroxybutyrate is above the reference range in plasma (0.5 mmol/L); therefore, cats are ketonemic well before ketones can be detected in urine with a dipstick.

    6. Cats with ketonemia but without significant acidosis usually appear as "healthy" diabetic cats.

    7. Fasting visible lipemia is detectable approximately 1 week before ketonuria is detectable on dipsticks.

B. It is essential that a **minimum data base** is obtained for **guiding treatment** which should include packed cell volume (PCV), white cell count (WCC), total protein, potassium, phosphorus, total carbon dioxide/bicarbonate, blood urea nitrogen (BUN), creatinine, and calcium, in addition to glucose and ketones:

    1. **Potassium, phosphate, and bicarbonate** must be measured on admission, and in critically ill cats, at least 2–3 times per day in the first 1–2 days. Although concentrations of potassium and phosphate may be elevated or normal (or subnormal) on admission, cats should be monitored frequently in the first 24–48 h as plasma concentrations of these electrolytes can drop rapidly once fluid and insulin therapy begins.

C. If intercurrrent disease is suspected, **ultrasonography** or other diagnostics such as **radiography** may be indicated, for example, to assist in identifying pancreatitis:

    1. **Urine sediment** should be examined for signs of infection.

V. Differential Diagnoses

A. Although diagnosis is rarely a problem in the severe form of DKA, identification of a precipitating comorbidity can be more difficult:

 1. Cats with acute **necrotizing pancreatitis, sepsis, acute renal failure,** and/or other life-threatening conditions need to be differentiated from those with uncomplicated DKA.

 2. Cats with DKA which do not respond within 1–2 days to fluid, electrolyte, and insulin therapy should be suspected of having underlying disease. Acute necrotizing pancreatitis was a frequent cause of death in one study.

B. **Hyperosmolar hyperglycaemic state (formally nonketotic hyperosmolar diabetes).** These cats have extreme hyperglycemia (>33 mmo/L [600 mg/dl], hyperosmolality (>350 mOsm/L), severe dehydration, and severe depression. In the classical form of nonketotic hyperosmolar diabetes, cats are not ketotic or acidotic; however, mixed forms occur with severe hyperosmolality compounded by ketoacidosis.

C. **Any severe illness resulting in severe depression, recumbency, and dehydration can clinically appear as DKA**, especially if there is preceding polyuria or polydipsia. However, these can be easily differentiated from DKA on the basis of the **absence of marked hyperglycemia, ketonuria, and glucosuria.**

D. Proximal tubulopathy (**Fanconi-like syndrome**) associated with dried meat treats that are flavored with "smoke flavor" has been reported in cats; typically cats have polyuria and polydipsia and glucosuria. **Ketonuria** can be present but **persistent hyperglycemia >12 mmol/L is not present.** Urinary fractional excretion studies show increased fractional excretion of phosphate with or without increases in fractional excretion of other electrolytes.

VI. Treatment

A. **Key points of treatment are correcting fluid and electrolyte imbalances and insulin therapy:**

 1. Appropriate **fluid and electrolyte replacement** is the number one priority when treating a DKA cat. Careful monitoring of serum potassium and phosphorus during fluid therapy is essential.

 2. **Insulin treatment** should begin 1–2 h after fluid and electrolyte therapy. If the cat is severely hypokalemic, delay insulin treatment to 3–4 h after the commencement of fluid therapy.

 3. As it is common to have **intercurrent disease** in DKA cats, appropriate diagnostics and management of other conditions may also be necessary.

B. Most DKA cats are **moderately to severely dehydrated (7–12% water loss)** on initial presentation; therefore, fluids are essential and lifesaving:

 1. Although both **0.9% or 0.45% intravenous saline** are used, 0.9% is more common and is advocated by the American Diabetes Association for human DKA patients. Use of hypotonic solutions (0.45%) is advocated by some because of the hyperosmolality of the plasma, but its use is controversial and there are no studies in cats to make evidence-based recommendations. Lactated Ringer's solution or Normosol-R are sometimes used because of their alkalizing effect.

 2. **Fluid rate administration** is dependent on clinical assessment of hydration status, degree of shock, and the presence of concurrent disease with the aim to **correct fluid deficits over 12–18 h using typical flow rates of 60–150 mL/kg/24 h.** Flow rates appropriate for shock therapy should be used for cats with severe signs of dehydration and poor perfusion. Reduce the flow rate if depression worsens, however, as cerebral edema is a possible complication. Despite significant plasma glucose elevations, many DKA cats are protected from marked hyperosmolality by whole body hyponatremia, because sodium rather than glucose is the major contributor to osmolality. This can be seen from the equation: **Osmolality = 2 (Na + K mE/L) + 0.05 (glucose mg/dL) + 0.33 (BUN mg/dL) [Normal range 290–310 mOsm/kg].** Hence many cats do not have severe hyperosmolality, with one study indicating only one third of sick diabetic cats were hyperosmotic (>350 mOsm/kg).

 3. Diabetic cats have relatively **high maintenance fluid requirements** due to high continual fluid losses secondary to glucosuria and ketonuria. **Careful monitoring of DKA cats is essential** to assess hydration status and adequacy of urine output. During hospitalization, continual monitoring of the cat's weight can help detect under- and overhydration. The estimated percent dehydration on admission can be used as a guide to calculating target body weight; account for 0.5–1% body weight loss per day associated with fasting.

Table 19.1 Potassium supplementation in hypokalemic cats.

Serum potassium (mmol/L [mEq/L])	Potassium (mmol or mEq) added to 250-mL fluid bag
<2.0	20
2.0–2.5	15
2.5–3.0	10
3.0–3.5	7

Infuse at a rate <0.5 mmol/kg/h (mEq/kg/h).

4. For cats with the **hyperosmolar hyperglycemic state, fluid replacement must be cautious to avoid adverse cerebral effects.** It is recommended that 60–80% of the deficit be replaced over 24 h and serum osmolarity should not be decreased by more than 0.5–1 osmol/h.

C. **Electrolytes:** Monitoring and correction of electrolyte abnormalities is an important component of therapy for DKA cats. It is essential that fluids are appropriately supplemented to replenish depleted electrolytes:

1. **Potassium:** If serum potassium concentrations are **initially normal or decreased,** immediate **supplementation is required:**

   a. Following initiation of fluid therapy and insulin treatment, **potassium levels will decrease and life-threatening hypokalemia can rapidly worsen.**

   b. Potassium supplementation at 40–80 mEq/L (40–80 mmol/L) may be required depending on the potassium concentration and rate at which it is falling.

   c. If **hyperkalemia** is present, **continual monitoring is essential** and potassium supplementation should be withheld until serum levels are within the normal range.

   d. Initial supplementation should be given at 30–40 mmol/L if serum potassium concentrations are not available; otherwise, supplement fluids using standard dosing protocols (Table 19.1).

2. **Phosphorus:** On initial presentation, plasma phosphorus levels may be **normal, decreased, or increased,** while **intracellular tissue phosphorus is usually depleted:**

   a. Subsequent correction of metabolic acidosis and commencement of insulin therapy results in a shift of extracellular phosphate to intracellular tissue causing **rapid and severe hypophosphatemia.**

   b. **Hypophosphatemia in cats should be considered life threatening** as it results in Heinz body formation and hemolytic anemia.

   c. **Excessive phosphorus** supplementation can cause iatrogenic **hypocalcemia** and its resultant signs, including neuromuscular signs, hypotension, and hypernatremia.

   d. **Normal or subnormal serum phosphorus** levels (<0.48 mmol/L; <1.5 mg/dL) require **supplementation** with **potassium phosphate** and careful monitoring of serum for hemolysis.

   e. Along with phosphorous, potassium is also usually depleted in DKA; therefore, one approach is to **divide potassium equally as potassium chloride and potassium phosphate.**

   f. Alternatively, phosphate can be added to a calcium-free fluid and infused at 0.01–0.03 mmol/L/kg/h (0.03–0.09 mg/dL/kg/h). If hemolysis is evident in conjunction with a decreasing PCV, provide a matched blood transfusion.

3. **Acidosis: Intravenous fluid therapy** and **insulin administration** usually **rapidly corrects acidosis** in DKA patients. Generally mild to moderately-severe acidosis ($HCO_{3-} \geq 7$ mmol/L; 7 mEq/L) resolves with fluid and insulin therapy alone, and **bicarbonate administration is only recommended** when HCO_3 is <7 mmol/L (7 mEq/L). This recommendation is also supported by the American Diabetes Association in human DKA patients with bicarbonate supplementation only indicated if arterial pH remains <7.0 after 1 h of fluid therapy:

   a. The **disadvantages of bicarbonate** therapy include accelerated development of hypokalemia and hypophosphatemia and **greatly outweigh the advantages.**

b. In cats where **severe acidosis** is associated with depression, decreased cardiac contractility, and peripheral vasodilatation, bicarbonate may need to be administered to avoid severe central nervous system acidosis; however, care must be taken to **correct the metabolic acidosis slowly.**

c. Add bicarbonate to fluids at the rate of: HCO_{3-} (mEq) = body weight (kg) $\times 0.4 \times (12 - \text{patient's } HCO_{3-}) \times 0.5$

D. Insulin: Insulin therapy is essential in the treatment of diabetic ketoacidosis because it is required to inhibit further ketone formation and promote glucose and ketone metabolism by insulin sensitive tissues:

1. Commence fluid and electrolyte replacement first, as insulin therapy will worsen hypokalemia and hypophosphatemia, sometimes markedly, resulting in possibly fatal electrolyte disturbances. While decisions on when to start insulin therapy vary with the experiences of the individual veterinarian, in general **wait 1–2 h after commencement of fluid therapy:**

   a. Insulin therapy can begin if serum potassium concentrations are within the normal range after 2 h of fluid therapy.

   b. Insulin therapy can be **delayed a further 1–2 h** if serum potassium is still **below 3.5 mmol/L (3.5 mEq/L),** allowing fluid therapy to replenish the potassium deficit.

   c. It is essential that **insulin therapy is initiated within 4 h** of starting fluids.

2. The aim with insulin treatment is to **gradually decrease blood glucose concentrations** by approximately 4 mmol/L/h (75 mg/dL/h) until 12–14 mmol/L (216–250 mg/dL) by increasing glucose uptake into cells for energy metabolism and reducing gluconeogenesis.

3. Route of administration of insulin can vary depending on protocol. Many practitioners find intermittent intramuscular (IM) and SC protocols easier to manage; however, most intensive-care hospitals use continuous intravenous protocols. While many protocols may be effective in reducing plasma glucose and ketone concentrations, there is debate regarding the most appropriate route for initial insulin administration.

4. Once the patient is rehydrated and serum glucose is reduced to 10–14 mmol/L (180–250 mg/dL), **regardless of initial protocol, change to SC insulin.** Use **SC regular insulin every 6–8 h or long-acting insulin (preferred) every 12 h** (glargine, detemir, or PZI) or porcine lente insulin where there is a legal requirement to first use a veterinary use insulin. Alternatively **maintain on regular insulin IM (q 4–6 h) until eating:**

   a. IM protocol: There are several methods in common use, including regular **insulin once every hour** or **once every 4 h** and **glargine administration every 4 h:**

      1) Regular insulin; hourly protocol: Give cats with severe DKA an **initial loading dose** of 0.2 U/kg followed by 0.1 U/kg hourly. Once blood glucose is 12–14 mmol/L (216–250 mg/dL), discontinue IM injections and change to SC insulin (either regular insulin every 6–8 h or standard maintenance insulin every 12 h). Dextrose can be added to fluids to maintain blood glucose concentration in the 12–14 mmol/L (216–250 mg/dL) range for the first 24 h.

      2) Regular insulin; 4-hourly protocol: Regular insulin can be administered IM every 4 h. While the 4-hourly protocol may seem appealing to many practitioners due to reduced labor, care must be taken as blood glucose concentration can occasionally drop precipitously presumably due to depots of insulin absorbed from previously poorly perfused muscles.

      3) Glargine protocol: Glargine has the same pharmacodynamic and pharmacokinetic effect as regular insulin when given IM or SC. An effective and simple protocol in cats is to initially give **glargine at 2 U/cat SC and 1 U/cat IM regardless of body weight,** and repeat the **IM dose 4 or more hours later if the blood glucose concentration is >14–16 mmol/L (250–290 mg/dL), and the decrease in glucose concentration has not exceeded 4 mmol/L/h; repeat SC administration every 12 h and adjust dose as necessary.**

      4) Add glucose to the fluids once blood glucose is 12–14 mmol/L (216–250 mg/dL).

      5) In one study, more than half the cats on this protocol were able to change to **SC insulin only within 24 h** after initiation of insulin. Cats respond remarkably well, with **most cats eating within 1–2 days** if there is no concurrent disease.

      6) This protocol has advantages of **reduced cost for the client, is less time-consuming, and is simple to follow.**

7) **Hyperosmolar hyperglycemic:** Delay insulin therapy for 2–4 h after initiation of fluid therapy. Give regular insulin at 0.2 U/kg initially and then at 0.05–0.2 U/kg every hour and ensure hyperglycemia is reversed slowly at around 3 mmol/L (54 mg/dL) per hour.

b. **Intravenous protocol:** There are two main methods for intravenous insulin administration:

1) To prepare the infusion add **25 U of regular crystalline insulin** (DO NOT USE lente or NPH) to a **500-mL bag of 0.9% saline.** This produces a concentration of **50 µ/mL** which is infused at **1 mL/kg/h.** Hourly blood glucose monitoring is essential and infusion rate can then be adjusted up or down accordingly to achieve a decrease in blood glucose concentration of 2.8–4.2 mmol/L/h (50–75 mg/dL/h).

2) Alternatively, if using a **250-mL bag of 0.9% saline, add 1.1 U/kg body weight** and infuse initially at **10 mL/h** to provide approximately **0.05 U/kg/24 h.** Adjustment to the rate of infusion can then be made based on subsequent blood glucose concentration.

3) An infusion or syringe pump should be used to administer insulin via a second infusion line attached by a Y piece to the maintenance fluid line. Alternatively two separate catheters can be used to provide both insulin and fluids separately. **Due to insulin's binding affinity to plastic and glass, the first 50 mL run through the line should be discarded.**

4) For both intravenous methods described above, infuse insulin until blood glucose concentration falls to 12–14 mmol/L (216–250 mg/dL), then halve the rate of flow or switch to IM administration of regular insulin every 4–6 h. Alternatively, if hydration status is good, switch to SC administration of regular insulin every 6–8 h or standard maintenance insulin SC.

5) Add 50% dextrose to the fluids to create a **5% dextrose** solution (e.g., **100 mL of 50% dextrose in 1 L of fluids**). This solution should be administered to prevent decreasing blood glucose concentration below 10–12 mmol/L (180–216 mg/dL) and to avoid hypoglycemia while enabling **insulin therapy** to be maintained to **reverse ketone production.**

D. **Food:** It is essential to get DKA cats to eat as soon as possible, as prolonged anorexia can result in further complications especially in obese cats. Preferably use a low carbohydrate food; however, palatable foods may be used initially to encourage eating. Force feeding may be necessary, but can lead to food aversion.

VII. Prognosis

A. Prognosis for cats with DKA is highly **dependent on presence and management of concurrent illness.**

B. Prognosis for recovery from DKA varies and **mortality rates** from tertiary referral hospitals range from **18–36%. Higher survival** rates (up to 100%) have been reported in **uncomplicated DKA cases.**

C. Survival rates are also affected by **delay in seeking treatment** and inability to provide intensive care for several ill cats.

D. Reports from one study indicate that diabetic cats with DKA are no less likely to achieve remission than diabetic cats without DKA. Another study reported that cats were **more likely to resolve their DKA and achieve remission** than to die from DKA.

VIII. Prevention

A. As risk factors for cats developing DKA include undiagnosed diabetes mellitus and inadequate insulin dose or frequency of administration, **early diagnosis of DM** and **appropriate insulin therapy** will decrease the incidence of DKA in cats.

B. Prevention and early intervention of disease concurrent with diabetes mellitus may also prevent complications such as DKA.

C. As **obesity and repeated glucocorticoid** administration are risk factors for diabetes, they should be avoided in cats 8 years of age or older.

References and Further Readings

DiBartola S, Panciera DL. Fluid therapy in endocrine and metabolic disorders. In: DiBartola S. ed. *Fluid, Electrolyte and Acid—Base Disorders in Small Animal Practice*, 3rd edn. Philadelphia, PA: Elsevier Saunders, 2006, pp. 478–489.
Feldman EC, Nelson RW. Diabetic ketoacidosis. In: Feldman EC, Nelson RW, eds. *Canine and Feline Endocrinology and Reproduction*, 3rd edn. Philadelphia, PA: Elsevier Saunders, 2004, pp. 580–615.

Hume DZ, Drobatz KJ, Hess RS, et al. *J Vet Intern Med.* 2006;20:547–555.

Koenig A, Drobatz KJ, Beale AB, King LG, et al. Hyperglycemic, hyperosmolar syndrome in feline diabetics: 17 cases (1995–2001). *J Vet Emerg Med Crit Care* 2004;14:30–40.

Marshall RD, Rand JS, Gunew MN, Menrath VH. Glargine administered intramuscularly is effective for treatment of feline diabetic ketoacidosis, 2010 ACVIM Forum Abstracts, *J Vet Intern Med* 2010;24:686–687.

Nelson R. Diabetes mellitus. In: *Textbook of Veterinary Internal Medicine*, 6th edn. St. Louis, MO: Elsevier Saunders, 2005, pp. 1563–1591.

Maintenance protocols for insulin administration are available. Available at: www.uq.edu.au/ccah/index.html?page=41544

CHAPTER 20

Equine Metabolic Syndrome/Insulin Resistance Syndrome in Horses

John Keen

Pathogenesis

- Equine metabolic syndrome (EMS) is a newly characterized syndrome of insulin resistance (IR) predisposing horses to laminitis.
- IR is reflected by subtle or more obvious changes to glycemic status.
- Obesity and genetic susceptibility play a key role in the EMS.
- The link between EMS and laminitis is not currently clear but may involve chronic low-grade inflammation and/or changes in vascular function.

Classical Signs

- Signs of EMS are similar to pituitary pars intermedia dysfunction (PPID) or equine Cushing's disease but lacking key crucial signs of PPID such as hirsutism.
- Overweight or obese (body condition score >3/5; >6/9) and/or accumulation of fat in specific sites such as the nuchal crest, rump, supraorbital region, and prepuce or mammary region.
- Repeated bouts of clinical laminitis.
- Signs of chronic low grade subacute laminitis such as divergent laminar rings, convex/flat sole, and widened white line.
- Infertility in mares.

Diagnosis

- Phenotype and clinical signs raise an index of suspicion.
- Assess glycemic status.
  - Resting metabolic profile.
  - Tests of glucose and insulin dynamics.
- Exclude PPID on the basis of clinical signs and tests.

Clinical Endocrinology of Companion Animals, First Edition. Edited by Jacquie Rand.
© 2013 John Wiley & Sons, Inc. Published 2013 by John Wiley & Sons, Inc.

Treatment

- Feed and exercise management.
- Some medications to improve insulin sensitivity and help weight loss are currently undergoing scrutiny.

I. Pathogenesis

The **Equine Metabolic Syndrome (EMS)** is a term used to define a complex metabolic disorder in horses and ponies which phenotypically is characterized by adiposity (either localized in specific regions or generalized obesity), insulin resistance (IR), and a predisposition to laminitis. Infertility in mares and an increased risk of developing pituitary pars intermedia dysfunction (equine Cushing's disease) may also be components of the syndrome. **IR appears to be a key factor** in the pathogenesis of the EMS, and IR may also represent a common factor increasing the risk of laminitis from a **variety of clinical risk factors** (Figure 20.1).

A. **Insulin sensitivity and IR: definitions and consequences:**
   1. Insulin sensitivity is defined as the glucose lowering effect of a given amount of insulin (pancreatic beta cell derived hormone). IR refers to markedly decreased insulin sensitivity:
      a. In a normal physiological state, the increase in glucose concentrations following a carbohydrate meal stimulates insulin secretion which maintains glucose concentrations in the normal range.
      b. In horses with IR, insulin concentrations are increased to compensate for the effects of reduced insulin sensitivity; when beta cells cannot adequately compensate, glucose concentrations also increase. IR is characterized by hyperinsulinemia, or abnormal glycemic and insulin responses to an oral or intravenous glucose and/or insulin challenge.
   2. In the earlier stages of dysregulation, resting glucose concentrations are normal (or slightly increased) but may be increased after a glucose challenge, termed **impaired glucose tolerance:**
      a. With **impaired glucose tolerance**, there is a **delayed return of glucose and insulin concentrations** to normal after a glucose challenge. The underlying IR results in resting insulin concentrations above the normal reference range and increased insulin secretion during the glucose tolerance test.
   3. As IR becomes more severe and beta cells are unable to fully compensate by secreting adequate amounts of insulin to maintain normoglycemia; concentrations of both insulin and glucose are increased at rest.

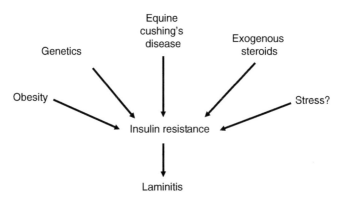

Figure 20.1   Clustering of clinical risk factors for equine laminitis. Insulin resistance is common to all of these risk factors. Genetic predisposition and obesity are currently thought to be key clinical components of the disorder termed equine metabolic syndrome (EMS).

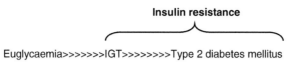

Insulin resistance

Euglycaemia>>>>>>>IGT>>>>>>>>Type 2 diabetes mellitus

Figure 20.2   Insulin resistance develops gradually, with impaired glucose tolerance preceding overt type 2 diabetes mellitus. Horses are rarely diagnosed with type 2 diabetes mellitus, but many are likely to demonstrate impaired glucose tolerance (IGT).

4. The ultimate event is marked hyperglycemia in the face of decreased insulin secretion as a result of pancreatic cell failure (i.e., decompensation) (Figure 20.2). **Resting glucose concentrations that are markedly increased signify the onset of type 2 diabetes mellitus.**

5. **More subtle alterations in glycemic status such as** impaired glucose tolerance **may be most relevant to the** situation **in horses and ponies, where overt type 2 diabetes mellitus is rarely detected clinically:**

    a. This highlights the importance of feeding appropriate low glycemic index (GI) feedstuffs to minimize postprandial glucose increases, particularly in at risk individual horses and ponies. Identifying these at risk horses is therefore crucial.

6. Strict criteria have been defined for normal glycemic status in humans. The situation is currently less clear in horses although many studies have started to define relevant criteria:

    a. Measuring compounds which reflect long-term glycemic status, such as **fructosamine or glycosylated hemoglobin**, may also be appropriate, although this has met with **limited success** in horses thus far.

7. The direct **consequences of IR** are not known. Studies in other species suggest that persistent hyperglycemia has **detrimental effects on vascular cell function, especially endothelial cells.** Furthermore insulin has direct vasoactive properties; in IR, persistent hyperinsulinemia may potentially be detrimental. Experimentally, **laminitis can be induced in horses and ponies with very high concentrations of insulin sustained over 48–72 h** while maintaining euglycemia.

B. The role of obesity:

The link between obesity, EMS and laminitis is unclear. While IR may promote fat deposition, obesity (particularly abdominal obesity) is likely a major contributor to IR. In addition to **producing the breakdown products of fat** (e.g., fatty acids) which themselves affect glucose metabolism, **adipocytes are metabolically active and appear to produce a number of hormones and cytokines that promote IR:**

1. Cytokines: for example, tumor necrosis factor (TNFα) and interleukins:

    a. Increased TNFα concentrations have been recorded in insulin resistant ponies predisposed to developing laminitis and in obese mares.

2. **Adipokines: these are secretory products of adipose tissue:**

    a. Some adipokines, for example, **resistin**, promote IR whereas others, for example, **adiponectin**, promote the actions of insulin.

    b. **Leptin** is a satiety hormone and leptin resistance (and therefore raised leptin concentration) is a feature of the human metabolic syndrome. Leptin concentrations are raised in obese horses.

    c. It is proposed that **in human metabolic syndrome**, an imbalance occurs, favoring production of the **hormones promoting IR.** This may be due to increased **deposition of certain types of fat** cells in certain locations.

    d. The potential role of adipokines in equine obesity and predisposition to laminitis is currently undergoing further scrutiny.

C. **The role of inflammation and vascular dysfunction:**

Chronic low-grade inflammation, particularly involving the vasculature, may be an important factor in the pathogenesis of the EMS:

1. As noted above, adipocytes release cytokines which are proinflammatory.

2. Furthermore, **in human metabolic syndrome** there is biochemical evidence of **vascular dysfunction** and **oxidative stress** prior to clinical signs of cardiovascular disease or the vascular complications of

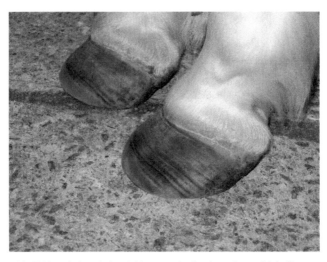

Figure 20.3   Foot of a pony with EMS and chronic laminitis; note the laminar rings which diverge toward the heel region.

diabetes. **Vasoconstrictor** mediators such as **endothelin** are **raised** while **vasodilator mediators are reduced.** Mediators involved in the coagulation cascade and cellular adhesion to endothelial cells are also raised. These factors may be related to hyperglycemia and/or hyperinsulinemia.

3. **No changes in such mediators** were noted in **preliminary studies of ponies** with EMS predisposed to laminitis or indeed in horses with pituitary pars intermedia dysfunction.

D. Other concepts:

1. **Diet has an important influence on the expression of EMS** and in affecting glucose and insulin dynamics. For example, **differences in glycemic status and blood pressure** between laminitis-prone and non-laminitis-prone ponies were most apparent when **grazing summer pasture.**

2. **Glucocorticoids:** the **similarities between pituitary pars intermedia dysfunction and EMS** are intriguing in terms of **fat distribution and predisposition to laminitis. Laminitis** has anecdotally been **linked to iatrogenic corticosteroid administration.** Furthermore, dexamethasone treatment can induce IR in horses. It has been proposed that local, tissue specific cortisol concentrations may be important in human metabolic syndrome and the same may be true of horses. The enzyme 11 beta-hydroxysteroid dehydrogenase type 1 (11beta HSD-1) which controls the intracellular concentration of active cortisol may be important in this regard.

II. Signalment

A. **Predisposed breeds** for the EMS include **UK native pony breeds** such as **Highland, Shetland, Welsh, Dartmoor ponies, etc.** and in the USA breeds such as **Morgan and Paso Fino.** These breeds are not however exclusively at risk. **Donkeys** may also be predisposed.

B. **All ages** of horse may be affected, including young adults, in contrast to PPID which is usually a disorder of aged horses.

C. **No sex predisposition** has been shown for EMS as yet:

1. In one study evaluating predisposition to laminitis in a closed herd of ponies at pasture, stallions were considerably less likely to become laminitic compared to mares.

2. Other studies of laminitis itself have not shown a sex predisposition; both sexes may be affected.

III. Clinical Signs

A. Repeated bouts of clinical **laminitis** and/or signs of chronic low-grade subacute laminitis such as **divergent laminar rings, convex/flat sole,** and **widened white line** are the most clinically important signs (Figure 20.3).

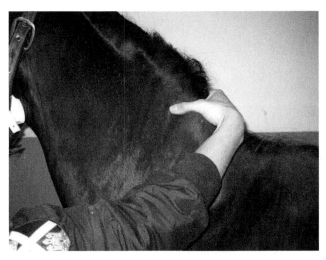

Figure 20.4   Increased fat deposition in the neck crest of a horse creating a mounded appearance and a neck that loses its sideways flexibility.

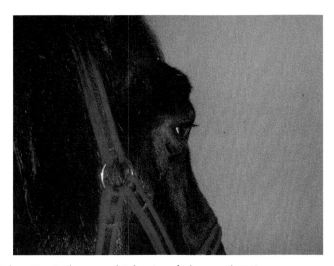

Figure 20.5   Increased fat deposition in the supraorbital region of a horse with EMS.

B. Affected cases are usually **overweight or obese** (body condition score >3/5 on the Carroll and Huntington scale or >6/9 on the Henneke scale) **and/or** show **accumulation of fat in specific depot sites** such as the nuchal crest (Figure 20.4), the rump, the supraorbital region (Figure 20.5), and the prepuce or mammary region (Figure 20.6):

1. **Subjective neck crest scores** (0–5) have been developed and correlate well with objective neck measurements as well as blood variables indicative of altered glycemic status.

C. **Chronic reproductive cycling abnormalities in mares** may occur with EMS, similar to obesity in other species such as dairy cattle.

D. One study showed that **relative hypertension may also be a feature** of the EMS although this is not otherwise clinically apparent:

1. As values for blood pressure vary widely in horses and will depend upon the method used, no recommendations for "cutoff" values indicating hypertension can be given at the present time.

2. The relative hypertension may reflect microvascular dysfunction which may predispose to laminitis.

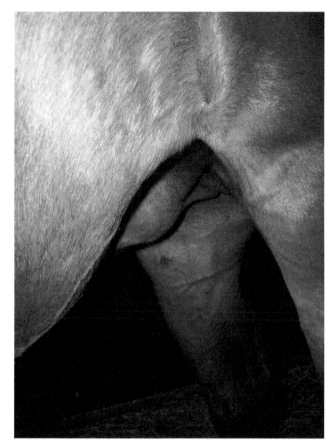

Figure 20.6 Fat deposition in the mammary region of a mare with EMS.

IV. Diagnosis

A. If a horse is **overweight/obese and suffers recurrent bouts of laminitis,** then it probably has underlying metabolic predisposition to obesity and laminitis and, in the absence of PPID, may be classified as suffering from EMS. Similarly any horse or pony with **unexplained laminitis** (e.g., no identifiable trigger such as severe colic, colitis, metritis, pleuritis, etc.) should be considered as **metabolically at risk** and therefore potentially classified as suffering from EMS:

    1. **Pasture associated laminitis, typically seasonal, is the most important group of horses in this regard.**

    2. Examples of horses with **unexplained laminitis** include those that develop laminitis **post vaccination** or **following exogenous steroid administration.**

B. Radiographic evaluation may reveal evidence of chronic laminar changes such as rotation, sinking, or tip remodeling of the pedal bone and laminar lucencies.

C. The **glycemic status** of such horses is worthy of further assessment, and if abnormal, it is likely an indicator of the degree of severity of IR and beta cell failure and also provides a benchmark to monitor response to any treatment regimen adopted. Evaluation of all variables must be taken in the clinical context. In many cases, "normal" reference ranges for different breed types and different body condition scores have not been established:

    1. Resting metabolic profiles:

        a. **Glucose and insulin.** The simplest approach is measurement of a **single resting glucose concentration** along with measurement of **serum insulin** concentration. This may be carried out in conjunction with tests to rule out PPID (see Chapter 11):

1) Water and a small amount of grass hay may be offered overnight without invalidating the test, but **concentrates must be excluded for 12 h prior to testing.**

Increased resting concentrations of **insulin (>139 pmol/L [20 mIU/L; 20 µIU/mL])** provide good supportive evidence of **IR.** Horses with normoglycemia and insulin concentrations **>694 pmol/L (100 mIU/L; 100 µIU/mL)** have more extreme evidence of IR and are at **high risk of laminitis.** It should be noted, however, that **insulin assays vary between laboratories,** and therefore using a **laboratory-specific reference range** for interpretation of results is essential:

   a) Note insulin conversion factors are as follows: Insulin (µU/mL)×6.945=(pmol/L); 1 mIU/L=1 µIU/mL).

2) Glucose concentrations are rarely above the upper limit of the reference range in EMS but often toward the upper end of the range (**upper limit of reference for glucose =6 mmol/L [108 mg/dL]).**

3) **High glucose concentrations** in a nonstressed resting horse **suggest severe IR** and some degree of **beta cell failure.** In a small minority of horses, this progresses to **type 2 diabetes** (diabetes mellitus in horses occurs most commonly **secondary to PPID** and would be classed as "**other specific type of diabetes**").

4) In humans, **impaired fasting glucose** is defined as **glucose concentrations above normal but less than diabetic.** Individuals with impaired fasting glucose are considered prediabetic and at increased risk of developing diabetes. Equivalent glucose concentrations for horses for **impaired fasting glucose in horses would be 7–10 mmol/L (126–180 mg/dL) and diabetic >10 mmol/L (>180 mg/dL).**

b. A mild increase in liver derived enzymes (e.g., gamma-glutamyl transferase and glutamate dehydrogenase) is often also apparent and likely to relate to the **mild triglyceridemia** (and therefore **triglyceride infiltration of the liver**) in these cases rather than primary liver dysfunction.

c. Since **dyslipidemia** is a feature of EMS, lipid profiles may also be useful, although this has not yet been fully evaluated clinically. **Triglyceride >0.64 mmol/L (57 mg/dL)** was used as one feature to **predict susceptibility to laminitis** in one study.

d. Other blood variables which have been shown to be abnormal in EMS cases (e.g., adipokines, markers of systemic inflammation), although of great interest from a research point of view, are unlikely to provide valuable and cost effective diagnostic use until considerable work has gone into assessing their sensitivity and specificity for diagnosing EMS.

2. **Proxies for measures of IR:**

a. Proxies (or surrogates) are **calculations based on resting blood concentrations of insulin and/or glucose.**

b. They are commonly used in large-scale human studies due to the ease of collection compared to dynamic profiles and their enhanced ability to detect IR compared to resting concentrations of insulin alone.

c. Two proxies that have been shown to be the **most accurate representation of dynamic insulin sensitivity status in horses** are:

   1) The **reciprocal of the square root of insulin (RISQI)** = $1/\sqrt{\text{insulin}}$ (mIU/L).

   2) **MIRG=modified insulin to glucose ratio**=[800 − 0.3 (insulin-50)^2] / glucose − 30 (mIU$_{\text{insulin}}^2$ / [10.l mg$_{\text{glucose}}$]) when glucose is measured in mg/dL and insulin in µIU/mL or mIU/L. Note that MIRG is not a useful proxy when resting insulin is >347 pmol/L (50 mIU/L).

d. These proxies have been used to **predict susceptibility to laminitis** in conjunction with **clinical (body condition score >6/9)** and biochemical [**triglyceride concentration >0.64 mmol/L (57 mg/dL)**] data:

   1) The reference values used for the proxies in that study were normal ≥0.32 (µIU/mL)$^{-0.5}$ for RISQI and normal <5.6 mIU^2 / (10.L.mg$_{\text{glu}}$) for MIRG.

   2) Note that these values indicated good accuracy for diagnosing predisposition to laminitis in a closed herd. The **cutoff values may not be appropriate** for all horses and ponies nor **if insulin is measured in other laboratories.** Nevertheless, differences in these proxies between normal and EMS horses have been noted in outbreed populations of horses.

e. Although more work is required to develop cutoff values for these **proxies** to determine IR versus non-IR, they may be **useful for monitoring response to therapeutic approaches adopted.**

Table 20.1   Dynamic tests for equine glycemic/insulin status applicable to clinical practice.

Test	Method	Interpretation
Oral glucose tolerance test (OGTT)	1 g/kg glucose is administered as a 20% solution Blood glucose and insulin levels are tested prior to administration and at 30, 60, 90, 120, 150, 180, 240 min	Blood glucose should double within 2 h and normalize within 6 h. Glucose (>11.1 mmol/L; 200 mg/dL) or delay to normal levels is indicative of insulin resistance. Beware of other conditions which could affect this test, for example, gastrointestinal dysfunction. Using the insulin levels as well as glucose gives more information. It has been suggested that an I:G at 90 min may be a convenient parameter to test for insensitivity. I:G >0.3–0.5 (insulin measured in mIU/L or µIU/mL and glucose in mg/dL) suggests relative insulin resistance. Total insulin secretion is also raised with insulin resistance. Note when also evaluating insulin, horses with type 2 diabetes mellitus (rare) may have low/normal insulin and high resting glucose and glucose responses
Intravenous glucose tolerance test (IVGTT)	0.5 g/kg dextrose as 50% solution IV following 12-h fast. Collect samples for glucose and insulin at 0, 0.25, 0.5, 1, 2, (3, 4, 5, 6) h	Normal is >300% increase in glucose at 15 min followed by rapid decrease; plus >600–700% increase in insulin at 15 and 30 min, followed by a decrease. Glucose and insulin concentrations should return to baseline within 1–2 h
Combined intravenous glucose and insulin tolerance test (CGIT)	Collect baseline blood sample for glucose and insulin. Infuse 50% dextrose (0.15 g/kg), immediately followed by 0.10 U/kg regular insulin. Further samples are collected for glucose at 1, 5, 25, 35, 45, 60, 75, 90, 105, 120, 135, and 150 min; and for insulin at 45 min	Impaired glucose tolerance is the maintenance of blood glucose above baseline for >45 min. Insulin levels should decline to <695 pmol/L (100 mIU/L; 100 µIU/mL) by 45 min; anything longer is suggestive of IR

3. **Dynamic assessment of glycemic status:**
   a. Dynamic tests are **more likely to detect subtle alterations in glycemic and insulinemic status.**
   b. These methods are however more complex, time consuming, and expensive.
   c. As with resting profiles, for all dynamic tests, horses are best **stabled overnight with no concentrate feed for 12 h** but a small amount of grass hay may be offered. Water should be removed 2 h prior to testing in oral tests.
   d. Table 20.1 describes the method and interpretation of four methods for dynamic assessment of glycemic status that have been evaluated in the horse. The more complex **hyperinsulinemic euglycemic clamp** method, deemed by many to be the gold standard for assessing insulin sensitivity, is not described as it is not applicable to general practice. Another useful research tool is the **frequently sampled intravenous glucose tolerance test (± insulin modification) with minimal model analysis.**
   e. Figures 20.7 and 20.8 show a schematic representation of the two commonly used tests: the oral glucose tolerance test and the combined intravenous glucose and insulin test. The latter has been recommended following a recent American College of Veterinary Internal Medicine consensus statement.

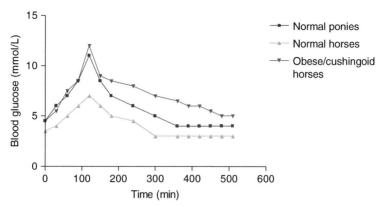

Figure 20.7   Schematic blood glucose curves following intragastric administration of 1 g/kg glucose (20% solution). Note the increased peak and longer duration of hyperglycemia in ponies and those considered insulin resistant (obese/EMS and pituitary pars intermedia dysfunction/Cushingoid).

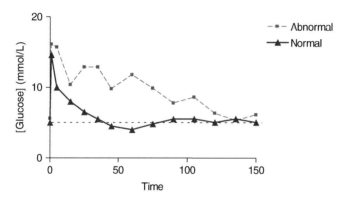

Figure 20.8   Schematic blood glucose curves following intravenous administration of glucose and insulin. Note that in the "normal" curve, the blood glucose quickly (<45 min) drops below the resting glucose level and is maintained at this level throughout the test. In contrast with the insulin resistant (abnormal) case, the glucose is maintained above the baseline for the duration of the test.

V.   Differential Diagnoses

A.   **Pituitary pars intermedia dysfunction (PPID)** is the most important clinical differential diagnosis for EMS and steps should be made to rule out this endocrine disorder, as treatment for PPID is well character-ized and effective. Since PPID develops insidiously, dynamic endocrine tests may be required to fully rule out this condition rather than relying on resting hormone analysis (see Chapter 11).

B.   **Hypothyroidism** is rare in horses. Despite the fact that ponies with EMS may have low T_4 concentra-tions, dynamic thyroid evaluation tests have shown that hypothyroidism is not the cause of EMS.

VI.   Treatment

At present, the major approach to managing the EMS is **control of energy intake combined with judicious exercise** in those individuals where this is possible. Some medical treatments under evaluation at the time of writing are also described.

A.   **Feeding and supplements:**

   1.   Feeds with a **low GI** should be chosen, that is, **low soluble carbohydrate and high structural carbohy-drate.** Complete starvation is not advised as this promotes a survival mode of increased IR, thus poten-tially exacerbating the EMS. Furthermore, many **donkeys and ponies** (especially the Shetland breed) are at **risk of hyperlipemia,** a **potentially life-threatening** condition.

2. **Grass should be avoided or restricted** in EMS horses since soluble (i.e., readily available) carbohydrate content can be unacceptably high, particularly during the growing seasons. **Restricted grazing practice must be balanced with the need for exercise;** therefore, the use of **grass muzzles or strip grazing** may be advantageous.

3. Fructans and other soluble carbohydrates (e.g., starch) are highest in the grass during the daytime therefore **early morning (except after frost) or night grazing may be preferable.**

4. **Grass hay** is a good source of preserved forage but may be **variable in soluble carbohydrate content** therefore best practice is to encourage owners to **have the quality analyzed.**

5. **Soaking hay** (12 h is suggested to be optimal) may reduce the soluble carbohydrate as it gets trapped in the water although the efficiency of this varies with the grass types and methods used. **Do not soak haylage.**

6. An amount of 1.5–2% of estimated ideal body weight of dry (presoaked) hay (i.e., **1.5–2 kg hay per 100 kg**) is recommended as an **initial ration for weight loss.** This may be reduced to a minimum of 1% of body weight but be aware that **unacceptable behavioral stereotypies** may develop at this ration level.

7. If further feeding is required in addition to forage, then other low GI foods may be acceptable. For example, **sugar beet (unmolassed) has a very low GI**, as does **alfalfa/lucerne chaff** which is often suitable for older ponies with bad dentition. Alternatively, there are good proprietary compounded feeds specially designed for laminitic horses.

8. Minerals, vitamins, and trace elements should be supplemented for those solely on a forage ration.

9. There is some evidence to suggest that **antioxidant therapies** protect against vascular dysfunction in human diabetics and others at risk of cardiovascular diseases; their usefulness in horses is unknown at present. Studies in ponies with a previous history of laminitis have shown conflicting evidence of redox dysfunction.

B. Exercise:

1. **Exercise is avoided in clinical laminitis** but, when the pony is clinically stable, exercise should be gradually built up and actively encouraged:

  a. **Exercise has been shown to improve insulin sensitivity in horses.**

  b. A recent study has shown that an increasing regimen of 2–4 h exercise per week (comprising a walking warm up, trotting, and a walking warm down) spread over 3 days combined with feed restriction improved insulin sensitivity and achieved beneficial weight loss.

  c. Others have suggested approximately 30 min/day of brisk walk or trot.

2. Placing an animal out to grass is beneficial to encourage exercise, but can be difficult at the high-risk times of year. Grazing muzzles which limit intake are useful in this regard.

C. Medications under investigation:

1. Humans with obesity and type 2 diabetes mellitus are often treated with oral hypoglycemic agents, for example, metformin, which improves insulin sensitivity and thereby enhances glucose uptake by cells, and unlike some other drugs used for human diabetes, will not cause hypoglycemia:

  a. Studies of **metformin** in horses have shown **mixed results** depending on the study type and dose used.

  b. One study using metformin doses of approximately 2.8–8.4 mg/kg PO BID in obese mares concluded that this drug showed no long-term improvement in insulin sensitivity.

  c. In a longitudinal intervention study of 18 horses and ponies, metformin administration at 15 mg/kg PO BID improved insulin sensitivity and decreased the secretion of insulin, as measured by proxy assessment from resting blood insulin and glucose values, at least in the short term.

  d. A recent controlled study however suggested that 15 mg/kg of metformin BID PO is not effective in improving insulin sensitivity in obese ponies.

  e. Other studies have shown that oral **bioavailability of metformin** at a dosage of 15 mg/kg PO BID is very poor, especially in fed horses (<5%) and that subtherapeutic concentrations (compared to those in humans) are detectable in plasma.

2. Thyroid supplementation has been administered to many obese laminitis in the belief that the horses were suffering from hypothyroidism. This is unlikely in the majority of cases. Nevertheless, it may be that **thyroid supplements could be an aid in the short term to help lose weight and increase insulin sensitivity:**

a. It has been shown that administration of 24–48 mg thyroxine per day can lead to weight loss and improve insulin sensitivity in normal horses. This has yet to be evaluated as a method of improving insulin sensitivity and reducing risk of laminitis in "at risk" horses.

3. There is great interest in human medicine in a group of compounds known as **thiazolidinediones** which lower IR (these are so-called insulin enhancers) by acting on nuclear receptor proteins known as PPARs. **Pioglitazone** administration to **lean healthy horses** did **not improve insulin sensitivity.**

4. In theory, considering its possible involvement in omental adiposity and the human metabolic syndrome, antagonism of cortisol activity may be advantageous. No such drugs are currently licensed for clinical use in the horse:

a. **Trilostane**, a 11betaHSD inhibitor licensed for canine Cushing's disease, has been used in EMS (approximate dose 1 mg/kg) and demonstrated **minimal beneficial effects**. Control animals were not evaluated.

5. In view of their currently questionable efficacy and lack of veterinary licensing, use of medications without also instituting management changes should be avoided.

VII. Prognosis

A. **Prognosis is good** in animals **without laminitis or overt diabetes provided successful weight loss** is achieved and soluble carbohydrate intake is controlled.

B. Prognosis is **guarded** in those cases with repeated bouts of **severe clinical laminitis** which are likely to have had irreparable damage to the laminar attachment or those with **overt diabetes**.

VIII. Prevention

A. **Devise dietary and exercise regimes** carefully for those breeds considered at risk of developing EMS and **feed to maintain an ideal body condition** (<6/9).

B. Early recognition of the condition and subsequent changes in management may reduce the risk of laminitis developing.

Further Readings

Asplin KE, Sillence MN, Pollitt CC, et al. Induction of laminitis by prolonged hyperinsulinaemia in clinically normal ponies. *Vet J* 2007;174:530–535.

Bailey SR, Habershon-Butcher JL, Ransom KJ, et al. Hypertension and insulin resistance in a mixed-breed population of ponies predisposed to laminitis. *American J Vet Res* 2008;69:122–129.

Carroll CL, Huntington PJ. Body condition scoring and weight estimation of horses. *Equine Vet J* 1988;20:41–45.

Carter RA, Geor RJ, Staniar WB, et al. Apparent adiposity assessed by standardised scoring systems and morphometric measurements in horses and ponies. *Vet J* 2009;179:204–210.

Durham AE, Rendle DI, Newton JR. The effect of metformin on measurements of insulin sensitivity and b cell response in 18horses and ponies with insulin resistance. *Equine Vet J* 2008;40:493–500.

Eiler H, Frank N, Andrews FM, et al. Physiologic assessment of blood glucose homeostasis via combined intravenous glucose and insulin testing in horses. *Am J Vet Res* 2005;66:1598–1604.

Frank N, Elliott SB, Boston RC. Effects of long-term oral administration of levothyroxine sodium on glucose dynamics in healthy adult horses. *Am J Vet Res* 2008;69:76–81.

Frank N, Geor RJ, Bailey SR, et al. Equine Metabolic Syndrome. *J Vet Intern Med* 2010;24:467–475.

Freestone JF, Beadle R, Shoemaker K, et al. Improved insulin sensitivity in hyperinsulinaemic ponies through physical conditioning and controlled feed intake. *Equine Vet J* 1992;24:187–190.

Geor RJ. Metabolic predisposition to laminitis in horses and ponies: obesity, insulin resistance and metabolic syndromes. *J Equine Vet Sci* 2008;28:753–759.

Gordon ME, Jerina ML, Raub RH, et al. The effects of dietary manipulation and exercise on weight loss and related indices of health in horses. *Compar Exerc Physiol* 2009;6:33–42.

Henneke DR, Potter GD, Kreider JL, et al. Relationship between condition score, physical measurements and body fat percentage in mares. *Equine Vet J* 1983;15:371–372.

Hoffman RM, Boston RC, Stefanovski D, et al. Obesity and diet affect glucose dynamics and insulin sensitivity in Thoroughbred geldings. *J Anim Sci* 2003;81:2333–2342.

Hustace JL, Firshman AM, Mata JE. Pharmacokinetics and bioavailability of metformin in horses. *Am J Vet Res* 2009;70:665–668.

Jeffcott LB, Field JR, McLean JG, et al. Glucose tolerance and insulin sensitivity in ponies and Standardbred horses. *Equine Vet J* 1986;18:97–101.

Johnson PJ. The equine metabolic syndrome peripheral Cushing's syndrome. *Vet Clin North Am Equine Pract* 2002;18:271–293.

Johnson PJ, Ganjam VK, Slight SH, et al. Tissue-specific dysregulation of cortisol metabolism in equine laminitis. *Equine Vet J* 2004;36:41–45.

Johnson PJ, Messer NT, Slight SH, et al. Endocrinopathic laminitis in the horse. *Clin Techn Equine Pract* 2004;3:45–56.

Johnson PJ, Slight SH, Ganjam VK, et al. Glucocorticoids and laminitis in the horse. *Vet Clin North Am Equine Pract* 2002;18:219–236.

Keen JA, McLaren M, Chandler KJ, et al. Biochemical indices of vascular function, glucose metabolism and oxidative stress in horses with equine Cushing's disease. *Equine Vet J* 2004;36:226–229.

Neville RF, Hollands T, Collins SN, et al. Evaluation of urinary TBARS in normal and chronic laminitic ponies. *Equine Vet J* 2004;36(3):292–294.

Tiley HA, Geor RJ, McCutcheon LJ. Effects of dexamethasone on glucose dynamics and insulin sensitivity in healthy horses. *Am J Vet Res* 2007;68:753–759.

Tinworth KD, Edwards S, Noble GK, Harris PA, Sillence MN, Hackett LP. Pharmacokinetics of metformin after enteral administration in insulin-resistant ponies. *Am J Vet Res* 2010;71:1201–1206.

Treiber K, Carter R, Gay L, et al. Inflammatory and redox status of ponies with a history of pasture-associated laminitis. *Vet Immunol Immunopathol* 2009;129:216–220.

Treiber KH, Kronfeld DS, Hess TM, et al. Evaluation of genetic and metabolic predispositions and nutritional risk factors for pasture-associated laminitis in ponies. *J Am Vet Med Assoc* 2006;228:1538–1545.

Vick MM, Adams AA, Murphy BA, et al. Relationships among inflammatory cytokines, obesity, and insulin sensitivity in the horse. *J Anim Sci* 2007;85:1144–1155.

Vick MM, Sessions DR, Murphy BA, Kennedy EL, Reedy SE, Fitzgerald BP. Obesity is associated with altered metabolic and reproductive activity in the mare: effects of metformin on insulin sensitivity and reproductive cyclicity. *Reprod Fertil Dev* 2006;18:609–617.

Walker BR. Glucocorticoids and cardiovascular disease. *Eur J Endocrinol* 2007;157:545–559.

CHAPTER 21

Insulinoma in Dogs

Rebecka S. Hess

Pathogenesis

- Most insulinomas are malignant carcinomas with local, vascular, lymphatic, hepatic, and other metastatic spread.
- Excess secretion of insulin leads to hypoglycemia which is the cause of most of the clinical signs.

Signalment

- The mean age of dogs with insulinoma is 9 years.
- There is no apparent sex or breed predilection.

Classical Signs

- Most clinical signs are due to the effect of hypoglycemia on the central nervous system (neuroglycopenia) and include seizures, collapse, weakness, ataxia, disorientation, mental dullness, and visual disturbances.
- Other clinical signs are related to excess catecholamine release and include tremors, hunger, and nervousness.
- Physical examination is unremarkable in most dogs. Some dogs may have weight gain, be postictal, or have a peripheral polyneuropathy.

Diagnosis

- A clinical suspicion of insulinoma is established with documentation of appropriate clinical signs, hypoglycemia, and concurrent absolute or relative hyperinsulinemia.
- The diagnosis of insulinoma is confirmed with histologic examination and immunohistochemical staining of the pancreatic mass.

Differential Diagnosis

- Differential diagnoses for hypoglycemia include insulinoma, extrapancreatic tumor, hypoadrenocorticism, liver dysfunction/failure, malnutrition, pregnancy, sepsis, extreme exercise, xylitol ingestion, and many drugs. Factitious hypoglycemia can also be considered.

Clinical Endocrinology of Companion Animals, First Edition. Edited by Jacquie Rand.
© 2013 John Wiley & Sons, Inc. Published 2013 by John Wiley & Sons, Inc.

Treatment

- The main component of treatment for an acute hypoglycemic crisis consists of IV dextrose administration.
- The long-term treatment of choice for insulinoma is surgical resection of the tumor and gross metastases.
- Long-term medical treatment may consist of dietary modification and treatment with prednisone, streptozocin, diazoxide, and synthetic somatostatin.

Prognosis

- Median survival time is about 1 year with a range of 0 days to 5 years.

I. Pathogenesis

A. Canine insulinoma is an **uncommon** condition. However, insulin-secreting beta cell neoplasia is the most common islet cell neoplasia in dogs, possibly due to the fact that **beta cells comprise approximately 70% of cells** in the islets of Langerhans.

B. Most canine insulinomas are **malignant**:

1. In two immunocytochemical reports, 25 of 26 insulinomas were **carcinomas** and only one was an adenoma.

2. About 80% of pancreatic tumors are **solitary** and most are located in one of the two limbs of the pancreas rather than in the body (Figure 21.1). **Occasionally, no discrete nodule or nodules are apparent during gross examination** of the pancreas, and histopathology is needed in order to identify the tumor.

3. The rate of **detected metastatic lesions at the time of initial diagnosis** in 187 dogs from different studies ranged from **45–75%** and is higher in studies based on necropsy than in those based on surgical biopsies.

4. **Clinical staging of pancreatic tumors** according to the **World Health Organization** defines three stages:

    a. **Stage I** as T1N0M0 (presence of a primary Tumor and absence of regional lymph Node and distant Metastases)

    b. **Stage II** as T1N1M0 (presence of a primary Tumor and regional lymph Node metastases with no distant Metastases).

    c. **Stage III** as T1N1M1 or T1N0M1 (presence of a primary Tumor with distant Metastases and with or without regional lymph Node metastases).

    d. Most dogs with insulinoma have stage II or stage III disease at the time of diagnosis. The most common sites of **metastases are regional lymph nodes, vasculature, and the liver**, although metastatic disease is possible anywhere.

C. While the **etiology of insulinoma is not known,** local growth hormone production, which is not associated with elevated plasma growth hormone concentration, has been documented in primary and metastatic canine insulinoma lesions. It is possible that local growth hormone affects insulinoma cell proliferation through paracrine or autocrine mechanisms.

D. Proliferation of beta cells results in **excess secretion of insulin and, therefore, hypoglycemia**. The most important compensatory mechanisms for hypoglycemia are inhibition of insulin secretion and stimulation of counter-regulatory hormone secretion:

1. **Glucose is the primary regulator of insulin secretion.** When glucose enters beta cells through the membrane-spanning helical glucose transporter GLUT2, it is metabolized to carbon dioxide and water with the formation of ATP. ATP, in turn, closes ATP-sensitive K^+ channels. Closure of the K^+ channels decreases K^+ efflux, resulting in depolarization of the beta cell and opening of voltage-sensitive Ca^{+2} channels. Increased cytoplasmic Ca^{+2} concentration results in insulin exocytosis.

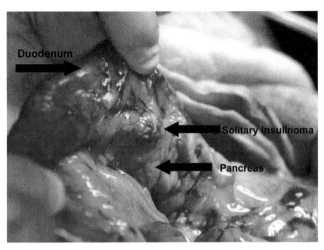

Figure 21.1 Most insulinomas are solitary nodules within one of the two pancreatic limbs. (Courtesy of Dr. Lillian Aronson.)

2. In normal animals, insulin secretion is completely inhibited when blood glucose is <80 mg/dL (4.4 mmol/L). However, **insulin secretion from neoplastic beta cells is independent of blood glucose concentration** and persists despite low blood glucose concentration. Therefore, one of the hallmarks of insulinoma is the finding of absolute or relative **elevations in blood insulin concentration despite low blood glucose concentration**.

3. The four **counter-regulatory hormones** secreted in response to hypoglycemia are **glucagon, catecholamines, growth hormone, and glucocorticoids**. Of these hormones, glucagon and catecholamines are most important in increasing blood glucose concentration.

II. Signalment
A. The **mean age** of dogs with insulinoma is **9 years**, with a range of 3–15 years.
B. Although any breed dog can develop insulinoma, it has been reported **mainly in medium to large breed dogs**. Controlled studies of breed risk for insulinoma have not been published.
C. There is **no apparent sex predilection** for the disease.

III. Clinical Signs
A. **Most clinical signs are due to the effect of hypoglycemia on the central nervous system (neuroglycopenia) or to hypoglycemia-induced catecholamine release:**
    1. Glucose is the single most important energy source in the brain, and carbohydrate storage in neural tissue is limited. Therefore, **brain function depends on a continuous supply of glucose. Clinical signs attributable to neuroglycopenia** include seizures, collapse, weakness, ataxia, disorientation, mental dullness, and visual disturbances.
    2. **Clinical signs related to excess catecholamine release** and stimulation of the sympathetic nervous system include tremors, hunger, and nervousness.
B. The severity of clinical signs increases as blood glucose decreases, and **severe hypoglycemia can ultimately result in coma and death**.
C. Clinical signs may also be **related to the duration and rate in which hypoglycemia develops**; a gradual decrease in blood glucose concentration may be less likely to stimulate catecholamine secretion.
D. **Clinical signs can be episodic** because secretion of counter-regulatory hormones increases blood glucose concentration and temporarily resolves neuroglycopenic clinical signs.
E. **Feeding can result in either alleviation or exacerbation of clinical signs:**
    1. If feeding restores blood glucose concentration to normal, clinical signs will resolve.
    2. However, feeding may also stimulate insulin secretion and exacerbate the hypoglycemia.

Table 21.1   Clinical signs reported in 206 dogs from several studies.

Clinical sign	Number of dogs (%)
Seizure	100 (49)
Collapse	84 (41)
Generalized weakness	79 (38)
Shaking/trembling/muscle twitching	45 (22)
Ataxia	45 (22)
Exercise intolerance	30 (15)
Hind limb weakness	28 (14)
Disorientation/bizarre behavior/hysteria	19 (9)
Polyphagia	16 (8)
Polyuria and polydipsia	16 (8)
Stupor/lethargy	12 (6)
Focal facial seizures	6 (3)
Obesity or weight gain	6 (3)
Blindness	5 (2)
Anorexia	5 (2)
Diarrhea	4 (2)
Head tilt	2 (2)
Nervousness	2 (2)

F.   **Fasting, exercise, or excitement can worsen clinical signs** by decreasing blood glucose concentration or increasing sympathetic stimulation.

G.   Clinical signs reported in 206 dogs from several studies are listed in Table 21.1. While most dogs have more than one of these clinical signs, **some dogs have none.** Reported **duration** of clinical signs prior to diagnosis **varies from 1 day to 3 years.**

H.   **Physical examination is unremarkable in most dogs with insulinoma:**

1.   Dogs may be **overweight** due to the anabolic effects of insulin.

2.   **Postictal findings** may be apparent if the dog had a recent seizure.

3.   A **peripheral polyneuropathy** characterized by tetraparesis and decreased or absent appendicular reflexes has been described in association with insulinoma in 13 dogs:

a.   The etiology of insulinoma-associated peripheral neuropathy is not known.

b.   It has been suggested that the polyneuropathy develops as a paraneoplastic immune-mediated disorder unrelated to the metabolic changes associated with insulinoma.

IV.   Diagnosis

A.   A **clinical suspicion** of insulinoma is established with documentation of:

1.   **Appropriate clinical signs as described in Table 21.1.**

2.   **Hypoglycemia** (i.e., blood glucose concentration <60 mg/dL; 3.3 mmol/L). It is important to note that many portable blood glucose meters tend to give a slightly lower blood glucose reading in dogs compared to commercially available analyzers that use a reference method based on the hexokinase reaction. However, meters calibrated for dogs such as the Abbott AlphaTRAK meter give more accurate readings, which can either over- or underestimate in comparison to the reference method.

3.   Concurrent **absolute or relative hyperinsulinemia:**

a. Blood for measurement of insulin concentration should only be collected when the blood glucose is <60 mg/dL (3.3 mmol/L).

b. Normal insulin concentrations can vary between laboratories and **must always be interpreted in consideration of the blood glucose concentration:**

1. **If insulin concentration is below the reference range,** a diagnosis of insulinoma is highly unlikely.

2. **If insulin concentration is within the reference range** when blood glucose concentration is low (i.e., **relative hyperinsulinemia**), a diagnosis of insulinoma should be considered possible, and testing should be repeated as described below.

3. **Absolute hyperinsulinemia,** that is, insulin concentration above the reference range, with concurrent hypoglycemia confirms a diagnosis of insulinoma.

4. Identification of a **pancreatic mass with imaging** studies may strengthen the suspicion for the presence of insulinoma.

B. The diagnosis of insulinoma is **confirmed with histologic examination and immunohistochemical staining** of a pancreatic mass.

C. Complete blood count, chemistry screen, and urinalysis are usually unremarkable aside from low blood glucose concentration:

1. While hypoglycemia is observed in most dogs with insulinoma, especially if the measurement is repeated on more than one occasion, it is important to remember that **some dogs with insulinoma may be euglycemic on repeated measurements.**

2. Mild **hypokalemia and elevations in alkaline phosphatase or alanine aminotransferase** have also been documented. Liver enzyme elevation is unrelated to the presence of metastases.

D. **If a dog suspected of having an insulinoma is euglycemic,** the following steps are followed in order to establish a diagnosis:

1. **The measurement of blood glucose concentration is repeated.**

2. **The dog is fasted under careful observation,** and blood glucose concentration is measured every 1–2 h. In most dogs with insulinoma, hypoglycemia will develop within 12 h of fasting. Blood for measurement of insulin concentration is collected when the animal is hypoglycemic, and the dog is then fed.

3. A small number of dogs will not exhibit hypoglycemia, even upon repeated measurements and after a prolonged (48–72 h) fast. Measurement of a **low fructosamine concentration** has been used to strengthen the clinical suspicion of insulinoma in several dogs with euglycemia.

4. **Glycosylated hemoglobin A1c** concentration has been low in some dogs with insulinoma, but not in all.

5. **Repeated measurements of fasted serum insulin concentration** may also aid in the diagnosis. One study of dogs with an insulinoma found that 76% of dogs had an absolute increase in fasted serum insulin concentration when it was measured once and 91% of dogs had an absolute increase when it was measured twice.

E. **Other tests** have been described for the diagnosis of insulinoma:

1. **Insulin-to-glucose and glucose-to-insulin ratios are not recommended** because of their low sensitivity, and the **amended insulin-to-glucose ratio is not recommended** because of its low specificity.

2. **Additional tolerance and stimulation tests** have been described but are **not advocated under any circumstance** because of questionable usefulness and potentially fatal side effects such as hypoglycemia and seizures.

F. Various **imaging modalities** may aid in establishing a clinical suspicion of insulinoma:

1. Most dogs with insulinoma have normal **abdominal and thoracic radiographs.**

2. When combining the results of several studies in which **abdominal ultrasound was performed in 87 dogs** with insulinoma, **a pancreatic mass was identified in 49 (56%)** dogs and abdominal metastasis was noted in 17 (19%). Thus, an abdominal ultrasound may be helpful in increasing the clinical suspicion of the presence of a pancreatic mass and metastases (Figure 21.2), but both **false positive and false negative results** have been described.

3. A single, optimal imaging technique for identifying insulinomas in **humans** has yet to be identified:

a. A **high-quality dual-phase thin-section multidetector-computed tomography (CT)** of the pancreas is effective in identifying a pancreatic mass in most affected humans.

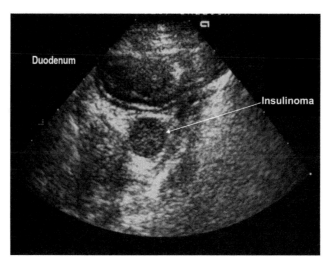

Figure 21.2   Abdominal ultrasound is helpful in detecting a pancreatic mass in about 50% of cases. (Courtesy of Dr. Gabriela Seiler.)

   b. **Intraoperative, intraductal ultrasonography**, which is not widely available, is more sensitive than CT in detecting small (1–3 mm diameter) insulinomas in humans.
   4. **CT has been reported in a small number of dogs with insulinoma, but its diagnostic sensitivity has yet to be determined. In one study in which 14 insulinomas were imaged by ultrasound, CT, and single-photon emission CT, CT correctly identified the highest number of tumors (10/14, 71%).**
   5. In another study utilizing **dual-phase computed tomographic angiography (CTA)** in three dogs with insulinoma, dual-phase CTA identified the insulinoma in all three, two of which did not have a pancreatic mass identified on ultrasound. In two dogs, strong enhancement of the insulinoma was noted during the arterial phase of the study only, suggesting the possible importance of CTA (Figures 21.3–21.5).
   6. Intravenous administration of radioactively labeled synthetic somatostatin followed by whole body **scintigraphy** is of limited value in imaging insulinomas in humans, likely because the number of somatostatin receptors expressed in human insulinomas is low. **Somatostatin receptor scintigraphy has been reported in a small number of dogs with insulinoma** and appears to have low specificity:
      a. **Abnormal foci of activity were observed in all dogs 1–24 h after administration of the radioligand.**
      b. **Accurate localization of the tumor was achieved in only 1 of 5 dogs.**

V. Differential Diagnoses
A. Differential diagnoses for **hy poglycemia** may be divided into those associated with excess secretion of insulin or insulin-like factors, decreased glucose production, excess glucose consumption, drug-associated, xylitol ingestion, or spurious causes:
   1. Disorders in which the most important mechanism for hypoglycemia is **excess secretion of insulin or insulin-like factors include insulinoma or extrapancreatic tumor, most commonly hepatoma or intestinal leiomyosarcoma.** Islet cell hyperplasia occurs in humans and may exist in dogs.
   2. Conditions associated with **decreased glucose production** include: **hypoadrenocorticism, hypopituitarism, growth hormone deficiency, liver dysfunction/failure and glycogen storage diseases.** Neonates of any breed and juveniles of toy breeds can easily become hypoglycemic if not eating adequately. Prolonged fasting, that is, >7–14 days except in toy breeds where shorter fasts can be an issue, malnutrition, or pregnancy may also result in hypoglycemia.
   3. **Excess glucose consumption may develop in sepsis or extreme exercise.**
   4. Some of the many **drugs** reported to induce hypoglycemia in human beings include: insulin, oral hypoglycemic agents (e.g., sulfonylurea), salicylates (e.g., aspirin), acetaminophen, beta-blockers (e.g., propranolol), beta-2 agonists, ethanol, monoamine oxidase inhibitors, tricyclic antidepressants

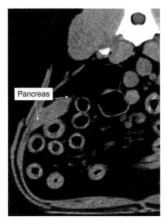

Figure 21.3 Dual-phase computed tomographic angiography prior to contrast administration. An insulinoma is not yet visible within the pancreas. (Courtesy of Dr. Wilfried Mai.)

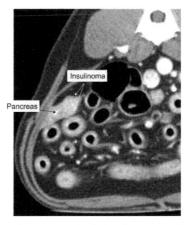

Figure 21.4 Dual-phase computed tomographic angiography during the venous phase of the study. Some enhancement of the insulinoma is apparent. (Courtesy of Dr. Wilfried Mai.)

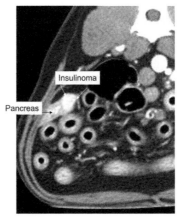

Figure 21.5 Dual-phase computed tomographic angiography during the arterial phase of the study. Strong enhancement of the insulinoma is apparent. (Courtesy of Dr. Wilfried Mai.)

(e.g., amitriptyline), angiotensin-converting enzyme inhibitors (e.g., captopril), antibiotics (e.g., tetracycline), lidocaine overdose, and lithium. The incidence of these toxicities in dogs is unknown.

5. **Xylitol** is a sweetening additive in some chewing gums, candy, diet foods, and dental products:
    a. It is a potent insulin secretagogue in dogs and can lead to profound hypoglycemia which may be associated with liver failure.
    b. Doses of xylitol >0.1 g/kg body weight have been associated with hypoglycemia, whereas doses higher than 0.5 g/kg body weight have been linked to liver failure.

6. **Factitious hypoglycemia** may occur when blood cells are not promptly separated from serum; in cases of severe polycythemia or leukocytosis, factitious hypoglycemia will develop because of cellular metabolism of glucose if serum separation is delayed by more than only 1 h.

VI. Treatment

A. Therapy for insulinoma can be **divided into treatment of an acute hypoglycemic crisis and long-term management.**

B. The main component of treatment for an **acute hypoglycemic crisis** consists of **IV dextrose** administration:
    1. Dextrose can be given as a **slow bolus** (0.5 g/kg IV, diluted in 0.9% sodium chloride at a ratio of 1:3).
    2. The bolus should be followed by an **IV continuous rate infusion** (CRI) of dextrose (2.5–5% in water). Dextrose must be **administered with caution** because it can stimulate insulin secretion and exacerbate hypoglycemia.
    3. Dextrose administration can be **discontinued when clinical signs resolve, even if mild hypoglycemia persists.** In most dogs, neuroglycopenia will resolve with administration of dextrose.

C. In the **unlikely event that the dog fails to respond to dextrose** administration alone, **dexamethasone** (0.1 mg/kg IV every 12 h) or **somatostatin analogue** (octreotide, 10–50 μg SC every 8–12 h) may be administered.

D. In severe cases, a dog may have to be **sedated with diazepam or pentobarbital** for several hours while the above treatment is continued and until seizures resolve.

E. Cerebral hypoxia may lead to **cerebral edema;** if cerebral edema is suspected, it can be treated with **mannitol** (1 g/kg IV given as a 20% solution at 2 mL/kg/h) and **furosemide** (1–2 mg/kg IV every 4 h).

F. Use of a **glucagon CRI** (5–13 ng/kg/min with or without a concurrent 10% dextrose infusion) has been reported in one dog with insulinoma-associated hypoglycemia:
    1. Clinical signs attributed to hypoglycemia resolved within 20 min and hypoglycemia resolved within 1 h.
    2. Glucagon increases blood glucose concentration by promoting glycogenolysis and gluconeogenesis. However, glucagon also directly increases insulin secretion, and animals should be monitored carefully for the **possibility of worsening hypoglycemia.**

G. The **long-term treatment of choice for insulinoma is surgical resection of the tumor and gross metastases:**
    1. Surgical exploration and biopsy of the pancreatic mass will also **confirm the diagnosis** and may help in estimating survival time.
    2. If **postoperative hyperglycemia develops, it is usually transient** and resolves once normal beta cells, which have been suppressed by excess insulin secretion from neoplastic cells, regain their function. Transient hyperglycemia may resolve with no exogenous insulin therapy within 24–72 h or require several days of insulin therapy.
    3. About 10% of dogs will develop **diabetes mellitus** and require treatment with exogenous insulin for 1–37 months.
    4. Other **postoperative complications** include acute pancreatitis, diabetic ketoacidosis, delayed wound healing, ventricular arrhythmias and cardiac arrest, hemorrhage, sepsis, and leukopenia. Death due to surgical manipulation of the pancreas has been reported infrequently in recent years.

H. **Medical treatment is indicated prior to surgery, postoperatively if needed, and in cases in which surgery is not performed.** Medical therapy can be **divided into cytotoxic treatment** directed at destroying insulin-secreting beta cells **versus treatment aimed at relieving the hypoglycemia:**
    1. **Streptozocin** is a nitrosourea antibiotic derived from the bacteria *Streptomyces achromogenes:*
        a. Streptozocin is a cytotoxic drug that **selectively destroys beta cells located in the pancreas or metastatic sites.**

b. The drug is **nephrotoxic** and has been reported to cause acute renal failure and renal tubular atrophy in dogs.

c. **Diuresis** with saline decreases contact time between the drug and renal tubular epithelial cells and **may reduce the risk of nephrotoxicity.**

d. **Successful use of streptozocin was reported in a study of 17 dogs**, most of which had surgery with incomplete resection of gross lesions:

  1) Dogs were treated with **0.9% sodium chloride (18 mL/kg/h IV) for 3 h prior to streptozocin administration, during two more hours of streptozocin treatment, and for 2 additional hours after treatment.**

  2) Streptozocin (500 mg/m^2) was given every 3 weeks.

  3) **Butorphanol** (0.4 mg/kg IM) was administered immediately following streptozocin therapy as an antiemetic, but vomiting still occurred in about 30% of treatments.

  4) Other **side effects included diabetes mellitus, transient hypoglycemia and seizures, transient hyperglycemia, transient elevations in alanine aminotransferase, azotemia, mild thrombocytopenia, or mild neutropenia.**

  5) **Although a few dogs appeared to have a prolonged survival due to streptozocin treatment, median duration of normoglycemia in streptozocin treated dogs was 163 days,** which was not significantly different than control dogs treated surgically or medically. Further studies are needed in order to determine if the benefits of streptozocin treatment outweigh its risks and costs.

2. The main modes of **relieving hypoglycemia,** typically added in a stepwise progress when blood glucose is no longer controlled, include dietary modification and treatment with prednisone, diazoxide, or synthetic somatostatin:

  a. **Small frequent meals** (every 4–6 h) of a **diet high in protein, fat, and complex carbohydrate** are recommended, and simple sugars (present in some soft moist dog foods) should be avoided.

  b. Glucocorticoids:

   1) They increase blood glucose concentration by increasing gluconeogenesis, elevating glucose 6-phosphatase activity, decreasing blood glucose uptake into tissues, and stimulating glucagon secretion.

   2) Glucocorticoids **can be administered intravenously during an acute hypoglycemic crisis** in the form of dexamethasone or can be given orally once the patient is stable.

   3) For long-term use, prednisone is given at a dose of 0.5–4 mg/kg/day PO beginning at the lower end of the dose, with gradual increases as needed.

   4) It is the **least expensive and most commonly used** drug for treatment of canine insulinoma.

  c. Diazoxide:

   1) Mechanism of action:

     It is a benzothiadiazine derivative whose main action is to **inhibit closure of ATP-dependent K$^+$ channels** in beta cells, preventing depolarization of beta cells and inhibiting opening of voltage-dependent Ca^{2+} channels. Decreased Ca^{2+} influx results in decreased exocytosis of insulin-containing secretory vesicles.

     a) Diazoxide also increases blood glucose concentration in depancreatized dogs by increasing **glycogenolysis and gluconeogenesis** and inhibiting tissue uptake of glucose.

   2) Diazoxide is administered at a dose of 10–40 mg/kg/day PO divided every 8–12 h, beginning at the lower end of the dose, with gradual increases as needed.

   3) **Approximately 70% of dogs with insulinoma respond** to treatment with diazoxide.

   4) **Side effects are uncommon** and include ptyalism, vomiting, and anorexia. However, in human beings, myocardial ischemia, salt and water retention, hyperglycemia, hypotension, and cerebral ischemia have been reported.

   5) Diazoxide is only available as a liquid and is **very costly**, especially in comparison to prednisone.

  d. Octreotide:

   1) It is a **long-acting synthetic somatostatin analogue** whose main mode of action is to inhibit insulin secretion.

2) In human beings, the action of octreotide is dependent on its binding affinity to any of the five somatostatin receptor subtypes present in the tumor. Despite the fact that dogs have only one somatostatin receptor subtype, their **response to octreotide treatment has been variable:**
   a) The lack of a dependable response to octreotide in dogs has been attributed to octreotide inhibition of glucagon and growth hormone secretion. If suppression of glucagon and growth hormone secretion is of greater magnitude and duration compared to suppression of insulin secretion, **octreotide may actually cause worsening hypoglycemia.**
   b) Additionally, some canine insulinomas may not have somatostatin receptors.
3) However, a study of 12 dogs with insulinoma found that when octreotide was administered to dogs at doses of 50 μg/dog SC (median dog weight was 23.3 kg) once, baseline plasma insulin concentrations decreased significantly but plasma concentrations of glucagon, GH, and ACTH were unchanged. These findings warrant longer term studies of a long-acting octreotide product in dogs with insulinoma.
4) **No adverse side effects have been reported** in dogs, but in humans they are mild and include pain at the site of injection (which can be reduced if octreotide is warmed to room temperature before administration), nausea, vomiting, abdominal pain, constipation, or steatorrhea.
5) Similar to diazoxide, octreotide is also **costly**, especially when compared to prednisone.

VII. Prognosis
A.   **Median survival time** of 142 dogs reported in different studies that underwent partial pancreatectomy was **12–14 months** with a range of 0 days to 5 years.
B.   While surgical intervention significantly improves survival as compared to medical management alone, most dogs die of metastatic disease, regardless of the type of treatment.
C.   Dogs with clinical **stage I of the disease have a significantly longer disease-free interval,** and about 50% are expected to be normoglycemic 14 months postoperatively compared to only 20% of dogs with clinical stage II or III.
D.   **Young dogs have a worse prognosis.**
E.   Dogs with **postoperative hyperglycemia or normoglycemia have a significantly better prognosis** than those with hypoglycemia.
F.   One study reported a median survival time of 2.1 years in 19 dogs with insulinoma that underwent partial pancreatectomy and a **median survival time of 3.6 years in the subgroup of dogs that received prednisone in addition to partial pancreatectomy.**
G.   A low mitotic rate within the tumor is strongly associated with survival of human beings with insulinoma. While a correlation between the number of mitotic figures per high power field and local invasiveness of the tumor has been documented in dogs, **a significantly worse prognosis in dogs with a high mitotic count has yet to be established.**
H.   Age (other the young dogs having a worse prognosis), sex, body weight, clinical signs and their duration, ultrasonographic detection of pancreatic mass, tumor location, gross presence of metastatic disease, and blood glucose or insulin concentration are not significantly associated with prognosis.

VIII. Prevention
No known prevention.

References and Further Readings

Caywood DD, Klausner JS, O'Leary TP, et al. Pancreatic insulin-secreting neoplasms: Clinical, diagnostic, and prognostic features in 73 Dogs. *J Am Anim Hosp Assoc* 1988;24:577–584.
Davison LJ, Podd SL, Ristic JME, et al. Evaluation of two point-of-care analysers for measurement of fructosamine or haemoglobin A1c in dogs. *J Small Anim Pract* 2002;43:526–532.
Dunayer EK, Gwaltney-Brant SM. Acute hepatic failure and coagulopathy associated with xylitol ingestion in eight dogs. *J Am Vet Med Assoc* 2006;229(7):1113–1117.

Feldman EC, Nelson RW. Hypoglycemia. In: Feldman EC, Nelson RW, eds. *Canine and Feline Endocrinology and Reproduction*, 1st edn. Philadelphia: WB Saunders, 1987, pp. 304–327.

Feldman EC, Nelson RW. Beta-cell neoplasia: Insulinoma. In: Feldman EC, Nelson RW, eds. *Canine and Feline Endocrinology and Reproduction*, 3rd edn. Philadelphia, PA: WB Saunders, 2004, pp. 616–644.

Fischer JR, Smith SA, Harkin KR. Glucagon constant-rate infusion: A novel strategy for the management of hyperinsulinemic-hypoglycemic crisis in the dog. *J Am Anim Hosp Assoc* 2000;36:27–32.

Garden OA, Reubi JC, Dykes NL, et al. Somatostatin receptor imaging in vivo by planar scintigraphy facilitates the diagnosis of canine insulinomas. *J Vet Intern Med* 2005;19:168–176.

Hawkins KL, Summers BA, Kuhajda FP, et al. Immunocytochemistry of normal pancreatic islets and spontaneous islet cell tumors in dogs. *Vet Pathol* 1987;24:170–179.

Iseri T, Yamada K, Chijiwa K, et al. Dynamic computed tomography of the pancreas in normal dogs and in a dog with pancreatic insulinoma. *Vet Radiol Ultrasound* 2007;48:328–331.

Kruth SA, Feldman EC, Kennedy PC. Insulin-secreting islet cell tumors: Establishing a diagnosis and the clinical course for 25 dogs. *JAVMA* 1982;181:54–58.

Lamb CR, Simpson KW, Boswood A, et al. Ultrasonography of pancreatic neoplasia in the dog: a retrospective review of 16 cases. *Vet Rec* 1995;137:65–68.

Leifer CE, Peterson ME, Matus RE. Insulin-secreting tumor: diagnosis and medical and surgical management in 55 dogs. *JAVMA* 1986;188:60–64.

Lester NV, Newell SM, Hill RC, et al. Scintigraphic diagnosis of insulinoma in a dog. *Vet Radiol Ultrasound* 1999;40:174–178.

Madarame H, Kayanuma H, Shida T, et al. Retrospective study of Canine insulinomas: Eight cases (2005–2008). *J Vet Med Sci* 2009;71(7):905–911.

Mai W, Caceres AV. Dual-phase computed tomographic angiography in three dogs with pancreatic insulinoma. *Vet Radiol Ultrasound* 2008;49:141–148.

Mellanby RJ, Herrtage ME. Insulinoma in a normoglycaemic dog with low serum fructosamine. *J Small Anim Pract* 2002;43:506–508.

Moore AS, Nelson RW, Henry CJ, et al. Streptozocin for treatment of pancreatic islet cell tumors in dogs: 17 cases (1989–1999). *JAVMA* 2002;221:811–818.

Polton GA, White RN, Brearley MJ, et al. Improved survival in a retrospective cohort of 28 dogs with insulinoma. *J Small Anim Pract* 2007;48:151–156.

Robben JH, Pollak YW, Kirpensteijn J, et al. Comparison of ultrasonography, computed tomography, and single-photon emission computed tomography for the detection and localization of canine insulinoma. *J Vet Intern Med* 2005;19:15–22.

Schrauwen E, Van Ham L, Desmidt M, et al. Peripheral polyneuropathy associated with insulinoma in the dog: Clinical, pathological, and electrodiagnostic features. *Prog Vet Neurol* 1996;7:16–19.

Tobin RL, Nelson RW, Lucory MD, et al. Outcome of surgical versus medical treatment of dogs with beta cell neoplasia: 39 cases (1990–1997). *JAVMA* 1999;215:226–230.

Trifonidou MA, Kirpensteijn J, Robben JH. A retrospective evaluation of 51 dogs with insulinoma. *Vet Q* 1998;20:S114–S116.

CHAPTER 22

Insulinoma in Cats

Danièlle Gunn-Moore and Kerry Simpson

Pathogenesis

- Functional tumor of pancreatic beta cells.

Classical Signs

- Typically attributable to hypoglycemia: seizures, lethargy, weakness, muscle twitching, and collapse.

Diagnosis

- Hyperinsulinemia in the face of hypoglycemia.
- Identification of mass.

Treatment and Prognosis

- Surgical resection with or without ad lib feeding and corticosteroid administration.
- Highly variable outcome.

I. Pathogenesis

A. The beta cells (located in the pancreatic islets) are responsible for monitoring and controlling blood glucose concentration. In the normal pancreas, these cells produce, store, and secrete insulin. Unlike the majority of cells, glucose uptake into beta cells is insulin independent. If the blood glucose concentration is elevated, the beta cells can detect this, with the predominant glucose "sensor" being glucokinase (GCK). This protein is coded for by the GCK gene in the pancreatic islet cells, and the expression of this gene is regulated by glucose concentration:

    1. It is the beta cells' ability to sense and uptake glucose in an insulin independent manner, and then release insulin in response to the blood glucose concentration, that allows the ratio of blood glucose concentration to insulin concentration to be kept relatively constant in a healthy animal, even during a prolonged fast.

B. Insulinomas are functional tumors of the pancreatic beta cells that autonomously synthesize and secrete insulin, even in the face of hypoglycemia. This predisposes animals to hypoglycemic crises during fasting and

---

Clinical Endocrinology of Companion Animals, First Edition. Edited by Jacquie Rand.
© 2013 John Wiley & Sons, Inc. Published 2013 by John Wiley & Sons, Inc.

exercise. These tumors retain some responsiveness to many of the normal stimuli for insulin secretion, but demonstrate an exaggerated response. Therefore, animals with insulinoma are at risk of hypoglycemia after eating or with the administration of glucose containing intravenous fluids:

1. Compared to normal pancreatic tissue, GCK expression may be elevated in insulinoma tissue from cats. As GCK is the predominant glucose "sensor" within the beta cells, this over expression may increase insulin secretion and glucose sensitivity.

II. Signalment

A. **Insulinomas are rare tumors in cats**; only 19 cases appear in the literature, and some only provide histology:

1. Where documented, the age of these cats ranged from 3 to 17 years, with only two <13 years of age.
2. Three cases have been reported in neutered female cats and seven in neutered male cats.
3. Six cases occurred in domestic short- or long-haired cats, **four in Siamese cats**, two in Persian cats; the breed was not reported in the other cases. The four cases in Siamese cats were among some of the earlier reports of insulinoma, and this has lead to the suggestion that this breed may be predisposed. However, whether or not this is true remains unknown.

III. Clinical Signs

A. **Clinical signs are generally present for weeks to months prior to investigation.** They typically included **seizures, lethargy, weakness, muscle twitching**, and **collapse**, although inappetence, diarrhea, and weight loss have also been reported:

1. One case had cervical ventroflexion and intermittent bouts of constipation, in addition to lethargy and exercise intolerance. However, this cat was diagnosed with multiple endocrine neoplasia type I (MEN I), having a concurrent aldosterone-secreting tumor within the adrenal gland and a functional parathyroid adenoma, which most likely account for these additional signs.

B. **Seizures** are commonly reported in cases of insulinoma. The central nervous system (CNS) is particularly susceptible to the effects of low blood glucose. This is because the carbohydrate reserves in neural tissue are limited and cellular metabolism is highly dependent on glucose supplies. In mammals, the cerebral cortex is typically most susceptible to decreased glucose concentrations so seizure activity is seen before other areas of the CNS and other organs, such as the heart, liver, and kidneys are affected.

C. **Hypoglycemia stimulates the release of counter-regulatory hormones, such as glucagon, catecholamines, cortisol, and growth hormone, which antagonize the effects of insulin** and so increase the blood glucose concentration. Release of these substances means that **seizure activity is generally short lived**:

1. In the reported cases, seizures generally lasted for a very short period and were either not treated or responded to oral glucose supplementation. However, one case remained disorientated between seizures and developed irreversible neurologic complications after surgical removal of the pancreatic mass, and one cat had seizures of 1–2 h duration.
2. Interestingly, seizure activity has only been reported associated with feeding in two cases. In dogs with insulinoma, it is recognized that feeding can trigger excessive insulin release and therefore perpetuate clinical signs. However, in the cat, postprandial glucose surges do not appear to occur in the same manner as in dogs. This species variation may therefore account for the lack of correlation between feeding and clinical signs.

D. **Reported findings on physical examination are highly variable.** Some cats have appeared relatively unremarkable, while others have been depressed, weak, disorientated, hypothermic, bradycardic, have a gallop rhythm, and variable menace response. One cat had previously had recurrent bouts of severe regenerative anemia, which was present at the time of referral.

IV. Diagnosis

A. **Hematological abnormalities** have rarely been reported in cases of insulinoma; those documented include anemia and mild thrombocytopenia. However, the latter result was obtained from an automated reader and a blood smear was not performed. A further case was leukopenic, with neutropenia and lymphopenia.

B. **Serum biochemistry demonstrates hypoglycemia**, with reported blood glucose concentrations ranging from 0.99 to 2.09 mmol/L (reference range: 3.5–5.0 mmol/L):

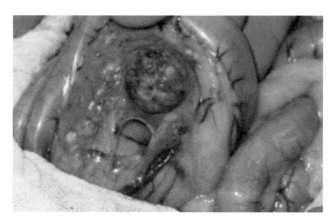

Figure 22.1   Insulinoma in a cat identified at exploratory laparotomy. This mass was not detected on abdominal ultrasonography. (From Reimer et al., 2005.)

1. In general, the remainder of the routine biochemistry is unremarkable, although two cats were mildly/moderately azotemic and one cat had elevated calcium and sodium concentrations and a decreased potassium concentration; however, that case also had concurrent elevations in aldosterone and parathyroid hormone and was diagnosed with MEN I.

C. **Urinalysis** is generally unremarkable or may demonstrate isosthenuria.

D. **Blood pressure**, when assessed, has been normal to slightly decreased.

E. **Thoracic radiography** has been normal in all reported cases.

F. **Abdominal ultrasonography** has only been reported in four cases, and a pancreatic mass was only identified in one, highlighting the fact that a **negative ultrasonographic examination does not rule out insulinoma** (Figure 22.1).

G. **Nuclear scintigraphy** using radiolabeled somatostatin analogs has been used in the assessment of islet cell tumors in people. This technique relies on the binding of analogs to somatostatin receptors, of which there are various types, with varying affinities for these analogs. This technology has been applied in some cases of canine insulinoma, but to date has not been assessed in feline insulinoma. However, its use may be limited in this species as immunohistochemical staining of insulinomas suggests that somatostatin receptors are not always present in cats.

H. **In order to diagnose an insulin-secreting tumor, blood insulin concentration should be assessed in the face of concurrent hypoglycemia.** In a normal animal, hypoglycemia suppresses insulin secretion, resulting in low insulin concentrations. However, if an insulinoma is present, the beta cells within the neoplasm tend to be less responsive to hypoglycemia so the insulin secretion is not suppressed and the insulin concentration is **normal or increased**:

1. The serum insulin levels have been reported in three cats diagnosed with insulinoma and have been inappropriately normal or increased.

I. **Histopathological assessment of resected tumors** should be performed. Chromogranin A is stored and co-released with insulin from beta cells and is a useful immunological marker which can be used to determine if the mass is neuroendocrine in origin; abundant Chromogranin A is consistently reported in insulinoma in cats (Figure 22.2). In addition, where immunohistochemical assessment has been reported, tumors have demonstrated patchy insulin staining, with >50% of cells staining positive in one report and no insulin staining in another. Similarly, somatostatin, glucagon, and pancreatic polypeptide immunoreactivity appear to vary between neoplasms.

V. Differential Diagnoses

A. There are several differentials for hypoglycemia in cats (Table 22.1). While evidence of an inappropriate insulin concentration in the face of hypoglycemia strongly supports the diagnosis of an insulin-secreting tumor, similar results can be obtained with **beta cell hyperplasia**. To date, this condition has not been reported in the cat; however, a single case has been identified in a Tajikistani street cat which was seen at the authors' hospital.

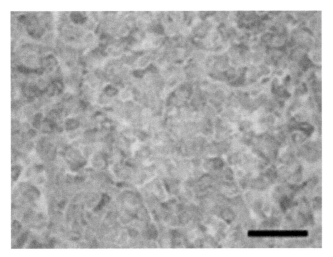

Figure 22.2   Insulinoma production of tumor markers and islet hormones was determined by immunohistochemistry. Chromogranin A, a marker for endocrine tumors, was expressed by 100% of tumor cells. (From Jackson et al., 2009.)

Table 22.1   Differential diagnosis for hypoglycemia.

Insulin overdose
Hepatic disease
Sepsis
Neonatal hypoglycemia
Insulinoma
Insulin-secreting neoplasm
Storage disease
Hypoadrenocorticism
Beta cell hyperplasia

VI. Treatment
A. **Surgical resection** is recommended as it may potentially cure cases with a solitary lesion:
   1. Surgical exploration of the abdominal cavity allows abnormal tissue to be identified and resected or, if a mass cannot be identified, some authors recommend partial pancreatectomy. However, this is problematic as there appears to be no predisposition for tumor location within the pancreas in cats, with masses having been reported in the left limb ($n = 3$), right limb ($n = 2$) and at the angle of the pancreas between the portal vein and the pancreatic duct ($n = 1$).
   2. In cases where the mass is nonresectable, surgery allows the mass to be debulked and this can aid in the stabilization of the patient. However, cases have not yet been managed like this in cats as the **masses have been small**, varying in size from **4 mm to 3 cm**.
   3. Surgical exploration of the abdominal cavity is also useful in the prognostic evaluation, allowing the clinician to assess the other organs for presence of metastases.
   4. The main **risks** associated with surgery are **pancreatitis** and postoperative **diabetes mellitus**, which can be transient or permanent.
B. **Medical therapy** has been limited in cats. Regular feeding of **small feeds** or **dried *ad lib*** food has been reported to be of some benefit. In addition, **glucocorticoids** can be used to antagonize the effects of insulin and stimulate hepatic glycogenolysis. Frequent feeding and glucocorticoid therapy have successfully palliated clinical signs for 8 and 17 months after the recurrence of clinical signs in cats which had previously had surgical resection of insulinoma:
   1. Other potential therapies which have been used in dogs include **octreotide** and **diazoxide**, but to date neither of these has been tried in the treatment of insulinoma in cats.

VII. Prognosis

A.   The prognosis for cats with insulinoma appears **highly variable**. Of the cats which have undergone surgical resection of the tumor clinical signs recurred in four of the six cats at 5 days, 7 days, 7 months, and 10 months. Of these cases, the first also received medical therapy and was euthanized 4 weeks later, the second was euthanized 1 month postoperatively for persistent neurological dysfunction despite normalization of the blood glucose concentration, the third also received medical therapy and survived for 2 years postdiagnosis, and the last represented with hypoglycemic crisis and died 18 months post surgical resection; postmortem examination revealed metastases in the liver and pancreatic lymph nodes. The two other cases where surgical resection was performed were alive and asymptomatic at the time that they were reported, 6 and 32 months postoperatively.

VIII. Prevention

No known prevention.

References and Further Readings

Carpenter JL, Andrews LK, Holzworth J. Tumors and tumorlike lesions. In: Holzworth J, ed. *Diseases of the Cat: Medicine and Surgery*. Philadelphia: W.B. Saunders, 1987.

Feldman EC, Nelson RW. Insulinoma. In: Feldman EC, Nelson RW, eds. *Canine and Feline Endocrinology and Reproduction*, 3rd edn. St Louis: WB Saunders, 2004.

Green SN, Bright RM. Insulinoma in a cat. *JSAP* 2008;49:38–40.

Hawks D, Peterson ME, Hawkins KL, Rosebury WS. Insulin-secreting pancreatic (islet cell) carcinoma in a cat. *JVIM* 1992;6:193–196.

Jackson TC, Debey B, Lindbloom-Hawley S, Jones BT, Schermerhorn T. Cellular and molecular characterization of a feline insulinoma. *JVIM* 2009;23:383–387.

Kraje AC. Hypoglycemia and irreversible neurological complications in a cat with insulinoma. *JAVMA* 2003;223:812–814.

McMillan F. Functional pancreatic islet cell tumor in a cat. *JAAHA* 1985;21:741–746.

Myers NC, Andrews GA, Chard-Bergstrom C. Chromogranin A plasma concentration and expression in pancreatic islet cell tumors of dogs and cats. *AJVR* 1997;58:615–620.

O'Brien TD, Norton F, Turner TM. Pancreatic endocrine tumour in a cat: Clinical, pathological and immunohistochemical evaluation. *JAAHA* 1990;26:453–457.

Reimer SB, Pelosi A, Frank JD, Steficek BA, Kiupel M, Hauptman JG. Multiple endocrine neoplasia type I in a cat. *JAVMA* 2005;227:101–104.

CHAPTER 23

Insulinomas in Other Species

Sue Chen and Michelle L. Campbell-Ward

Pathogenesis

- Insulinomas are pancreatic beta cell tumors that overproduce insulin despite inhibitory stimuli and may release excessive amounts of insulin with provocative stimuli.
- Hypoglycemia ensues due to the inappropriate elevations of insulin.
- Although insulinomas are one of the most common neoplasms noted in ferrets, they are rarely reported in other species except dogs.

Classical Signs

- Affected ferrets are usually between 4 and 6 years of age.
- Lethargy, weakness, and ataxia with progression of signs if left untreated.
- Signs can be intermittent, with normal activity between bouts of weakness.

Diagnosis

- Persistent hypoglycemia.

Treatment

- Surgical excision of the insulinoma; medical management of hypoglycemia with prednisone or diazoxide.

With the exception of ferrets, dogs, and cats, insulinomas have not been reported in other species other than in two case reports: one describing insulinoma in two guinea pigs identified postmortem and one in which the cause of episodic seizure in a 12-year-old Shetland pony broodmare was attributed to a pancreatic adenoma. In the author's practice (Chen), we believe we had a rabbit with insulinoma based on clinical symptoms and response to diazoxide. This chapter will focus primarily on the disease in ferrets since information on insulinomas in other species is limited.

Clinical Endocrinology of Companion Animals, First Edition. Edited by Jacquie Rand.
© 2013 John Wiley & Sons, Inc. Published 2013 by John Wiley & Sons, Inc.

I. Pathogenesis
A. Insulinomas produce their effects through **secretion of an excessive amount of insulin:**
1. **Insulin is secreted indiscriminately** and the tumors are **not responsive to normal inhibitory stimuli** such as low blood glucose or elevated insulin levels.
2. **Provocative stimuli,** such as a rapidly increasing glucose level, can **stimulate excessive insulin secretion** from these tumors causing a profound **rebound hypoglycemia.**
3. Insulin decreases circulating blood glucose levels by a number of methods:
    a. Inhibition of hepatic gluconeogenesis and glycogenolysis.
    b. Rapid uptake of glucose into peripheral tissues.
    c. Promotes the storage of glucose as glycogen in the muscle and liver.
    d. Promotes the conversion of excess glucose into fatty acids.
B. Insulinomas are **one of the most commonly diagnosed neoplasms seen in middle-aged to older ferrets** with a reported incidence of 25% (382 of 1525) and 21.7% (139 of 574) of neoplasms diagnosed in two large retrospective studies.
C. A majority of these tumors occur in North America. A few cases of beta cell tumors have been reported in the Netherlands, Australia, Japan, and the United Kingdom, though they are still exceedingly rare as compared to in North America:
1. Ferrets in the United States are supplied by a small number of breeders, thus limiting their genetic diversity. It is thought that there may be a genetic component in the development of insulinomas.
D. An inappropriate diet may be a contributing factor in the development of insulinomas in ferrets:
1. Most ferrets in the United States are fed a commercial kibble diet, which is higher in carbohydrates than the whole prey diet commonly fed in the United Kingdom.
2. Diets that are high in carbohydrates may have a negative effect on glucose metabolism in ferrets (a strictly carnivorous species).
E. Insulinomas usually range in size from **microscopic to small nodules,** though larger tumors are occasionally noted.
F. Multiple pancreatic nodules due to local recurrence is **a common finding:**
1. Metastasis to other organs is uncommon. When it does occur, the regional lymph nodes, liver, and the spleen are the most commonly involved.

II. Signalment
A. Most ferrets begin exhibiting clinical signs around 4–6 years of age, although it appears that younger ferrets are increasingly being affected.
B. There are conflicting reports on whether males are slightly overrepresented over females.
C. Ferrets with insulinomas can have varying body conditions especially if they have concurrent diseases (e.g., adrenal disease, lymphoma).

III. Clinical Signs
A. Clinical signs include **mental dullness, irritability,** and **lethargy.** Owners often assume the behavior is a slowing down due to old age (Figure 23.1).
B. **Nausea** can result in **ptyalism** or pawing at the mouth.
C. **Stargazing, hindlimb weakness,** and **ataxia** are often noted as the hypoglycemia worsens.
D. Severely hypoglycemic ferrets may exhibit **generalized seizures** or may be **comatose** on presentation.
E. Clinical signs are often **episodic,** with bouts of normal activity between periods of lethargy.
F. Progression of clinical signs can extend over a period of days, weeks, or months. Severity and frequency of clinical signs often progresses if left untreated.

IV. Diagnosis
A. A presumptive diagnosis of insulinoma is made in ferrets when they demonstrate **a fasting blood glucose <60 mg/dL (<3.2 mmol/L),** especially in the presence of clinical symptoms and these symptoms cease after a feeding or intravenous administration of glucose. (Figure 23.2):
1. In patients where an insulinoma is suspected but the fasting blood glucose is within normal limits 90–125 mg/dL (5.0–7.0 mmol/L), **a carefully monitored 3–4 h fast may be required to confirm hypoglycemia.**

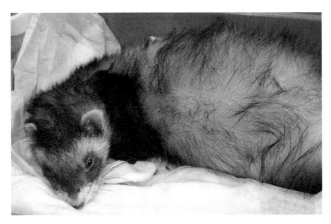

Figure 23.1   Most ferrets with insulinoma are presented for lethargy and weakness that may wax and wane, but is often progressive. Owners may also report the ferret seems to be sleeping more or is not as easily rousable.

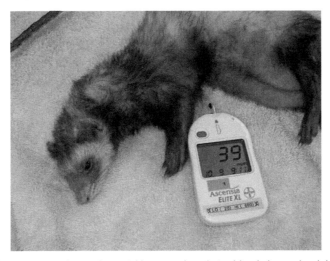

Figure 23.2   Handheld glucometers can be used to quickly assess the relative blood glucose level; however, it should be noted that many handheld glucometers are not validated for ferrets.

B. **Elevated insulin levels >108 μU/mL (>773 pmol/L) with concurrent hypoglycemia** supports the diagnosis of an insulinoma:
   1. A normal or even low insulin level does not necessarily rule out the presence of an insulinoma due to a presumed erratic insulin secretion by some insulinomas.
C. Diagnostic imaging, such as radiography and ultrasonography, is usually unrewarding as **a majority of the nodules are only a few millimeters in diameter.**
D. **Histology of surgical biopsies is required for definitive diagnosis:**
   1. Most insulinomas are composed of **cords and nests of eosinophilic polyhedral cells** on a fine fibrovascular stroma.
   2. Though most are **usually well circumscribed,** some tumors can be infiltrative.
   3. The tumor cells may be described as **hyperplasia, adenomas,** or **carcinomas** and a specific nodule **may have a combination** of any of these processes.
   4. Most islet cell tumors express strong immunoreactivity for insulin, though immunostaining for peptide hormones such as glucagon, somatostatin, and pancreatic polypeptide has been occasionally noted.

V.   Differential Diagnoses
A. Increased glucose utilization and impaired hepatic function during **sepsis** can lead to hypoglycemia.

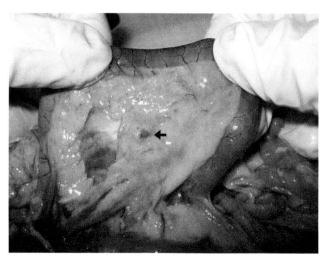

Figure 23.3 Evaluate both limbs of the pancreas for insulinomas (arrow). Most insulinomas are no more than a few millimeters in diameter and gentle palpation of the pancreas may be required to identify some nodules.

B. **Hepatic insufficiency** (e.g., hepatic neoplasia, cirrhosis, portal caval shunts) can result in hypoglycemia due to impaired hepatic gluconeogenesis and glycogenolysis.

C. Decreased intake of nutrients from **prolonged starvation** may impair hepatic gluconeogenesis and may result in hypoglycemia.

D. Improper prolonged storage of blood samples can artifactually decrease blood glucose levels.

E. Generalized weakness, lethargy, and hindlimb ataxia can also be seen in ferrets with **cardiac disease** (e.g., canine heartworm *Dirofilaria immitis*), **renal disease** (e.g., urinary blockage from prostatomegaly), **gastrointestinal disease** (e.g., gastric foreign body, enteritis), and other **neoplasms** (e.g., lymphosarcoma). These diseases should be considered in any weak ferret especially if the blood glucose is within normal limits.

VI. Treatment

A. **Surgical therapy:**

　1. **Surgical excision** of the insulinomas is considered the **treatment of choice.** (Figure 23.3). However, due to the high incidence of local recurrence, surgery is **rarely curative** long term.

　2. Improved clinical signs and longer survival times have been noted for ferrets that have had their insulinomas removed:

　　a. Reported disease-free intervals have ranged from 0 to 23.5 months (medians of 234 days, 240 days, and 10.6 months).

　　b. Owners should be advised that surgery should not be considered curative, but that it may temporarily stop or slow the progression of disease for a longer disease-free interval.

　　c. Incomplete resolution of clinical signs may be due to remaining microscopic diseased islet cells. One case study demonstrated as many as 52% (26 out of 50) of ferrets remained hypoglycemic after surgery. However, these ferrets may require lower doses of medication to be symptom free than before the surgery.

　　d. Some ferrets may have a transient hyperglycemia after removal of an insulinoma. Most of these resolve on their own within a few weeks.

　3. To prevent a hypoglycemic crisis, an intravenous catheter should be placed preoperatively to **administer a constant rate infusion of a balanced electrolyte solution supplemented with 2.5–5% dextrose** pre-, peri-, and postoperatively.

　4. **Careful visualization** and **gentle palpation** of both limbs of the pancreas is performed to locate pancreatic nodules. Pancreatic nodules can be individually removed or in the case of multiple nodules, a partial pancreatectomy can be performed.

Table 23.1 Drug dosages for treating hypoglycemia in ferrets.

Drug	Dosage
Prednisolone	0.25–2 mg/kg PO q 12 h
Diazoxide	5–30 mg/kg PO q 12 h
Octreotide	1–2 µg/kg q 8–12 h; equivocal results noted
Dextrose 50%	To be given during a hypoglycemic crisis; 0.25–2 mL of 50% dextrose diluted 1:1 with LRS or saline. Administer as a slow intravenous bolus to effect.

Start at the low end of the dose range when starting palliative therapy. Check the blood glucose level every 5–7 days and increase the dosage incrementally as needed to manage the hypoglycemia and clinical symptoms.

5. A full abdominal exploratory is highly recommended to evaluate **areas of potential metastasis** and to evaluate for any **concurrent conditions such as adrenocortical neoplasia** or **lymphoma**.

6. Postoperative complications such as pancreatitis appear to be uncommon in ferrets.

B. **Medical (palliative) therapy** (Table 23.1):

1. The goal of medical therapy is to increase blood glucose levels to the point where clinical signs are abated, but not necessarily to reestablish normoglycemia. Most ferrets enjoy an **improved quality of life** with palliative therapy; however, the owners must be advised that it **does not provide a cure for insulinomas** and increasing doses may be needed over time.

2. **Glucocorticoids** (i.e., prednisone and prednisolone) increase a patient's blood glucose level by **increasing hepatic gluconeogenesis, decreasing glucose uptake by peripheral tissues, and inhibiting insulin binding to insulin receptors:**

   a. Doses range from 0.5 to 2 mg/kg PO q 12 h. Start at a low dose and increase the dose incrementally as needed to control clinical symptoms.

   b. Initially, the blood glucose should be rechecked within 5–7 days to assess if the dose needs adjusting.

   c. **Most ferrets are relatively resistant to the immunosuppressive effects of prednisolone.** However, possible side effects of long-term glucocorticoid therapy include polyuria and polydipsia, abdominal weight gain, and slow or impaired hair growth in any shaved areas.

3. **Diazoxide**, a nondiuretic benzothiadiazine, increases blood glucose levels by directly **inhibiting pancreatic insulin secretion by preventing the release of insulin** from insulin granules. Additionally, diazoxide stimulates the release of epinephrine which in turn **promotes hepatic gluconeogenesis and glycogenolysis and decreases cellular uptake of glucose.** It does not possess any antineoplastic activity:

   a. Dosing starts at 5–10 mg/kg q 12 h PO and is gradually increased to a maximum of 30 mg/kg q 12 h if lower doses do not control clinical signs adequately.

   b. Diazoxide can be added to the treatment regimen when glucocorticoids alone no longer control clinical symptoms or can be used by itself.

   c. Adverse side effects are not commonly noted, but can include anorexia and vomiting.

   d. Diazoxide should be used cautiously in patients with renal disease or congestive heart failure as it can cause sodium and fluid retention.

4. Octreotide, a synthetic long-acting analog of somatostatin, inhibits the secretion of insulin, glucagon, secretin, gastrin, and motilin. Limited use of this drug has been reported in the veterinary literature, and the **sporadic use of octreotide in ferrets has produced equivocal results:**

   a. This medication may be useful in some insulinoma patients that are refractory to other types of treatment. However, not all insulinomas are responsive to this medication because pancreatic islet cell tumors have varied expression of somatostatin receptors.

   b. If somatostatin receptors are lacking, administration of octreotide may exacerbate hypoglycemia due to suppression of glucagon.

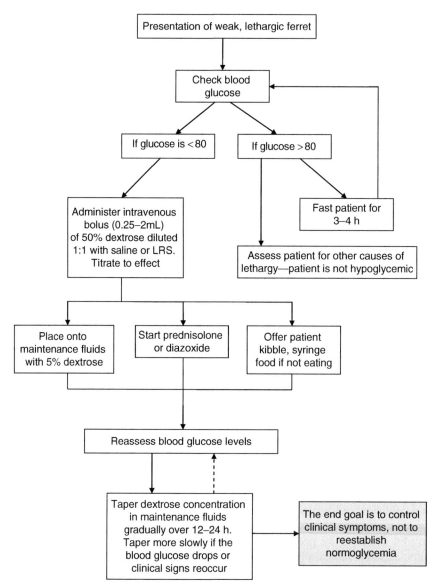

Figure 23.4   Management of a hypoglycemic crisis. Note that glucose units refer to measurement in micrograms per deciliter.

   c. Reported dosage is 1–2 µg/kg q 8–12 h subcutaneously.

C. **Management of a hypoglycemic crisis** (Figure 23.4):

   1. If a ferret is lethargic or comatose on presentation to the clinic, quickly assess the blood glucose level to confirm that hypoglycemia is the cause of the clinical signs.

   2. Administer intravenously *slowly* 0.25–2 mL of 50% dextrose diluted 1:1 with saline or Lactated ringer's and titrate to effect:

      a. If a ferret continues to seizure despite an intravenous dextrose bolus, diazepam (1 mg/kg IV) may be administered.

   3. After the initial dextrose bolus, the patient should be placed on maintenance fluids supplemented with 5% dextrose to prevent a rebound hypoglycemic episode.

   4. Oral medications that increase the blood glucose level (i.e., prednisolone or diazoxide) and small feedings should be initiated once the ferret is able to swallow.

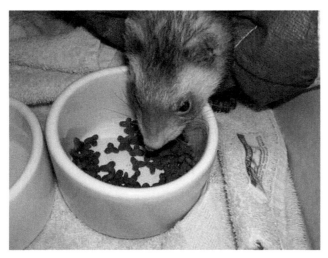

Figure 23.5   Kibble should be available at all times and in easily accessible places. A kibble that is high in protein and low in carbohydrates is recommended to prevent dramatic swings in blood glucose.

5. As the blood glucose stabilizes through oral medications and feedings, the patient should be gradually weaned off intravenous dextrose and fluids.

D.   **Home management of insulinomas:**

1. Owners should be counseled on the clinical signs of hypoglycemia, such as lethargy, ataxia, or drooling (nausea). Changes in diet and management of hypoglycemic episodes must be discussed with the owner if the ferret is to have any quality of life.

2. **Diet modification** to **a high-protein, low-carbohydrate kibble** helps decrease the consumption of simple carbohydrates which can induce a rebound release of insulin, thus triggering a hypoglycemic episode. (Figure 23.5):

    a. Owners should be instructed to **discontinue all treats that are high in simple sugars,** including raisins, peanut butter, and any ferret supplements containing corn syrup or dextrose.

    b. When changing brands of kibble, make sure the ferret accepts the new diet as some ferrets can be picky eaters and may inadvertently go into a hypoglycemic crisis from not eating. Owners may consider gradually mixing the new food in with the old kibble to improve acceptance.

3. **Kibble should be available to the ferret at all times.** In homes where ferrets are allowed to run free in a ferret-proofed area, instruct owners to provide **multiple feeding stations** so that food is easily accessible.

4. If mild clinical signs are noted, owners should feed the ferret immediately. Oftentimes mild clinical signs improve once the ferret is fed.

5. If the owner finds their ferret comatose or exhibiting seizures, owners should **drip corn syrup (e.g., Karo®) or a sugar solution on the mucous membranes.** This provides temporary relief for the hypoglycemia until the ferret can be transported to a veterinary facility for supportive care.

VII. Prognosis

A.   The prognosis is good to excellent for an improved quality of life with palliative care, but the owners must be informed that the medicines are only controlling the clinical signs and not providing a cure for the insulinoma. The dose of medications may need to be increased over time as needed to help control clinical symptoms.

B.   Because of the high rate of local recurrence, the prognosis for a long-term cure is guarded to poor. Surgical excision is required for any cessation of clinical signs though the disease-free period can vary greatly.

VIII. Prevention

A.   It is thought that diets high in sugar or simple carbohydrates are believed to be risk factors in the development of insulinomas. A high-quality kibble that is high in protein and low in carbohydrates may be beneficial.

References and Further Readings

Antinoff N, Hahn K. Ferret oncology: Diseases, diagnostics, and therapeutics. *Vet Clin North Am Exot Anim Pract* 2004;7(3):579–625.

Antinoff N, Williams BH. Neoplasia. In Quesenberry KE, Carpenter JW, eds. *Ferrets, Rabbits, and Rodents: Clinical Medicine and Surgery*, 3rd edn. St. Louis: Elsevier Saunders, 2012, pp. 104–105.

Caplan ER, Petereon ME, Mullen HS, et al. Diagnosis and treatment of insulin-secreting pancreatic islet cell tumors in ferrets: 57 cases (1986–1994). *J Am Vet Med Assoc* 1996;209(10):1741–1745.

Chen S. Pancreatic endocrinopathies in ferrets. *Vet Clin North Am Exot Anim Pract* 2008;11(1):107–123.

Ehrhart N, Withrow SJ, Ehrhart EJ, et al. Pancreatic beta cell tumor in ferrets: 20 cases (1986–1994). *J Am Vet Med Assoc* 1996;209(10):1737–1740.

Lewington JH. Endocrine diseases. In: Lewington JH, ed. *Ferret Husbandry, Medicine and Surgery*. Edinburgh: Elsevier Science Limited, 2000, pp. 211–222.

Li X, Fox JG, Padrid PA. Neoplastic diseases in ferrets: 574 cases (1968–1997). *J Am Vet Med Assoc* 1998;212(9):1402–1406.

Rosenthal KL, Wyre NR. Endocrine diseases. In: Quesenberry KE, Carpenter JW, eds. *Ferrets, Rabbits, and Rodents: Clinical Medicine and Surgery*, 3rd edn. St. Louis: Elsevier Saunders, 2012, pp. 92–102.

Rosenthal KL. Ferret and rabbit endocrine disease diagnosis. In: Fudge AM, ed. *Laboratory Medicine: Avian and Exotic Pets*. Philadelphia: WB Saunders, 2000, pp. 319–24.

Ross MW, Lowe JE, Cooper BJ, et al. Hypoglycemic seizures in a Shetland pony. *Cornell Vet* 1983;73:151–169.

Vannevel JY, Wilcock B. Insulinoma in 2 guinea pigs (Cavia porcellus). *Can Vet J* 2005;46(4):339–341.

Weiss CA, Williams BH, Scott MV. Insulinoma in the ferret: Clinical findings and treatment comparison of 66 cases. *J Am Vet Med Assoc* 1998;34(6):471–475.

CHAPTER 24

Gastrinoma, Glucagonoma, and Other APUDomas

Craig Ruaux and Patrick Carney

Pathogenesis

- Neoplastic transformation of neuroendocrine (**A**mine **P**recursor **U**ptake and **D**ecarboxylation [APUD]) cells.
- Clinical syndromes generally caused by elevated secretion of functional endocrine products.
- May be orthoendocrine (i.e., produce the same hormone as the cell type of tumor origin) or paraendocrine (i.e., produce a hormone not normally made in the cell type of origin).
- Majority are malignant, but adenomas do occur.
- Chemodectoma (dog), medullary thyroid carcinoma (dog), gastrinoma, and carcinoid are the most commonly reported; glucagonoma is less frequent in dogs and has not been reported in cats.
- Somatostatinoma and pancreatic polypeptidoma have been reported in one dog each.

Classical Signs

- Vary with tumor type and hormone(s) elaborated.
- Gastrinoma: Most dogs are >8 years old and feline cases have been 8–12 years of age; vomiting, weight loss, decreased appetite, diarrhea (dog), gastric mucosal hypertrophy, and duodenal ulcerations.
- Glucagonoma: Most reported cases in older adults to geriatric; characteristic crusting, ulcerative lesions of extremities, pressure points, and mucocutaneous junctions; lack of appetite, lethargy.
- Somatostatinoma: weight loss.
- Pancreatic polypeptidoma: signs similar to gastrinoma.

Diagnosis

- Presumptive based on clinical signs and elevated serum/plasma hormone assay.
- Definitive diagnosis via immunohistochemistry of tumor.

Treatment

- All tumors: surgical resection/debulking and supportive care.
- Gastrinoma: proton pump inhibitors, somatostatin analogues.
- Glucagonoma: amino acid supplementation.

Clinical Endocrinology of Companion Animals, First Edition. Edited by Jacquie Rand.
© 2013 John Wiley & Sons, Inc. Published 2013 by John Wiley & Sons, Inc.

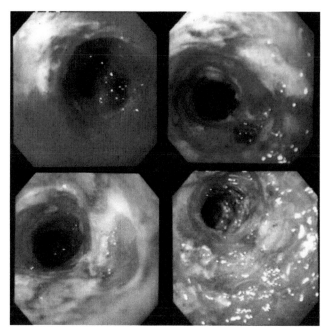

Figure 24.1   Composite of four endoscopic images showing severe duodenal ulceration in a dog with gastrinoma. (Images courtesy of Dr. C. Ludlow, Animal Specialty Hospital, Rockledge, FL.)

I. Pathogenesis

A. APUDomas **arise from neoplastic transformation of neuroendocrine (APUD) cells** with similar biosynthetic pathways and ultrastructural characteristics; these include:

    1. Pituitary corticotrophs producing **ACTH** (see Chapters 5 and 7) give rise to hyperadrenocorticism.

    2. Pancreatic islet β cells producing **insulin** (see Chapters 21–23) which give rise to **insulinomas**.

    3. Pancreatic islet α cells producing **glucagon** give rise to **glucagonomas**.

    4. Thyroid C-cells producing **calcitonin** give rise to **medullary thyroid carcinomas**.

    5. Gastric and duodenal G-cells producing **gastrin** give rise to **gastrinomas**:

        a. Gastrin is not produced in the normal adult canine pancreas.

        b. While the origin of **pancreatic gastrinomas** has not been identified, they may arise as paraendocrine tumors of islet cells or from persistence and transformation of fetal islet cells, which do express gastrin.

    6. Adrenal medullary chromaffin cells producing **epinephrine** and **norepinephrine** give rise to **pheochromocytomas** (see Chapters 13 and 14).

    7. Chemoreceptor (carotid, aortic body) cells with no known endocrine function give rise to **chemodectomas**.

    8. Pancreatic islet, gastric, and small intestinal cells producing **vasoactive intestinal peptide (VIP)** give rise to **VIPomas**.

    9. Pancreatic islet δ (delta) cells producing **somatostatin** give rise to **somatostatinomas**.

    10. Pancreatic PP cells producing **pancreatic polypeptide** give rise to **pancreatic polypeptidomas**.

    11. Gastrointestinal and respiratory enterochromaffin cells producing **serotonin, histamine**, and **kallikrein** give rise to **carcinoids**.

B. **Secretion of active hormones** or hormone derivatives/analogues is **responsible for the majority of clinical signs observed with gastrinoma, glucagonoma, and VIPoma**:

    1. **Gastrinoma:**

        a. Gastrin stimulates gastric acid secretion.

        b. The presence of excess gastric acid leads to greatly reduced gastric pH, causing **gastroduodenal ulceration** (Figure 24.1) that **may progress to perforation, gastric mucosal hypertrophy, mucosal**

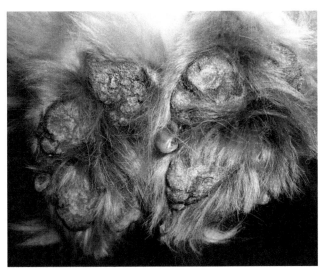

Figure 24.2   Footpads of a dog showing characteristic skin lesions of hepatocutaneous syndrome. Note marked hyperkeratosis and crusting of foot pads with deep ulcerative fissures. (Image courtesy of Dr. Oliver Garden, Royal Veterinary College, London.)

irritation, **altered gastrointestinal motility,** and **inactivation of pH-sensitive digestive enzymes** such as trypsin, pancreatic lipase, and amylase.

c. **Malabsorptive diarrhea** develops secondary to enzyme inactivation and altered motility, contributing to **weight loss.**

d. Gastric hyperacidity, mucosal irritation, and mucosal (antral/pyloric) hypertrophy contribute to **emesis.**

2. Glucagonoma:

a. **Glucagon stimulates both breakdown of glycogen and gluconeogenesis** within the liver while signaling for **insulin release** from the pancreas. The end result of normal glucagon secretion is to elevate blood glucose concentrations and allow peripheral tissues to utilize the glucose.

b. In excess, glucagon may lead to **insulin-resistant diabetes mellitus, hypoaminoacidemia** (perhaps due to gluconeogenesis), and nonspecific secondary vacuolar hepatopathy.

c. The pathogenesis of the **characteristic skin lesions** seen in patients with glucagonoma (variously called **superficial necrolytic dermatitis [SND],** necrolytic migratory erythema [NME], or metabolic epidermal necrosis [MEN]; Figure 24.2) is poorly understood:

   1) Lesions may relate to persistent hypoaminoacidemia resulting in depletion of epidermal protein.

   2) A direct effect of glucagon, zinc deficiency, hypoalbuminemia, or essential fatty acid deficiency have all been postulated to cause the skin lesions, but objective evidence in support of any possibility is lacking in the literature.

3. VIPoma:

a. Causes Verner–Morrison syndrome, **characterized by profuse watery diarrhea, hypokalemia, and achlorhydria** (hence its other name, WDHA syndrome).

b. It has **not been identified in companion animals.**

C. Carcinoids, chemodectomas, medullary thyroid carcinomas, somatostatinomas, and pancreatic polypeptidomas **usually do not cause clinical signs due to an endocrine product;** clinical signs generally relate to tumor location, size, presence of any metastases, and interference with adjacent organ function:

1. Carcinoids:

a. Occur primarily throughout the **gastrointestinal tract,** with less common occurrences in the liver, gallbladder, and lungs.

b. They produce a characteristic hormone-driven syndrome of torso and facial flushing and diarrhea in 10% of affected humans but seem to primarily **produce nonspecific clinical signs (e.g., anorexia, vomiting, dyschezia, weight loss)** in animals:

1) It is unclear if this is due to lack of release of serotonin, histamine, and kallikrein or to the difficulty of assessing clinical signs of flushing in veterinary patients.

2) **Diarrhea occurs in 32% of affected dogs** but may be caused by the physical presence of the tumor rather than hormone elaboration, particularly given that diarrhea is rare in extraintestinal carcinoids. The incidence of diarrhea in cats with carcinoids is unclear.

  c. One case of a carcinoid in a dog that was presumed to secrete ACTH, leading to Cushing's syndrome, has been reported. However, the presence of ACTH could not be demonstrated in the carcinoid.

2. Chemodectomas:

  a. Have been reported in dogs and cats, but are more common in dogs.

  b. They have not been documented to actively secrete neurotransmitters or hormones. **Clinical signs arise from tumor location and interference with the function of adjacent organs.**

  c. **Aortic body tumors account for 83% of chemodectomas,** carotid body tumors account for 15.5%, 2.5% occur in both locations simultaneously, and <0.2% occur elsewhere.

  d. **Aortic body tumors** may lead to **heart failure, pericardial effusion/cardiac tamponade, ascites, and/ or pleural effusion** by compressing the heart or great vessels, rupturing with subsequent hemorrhage into the pericardium or thorax, or generating malignant effusion.

  e. **Carotid body tumors** may cause the **same clinical signs and complications** as aortic body tumors, but they **also commonly compress or infiltrate cervical structures.**

  f. **Metastases** may occur to virtually any location, although the **majority of chemodectomas (roughly 75%) are benign.**

  g. **Boxers and Boston terriers** are markedly overrepresented:

    1) Account for 39% and 17% of cases, respectively, resulting in a relative risk (risk ratio) of 9.3–26.3 for Boxers and 8.8–19.2 for Boston terriers.

    2) While unproven, it is hypothesized that a combination of genetics and stimulation of chemoreceptors due to chronic hypoxia leads to malignant transformation of cells within the aortic and carotid bodies.

  h. Chemodectomas **will not be discussed further** in this chapter as they do not result in an endocrinopathy.

3. **Medullary thyroid carcinomas are rare tumors of calcitonin-secreting cells,** accounting for 36% of canine thyroid carcinomas. They have **not been reported in cats:**

  a. **Sporadic and familial** canine cases have been reported, indicating both spontaneous oncogenesis and genetic influence may play a role in tumoral etiology. While human familial medullary carcinoma is almost invariably linked to mutations in the proto-oncogene *RET*, similar mutations were not identified in the one reported pedigree of a canine family with medullary thyroid carcinoma.

  b. Up to 100% of canine medullary thyroid carcinomas are **immunohistochemically positive for the presence of calcitonin. No assay is commercially available** for measuring circulating serum calcitonin concentrations, which might help as a serum biomarker to distinguish medullary from follicular thyroid tumors.

  c. Despite secreting excessive amounts of calcitonin, human medullary thyroid carcinomas are **not associated with a calcitonin-induced syndrome, that is, signs associated with hypocalcemia.** The same is thought to be true of dogs. Because the endocrine component of this tumor is believed to be clinically silent, medullary carcinomas **will not be discussed further.**

4. **The normal role of somatostatin is to inhibit the release of virtually all pancreatic and digestive hormones:**

  a. **"Somatostatin syndrome" in humans** includes hypogastrinemia-mediated reduction in gastric acid secretion, gallbladder disease attributed to lack of regular contraction, and diarrhea and steatorrhea due, in part, to ineffective digestion in the face of altered gastrointestinal pH. However, the syndrome is extraordinarily rare in humans with a somatostatinoma.

  b. **Compatible findings were not reported in the one affected dog.**

5. **Pancreatic polypeptide has a biphasic effect on digestive secretions,** initially stimulating digestive enzyme release and gallbladder contraction, then inhibiting both. It also promotes satiety and gastric emptying:

  a. Little is known about the clinical syndrome(s) associated with excessive production in humans.

  b. The **single affected dog reported experienced vomiting and gastrointestinal ulceration,** which are rare in human cases.

II. Signalment
A. **Gastrinoma:**
1. **Dogs:**
    a. **Median age of 10 years** at diagnosis with a range of 3.5–12 years.
    b. Of the 21 dogs with gastrinoma, 3 were German shepherds, 2 were Shih-tzus, and 5 were mixed breeds; **no breed predisposition can be inferred** from the limited number of reported cases.
    c. **No sex bias** is evident.
2. **Cats** (*n* = 4):
    a. **Median age of 10 years** at diagnosis with a range of 8–12 years.
    b. Three were domestic shorthair cats, while one cat's breed was not reported.
    c. Only one cat was male, but the number of reported cases is too small to draw any conclusion about sex distribution.
B. **Glucagonomas** have been reported in nine dogs and no cats:
1. **Median age is 9 years old,** with a range of 5–13 years.
2. No purebred was represented more than once, with three mixed breeds.
3. Males outnumber females by 2:1, but the small sample size makes this difficult to extrapolate.
C. **Carcinoids** have been reported in at least 35 dogs and 5 cats:
1. **Dogs:**
    a. Average age of 9.3 years, with a peak at 10 years of age.
    b. No sex or breed predisposition is evident, although 4 of 18 were German shepherds and 2 of 18 were whippets.
2. **Cats:**
    a. Affected cats ranged from 9 to 15 years old.
    b. Insufficient information is available with respect to sex or bred predisposition.
D. **Somatostatinoma** has been reported in only one dog, a 10-year-old spayed female Portuguese water dog with a concurrent metastatic hepatic gastrinoma.
E. **Pancreatic polypeptidoma** has been reported in only one dog, a 7-year-old spayed female cocker spaniel.

III. Clinical Signs
A. **Gastrinoma:**
1. **Dogs:**
    a. **Vomiting** (90%), **weight loss** (81%), and **inappetence** (62%) are most common, with **diarrhea** occurring in slightly less than half.
    b. **Melena, hematochezia, hematemesis, and pyrexia** are infrequent presenting complaints, but **may indicate more emergent disease.**
    c. **Emaciation, thin body condition, or weight loss** noted in 62%.
    d. **Pale mucous membranes** noted in 24%, and cranial **abdominal pain** found on examination in 14%.
2. **Cats:**
    a. Of the four cats reported, all presented with **vomiting,** two with **weight loss,** and one each with inappetence and polyuria/polydipsia.
    b. **Physical examination findings varied,** with the most fully documented case noted as thin with a poor hair coat and having pale mucous membranes and a systolic heart murmur.
B. Glucagonoma:
1. **Marked ulcerative, crusted lesions** of the distal extremities, pressure points (hocks, elbows), and/or mucocutaneous junctions occur in **100%:**
    a. **Often begins on distal extremities,** particularly on **footpads,** which develop **marked hyperkeratosis and fissures (Figure 24.2).**
    b. **Digital lesions** may lead to overt lameness or a mincing gait.
    c. **Truncal lesions** tend to lag behind, generally first appearing on the ventrum.
2. Nondermatologic signs are vague and nonspecific, with **decreased appetite** (44%) and **lethargy** (33%) being most common.

3. On **physical examination, muscle atrophy** (33%) and depressed mentation (22%) were the only nondermatologic signs.

C. Carcinoid:

1. **Dogs**—Perhaps reflecting the wide anatomic distribution of carcinoids and the lack of a common syndrome, **no single clinical sign is present in >33% of patients:**

a. **Diarrhea** (32%), **weight loss** (32%), **vomiting** (29%), **and inappetence** are most common.

b. Two patients presented for evaluation of visible anorectal masses, and one (pulmonary) carcinoid was considered an incidental finding.

2. **Cats**—Chronic vomiting reported in one case of gastric carcinoid.

D. **Somatostatinoma:** The sole reported case presented with a 2-month history of weight loss and historically elevated liver enzymes. Physical examination findings were not reported.

E. **Pancreatic polypeptidoma:** The sole reported case presented with a 6-week history of progressive disease that included vomiting, anorexia, lethargy, and weight loss. Physical examination was unremarkable.

IV. Diagnosis

A. **Gastrinoma—Presence of an elevated fasting serum gastrin concentration along with appropriate clinical signs** should raise clinical suspicion of the presence of a gastrinoma:

1. A blood sample for **measurement of serum gastrin concentration** is often only submitted upon discovery of gastroduodenal ulceration, but evaluation should be considered in any patient with evidence of unexplained gastrointestinal hemorrhage:

a. Elevations in gastrin concentrations reported in veterinary gastrinoma patients have ranged from twofold increase to >200-fold.

b. For patients with smaller relative gastrin elevations, **provocative testing with 2–4 U/kg secretin** IV and evaluation of serum gastrin at 0, 2, 5, 10, 15, and 20 min postinjection is recommended. Secretin should not cause a rise if the hypergastrinemia is not due to a gastrinoma. At least doubling of the presecretin gastrin value or an absolute value over 200 pg/mL are both positive results for the presence of a gastrinoma.

c. **Other causes of hypergastrinemia exist besides gastrinoma,** for example, administration of proton pump inhibitors or H2 receptor antagonists and other diseases (see section on Differential Diagnoses below).

2. Patients have often failed to respond to **empirical symptomatic therapy** for gastritis, although marked improvement may be seen in some with proton pump inhibitors.

3. **Diagnostic imaging:**

a. **Barium contrast radiographic studies** of the stomach or **abdominal ultrasound** may identify gastric mucosal defects consistent with ulceration.

b. **Abdominal ultrasound** failed to identify a discrete pancreatic tumor in five of five dogs and one of two cats.

c. **CT and MRI** may be used to attempt to localize a tumor, but pancreatic islet cell tumors of the size range reported for gastrinomas are typically not identified.

d. **Nuclear scintigraphy** using a radiolabeled somatostatin analogue (Octreoscan) is commonly used in human medicine and accurately identified a gastrinoma in one dog.

4. **Gastroduodenoscopy** is the preferred diagnostic modality for identification of characteristic gastric mucosal thickening and gastric and duodenal ulceration (Figure 24.1):

a. While **ulceration most commonly involves the stomach and/or duodenum,** ulcers involving the esophagus, stomach, duodenum, and (rarely) jejunum may occur in any combination or singly. Duodenal ulcers tend to be large, multifocal lesions, commonly visualized immediately after the pylorus (i.e., cranial to the major duodenal papilla).

b. Endoscopy is **contraindicated if a perforating ulcer is suspected** (e.g., presence of pyrexia, severe abdominal pain, marked left shift, etc.).

c. The overwhelming majority (10 of 13 in which gastrointestinal biopsy results were reported) have **inflammatory infiltrates identified on biopsy,** but do not respond as expected with treatment. **No specific infiltrate type** predominated.

5. Definitive diagnosis relies on histopathology and immunohistochemistry from a primary or metastatic tumor.

B. **Glucagonoma** is presumptively diagnosed by demonstration of compatible clinical signs (dermatologic) combined with skin biopsy and measurement of plasma glucagon concentration:

1. **Skin biopsy reveals a marked parakeratotic hyperkeratosis,** varying degrees of epidermal edema and hyperplasia, and extensive crusting. Evidence of secondary infection is common and should be addressed but will not lead to resolution of the lesions:

a. Within the veterinary literature, the skin lesions are identified in dogs with liver disease approximately four times as commonly as in dogs with identified glucagonoma.

b. Many reported cases (approximately 1/3), however, did not document exhaustive examination of the pancreatic parenchyma for small tumors or plasma glucagon determination; thus the true relationship between glucagonoma and the skin lesions in dogs may be underestimated.

2. **Plasma glucagon concentration is typically elevated despite normoglycemia or hyperglycemia.** Reported glucagon concentrations have been 1.6–7.5 times higher than the reference range.

3. Specific **serum amino acid concentrations,** when measured, are **generally below the reference range:**

a. In the few reported cases ($n = 3$) where circulating amino acids were measured and reported, most measured amino acid concentrations have been low; of 22, 5, and 24 amino acids measured, concentrations of 22, 4, and 20 were below the reference range, respectively.

b. In general, the ratio of branched chain to aromatic amino acids is decreased.

c. Determination of serum amino acid concentrations **requires specialized laboratory services** (e.g., the Amino Acid Laboratory at UC Davis School of Veterinary Medicine, see http://www.vetmed.ucdavis.edu/VMB/aal/index.cfm) and is not routinely available.

4. **Diagnostic imaging:**

a. **Ultrasound, CT, or MRI** may be used to localize the tumor, but, as with gastrinomas, the **majority of tumors will not be detected.**

b. Octreoscan has not been used for diagnosis of canine glucagonoma, but likely has utility.

5. **Histopathologic and immunohistochemical identification is required for definitive diagnosis.**

C. **Carcinoids** are most often detected via common imaging modalities such as plain abdominal radiographs or ultrasound examination. Fine needle aspirates may provide some information, but definitive diagnosis relies on biopsy.

D. **Somatostatinoma** has only been diagnosed via surgical excisional biopsy.

E. **Pancreatic polypeptidoma** was presumptively diagnosed in one dog based on profoundly elevated fasting serum pancreatic polypeptide concentration; the diagnosis was confirmed at necropsy:

1. Fasting hypergastrinemia was also found, but provocative testing with secretin did not result in further elevation of gastrin, effectively ruling out gastrinoma.

2. A pancreatic mass was visualized via transabdominal ultrasonography.

V. Differential Diagnoses

A. **Gastrinoma:**

1. **Any cause of acute or chronic vomiting should be considered,** including inflammatory bowel disease, infiltrative neoplasia (e.g., gastrointestinal lymphoma), dietary indiscretion, foreign body ingestion, mast cell disease, gastroduodenal neoplasia, gastric hamartoma, *Physaloptera* spp. (cat, dog) or *Ollulanus tricuspis* (cat) infestation, *Helicobacter*-associated gastritis, hypertrophic pyloric gastropathy, gastric pythiosis, irritant toxin ingestion, acute or chronic pancreatitis, hepatobiliary disease, renal disease, intracranial disease (neoplastic, inflammatory, or infectious), atrophic gastritis, Basenji enteropathy, hypoadrenocorticism, and hyperthyroidism (cat).

2. **Presence of an elevated serum gastrin concentration is not considered diagnostic for gastrinoma:**

a. It is particularly important to realize that **administration of proton pump inhibitors or H2 receptor antagonists will elevate serum gastrin concentrations.**

b. **Other causes of hypergastrinemia** include lack of appropriate fasting (a minimum 12-h fast is required), renal failure, hypo/achlorhydria, hepatic disease, Basenji enteropathy, and hypertrophic pyloric gastropathy.

B. **Glucagonoma must be differentiated from nonglucagonoma SND also called hepatocutaneous syndrome,** which shares apparently identical gross and histopathologic dermatological findings:

1. Measurement of plasma glucagon concentration, identification of a pancreatic tumor, and liver function testing should help to distinguish between the two, with glucagon concentrations elevated in patients with glucagonoma and within the reference range in those with liver disease as the cause of SND.

2. **Plasma glucagon assay is available from a limited number of specialist laboratories.** Sample handling and storage conditions are stringent.

3. While glucagonomas may lead to persistently elevated blood glucose concentration or overt insulin-resistant diabetes mellitus, it should be remembered that a significant proportion of nonglucagonoma SND patients have concurrent diabetes mellitus.

4. **Differential diagnoses for the characteristic skin lesions** include ectoparasitism, canine distemper (footpad hyperkeratosis), chemical/irritant injury, folliculitis/furunculosis, zinc deficiency, and immune-mediated dermatopathies.

C. **Carcinoid tumors may mimic a variety of diseases** depending on the tumor location:

1. Once a tumor is identified, it should be **distinguished from other neoplasms, granulomas, abscesses, and cysts** via fine needle aspiration, incisional biopsy, or excisional biopsy.

2. Cytology of a carcinoid will reveal characteristic bare nuclei against a background of cytoplasm, typically without marked criteria of malignancy (i.e., appear neuroendocrine).

3. Cytology can differentiate a carcinoid from non-neuroendocrine tumors, but will be unable to distinguish carcinoids from other neuroendocrine tumors.

D. **Somatostatinoma and pancreatic polypeptidoma:**

1. Should be considered when a pancreatic tumor is identified in association with consistent clinical signs.

2. These tumors can only be differentiated from other islet cell tumors (e.g., insulinoma, gastrinoma) immunohistochemically.

VI. Treatment

A. **General principles:**

1. **Surgical resection** of tumor and metastases, if present, is the **only definitive treatment** and should be attempted if feasible.

2. Local invasion, high rates of metastasis, and difficulty in locating the tumor pre- or intraoperatively all severely **limit the likelihood of curative surgery.**

B. **Gastrinoma:**

1. In patients with unresected, partially resected, or metastatic disease, **simultaneous aggressive antacid and gastroprotective therapy is indicated:**

   a. **Omeprazole** (1 mg/kg PO q 24 h) is preferred due to noncompetitive inhibition of gastric acid secretion.

   b. **H2 antagonists** (famotidine 0.5–1.0 mg/kg IV/SC/PO q 24 h, ranitidine 2 mg/kg IV/SC/PO q 12 h) may be used, but are less effective than proton pump inhibitors due to the competitive mode of action.

   c. **Sucralfate** 0.5–1.0 g PO as a liquid slurry q 8 h.

2. **Octreotide,** a somatostatin analogue that inhibits secretion by pancreatic islet cells and gastric cells, has been used in a small number of cases and appears effective:

   a. Initial dose is 2–20 µg/kg SC q 8–12 h. In two cases, repeated dose escalation was required.

   b. Cost may limit use, particularly in larger patients.

3. In patients with **actively bleeding ulcers:**

   a. **Intervention with fluid therapy, blood product administration, and intensive monitoring** may be required.

   b. **Sucralfate** may be given at an increased frequency (e.g., q 30 min) or at an initially increased dose (up to 10 g) to help stop acute hemorrhage.

4. **Perforated ulcers are a surgical emergency.**

5. **Total gastrectomy** is used in humans with nonresectable or metastatic gastrinomas, removing the target organ of the excess gastrin. It has not been reported in any veterinary gastrinoma patients, likely due to the difficulties of managing such a patient long term.

6. **Chemotherapy** is also used in some human patients:

    a. Most protocols incorporate streptozotocin, dacarbazine, and/or 5-flurouracil and show a modest benefit.

    b. Concerns about the toxicity of streptozotocin in companion animals have limited its use in the past. However, use with a diuresis protocol greatly improves safety.

    c. To our knowledge, no veterinary gastrinoma patient has been treated with chemotherapy to date.

C. **Glucagonoma:**

1. In patients with unresected, partially resected, or metastatic tumors, **no proven treatments exist**.

2. Octreotide may decrease the amount of glucagon secreted, and chemotherapy protocols like those proposed for gastrinoma may be of limited benefit.

3. **Intravenous amino acid supplementation** may alleviate dermatologic signs, and dietary supplementation with protein of high-biological value, zinc, and essential fatty acids has been proposed.

D. **Carcinoids** are treated with surgical resection and/or chemotherapy as above.

E. The one dog with **somatostatinoma** was treated with an H2 antagonist, omeprazole, metoclopramide, and metronidazole:

1. Treatment efficacy and survival cannot be evaluated in the one reported case because the somatostatinoma was a comorbid condition (concurrent gastrinoma).

2. If curative surgery cannot be performed, chemotherapy with streptozotocin, doxorubicin, and/or dacarbazine could be considered.

F. Given that the majority of clinical signs with **pancreatic polypeptidoma** in humans are related to mass effect, surgical resection/debulking should be considered. Symptomatic therapy with the possible addition of octreotide may help palliatively.

VII. Prognosis

A. **Gastrinoma:**

1. **In dogs, overall prognosis is poor**, with a **median survival of approximately 2 months**. Of 15 dogs, 5 were reported to have died or been euthanized within a week of presentation. Two dogs were alive at >2 years.

2. In contrast to dogs, **prognosis in cats is fair** based on the limited number of cases reported. Three of the four cats were alive at 1 year, with the fourth cat surviving only 3 weeks. One cat died at 18 months, and one was alive at 17 months.

B. **Glucagonoma:**

1. **Grave prognosis**, with a median survival time of less than a week from the time of diagnosis.

2. One patient with a primary pancreatic tumor and pancreatic lymph node metastasis removed surgically appeared to have complete resolution; however, the case is unusual for the length of time clinical signs were noted (16 months) prior to diagnosis, perhaps suggesting a more indolent tumor despite the presence of local metastasis.

C. **Carcinoid:**

1. For **dogs**, prognosis appears to **depend largely upon the presence or absence of metastases**:

    a. Median survival reported to be <1 week for patients with metastases.

    b. Patients without metastases tended to be alive at the time of last follow-up (times vary widely from months to years) in the majority of reports.

2. For **cats, prognosis appears grave**, but is likely biased by the small number of cases:

    a. Four of the five cases died or were euthanized within a very short period after presentation. All four had multiple metastases.

    b. The one cat without observable metastases was lost to follow-up 21 weeks postsurgery.

D. The dog with a **somatostatinoma** was euthanized 2 months postoperatively for esophageal stricture.

E. The dog with **pancreatic polypeptidoma** was euthanized intraoperatively.

VIII. Prevention

A. With the exceptions of chemodectoma in Boxers and Boston terriers (and certain familial multiple endocrine tumor presentations), no risk factors for the development of APUDomas have been identified.

B. If breed or familial disposition is present, selective breeding and further elaboration of possible genetic underpinnings may prove useful in reducing incidence.

References and Further Readings

Allenspach K, Arnold P, Glaus T, Hauser B, Wolff C, Eberle C, Komminoth P. Glucagon-producing neuroendocrine tumour associated with hypoaminoacidaemia and skin lesions. *J Small Anim Pract* 2000;41(9):402–406.

Altschul M, Simpson KW, Dykes NL, Mauldin EA, Reubi JC, Cummings JF. Evaluation of somatostatin analogues for the detection and treatment of gastrinoma in a dog. *J Small Anim Pract* 1997;38(7):286–291.

Diroff JS, Sanders NA, McDonough SP, Holt DE. Gastrin-secreting neoplasia in a cat. *J Vet Intern Med* 2006;20(5):1245–1247.

Hoenerhoff M, Kiupel M. Concurrent gastrinoma and somatostatinoma in a 10-year-old Portuguese water dog. *J Comp Pathol* 2004;130(4):313–318.

Langer NB, Jergens AE, Miles KG. Canine glucagonoma. *Compend Contin Vet* 2003;25(1):56–63.

Lurye JC, Behrend EN. Endocrine tumors. *Vet Clin North Am Small Anim Pract* 2001;31(5):1083–1109.

Papadogiannakis E, Frangia K, Matralis D. Superficial necrolytic dermatitis in a dog associated with hyperplasia of pancreatic neuroendocrine cells. *J Small Anim Pract* 2009;50(6):318.

Simpson KW, Dykes NL. Diagnosis and treatment of gastrinoma. *Semin Vet Med Surg (Small Anim)* 1997;12(4):274–281.

Torres SMF, Caywood DD, O'Brien TD, O'Leary TP, McKeever PJ. Resolution of superficial necrolytic dermatitis following excision of a glucagon-secreting pancreatic neoplasm in a dog. *J Am Anim Hosp Assoc* 1997;33(4):313–319.

CHAPTER 25

Hypothyroidism in Dogs

David Panciera

Pathogenesis

- Primary hypothyroidism resulting from gradual destruction of the thyroid gland by autoimmune lymphocytic thyroiditis or idiopathic atrophy is responsible for the vast majority of cases.
- Secondary, tertiary, and congenital hypothyroidism are rare.

Classical Signs

- Occurs most commonly in middle-aged purebred dogs.
- Weight gain, lethargy, and exercise intolerance.
- Dermatologic abnormalities, including alopecia, poor hair coat, seborrhea, and hyperpigmentation.
- Generalized or focal peripheral neuropathy is a less common neurologic complication of hypothyroidism.

Diagnosis

- Hypercholesterolemia, hypertriglyceridemia, and mild nonregenerative anemia are common but not diagnostic for hypothyroidism.
- Diagnosis is confirmed by the presence of appropriate clinical signs and some combination of serum thyroxine and free thyroxine concentrations below and thyroid-stimulating hormone (TSH) concentration above their respective reference ranges.

Treatment

- Levothyroxine supplementation results in rapid complete resolution of most clinical signs; some signs, for example, dermatologic, may take a few months.

I. Pathogenesis

A. The **vast majority of dogs with hypothyroidism have primary hypothyroidism,** that is, the disease originates in the thyroid gland:

Clinical Endocrinology of Companion Animals, First Edition. Edited by Jacquie Rand.
© 2013 John Wiley & Sons, Inc. Published 2013 by John Wiley & Sons, Inc.

1. **Primary hypothyroidism** is due to an **immune-mediated lymphocytic thyroiditis or idiopathic follicular atrophy.** Follicular atrophy is likely end-stage thyroiditis. Autoantibodies to thyroglobulin (TgAA), the major follicular colloid protein in the thyroid gland, are a marker of autoimmune thyroiditis.
2. **A hereditary component to hypothyroidism is likely in many purebred dogs.** Golden Retrievers and Doberman Pinschers have been shown to be at increased risk for developing hypothyroidism, and Beagles and Borzois have been shown to have heritable lymphocytic thyroiditis. Other breeds with a high incidence of TgAA and thus at risk for hypothyroidism include English Setters, Old English Sheepdogs, Boxers, Giant Schnauzers, Dalmatians, Maltese, and many others.
3. **Thyroiditis results in gradual destruction of the thyroid gland**, with progression of thyroid gland dysfunction likely occurring **over many months to even years.**
4. **No other risk factor, including vaccination, has been identified** as a factor in development of canine hypothyroidism.

B. A deficiency in secretion of pituitary TSH (**secondary hypothyroidism**) or hypothalamic thyrotropin-releasing hormone (**TRH, tertiary hypothyroidism**) account for **<5% of cases** of canine hypothyroidism. **Most dogs with these forms of hypothyroidism have clinical signs associated with pituitary, hypothalamic, or midbrain dysfunction** in addition to those attributable to hypothyroidism.

C. **Congenital hypothyroidism** is a **rare** disorder resulting from any of a number of defects in hormone synthesis, TSH secretion, or iodine deficiency.

II. Signalment

A. The **average age at diagnosis is about 7 years,** with a range of 0.5–15 years.

B. **Golden Retrievers and Doberman Pinschers** have been shown to be at increased risk, but many **other breeds as mentioned above are also likely predisposed.** There is no important predisposition based on gender.

C. **Congenital hypothyroidism is very rare** in dogs. It has been reported as an inherited disease in toy fox terriers, as well as in litters of boxers, giant schnauzers, and Scottish deerhounds.

III. Clinical Signs

A. The decrease in metabolic rate with thyroid hormone deficiency is reflected by **weight gain** and **obesity** that is present in about **50% of cases** (Table 25.1).

B. **Lethargy and exercise intolerance** are common, but **often noted only in retrospect** by many owners after initiation of thyroid hormone supplementation because of their **gradual onset and mild nature.** The exercise intolerance and weakness result from a combination of the global effects of hypothyroidism on metabolism as well as a myopathy that is frequently present, albeit mild.

C. **Dermatologic abnormalities,** including **alopecia, seborrhea or dry, scaly skin,** and **poor hair coat** occur in **60–80%** of affected dogs. Alopecia **often begins in areas of friction** such as the tail or neck (Figure 25.1) and can progress to **bilateral symmetrical truncal alopecia,** often with **hyperpigmentation** in areas of alopecia (Figure 25.2). **Pyoderma, otitis externa,** *Malassezia* **dermatitis,** and **comedones** can also occur. **Myxedema,** a nonpitting thickening of the skin associated with hyaluronic acid deposition in the dermis, occasionally is of sufficient magnitude to results in a "tragic" facial expression (Figure 25.3).

D. **Peripheral neuropathy** is an **uncommon** manifestation of hypothyroidism (**5–10%** of cases) and may be localized or generalized. In many cases, other clinical signs of hypothyroidism may not be recognized:
1. **Generalized peripheral neuropathy** is manifested by generalized weakness, ataxia, hyporeflexia, proprioceptive deficits, similar to other causes of neuropathy.
2. **Localized peripheral neuropathy** most commonly involves the **vestibulocochlear nerve,** resulting in head tilt, nystagmus, strabismus, ataxia, and circling, or the **facial nerve** with subsequent loss of motor function to facial muscles.
3. **Megaesophagus and laryngeal paralysis** have been diagnosed in dogs with hypothyroidism, but it **remains to be established that hypothyroidism causes these abnormalities.** Resolution of megaesophagus or laryngeal paralysis following levothyroxine supplementation is poorly documented.

E. **Myopathy** is probably a common consequence of hypothyroidism, but **rarely results in overt clinical abnormalities.** However, the improvement in activity and exercise tolerance after supplementation with thyroid hormones may in part result from resolution of the myopathy.

F. **Central nervous system involvement** has been **identified infrequently** in hypothyroid dogs:

Table 25.1   Clinical findings in dogs with hypothyroidism.

Historical or physical examination abnormality	Percent affected
Dermatologic abnormalities	88
Alopecia	40
Flaky skin or seborrhea	22
Pyoderma	14
Dry or poor hair coat	9
Obesity	49
Lethargy	48
Weakness	12
Bradycardia	10
Facial nerve paralysis	4
Peripheral vestibular disease	3
Generalized polyneuropathy	2
Central vestibular disease	Unknown
Infertility	Unknown
Clinical pathology abnormality	
Hypercholesterolemia	75
Anemia	36

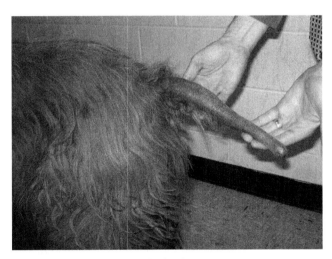

Figure 25.1   Alopecia of the tail ("rat tail") in a hypothyroid Labrador Retriever.

1. Disease has been localized to the myelencephalon or vestibulocerebellum on neurologic examination and some cases have had documented infarction.
2. **Nystagmus that is vertical or alters direction with change in body position, abnormal postural reactions, paresis, and altered consciousness may be seen.**

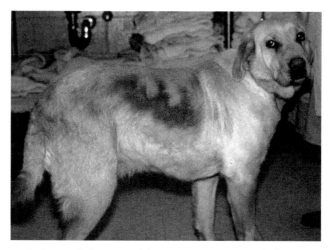

Figure 25.2   Bilaterally symmetrical, truncal alopecia with hyperpigmentation typical of hypothyroidism.

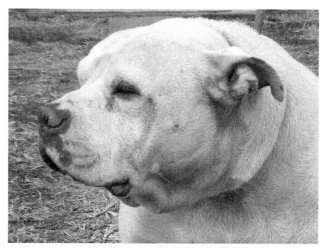

Figure 25.3   Myxedema in an American Pit Bull resulting in thickening of the subcutis of the face. The "puffy" appearance and "tragic facial expression" are typical.

    3. Affected dogs often do not have other signs of hypothyroidism.
    4. Clinical signs are largely reversible with thyroid hormone replacement therapy.
G. **Cardiovascular** abnormalities in hypothyroid dogs include **bradycardia, weak pulses, low voltage ECG complexes, first-degree atrioventricular block, and decreased myocardial contractility.** Rarely, myocardial dysfunction can result in congestive heart failure that is reversible with levothyroxine treatment.
H. **Reproductive abnormalities can occur:**
    1. **Infertility** in bitches can result from prolonged, severe hypothyroidism.
    2. Parturition may be prolonged and uterine contractions weak. **Puppies born to hypothyroid bitches are likely to be weak and have a low body weight** and are more likely to be stillborn than those born to euthyroid bitches.
    3. The **estrous cycle is not altered by hypothyroidism.**
    4. Hypothyroidism has **no important negative effects on reproduction in males.**
I. **Ocular abnormalities** attributed to hypothyroidism include corneal lipid dystrophy, corneal ulcers, and anterior uveitis, although little evidence supports an association. Tear production has been shown to be normal or reduced in hypothyroid dogs, but overt keratoconjunctivitis sicca has not been attributed to hypothyroidism.

J. While hypothyroidism has been suggested to cause bleeding in dogs as a result of von Willebrand factor deficiency, **numerous studies have documented normal von Willebrand factor concentrations and normal hemostasis in hypothyroid dogs.**

K. **Myxedema stupor or coma** is a **rare** manifestation of hypothyroidism:

1. Characterized by mental dullness or coma, hypothermia without shivering, proprioceptive deficits, bradycardia, hypotension, and nonpitting edema. Other signs of hypothyroidism may also be present.

2. Rottweilers and Doberman Pinschers may be predisposed.

3. Concurrent illness is common.

4. Hypercholesterolemia, hyponatremia, lipemia, and normocytic normochromic anemia are frequently present.

L. **Secondary and tertiary hypothyroidism** can result in **clinical signs due to hypothyroidism** as described above **or signs due to local disease:**

1. **Deficiencies of other hypophyseal hormones** can result in diabetes insipidus, secondary hypoadrenocorticism, or growth hormone deficiency arising from destruction of normal pituitary gland.

2. **Neurologic signs** can result if the underlying disease, that is, trauma, neoplasia, or vascular abnormalities result in damage to the hypothalamus or midbrain.

M. **Congenital hypothyroidism** is a rare disease that can be caused by a variety of defects in iodine uptake or hormone synthesis in the thyroid gland or can result from pituitary or hypothalamic dysfunction:

1. **Disproportionate dwarfism** results in slow growth, short limbs, and delayed skeletal maturation due to epiphyseal dysgenesis.

2. **Broad head, macroglossia, delayed dental eruption, abdominal distension, constipation, and ataxia are typically present.**

3. Depending on the etiology, some affected pups **may have a goiter.**

4. Effects on the **central nervous system development** cause mental retardation, difficulty training, and, possibly, obtundation. The disease can be fatal in severely affected pups.

Clinicopathologic Findings

A. **Hypercholesterolemia** is present in approximately **75% of cases,** and hypertriglyceridemia is also common.

B. **Mild elevation of creatine kinase** and **hyponatremia** can occur occasionally. Elevated alkaline phosphatase and alanine aminotransferase activities have been reported but are not clearly associated with hypothyroidism.

C. **A mild, normocytic, normochromic, nonregenerative anemia is present in 25–40%** of dogs.

D. Serum fructosamine can be mildly elevated.

IV. Differential Diagnoses

A. **Alopecia** in hypothyroidism must be differentiated from other endocrine disorders such as hyperadrenocorticism and alopecia X, follicular dysplasia, telogen effluvium, flank alopecia, and infectious diseases. **Poor hair coat, seborrhea, and recurrent bacterial and yeast cutaneous infections** can occur as a result of numerous other disorders.

B. **Obesity** or weight gain results most commonly from overfeeding but can also occur in hyperadrenocorticism.

C. **Lethargy** and **exercise intolerance** can occur as a result of numerous metabolic, neurologic, or cardiovascular disorders.

D. **Peripheral neuropathy** can be due to a primary neurologic disorder (e.g., congenital, immune-mediated, neoplastic, paraneoplastic, infectious, idiopathic) or can occur secondary to metabolic diseases (e.g., insulinoma, diabetes mellitus), neoplasia, toxins, or trauma.

E. **Central vestibular disease** may result from neoplasia, inflammatory disorders (granulomatous meningoencephalitis, vasculitis), cerebrovascular disease, or infection.

F. **Infertility** in bitches could be caused by numerous hormonal, infectious, or primary uterine disorders.

G. **Bradycardia** may result from other metabolic disorders including hyperkalemia and hypoglycemia or due to primary cardiac disease.

H. **Hypercholesterolemia** can be a postprandial change or be caused by hyperadrenocorticism, diabetes mellitus, cholestasis, pancreatitis, protein-losing nephropathy, or primary hyperlipidemia disorders.

V. Diagnosis

A. Diagnosis of hypothyroidism is **made on the basis of abnormal thyroid function tests and appropriate clinical signs.** Serum free thyroxine (fT4) measured using the equilibrium dialysis method is the best single test for diagnosis of hypothyroidism. However, serum total thyroxine (T4) is most commonly used for routine testing because of availability, rapid turnaround time, and cost. Concurrent measurement of serum TSH increases the accuracy of both T4 and fT4. **Serum total thyroxine (T4) concentration** is the most practical single test for diagnosis of hypothyroidism in the dog:

1. **Serum T4 is below the reference range in over 90% of hypothyroid dogs.** A T4 concentration above the lower end of the reference range eliminates hypothyroidism as a diagnosis in most cases:

   a. Dogs with **early hypothyroidism** may have clinical signs of hypothyroidism yet have a low normal serum T4 concentration.

   b. **Autoantibodies to T4** may interfere with the T4 assay and **result in a false increase in T4 concentration** to a level above or within the reference range.

2. **Serum T4 is below normal in 20–25% of euthyroid dogs** with clinical signs that could be consistent with hypothyroidism:

   a. The lack of specificity is why **a diagnosis of hypothyroidism should be made with caution when T4 is used as the sole test of thyroid function.**

   b. **Routine screening of dogs without clinical signs of hypothyroidism,** for example, geriatric profiles, **is not recommended and will result in frequent false positive tests.**

3. **Good quality control is essential** for accurate measurement of T4, including in-hospital assays.

4. **Factors that frequently result in serum T4 concentrations being below the reference range** in euthyroid dogs include **breed-specific normal variations, nonthyroidal illness, and administration of some drugs:**

   a. **Sight hounds,** including Greyhounds, Whippets, Scottish Deerhounds, Basenji, and Sloughis, have a significantly lower normal range for serum T4 concentration than other breeds, with values often falling below the reference range of most laboratories.

   b. **Nonthyroidal illness** frequently induces a low T4 concentration and is more likely to happen with more severe illness or specific diseases such as hyperadrenocorticism. **Serum total T4 is not a reliable test for hypothyroidism in such cases.**

   c. **Drugs,** including **sulfonamides, glucocorticoids, phenobarbital, clomipramine,** and, to a much lesser degree, **aspirin and carprofen,** can decrease serum T4 concentration. Chronic administration of sulfonamides (>2–4 weeks) can induce clinical hypothyroidism. Chronic phenobarbital administration and treatment with high doses of corticosteroids frequently decreases serum T4 below the reference interval and may do the same to free T4.

B. **Serum fT4 concentration is the most accurate single test for diagnosing hypothyroidism,** with higher sensitivity and specificity than any other test:

1. T4 is highly bound to transport proteins, with only 0.1% unbound or "free". Only unbound T4 is able to leave the circulation and enter cells, thus it represents the **metabolically active form of circulating T4.**

2. **FT4 can only be measured accurately using an equilibrium dialysis assay.** Other assays for fT4 provide little if any advantage over measurement of total T4.

3. **Serum fT4 is below the reference range in up to 98% of hypothyroid dogs:**

   a. Thus, measurement of serum fT4 is a **more sensitive test for diagnosis of hypothyroidism** than is measurement serum total T4.

   b. FT4 measured by equilibrium dialysis is not affected by T4 autoantibodies, accounting for much of the improved sensitivity over serum T4.

4. **Serum fT4 is more specific than measurement of T4** because many of the factors that lower serum T4 concentrations have less effect on fT4:

   a. **Nonthyroidal illness alters fT4 concentrations less frequently than it does serum T4.** However, more severe nonthyroidal illness and some specific diseases, such as hyperadrenocorticism, can cause a decrease in fT4 to below the reference range.

   b. While some drugs have less effect on fT4 than T4, **sulfonamides, glucocorticoids, and phenobarbital** administration result in reduction of fT4 similar to T4.

c. **Greyhounds** and Salukis have lower fT4 concentrations than typically noted in other breeds, but similar changes have not been found in other sight hound breeds.

5. **Measurement of fT4 by equilibrium dialysis is recommended in cases where nonthyroidal illness or drug administration that may alter thyroid function is present and diagnostic testing cannot be delayed until these factors are resolved.** In addition, fT4 is an important diagnostic tool in cases of suspected hypothyroidism where serum T4 is normal or T4 autoantibodies are present.

C. **3,5,3′-triiodothyronine (T3)** is the **metabolically active form** of thyroid hormone. The circulating T3 concentration is equally derived from secretion by the thyroid gland and from deiodination of T4 in peripheral tissues. Thus, because it is primarily an intracellular hormone, **serum T3 concentrations frequently do not accurately reflect thyroid function:**

1. Measurement of serum T3 is, **in general, not a useful test** since it has poor sensitivity and specificity for the diagnosis of hypothyroidism.

2. Serum T3 **may be useful in diagnosis of hypothyroidism in sight hounds,** particularly greyhounds where both serum T4 and fT4 concentrations are normally below the standard reference ranges.

D. **TSH (thyrotropin)** is a glycoprotein produced by the pituitary gland that is the **primary stimulus for secretion of T4 and T3** from the thyroid gland. It is controlled primarily by stimulation from hypothalamic secretion of **TRH** and by negative feedback inhibition from circulating thyroid hormones, particularly fT4:

1. TSH concentration **increases as thyroid hormone concentrations decrease** during development of primary hypothyroidism. Because the majority of cases of hypothyroidism in dogs are primary, TSH would be expected to be elevated.

2. However, measurement of serum TSH concentration is **not very sensitive** for diagnosis of hypothyroidism, being **elevated in 65–75% of dogs with hypothyroidism:**
    a. The reason for the insensitivity of TSH measurement is not clear.
    b. It may be related to exhaustion of pituitary secretion of TSH with prolonged hypothyroidism or altered posttranslational glycosylation of TSH in hypothyroid dogs so the hormone is not detected by the current assay.

3. The **combination of elevated serum TSH and decreased T4 or fT4 has a specificity of 98% for diagnosis of hypothyroidism:**
    a. Measurement of TSH with T4 or fT4 is very useful because of the high specificity of this test combination.
    b. Therefore, it is **recommended that TSH be measured routinely** in the diagnosis of hypothyroidism.

4. **Nonthyroidal illness can cause an increase in serum TSH concentration,** but infrequently (3–15%).

5. **Drugs that decrease T4 and fT4, including sulfonamides and phenobarbital, can increase serum TSH concentration.** Elevated TSH is not typically found in dogs administered glucocorticoids despite the decrease in thyroid hormone concentrations.

6. The **reference range of TSH is similar in sight hounds** and other breeds.

E. **Other tests of thyroid function are used infrequently or in special circumstances,** such as in dogs with nonthyroidal illness or when results of standard tests are conflicting:

1. **TSH response test** evaluates the reserve function of the thyroid gland. It is **more accurate than basal thyroid function tests,** but results **can still be affected by nonthyroidal illness and drug administration:**
    a. **Protocol:** Obtain blood sample for serum T4 concentration before and 6 h after intravenous administration of 150 µg human recombinant TSH.
    b. A post-TSH T4 concentration < 19 nmol/L is diagnostic of hypothyroidism while a T4 > 30 nmol/L is consistent with normal thyroid function.
    c. Human recombinant TSH is **very costly.** Once reconstituted, it can be stored frozen for at least 8 weeks without loss of activity.

2. The **TRH response test** is performed by measuring either T4 or TSH after TRH administration. Because the T4 response is small and inconsistent and measurement of TSH concentration does not reliably distinguish euthyroid and hypothyroid states, this test is **not recommended.**

3. **Thyroid scintigraphy** using radioactive sodium pertechnetate has been shown to be the **most accurate method for differentiating hypothyroidism from euthyroidism in dogs with decreased serum T4**

concentrations. Because access to this test is limited, it requires anesthesia, a period of isolation after the test, and is costly, the use of thyroid scintigraphy for diagnosis of hypothyroidism will be infrequent.

4. **Thyroid gland ultrasound** examination has been used in an attempt to differentiate hypothyroidism from nonthyroidal illness in dogs with serum T4 concentration below the reference range. Thyroid gland size and echogenicity are decreased in hypothyroid dogs, the parenchyma may be heterogenous, and the margins of the thyroid gland are irregular compared with euthyroid dogs. Ultrasonography **may be useful in dogs with nonthyroidal illness if testing cannot be delayed until resolution of the illness.** Thyroidal ultrasonography, however, requires great skill and practice.

F. **Tests of thyroid autoimmunity** are useful for diagnosis of autoimmune thyroiditis, but are **not measures of thyroid function:**

   1. **Antithyroglobulin antibodies** are formed as a result of an autoimmune response to thyroglobulin, the major protein in the colloid of the thyroid gland:

      a. As a marker of thyroiditis, antithyroglobulin antibodies are **present in about 50% of hypothyroid dogs,** with a prevalence that is highly variable amongst specific breeds.

      b. Antithyroglobulin antibody results are **useful for interpreting thyroid function tests that are equivocal or discordant** (such as decreased T4 and normal TSH); a positive autoantibody test would be supportive of thyroid disease.

      c. **Dogs with a positive antithyroglobulin antibody test and normal thyroid function test results are at increased risk for developing hypothyroidism,** and annual testing of thyroid function is recommended.

   2. **Anti-T4 and anti-T3 antibodies** occur in some dogs with autoimmune thyroid disease:

      a. Their importance lies primarily in their interference with assays of T4 and T3:

         1) The presence of anti-T4 antibodies results in a **false elevation of the measured hormone concentration.**

         2) The presence of anti-T3 antibodies results in **false elevation of the measured hormone concentration in the vast majority of laboratories**; in some laboratories, anti-T3 antibodies cause the apparent serum T3 concentration to be falsely low:

           a) Approximately 15% of hypothyroid dogs have anti-T4 antibodies. Some of these dogs have markedly elevated measurements of serum T4 and are easily identified as having anti-T4 antibodies. **Up to 10% of hypothyroid dogs may have lower antibody levels that result in an elevation of T4 into the reference range,** making diagnosis of hypothyroidism challenging.

           b) While some laboratories estimate anti-T4 antibody levels, measurement of fT4 by equilibrium dialysis is the most effective method to diagnose hypothyroidism in these cases.

G. Therefore, **recommendations for routine testing of thyroid function** are as follows:

   1. Measure serum T4 and TSH in all cases; a diagnosis of hypothyroidism is nearly certain if T4 is decreased and TSH is elevated. Alternatively, fT4 concentration can replace the T4 concentration with a slight increase in accuracy.

   2. Serum fT4 concentration should be measured in cases where T4 and TSH are either inconclusive, anti-T4 antibodies are suspected or known to be present, or nonthyroidal illness exists. While serum fT4 may be more accurate when dogs are receiving some medications such as carprofen or corticosteroids, most drugs that have the potential to lower T4 can lower fT4 as well.

   3. Be **aware of the effects that nonthyroidal illness and medications have on thyroid function tests. When** possible, delay testing until these confounding factors can be alleviated.

   4. Appropriate response to levothyroxine administration should confirm diagnosis.

VI. Treatment

A. **Levothyroxine is the only thyroid hormone that is indicated for treatment of hypothyroidism.** Other preparations, including dessicated thyroid, liothyronine, and combinations of T4 and T3 have no place in the management of hypothyroidism in dogs. There is no evidence that name brand products offer an advantage over generic preparations.

B. Treatment can be administered at 0.02 mg/kg once daily with resolution of clinical signs in most cases. In dogs >40 kg, a dose based on body surface area (0.5 mg/m^2) should be considered to avoid oversupplementation. It is recommended to not exceed a dose of 0.8 mg when instituting treatment regardless of body weight. However, if adequate post-pill concentrations are not achieved, the dose can be raised. Subsequent alterations in dose should be made based on therapeutic monitoring:

1. There is considerable variability in hormone absorption and serum half-life between individuals, so it is important to monitor clinical response and post-pill serum T4 concentrations.

2. Some dogs may require twice daily treatment; if the response to once daily supplementation is incomplete, consider increasing the frequency of administration to q 12 h.

3. The **initial dosage should be decreased to 0.005 mg/kg if the dog has concurrent diabetes mellitus, hypoadrenocorticism, renal failure, hepatic insufficiency, or congestive heart failure.** The dosage can be increased by approximately 0.005 mg/kg every 2 weeks until an adequate clinical response and therapeutic serum T4 concentration are reached. Because hypothyroidism induces insulin resistance, the insulin dosage will have to be reduced during initiation of levothyroxine administration in many diabetic dogs, and careful monitoring for hypoglycemia should be instituted.

4. A **commercially available liquid levothyroxine** preparation has higher bioavailability than tablets, but the recommended **initial dosage is the same.**

5. **Administration with food may decrease bioavailability.**

C. **Treatment of a dog with evidence of autoimmune thyroid disease** is not indicated unless hypothyroidism is present.

D. **Treatment of a dog with myxedema stupor or coma** should consist of passive warming to prevent cutaneous vasodilation and worsening of hypotension, judicious fluid therapy, treatment of any concurrent disease, and, ideally, intravenous administration of levothyroxine.

E. **Response to treatment typically occurs within the first 1–2 weeks of treatment,** manifested initially as an increase in activity and attitude in most dogs. Weight loss should begin within the first few weeks of treatment. Both peripheral and central neurologic signs typically improve within the first few days of treatment with complete resolution within 4–6 weeks. However, some dogs require up to 12 weeks for resolution and a few may have long-term residual neurologic deficits such as head tilt or partial facial nerve deficits. **Hair regrowth may require several months** to be complete.

F. **Therapeutic monitoring should be performed after 6–8 weeks of treatment,** even though steady state is reached within 1–2, in order to allow sufficient time to assess both thyroid hormone concentrations and the clinical response:

1. The clinical response is the most important parameter to monitor.

2. Serum T4 concentration should routinely be measured, while the value of measuring serum TSH has not been determined.

3. The maximum serum T4 concentration after oral administration occurs approximately 4 h after administration. The desired "post-pill" serum T4 concentration 4 h after administration in most laboratories is 40–70 nmol/L.

4. If monitoring is performed 24 h after administration of the previous dose of levothyroxine, the serum T4 should be within the lower 25–50% of the reference range.

5. If serum TSH is measured, it should be suppressed to within or below the reference range. Because of the relatively poor sensitivity of the current TSH assay, it is not possible to use serum TSH concentration as a measure of oversupplementation.

6. If a good clinical response to treatment has occurred and the serum T4 is below the therapeutic target, consideration to factors that could have decreased the serum T4 on that day (failure of levothyroxine administration) should be considered prior to any dosage increase.

7. A good clinical response with a post-pill serum T4 above the therapeutic range should prompt a reduction in the levothyroxine dosage.

8. If treatment of a concurrent illness is undertaken at the same time as initial levothyroxine administration, any clinical improvement noted could be due to treatment of the concurrent disease rather than resolution of hypothyroidism. This is of particular importance if the initial diagnosis of hypothyroidism was tentative.

9. If improvement **in clinical signs has not occurred within 8 weeks** of beginning treatment and the post-pill serum T4 is in the desired range, either an alternative diagnosis to hypothyroidism or the presence of a concurrent disease should be considered.

10. **Failure to achieve both therapeutic serum T4 concentrations and a good clinical response** may be the result of poor bioavailability. While no consistent difference has been documented between specific brands of levothyroxine, failure to respond to one preparation should prompt consideration of administration of levothyroxine from a different manufacturer.

G. **Complications of treatment, namely clinical hyperthyroidism** due to oversupplementation, are **uncommon**:

1. Clinical signs of hyperthyroidism include polydipsia, polyuria, hyperactivity, panting, tachycardia, weight loss, and vomiting.

2. If hyperthyroidism is suspected, a serum T4 should be measured and levothyroxine treatment discontinued pending results.

3. After cessation of levothyroxine administration for 2–3 days, therapy should be reinstituted with at least a 25% reduction in dosage. Follow-up evaluation for resolution of clinical signs of hyperthyroidism and serum T4 measurement should be performed in 1–2 weeks.

VII. Prognosis

A. The prognosis for complete recovery is **excellent in most cases** of hypothyroidism.

B. The prognosis for dogs with **myxedema coma is guarded.**

C. Dogs with **congenital hypothyroidism** may have residual mental retardation and skeletal abnormalities including degenerative arthropathy.

VIII. Prevention

A. No known prevention.

References and Further Readings

Diaz-Espineira MM, Mol JA, Peeters ME, et al. Assessment of thyroid function in dogs with low plasma thyroxine concentration. *J Vet Intern Med* 2007;21:25–32.

Dixon RM, Reid SWJ, Mooney CT. Epidemiological, clinical, haematological and biochemical characteristics of canine hypothyroidism. *Vet Rec* 1999;145:481–487.

Dixon RM, Reid SWJ, Mooney CT. Treatment and therapeutic monitoring of canine hypothyroidism. *J Small Anim Pract* 2002;43:334–340.

Ferguson DC. Testing for hypothyroidism in dogs. *Vet Clin N Am Small Anim* 2007;37:647–669.

Gulikers KP, Panciera DL. Influence of various medications on canine thyroid function. *Compend Contin Educ Pract Vet* 2002;24:511–523.

Mooney CT, Siel RE, Dixon RM. Thyroid hormone abnormalities and outcome in dogs with nonthyroidal illness. *J Small Anim Pract* 2008;49:11–16.

Panciera DL. A retrospective study of 66 cases of canine hypothyroidism. *J Am Vet Med Assoc* 1994;204:761–767.

Peterson ME, Melian C, Nichols R. Measurement of serum total thyroxine, triiodothyronine, free thyroxine, and thyrotropin concentrations for diagnosis of hypothyroidism in dogs. *J Am Vet Med Assoc* 1997;211:1394–1402.

Scott-Moncrieff JC. Clinical signs and concurrent diseases of hypothyroidism in dogs and cats. *Vet Clin N Am Small Anim* 2007;37:709–722.

CHAPTER 26

Hypothyroidism in Cats

Danièlle Gunn-Moore

Pathogenesis

- Most cases are iatrogenic, following treatment for hyperthyroidism.
- There has been one case of adult-onset primary hypothyroidism due to immune-mediated thyroiditis.
- A small number of congenital cases have resulted from a variety of different underlying defects; most have been genetic and one was due to head trauma.

Classical Signs

- Iatrogenic cases may show weight gain, lethargy, inappetence, an ill-kempt coat, and alopecia of the pinnae.
- Congenital hypothyroidism varies depending on the underlying defect. Kittens typically develop disproportionate dwarfism, appear mentally dull, retain deciduous teeth, have constipation, a soft "kitten coat," and may have a goiter.

Diagnosis

- Circulating thyroxin (T_4) and free T_4 concentrations should be low or low normal. Confirmation usually relies on thyroid-stimulating hormone (TSH) or thyrotrophic-releasing hormone (TRH) response tests or measurement of baseline TSH concentration.
- Kittens may have radiographic changes including delayed closure of ossification centers in long bones.

Treatment

- Oral levothyroxine (L-T_4) (0.05–0.1 mg/cat 24 h).

I. Pathogenesis
A. Hypothyroidism is a relatively rare condition of cats:
   1. **Most cases are iatrogenic,** and occur following treatment for hyperthyroidism, either by bilateral thyroidectomy, I^{131} treatment, or an overdose of antithyroid drugs.

Clinical Endocrinology of Companion Animals, First Edition. Edited by Jacquie Rand.
© 2013 John Wiley & Sons, Inc. Published 2013 by John Wiley & Sons, Inc.

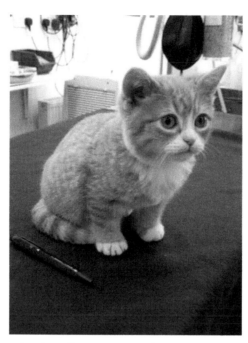

Figure 26.1 Five-month-old domestic short-haired kitten with congenital hypothyroidism. Total T_4 level 0.6 nmol/L. Note the small stature and signs of disproportionate dwarfism characterized by short limbs, a round body, and an enlarged broad head (Picture by Sarah Roberts.)

2. **Adult-onset primary hypothyroidism appears to be very rare in cats**. It has been well described in a single 5-year-old domestic cat (resulting from immune-mediated thyroiditis) and in a single 19-year-old Lynx (where 60–90% of its thyroid gland had been replaced with adipose tissue).

3. **Congenital hypothyroidism has been recognized** more frequently, not only in domestic short-haired cats (Figure 26.1) but also in cats of the Abyssinian breed. The condition has resulted from a number of different causes, including defective thyroid hormone synthesis (presumably related to abnormal peroxidase activity); thyroid dysgenesis; an inability of the thyroid gland to respond to TSH; and juvenile-onset immune-mediated thyroiditis:

    a. Most of these cases appear to have been inherited as autosomal recessive traits.

    b. Feeding kittens on an all-meat diet may, very occasionally, result in hypothyroidism.

    c. One case of secondary hypothyroidism (with concurrent central diabetes insipidus) resulted from head trauma.

II. Signalment

A. **Acquired iatrogenic hypothyroidism** is seen in cats that have been treated for hyperthyroidism. These cats are typically over 8 years of age.

B. **Congenital hypothyroidism** has been seen in domestic short-haired cats and Abyssinian cats, with no sex predisposition.

C. **Spontaneous acquired hypothyroidism was reported in a 5-year-old domestic short-haired cat.**

III. Clinical Signs

A. **Many iatrogenic cases remain subclinical.** However, when they do have clinical signs, affected cats tend to show **marked weight gain, lethargy, inappetence**, and, occasionally, hypothermia and bradycardia. Skin changes may include a dull, dry, ill-kempt hair coat, with matting and seborrhea, and affected cats may develop **alopecia of the pinnae,** which in some cases may also affect the pressure points, tail-base, and caudal flanks. Since acquired hypothyroidism predisposes to renal insufficiency, polyuria and polydipsia may also be present.

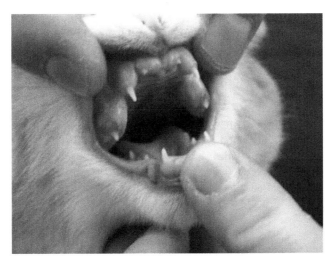

Figure 26.2   Same kitten as in Figure 26.1. Note the retained deciduous teeth (Picture by Sarah Roberts.)

B. The cat with adult-onset hypothyroidism presented with extreme lethargy, hypothermia, poor hair regrowth after clipping, seborrhea, and puffy facial features (presumable resulting from myxedema).
C. **Congenital hypothyroidism**—The clinical signs depend on the type and severity of the underlying defect:
1. Affected kittens typically appear normal at birth, but by 4–8 weeks of age their growth rate slows down. Signs of **disproportionate dwarfism** develop by the time the kittens are 6–9 months old. This is characterized by short limbs, a round body, and an enlarged broad head:
a. However, an 18-month-old cat with secondary hypothyroidism that had developed after head trauma was poorly grown for its age, but had normal head and limb proportions (this may have been because the trauma occurred when the cat was already 8 weeks of age, rather than earlier).
Affected kittens are generally **mentally dull and lethargic**, they become hypothermic and bradycardic, and may suffer recurrent episodes of **severe constipation. Deciduous teeth are usually retained** until 12–18 months of age (Figure 26.2), and the coat may either have only a few guard hairs and retain its undercoat or become very shaggy. Seizures have been seen in occasional cases. In cats with thyroid dyshormonogenesis defects, goiter is evident from 6 months of age:
a. Kittens with immune-mediated thyroiditis typically die within 1–2 weeks of developing clinical signs at 1–2 months of age; kittens with TSH resistance usually die by 16 weeks of age, while the changes in kittens with thyroid peroxidase defects may become less pronounced with time.

IV. Diagnosis
A. Routine hematology may demonstrate mild anemia, while serum biochemistry may show hypercholesterolemia and/or indication of renal insufficiency (particularly in iatrogenic cases).
B. In affected kittens, radiographic changes may include delayed closure of ossification centers in long bones, plus shortening and scalloping of the ventral borders of the vertebral bodies.
C. **Circulating T_4 and free T_4 concentrations should be low or low normal in all cases:**
1. However, care is required with interpretation as low T_4 concentrations are commonly associated with nonthyroidal illness.
2. Concurrent assessment of free T_4 concentration may improve the sensitivity and specificity of diagnosis.
3. While the thyroid-suppressive effects of certain drugs (e.g., glucocorticoids, anticonvulsants, sulfonamide antibiotics, and some nonsteroidal anti-inflammatory agents) are well known in dogs, their effects in cats have generally been less well studied.
D. Confirmation usually relies on results from **TSH or TRH response tests:**
1. The TSH test is performed by collecting a blood sample for a basal total T_4 determination, giving 0.1 IU of TSH/kg body weight IV, then collecting a second blood sample for repeat total T_4 assessment after 6 h. In a hypothyroid cat there should be no stimulation.

2. The TRH test is performed in the same manner as described in the section on hyperthyroidism. However, the total T_4 increase is less than that seen following TSH administration and is more prone to being complicated by severe nonthyroidal illness.

E.   Other tests can also be considered: These include assessing a **baseline TSH concentration**. While feline specific reagents are not currently available, studies using canine reagents for the detection of endogenous TSH and antithyroglobulin look promising (http://www.animalhealth.msu.edu/Sections/Endocrinology/Thyroid_Feline.php):

1. Cats with hypothyroidism should have an increased TSH concentration, and the presence of circulating thyroglobulin and thyroid hormone antibodies may help in confirming lymphocytic thyroiditis.

2. A diagnosis of lymphocytic thyroiditis has previously been confirmed by thyroid biopsy in an adult cat and some kittens.

3. Diagnosis of the precise underlying genetic defects requires specific investigations.

4. Brain damage resulting in secondary hypothyroidism may be evident on MRI or CT.

V.   Differential Diagnoses

A.   The major differential diagnoses for congenital hypothyroidism include a number of lysosomal storage diseases (e.g., mucopolysaccharidosis) and possibly, chondrodysplasia, congenital hyposomatotropism, or even a congenital portosystemic liver shunt. However, diagnosis is not always straightforward as one case of congenital hypothyroidism was found to have a reduced serum concentration of insulin-like growth factor (IGF-1) plus abnormal liver function tests, all of which resolved on treatment for congenital hypothyroidism.

VI.   Treatment

A.   Treatment requires giving oral levothyroxine (0.05–0.1 mg/cat q 24 h) then adjusting the dose based on the clinical response after 4–6 weeks; twice daily dosing may be needed in some cats.

VII.   Prognosis

A.   In iatrogenic and adult-onset hypothyroidism, the response to treatment is usually excellent and the prognosis very good.

B.   Without treatment, kittens with TSH resistance usually die by 16 weeks of age:

1. Giving prophylactic levothyroxine to kittens genetically at risk of developing immune-mediated thyroiditis may reduce the severity of the disease.

2. In general, the response to treatment in congenitally affected kittens has been variable, often with incomplete resolution of clinical signs.

3. That said, even late detection is not necessarily deleterious: for example, a female cat presented at 18 months of age with acute renal failure and a 3-year-old male cat presented with constipation, both responded well to supplementation with levothyroxine and lived for a number of years on medication. Interestingly, when the kitten with renal failure had follow-up radiographs taken 1 year later, all the ossification centers had closed.

VIII.   Prevention

Spontaneous hypothyroidism cannot be prevented. Iatrogenic hypothyroidism can be prevented by close monitoring and dose adjustment when using anti-thyroid medication, by using lower doses of radioactive iodine, and by not performing bilateral thyroidectomies.

References and Further Readings

Feldman EC, Nelson RW. Hypothyroidism. In: Feldman EC, Nelson RW, eds. *Canine and Feline Endocrinology and Reproduction*, 3rd edn. St. Louis: WB Saunders, 2004, pp. 86–151.

Greco DS. Diagnosis of congenital and adult-onset hypothyroidism in cats. *Clin Tech Small Anim Pract* 2006;21(1):40–44.

Greer LL, Troutman M, McCracken MD, Ramsay EC. Adult-onset hypothyroidism in a lynx (*Lynx canadensis*). *J Zoo Wildl Med* (2003;34(3):287–291.

Jones BR, Gruffydd-Jones TJ, Sparkes AH, Lucke VM. Preliminary studies on congenital hypothyroidism in a family of Abyssinian cats. *Vet Rec* 1992;131:145–148.

Mellanby RJ, Jeffery ND, Gopal MS, Herrtage ME. Secondary hypothyroidism following head trauma in a cat. *J Feline Med Surg* 2005;7:135–139.

Nykamp SG, Dykes NL, Zarfoss MK, Scarlett JM. Association of the risk of development of hypothyroidism after iodine 131 treatment with the pretreatment pattern of sodium pertechnetate Tc 99 m uptake in the thyroid gland in cats with hyperthyroidism: 165 cases (1990–2002). *J Am Vet Med Assoc* 2005;226(10):1671–1675.

Peterson ME. Feline hypothyroidism. In: Kirk RW, eds. *Current Veterinary Therapy X.* Philadelphia: WB Saunders, 1989, pp. 1000–1001.

Peterson ME, Ferguson DC. Thyroid disease. In: Ettinger SJ, ed. *Textbook of Veterinary Internal Medicine.* Philadelphia: WB Saunders, 1989, pp. 1654–1667.

Peterson ME, Randolf JH. Endocrine diseases. In: Sherding RG, ed. *The Cat: Diseases and Clinical Management.* New York: Churchill Livingston, 1989, pp. 1101–1103.

Rand JS, Levine J, Best SJ, Parker W. Spontaneous adult-onset hypothyroidism in a cat. *J Vet Intern Med* 1993;7(5):272–276.

Sjollema BE, den Hartog MT, de Vijlder JJ, van Dijk JE, Rijnberk A. Congenital hypothyroidism in two cats due to defective organification: Data suggesting loosely anchored thyroperoxidase. *Acta Endocrinol (Copenh)* 1991;125(4):435–340.

Sparkes AH, Jones BR, Gruffydd-Jones TJ, Walker MJ. Thyroid function in the cat: Assessment by the TRH response test and the thyrotrophin stimulation test. *J Small Anim Pract* 1991;32:59–63.

Szabo SD, Wells KL. What is your diagnosis? *J Am Vet Med Assoc* 2007;230(1):29–30.

Tanase H, Kudo K, Horikoshi H, Mizushima H, Okazaki T, Ogata E. Inherited hypothyroidism with thyrotropin resistance in Japanese cats. *J Endocrinol* 1991;129(2):245–251.

Traas AM, Abbott BL, French A, Giger U. Congenital thyroid hypoplasia and seizures in 2 littermate kittens. *J Vet Intern Med* 2008;22:1427–1431.

Quante S, Fracassi F, Gorgas D, Kitcher PR, Boretti FS, Ohlerth S, Reusch CE. Congenital hypothyroidism in a kitten resulting in decreased IGF-1 concentration and abnormal liver function tests. *J Feline Med Surg* 2010;12:487–490.

Williams TL, Elliott J, Syme HM. Association of iatrogenic hypothyroidism with azotemia and reduced survival time in cats treated for hyperthyroidism. *J Vet Intern Med* 2010;2:1086–1092.

CHAPTER 27

Hypothyroidism in Other Species

Janice Sojka Kritchevsky

Hypothyroidism in Foals

Pathogenesis

- Results from a deficiency in thyroid hormone in utero.
- The most common presentation is as part of the thyroid gland hyperplasia and musculoskeletal deformities (TS-MSD) syndrome; the exact etiology of this condition remains unknown.
- Hypothyroidism occurs when the diet of the dam has a deficient or excess iodine concentration.

Classical Signs

- No breed or sex predilection.
- Dysmaturity despite prolonged gestation (340 days or greater).
- Musculoskeletal abnormalities—particularly failure of the cuboidal bones of the carpus and tarsus to ossify and mandibular prognathism.

Diagnosis

- Thyroid-releasing hormone (TRH) response test to document low baseline levels of thyroxine (T4) and triiodothyronine (T3) and failure of T3 to increase after TRH administration.

Treatment

- Thyroid hormone supplementation.
- Removal of excess iodine source if present.
- Treatment of TS-MSD is often unsuccessful due to the severity of musculoskeletal deformities.

I. Pathogenesis

A. **Iodine deficiency or excess** can cause congenital goiter and hypothyroidism. The dam is invariably unaffected. This is due to two reasons:

  1. The thyroid gland in a healthy adult possesses the ability to **autoregulate** when presented with abnormally high iodine concentrations. **The fetal thyroid gland does not autoregulate.**

Clinical Endocrinology of Companion Animals, First Edition. Edited by Jacquie Rand.
© 2013 John Wiley & Sons, Inc. Published 2013 by John Wiley & Sons, Inc.

Thyroid function is permanently altered if abnormal iodine intakes are present and congenital hypothyroidism will result.

1. The euthyroid state is not necessary to maintain relatively normal function in the adult horse, but it is **crucial in the fetus and neonate** for the development of the normal skeleton and nervous system. Thus, the effects of hypothyroidism in the developing foal are much more severe than those seen in an adult animal.

B. Daily iodine intake in horses in North America is typically 2 mg, which is twice the requirement for the average horse.

C. Pregnant mares fed an **iodine-deficient** diet will have weak or dead foals with goiter and alopecia.

D. **Goiter and hypothyroidism occurs in foals if the dam ingests high iodine levels** in the diet:

1. Congenital goiter has been reported in foals when mares have been supplemented with as little as **35 mg/day** of iodine.

2. Any time a foal with an abnormal thyroid gland is observed, it should prompt the practitioner to take a **detailed dietary history** of the dam.

3. If a high iodine product such as **natural seaweed extract** is being fed, feed analysis that determines the total iodine concentration in the diet should be performed.

E. **TH-MSD** has been reported in the **Pacific Northwest region of the North American** continent although it occurs sporadically in other geographic areas:

1. In some instances, **multiple cases occur on one farm** in a season. Dams have normal thyroid function at the time of parturition and are asymptomatic.

2. The exact cause of TH-MSD is still not determined. An epidemiologic study of foals with this syndrome revealed that **pregnant mares that were fed green feed, did not receive supplemental mineral, or grazed irrigated pastures had an increased risk of producing foals with the syndrome.**

3. A combination of **nitrate ingestion and low iodine levels** in the feed may be responsible for the condition.

II. Signalment

A. Neonatal and congenital; problems associated with hypothyroidism are present from birth.

B. TS-MSD often presents as a **herd problem** with multiple foals from the same farm affected. The problem may be present in a particular year and then not reoccur despite no obvious change in management.

III. Clinical Signs

A. The most frequent clinical signs of hypothyroidism in foals include goiter (enlarged thyroid gland), ruptured common digital extensor tendon, failure of the cuboidal bones of the carpus and tarsus to ossify, and mandibular prognathism.

B. Affected foals are delivered after **prolonged gestation** (340–400 days). Despite the prolonged gestation foals are dysmature with **short, silky hair coat, pliable ears, muscle weakness, and incomplete skeletal development.**

C. **Less commonly reported clinical signs** include dry hair coat, poor suckle reflex, angular limb deformities, subnormal temperature, anemia, persistent lipemia, and listlessness.

D. Foals often **require assistance** to stand and suckle.

E. Muscle weakness may result in **respiratory distress** without other clinical signs.

IV. Diagnosis

A. **Histopathology** of the thyroid gland in foals with TH-MSD reveals colloid goiter with a large variation in follicular size or thyroid hyperplasia with small, crowded, irregular follicles.

B. The circulating blood concentrations of total and **free T3 and T4 are quite elevated in normal neonatal foals when compared to adult horses**—and can be up to ten times normal adult values:

1. **Serum thyroxine levels reach adult values by 16 days of age,** but free T4 and T3 and total T3 remain above adult levels at 3 months of age.

2. **Serum T3 levels rise in the first hours after birth as T4 levels fall, suggesting that T4 is being converted to T3** at this time. The need of foals for high thermogenic capacity and rapid bone and nervous system growth has been postulated as the reason for increased thyroid hormone values.

3. Because of the neonate's high circulating T3 and T4 concentrations and the rapid fall in these values after birth, **it is important to know a foal's exact age when evaluating blood hormone values.**

C. Results of thyroid function testing differ between neonates and adult horses:

Table 27.1   Flow chart for evaluating a foal with suspected hypothyroidism.

Clinical signs	Nonthyroid disease rule outs
Prolonged gestation	Evaluate mare's diet for presence of fescue Evaluate mare's history; some mares have prolonged gestational lengths Mule foals have prolonged gestation compared to horses
Signs of dysmaturity—silky hair coat, floppy ears, weakness	Placental insufficiency Fescue toxicosis Sepsis
Weakness, unable to stand	Sepsis, prematurity
Poor suckle reflex	Sepsis, ischemic encephalopathy
Angular limb deformities	Uterine malposition Prematurity
Incomplete ossification of carpal or tarsal bones	Prematurity, dysmaturity
Prognathism	Poor conformation
Goiter	Excess or deficient iodine during gestation

   1. **T3 increases after thyroid-stimulating hormone (TSH) administration in 1-day-old foals while the response of T4 is quite variable.** This suggests that a rise in T3 concentrations is a better measure of thyroid function than T4 in neonates.
   2. Determining thyroid hormone concentrations in **age-matched controls** may assist in the evaluation of test results.
D.   Characteristic musculoskeletal lesions can be detected via careful physical examination and radiography.
   1. Radiographs of carpi and tarsi will reveal characteristic **lack of calcification of cuboidal bones.**

V.   Differential Diagnoses
A.   Differential diagnosis for dysmaturity after prolonged gestation includes ingestion of *Acremonion coenophialum*-infected fescue during gestation. **Fescue toxicosis** produces multiple abnormalities such as dysmaturity, weakness at birth, and prolonged gestation that are also seen in TH-MSD.
B.   Differential diagnoses for weakness and poor ventilation include **prematurity and placental insufficiency.**
C.   **Sepsis, either bacterial or viral,** is always a possibility when presented with a weak neonatal foal that is unable to stand without assistance. (Table 27.1).

VI.   Treatment
A.   Remove foal from excess iodine source if present. **Iodine is concentrated in mare's milk,** thus lactating mares need to be on proper iodine levels in their diet to avoid exposing the foal to high levels of the element.
B.   Iodine supplementation is indicated if a deficiency exists.
C.   Thyroid hormone supplementation: **synthetic thyroxine administered at a dose of 20 μg/kg.**

VII.   Prognosis
A.   **Prognosis for foals with TS-MSD is extremely poor** due to the extensive skeletal lesions.
B.   **Prognosis for foals that suffer from hypothyroidism due to other causes is good** with proper thyroxine supplementation and correction of dietary iodine levels.

VIII.   Prevention
A.   The diets of pregnant mares should be evaluated to ensure an appropriate amount of iodine is provided and that there is not an excessively high nitrate level.

Hypothyroidism in Adult Horses

Pathogenesis

- Hypothyroidism in adult horses is caused by a decrease in circulating thyroid hormone concentrations and an inability of the thyroid gland to respond in an appropriate fashion to stimulation.

Classical Signs

- Documented thyroid deficiency in adult horses is extremely rare; most horses that fit the "classical" definition of thyroid disease actually suffer from equine metabolic syndrome due to insulin resistance.
- Hypothyroidism can lead to parasympathetic dysfunction of the face resulting in keratoconjunctivitis sicca.
- Poor hair coat, exercise intolerance, and agalactia may be the result of hypothyroidism in adult horses.

Diagnosis

- Exclusion of nonthyroidal illness.
- Evocative testing with TSH or TRH.

Treatment

- T4 administered at a dose of 20 µg/kg.

I. Pathogenesis

A. Biologically active thyroid hormone, primarily in the form of **free T3 (fT3)**, binds receptors within the cell nucleus. These stimulate transcription factors to act upon DNA response elements to enhance the expression of genes:

    1. Increased enzyme synthesis **accelerates cellular energy production and heat is generated** as a result.

    2. In addition to its effects on energy metabolism, **thyroid hormone is essential for both prenatal and postnatal developmental events including organ formation and skeletal maturation.**

    3. **T4 may have some direct physiologic effects as well**, particularly in maintaining neuronal integrity.

B. The majority of circulating thyroid hormone is **bound to thyroid hormone–binding globulin and other blood proteins.**

C. Unbound hormone is also referred to as free hormone and is the **biologically active form.**

D. Free T3 is supplied from both circulating bound T3 and thyroxine (T4):

    1. Small quantities of free T4 (fT4) are also produced and enter tissues, but the **biological activity of this hormone is estimated to be one-fifth that of fT3.**

    2. The action of 5′-monodeiodinase generates T3, while 5-monodeiodinase activity results in the synthesis of inactive **reverse T3.**

E. Thyroid hormone secretion is dependent upon adequate blood concentrations of TSH, also referred to as thyrotropin, and an appropriate supply of iodine:

    1. **TSH originates from the pars anterior** of the pituitary gland.

    2. Central nervous system **tissues including the hypothalamus monitor blood concentrations of free thyroid hormone,** particularly fT4.

    3. **Detection of low thyroid hormone concentrations elicits a rise in TRH secretion by the hypothalamus.** Release of TSH from the anterior pituitary gland is stimulated by TRH.

F. **Iodide is actively transported into the colloid of thyroid follicles** and rapidly oxidized to iodine by hydrogen peroxide. **Thyroperoxidase catalyzes the oxidation of iodide and mediates the subsequent iodination of tyrosine residues within thyroglobulin.**

G. This enzyme uses **selenium as a cofactor,** and selenium deficiency may result in a secondary decrease in circulating thyroid hormone levels.

H. **Thyroglobulin is secreted by follicular cells and accumulates within the colloid.**

I. Monoiodotyrosines located on adjacent thyroglobulins couple together, follicular cells internalize thyroglobulin by pinocytosis, and **T3 and T4 are liberated through the action of lysosomal proteases.**

J. In adult horses, however, **there does not appear to be a clear relationship between dietary iodine and hypothyroidism** due to the adult horse thyroid's ability to **auto regulate** and maintain normal function despite a wide range of iodine intake.

II. Signalment

A. The typical age range of horses described as hypothyroid is 6–13 years.

B. No breed or sex predilection has been identified.

III. Clinical Signs

A. Hypothyroidism can lead to **parasympathetic nerve dysfunction:**
1. This, in turn, can lead to **keratoconjunctivitis sicca, hyperemic and edematous conjunctiva,** dull cornea, decreased tear production, blepharospasm, dry nasal mucosa, **head shaking and rubbing,** and excess Flehmen response.
2. **Obesity** and fat deposits along the body may also be present.

B. Clinical signs of horses with experimentally induced hypothyroidism include: hypothermia, facial swelling, poor quality hair coat, limb edema, cold intolerance, bradycardia, alopecia, anemia, decreased cardiac output, and increased plasma and blood volumes. Also observed are increased blood cholesterol, failure of growth plates to close, and stunting in growing animals.

C. Incremental treadmill exercise challenges reveal that hypothyroid horses have reduced distances to fatigue and lower maximal oxygen, maximal heart rate, and maximal velocity parameters.

D. True **hypothyroidism that is documented via evocative testing in adult horses has been described but is extremely rare:**
1. Clinical signs reported from poorly documented cases of naturally occurring thyroid disease include decreased libido, lethargy, muscle disease, anhidrosis, agalactia, poor performance, and infertility.

E. It is now known that the **"classic" clinical presentation of hypothyroidism in adult horses;** cresty neck, increased adipose deposition, laminitis, and infertility, **is actually that of idiopathic insulin resistance or equine metabolic syndrome** (see Chapter 20):
1. The distinction between equine metabolic syndrome and hypothyroidism can be confusing because T4 administration as a **pharmacologic** agent has been advocated in the treatment of equine metabolic syndrome.
2. In these instances, T4 is believed to increase overall metabolic rate and enhance fat metabolism leading to increased insulin sensitivity.
3. The administered **thyroid hormone is not replacing an endogenous deficiency.**

F. Tumors, primarily **adenomas,** are relatively common in aged horses. They often produce goiter, or enlargement of the thyroid gland, but **do not result in hypothyroidism.**

IV. Diagnosis

A. **Endogenous T4 and T3 assays** are often the first step in establishing a diagnosis. Free hormone is the biologically active form of both hormones.

B. **Determination of the concentrations of free T3 and T4 using equilibrium dialysis will produce the most accurate indication of thyroid status:**
1. There is **no documentation in the horse that determining free thyroid hormone values, by any method, leads to a superior diagnostic accuracy** of hypothyroid or euthyroid states.
2. This is even true in instances when phenylbutazone or other highly protein-bound substances have been administered.
3. Normal range for equine free T4 via equilibrium dialysis is **7–47 pmol/L** (0.54–3.65 ng/dL).

C. Because of the large number of factors that affect resting T4 and T3 levels (Table 27.2), low blood concentrations on onetime testing is not sufficient to make a diagnosis of hypothyroidism:
1. **Factors that will result in decreased thyroid hormone concentrations** include: high energy diets, concurrent disease, particularly pituitary pars intermedia dysfunction (PPID) or other endocrine

Table 27.2   Factors that affect thyroid hormone values in horses.

Age—Thyroid concentrations decrease over the life of an animal

Ambient temperature—Decreased temperatures stimulate higher thyroid hormone concentrations

Diet—Particularly abnormal iodine concentrations or increased dietary carbohydrate or protein concentrations

Diurnal variation—T4 is highest in the evening while T3 is highest in the morning

Training—Thyroid hormone values decrease with training

Pregnancy—Thyroid hormone values increase slightly

Ovulation—T4 decreases on the day after ovulation

Illness—Euthyroid sick syndrome may result in decreased thyroid hormone concentrations in animals that are ill or in negative energy balance

Other endocrine diseases—Thyroid hormone concentrations can be decreased in horses with equine metabolic syndrome and pituitary pars intermedia dysfunction

Therapeutic agents—A large number of therapeutic agents can decrease thyroid hormone concentrations. These include:

Phenylbutazone   Diphenylhydantoin
Glucocorticoids   Phenobarbital
Sulfa antibiotics   Furosemide
Insulin
Radio-contrast agents
Halothane

A wide variety of factors can affect thyroid hormone concentrations in a euthyroid animal. For this reason, evocative testing is always preferred when making a diagnosis of thyroid dysfunction.

abnormalities, age, diurnal variation, climate, stage of estrus cycle, pregnancy, level of training, and dietary iodine.

2. **Therapeutic agents** that may cause decreased thyroid hormone levels include: phenylbutazone, sulfa antibiotics, glucocorticoids, insulin, radio contrast dyes or other iodine-containing products, halothane, diphenylhydantoin, phenobarbital, and furosemide.

D. **Any horse with a suspected endocrine problem should be tested for both insulin resistance and equine PPID in addition to having their thyroid function evaluated.**

E. **TRH and TSH response testing is the best way to establish a diagnosis of hypothyroidism:**

1. **TRH is currently unavailable except as a reagent grade chemical.** It will produce increases in thyroid hormone levels in horses, but its use in client-owned animals is problematic.

2. **Administration of TSH may not be practical due to difficulty in locating an affordable source of the compound.** However, the best means to determine if the thyroid gland is functioning is to perform a response test.

3. After a baseline determination of T3 and T4, either 0.5–1 mg TRH or 5 IU TSH is given intravenously and blood collected again at 2 and 4 h. **In normal horses, the T3 value will be double baseline at the 2-h collection point and the T4 value will be double the baseline concentration at the 4-h point** (see Table 27.3).

4. Because of the expense of TRH and likelihood that other endocrinopathies exist, **evaluating both pars intermedia function (by assessing blood ACTH before and 30 min after TRH administration) and thyroid function after TRH administration is often indicated.**

V. Differential Diagnoses

A. The classic "hypothyroid" cresty necked, laminitic horse probably has **equine metabolic syndrome** (Table 27.4; see Chapter 20).

B. **Equine Pituitary Pars Intermedia Dysfunction** (see Chapter 11).

C. Any illness may result in **euthyroid sick syndrome.** Thyroid disease should not be diagnosed if any other debilitating disease is present.

Table 27.3   Protocol for evocative testing using TSH and TRH in horses and foals.

	TSH adult	TSH foal	TRH
Dose	2.5–5.0 IU	5.0 IU	0.5–1.0 mg
Route	IV	IV	IV
Time of sample	0, 2, and 4 or 6 h	0 and 3 h	0, 2, and 4 h
Expected T4 results	2×baseline at 4 or 6 h	Inconsistent	2×baseline at 4 h
Expected T3 results	2×baseline at 2 h	>50% of baseline at 3 h	2×baseline at 2 h

Source: Sojka JE. Hypothyroidism in horses. *Compend Contin Educ Pract Vet* 1995;17:845–852.
TSH=thyroid-stimulating hormone; TRH=thyroid-releasing hormone. TRH is commercially available but quite expensive. TRH that is not used once reconstituted can be kept frozen until needed; this will prolong its useful "shelf life." TSH is not available in a form that is labeled for parenteral administration. It can be obtained from chemical companies and administered after being passed through a Millipore filter. This is appropriate in a research setting, but may not be in the context of a client–patient–clinician relationship.

Table 27.4   Flow chart for evaluating a horse with T4 and T3 blood concentrations below the reference range.

Clinical signs or clinical pathology findings	Assessment
Cresty neck, increased adiposity, laminitis	Horse suffers from either equine metabolic syndrome or PPID; test for these conditions
Concurrent disease present	Euthyroid sick syndrome
Horse receiving medications, particularly sulfa antibiotics or phenylbutazone	Suppression due to medication
Horse tested after ingesting meal high in carbohydrate, protein, zinc, or copper	Balance diet; retest after fasting or ingestion of grass hay
Presence of goitrogens in the feed or endophyte-infected fescue	Remove from diet
Diet too high or low in iodine	Balance diet
Horse presents with keratoconjunctivitis, alopecia, or cold intolerance	Consider hypothyroidism if other causes ruled out

Because primary hypothyroidism is so rare in adult horses, every attempt should be made to rule out other causes of low thyroid hormone values.

VI.   Treatment
A.   Synthetic **thyroxine administered at a dose of 20 µg/kg** (10 mg for a 500-kg horse) maintains normal T3 and T4 concentrations for 24 h.
B.   **Manufacturer's instructions** should be consulted and serum thyroid hormone measurements repeated every 6–8 weeks to ensure adequate dosing.
C.   As with other hormone therapies, **gradual weaning is recommended if therapy is discontinued.**

VII.   Prognosis
A.   Hypothyroidism is not a life-threatening condition in adult horses. Hormone supplementation should be effective if patients are assessed and monitored appropriately.

VIII.   Prevention
A.   No specific preventative measures for this condition have been identified although ensuring a balanced diet is provided is prudent.

Hypothyroidism in Ferrets, Rabbits, and Rodents

Pathogenesis

- Decrease in circulating thyroid hormone concentrations and inability of the thyroid gland to respond in an appropriate fashion to stimulation.

Classical Signs

- Thyroid enlargement (goiter) can develop in rabbits and other herbivorous species ingesting plants high in goitrogenic substances.
- Disease of the thyroid gland in ferrets and rats has been limited to neoplastic diseases. Clinical signs such as weight loss and anorexia are referable to the neoplastic condition.

Diagnosis/Treatment

- Naturally occurring, clinical hypothyroidism has not been reported in these species.

I.   Pathogenesis
A.   **Herbivorous animals are susceptible to the effects of goitrogenic plants** (Table 27.5) if they are fed as a high enough percent of the total diet:
   1.   **Rabbits on a cabbage diet develop goiter.**
   2.   Signs referable to hypothyroidism are not present.
B.   Although thyroid disease has not been described in **ferrets, normal thyroid hormone values and response to TRH and TSH testing have been reported.**

II.   Signalment
A.   Herbivorous species may be susceptible to the effects of goitrogenic substances in certain plants.
B.   Adult rabbits consuming diets a large percentage of which consists of cruciferous plants such as broccoli, cabage, and mustard greens.

III.   Clinical Signs
A.   An enlarged thyroid gland in a rat or ferret would be consistent with neoplastic disease.
B.   Thyroid problems may be an incidental finding at post mortem, but could result in premortem disease such as weight loss, alopecia, and anorexia.

IV.   Diagnosis
A.   There is **no commercially available assay for endogenous TSH in these animals.** Because TSH is an extremely species-specific compound, using assays designed for other species is not a valid means of assessing thyroid function.
B.   There is a range in normal ferret thyroid hormone values which may be due to seasonal influences, sex, or diet:
   1.   Resting T4 values range between 19.3 and 38.6 nmol/L (1.5 and 3 µg/dL).
   2.   Resting T3 values range from between 0.9 and 1.5 nmol/L (60 and 95 g/dL).
   3.   After administration of 500 µg TRH to adult male ferrets, T4 doubled over baseline at 6 h. After administration of 1 IU TSH, T4 doubled over baseline at the 2-, 4-, and 6-h time points post injection.
   4.   There was **no change in T3** at any time point after TRH or TSH administration.

Table 27.5   Goitrogen-containing plants.

Chard	Bok choy
White mustard seed	Cauliflower
Flixweed	Strawberries
Tansy mustard	Spinach
Kohlrabi	Pears
Rape seed and meal	Peaches
Kale	Sweet potatoes
Broccoli	Collard greens
Cabbage	Horseradish
Brussel sprouts	Millet
Rutabaga (Swede)	Peanuts
Chinese cabbage	Pine nuts
Turnip root	Bamboo shoots
Flax	Radish
Soybean	

Many of the plants that inhibit iodine absorption are members of the genus *Brassica*. These contain L-5-vinyl-2-thiooxazolidone, which has been determined to be the primary goitrogenic factor. Other compounds in plants that prevent thyroid hormone formation include cyanides, thiourea, thiouracil, thiocyanate, and sulfonamides. Some products, such as rapeseed, can be fed safely if they have been processed to remove the goitrogenic substances.

   5. TRH administration resulted in transient salivation, hyperventilation, vomiting, and depression in male ferrets. For this reason, TSH is the preferable compound to use in evocative testing of thyroid function.

C.   **TSH is not available in a form labeled for medical use.** Reagent grade TSH is available for purchase and has been used in experimental studies. Its use on client-owned animals is problematic.

V.   Differential Diagnoses

A.   Rabbits may suffer from disease of the **thymus**.

B.   Other, more common, neoplastic conditions should be considered in ferrets with swelling of the cervical region.

VI.   Treatment

A.   **Remove goitrogens** from the diet if they are identified in a dietary history.

B.   Feed a **balanced diet that has adequate iodine** content.

VII.   Prognosis

A.   No data is available with respect to prognosis.

VIII.   Prevention

A.   No specific preventative measures for this condition have been identified although ensuring the diet contains sufficient iodine is prudent, as well as limiting the amount of goitrogenic plants offered.

Hypothyroidism in Pet Birds

Pathogenesis

- Iodine deficiency—either absolute or relative causes decreased circulating thyroid hormone concentrations.
- Consuming goitrogenic substances binds iodine and makes it unavailable for metabolic needs.

Classical Signs

- Nonpruritic feather loss, with no skin inflammation.
- Increased body weight.
- Goiter is most commonly observed in budgerigars and pigeons.

Diagnosis

- Total T4 values below reference ranges.
- No response to TRH administration.

Treatment

- Correct diet if goitrogens are present or iodine deficiency exists.
- T4 supplementation.

I. Pathogenesis
A. **T3 has a shorter half-life in birds** than in mammals.
B. Thyroid hormone secretion is **directly influenced by ambient temperature, photoperiod, and dietary protein.**

II. Signalment
A. **Macaws,** particularly blue and gold macaws—represented half of all cases of hyperplastic goiter in over 12 000 avian accessions in one survey.
B. **Functional hypothyroidism is uncommon in birds.** It has been documented in a single case report describing disease in a scarlet macaw.
C. No known sex predilection.

III. Clinical Signs
A. In one case report, the presenting clinical sign was **feather loss without pruritus:**
  1. **Contour feathers** were lost primarily rather than other feather types.
  2. Also described was **increased subcutaneous fat and epidermal atrophy with no evidence of inflammation.**
B. Birds with enlarged thyroid glands may have difficulty swallowing or breathing if the goiter presses on cervical tissue.
C. Less well-documented clinical signs include docile nature, **atherosclerosis, and obesity.**

IV. Diagnosis
A. **Scintigraphy using Tc99m pertechnetate** can detect hypothyroidism, but is not clinically available.
B. Serum total T4 concentrations can be determined, but **a onetime measurement is not diagnostic of a hypothyroid or euthyroid state.** Clinical signs and other findings must also be taken into consideration as well.
C. **Sample must be submitted to a laboratory that can accurately measure avian samples.**
D. Thyroid hormone concentrations are quite a bit lower in birds compared to mammals, and **many diagnostic laboratories cannot measure avian samples** with sufficient accuracy:
  1. **Radioimmunoassay (RIA) for total T4** has been recently developed for psittacine birds and is considered the most accurate measure.
E. As in mammals, the **TSH response test is the best way to document hypothyroidism:**
  1. It is difficult to locate a source of pharmaceutical grade TSH, limiting the usefulness of this test.

Table 27.6 Resting thyroxine values and results of TSH testing in selected species of birds.

	T4 baseline	T4 post TRH	T3 baseline	T3 post TRH
Cockatoos	17.5 (13.6)	45.2 (35.1)	1.88 (1.22)	2.57 (1.67)
Parrots	10.5 (8.19)	35.3 (27.4)	1.94 (1.26)	2.48 (1.61)
Scarlet Macaw	1.7 (1.34)	8.3 (6.46)	1.29 (0.84)	1.06 (0.69)
Blue and Gold Macaw	4.4 (3.41)	15.9 (12.36)	1.16 (0.75)	1.08 (0.70)
African Grey Parrot	1.8 (1.42)	12.0 (9.3)	2.02 (1.31)	2.26 (1.47)
Conure	2.3 (1.76)	17.4 (13.5)	1.29 (0.84)	1.77(1.15)
Cockatiel	15.2 (11.83)	50.2 (39.0)	2.31 (1.45)	2.57 (1.67)

Source: Lothrop CD, Loomis MR, Olsen JH. Thyrotropin stimulation test for evaluation of thyroid function in psittacine birds. *JAVMA* 1985;186:47–48.
All values are in nmol/L. (Conventional values in ng/mL are given in parenthesis); post TRH samples were collected 6 h after administration of TSH.

2. Serum thyroid hormone concentrations before and after thyroid-stimulating hormone administration have been published (Table 27.6).
3. Serum **T3 concentration did not increase significantly after TSH** stimulation.

V. Differential Diagnoses
A. Feather loss is most commonly attributable to **feather plucking** which has a host of causes including behavioral, infectious, and reproductive disorders.
B. Obesity due to **overfeeding and inadequate exercise** is common in cage and aviary birds.
C. Dyspnea or difficulty swallowing may indicate **respiratory or upper alimentary tract disease.**

VI. Treatment
A. Evaluate diet and **ensure adequate iodine. Eliminate potential goitrogens** (Table 27.5).
B. In one report, a scarlet macaw received **0.02 ng thyroxine PO q 12 h for 5 months**, then q 24 h until signs of hypothyroidism resolved.

VII. Prognosis
A. Limited data is available regarding prognosis.

VIII. Prevention
A. Ensure diet provides sufficient iodine and does not contain excessive amounts of goitrogen-containing plants.

Hypothyroidism in Pet Reptiles

Pathogenesis

● A variety of improper management and dietary factors can cause thyroid gland dysfunction.

Classical Signs

● Goiter.
● Anorexia, lethargy, depression, obesity, and stunting may also be present.

Diagnosis

● Careful history of animal husbandry practices and diet to rule out goitrogens or iodine imbalance.
● Low total thyroxine concentrations.

Treatment

- Feed balanced diet.
- Maintain proper thermal gradients and light cycles in the animal's environment.

Table 27.7   Total T4 values in selected species of reptiles.

Species	Total T4
Green iguana	3.81±0.84 (0.3±0.07)
Fence lizard	4.81 – 6.78 (0.37 – 0.53)
Garter snake	0.90 – 1.67 (0.07 – 0.13)
Corn snake	0.45 – 6.06 (0.035 – 0.47)
Ball python	0.93 – 4.79 (0.072 – 0.37)
Red-tailed boa	≤0.24 – 3.98 (≤0.02 – 0.31)
Milk snake	0.27 – 2.94 (0.021 – 0.23)
Desert tortoise	0.35 – 4.0 (0.027 – 0.31)

Source: Rivera S, Lock B. The reptilian thyroid and parathyroid glands.
Vet Clin North Am Exot Anim Pract 2008;11(1):163–176.
All values in nmol/L (Conventional values in µg/dL given in parenthesis).

I.   Pathogenesis
A.   Thyroid hormone maintains **ecdysis, reproduction, tail regeneration, growth, and metabolic rate.**
B.   **Abnormal light cycles, temperature gradients, or hibernation conditions** will affect reptilian thyroid hormone concentrations.
C.   **Goiter** will develop if excess or deficient iodine is fed in the diet:
   1. **Herbivorous reptiles will develop goiter if goitrogenic plants are fed as a significant part** of the diet.
D.   **Over supplementation of iodine interferes with production of thyroxine** resulting in hypothyroidism.

II.   Signalment
A.   Herbivorous reptiles, particularly iguana.
B.   Iguana ingesting cruciferous plants as a large percent of their total diet.

III.   Clinical Signs
A.   **Goiter.**
B.   Hypothyroidism in iguanas leads to **lethargy, weight gain, obesity, decreased rate of growth, and increased docility.** Signs resolve within a couple of weeks after goitrogenic foods are eliminated from the diet.

IV.   Diagnosis
A.   **RIA to measure total T4 is the most sensitive assay.** Blood values for total T4 in a variety of reptilian species is given in Table 27.7.
B.   Circulating thyroid hormone **concentrations in reptiles are lower than in mammalian species** and are **often outside the detectable range of many clinical pathology laboratories.**
C.   **Anatomic location and appearance of the thyroid gland varies greatly among reptilian species,** making detection of thyroid enlargement difficult in some species.

V.   Differential Diagnoses
A.   Lethargy, decreased rate of growth, and increased docility are more often directly attributable to general husbandry-related issues such as inappropriate temperature and light provision, and malnutrition.

Hypothyroidism is rarely diagnosed in reptiles; as such thorough evaluation of patients with nonspecific clinical signs is essential to rule out more common health problems.

B. Weight gain is usually due to overfeeding.

VI. Treatment

A. Feed a balanced **diet appropriate for the reptile species in question.**

B. **Eliminate or greatly reduce the number of goitrogenic foods** offered.

C. **Ensure overall husbandry is appropriate for the affected species.**

VII. Prognosis

A. The prognosis should be good if diet and other husbandry changes are made.

VIII. Prevention

A. Ensure the environment and diet are appropriate for the given species.

B. For herbivorous species, limit the amounts of goitrogenic plants offered.

References and Further Readings

Allen AL, Doige CE, Fretz PB, et al. Hyperplasia of the thyroid gland and concurrent musculoskeletal deformities in western Canadian foals: Reexamination of a previously described syndrome. *Can Vet J* 1994;35:31–38.

Breuhaus BA, Refsel KR, Beyerlein SL. Measurement of free thyroxin concentration in horses by equilibrium dialysis. *J Vet Intern Med* 2006;20:371–376.

Fox JG, Dangler CA, Snyder SB, et al. C-cell carcinoma (medullary thyroid carcinoma) associated with multiple endocrine neoplasms in a ferret (*Mustela putorius*). *Vet Pathol* 2000;37:278–282.

Frank N, Sojka J, Messer NT. Equine thyroid dysfunction. *Vet Clin North Am Equine Pract* 2002;18(2):305–320.

Heard DJ, Collins B, Chen DL, et al. Thyroid and adrenal function tests in adult male ferrets. *Am J Vet Res* 1990;51:32–35.

Lothrop CD, Loomis MR, Olsen JH. Thyrotropin stimulation test for evaluation of thyroid function in psittacine birds. *J Am Vet Med Assoc* 1985;186:47–48.

Oglesbee BL. Hypothyroidism in a scarlet macaw. *J Am Vet Med Assoc* 1992;201:1599–1601.

Rivera S, Lock B. The reptilian thyroid and parathyroid glands. *Vet Clin North Am Exot Anim Pract* 2008;11(1):163–176.

Schmidt RE, Reavill DR. The avian thyroid gland. *Vet Clin North Am Exot Anim Pract* 2008;11(1):15–24.

Schwarz BC, Sallmutter T, Nell B. Keratoconjunctivitis sicca attributable to parasympathetic facial nerve dysfunction associated with hypothyroidism in a horse. *J Am Vet Med Assoc* 2008;233:1761–1766.

Sojka JE. Hypothyroidism in horses. *Compend Contin Educ Vet* 1995;17:845–852.

CHAPTER 28

Hyperthyroidism in Dogs

David Panciera

Pathogenesis

- Hyperthyroidism is caused by excessive thyroid hormone secretion by a functional thyroid tumor, usually a malignant thyroid carcinoma.

Classical Signs

- Older dogs, particularly boxers, beagles, and golden retrievers are affected.
- Weight loss, polyphagia, polydipsia, polyuria, panting, muscle wasting, tachycardia, dyspnea, and a mass in the ventral cervical area are the most common findings.

Diagnosis

- Elevated serum T4 concentration confirms hyperthyroidism, while incisional or excisional biopsy of the cervical mass confirms the diagnosis of thyroid carcinoma.

Treatment

- Surgical excision of the tumor, radioiodine administration, or external beam radiation therapy are effective for control or cure of thyroid carcinoma and control of signs of hyperthyroidism.

I. Pathogenesis
A. Hyperthyroidism is caused by thyroid neoplasia:
   1. **Thyroid carcinoma** is the cause of the **vast majority** of cases of canine hyperthyroidism.
   2. Rare causes of canine hyperthyroidism include benign adenoma and struma cordis (ectopic thyroid tissue in the heart).
   3. Tumor **location ranges from the base of the heart to the base of the tongue.**
   4. **Only 10–20% of thyroid carcinomas result in hyperthyroidism,** while the remainder are nonfunctional.
   5. The cause of thyroid neoplasia in the dog is not known.

Clinical Endocrinology of Companion Animals, First Edition. Edited by Jacquie Rand.
© 2013 John Wiley & Sons, Inc. Published 2013 by John Wiley & Sons, Inc.

II. Signalment

A. The **median age** at diagnosis of dogs with thyroid tumors is **9–10 years**.

B. **Boxer, beagle, and golden retrievers are predisposed** to develop thyroid tumors.

C. There is **no gender predilection**.

III. Clinical Signs

A. Clinical signs of thyroid neoplasia **result from either thyroid hormone excess, local effects of the tumor, or metastasis.**

B. **Signs of hyperthyroidism** are similar to those in cats:

  1. The **most common historical complaints** present in **>50% of cases** include:

    a. **Weight loss despite normal or increased food intake** caused by increased metabolic rate.

    b. **Polyuria and polydipsia** due largely to increased cardiac output and renal blood flow.

    c. **Increased activity or restlessness and panting.**

  2. May cause tachycardia, cardiac arrhythmias, hypertension, thin body condition, muscle wasting, and panting.

C. **The mass** is frequently found by the owner, and **can result in dysphagia, dyspnea or cough, and dysphonia** due to compression or invasion of the esophagus, trachea, or recurrent laryngeal nerve, respectively.

D. **Regional lymph node enlargement**, including nodes both cranial and caudal to the mass, may be present in dogs **with metastasis**.

E. The **most common physical examination finding is a palpable ventral cervical mass**, present in **over 75% of cases**, regardless of the functional nature of the tumor:

  1. **It can be difficult to determine if the tumor is unilateral or bilateral** in many cases.

  2. Small thyroid masses **may require careful, deep palpation of the entire ventral cervical area** for detection.

F. Thyroid **tumors infrequently occur at the base of the tongue, in the cranial mediastinum or at the heart base** with a resultant oral mass, pleural effusion, or edema of the head and front limbs, respectively.

IV. Diagnosis

A. **Clinicopathologic findings:**

  1. **Routine complete blood count, serum chemistries, and urinalysis** are usually normal.

  2. **Elevated liver enzyme activity and azotemia are occasionally present** in dogs with thyroid carcinoma independent of the functional status of the thyroid tumor and are **not related to hyperthyroidism or the presence of metastasis to the liver or kidneys.**

B. **Hyperthyroidism is confirmed by finding an elevated serum total T4 concentration in a dog** with appropriate clinical signs and a mass consistent with thyroid neoplasia.

C. **Diagnosis of a thyroid neoplasm is determined by biopsy:**

  1. **Fine needle aspirate** is an effective method of confirming that the thyroid gland is the origin of the mass, but it is difficult in most cases to determine if the tumor is benign or malignant:

    a. Hemodilution of aspiration samples sometimes results in nondiagnostic cytology.

    b. **If the sample is contaminated with a large amount of blood,** preparing the smear using a technique similar to a complete blood count might result in **identification of malignant cells at the feathered edge of the smear.**

    c. **Significant hemorrhage can occur** after fine needle aspiration.

  2. **Surgical incisional biopsy to obtain a wedge of tissue is recommended** because surgery allows the best chance to control the potential severe hemorrhage due to biopsy.

  3. **Percutaneous needle core biopsy is *not* recommended** because of the risk of hemorrhage.

D. **Staging of thyroid carcinoma is important** because metastasis is present at diagnosis in 35–40% of dogs and develops in up to 80% eventually:

  1. The **lungs are most commonly affected and metastatic lesions are often small, indistinct, and numerous** rather than the more typical metastatic pattern.

  2. **Lymph node metastasis** is also common.

  3. Staging to detect metastasis should **include fine needle aspiration of retropharyngeal, submandibular and cervical lymph nodes, and thoracic radiographs.**

E.   **Cervical radiographs** may allow documentation of a mass and displacement of surrounding structures, but are rarely necessary.

F.   **Ultrasound examination of the tumor and neck** is useful in determining if the mass is unilateral or bilateral and extent of invasion of surrounding tissue (important prognostic indicators). Ultrasound may also be useful in **guiding fine needle aspirates** in an attempt to minimize hemorrhage.

G.   **Thyroid scintigraphy** with ^{99m}technetium pertechnetate may be useful in detecting ectopic tissue or metastasis to lymph nodes, but is not necessary in most cases. Thoracic radiographs may be more sensitive than scintigraphy for detection of pulmonary metastasis, although scintigraphy can rarely identify metastasis not visible on thoracic radiographs.

H.   Cardiac arrhythmias and hypertension may be present, so an **ECG and measurement of systemic arterial blood pressure** should be considered.

V.   Differential Diagnoses

A.   Possible causes of a **ventral cervical mass** other than thyroid neoplasia include abscess, salivary mucocele, sialadenitis, foreign body, or granuloma. Nonthyroid neoplasia in the soft tissues of the neck (e.g., lymphoma, salivary neoplasia, rhabdomyosarcoma, and leiomyosarcoma) or metastasis to lymph nodes from tumors of the head and neck are other causes.

B.   **Weight loss and polyphagia** could be caused by diabetes mellitus, maldigestion, or malabsorption.

C.   The causes of **polyuria and polydipsia** are numerous (see Chapter 42), but diabetes mellitus should be considered along with hyperthyroidism given the other signs that are usually present.

VI.   Treatment

A.   Treatment **largely targets management of the malignancy,** often without specific treatment of the hyperthyroidism.

B.   **Treatment of the thyroid hormone excess** can be accomplished in some dogs by administration of methimazole or propylthiouracil:

    1.   While **efficacy and dosages have not been well established** in dogs, **methimazole** should be initiated at 5–10 mg q 12 h and dosage adjusted based on clinical response and serum T4 concentration after 2–4 weeks of treatment.

    2.   If methimazole is not effective, **propylthiouracil** (3 mg/kg q 8 h) can be used with similar monitoring.

C.   **Sinus tachycardia and other cardiac arrhythmias** may be managed by administration of **a β-adrenergic antagonist** such as atenolol or propranolol.

D.   **Hypertension** is usually most effectively treated with an angiotensin-converting enzyme inhibitor such as enalapril or benazepril.

E.   Surgical excision of the neoplasm:

    1.   Treatment of choice when the tumor is not deeply attached (mobile on palpation) and is unilateral.

    2.   **Complications:**

        a.   Because of the vascular nature of thyroid carcinomas, **hemorrhage can be severe** and is the most common complication.

        b.   **Hypoparathyroidism** can occur as a consequence of parathyroidectomy if bilateral thyroidectomy is attempted.

        c.   Damage to the recurrent laryngeal nerve or vagosympathetic trunk can result in **laryngeal paralysis or megaesophagus.**

        d.   General anesthesia may exacerbate **cardiac arrhythmias** due to hyperthyroidism.

F.   Radioactive iodine (^{131}I):

    1.   **Highly effective in treatment of hyperthyroidism** and results in resolution of the hyperthyroidism within 2 weeks of administration.

    2.   A very **high dose of** ^{131}I **must be administered,** so time in isolation is much longer posttreatment and availability of treatment is much more limited than that for hyperthyroidism in cats.

    3.   **Fatal myelosuppression** has been reported in a few dogs treated with radioiodine for thyroid cancer.

    4.   The **optimal dosage of radioiodine has not been determined.**

    5.   **May be useful to downsize tumor** prior to surgery or as an adjunct following incomplete surgical resection.

G. **External beam radiation therapy** is effective:
   1. Should be **considered particularly in dogs with invasive thyroid carcinomas.**
   2. The reduction in tumor size may occur slowly, with a maximum effect requiring several months to over 1 year.
H. **Chemotherapy:**
   1. Should be considered in cases where **distant metastasis** is present and **possibly following surgery or radiation therapy if the tumor has characteristics that indicate a high risk for metastasis** (large size, bilateral, and vascular invasion) or **when resection is incomplete.**
   2. Has **limited efficacy** in treatment of thyroid carcinoma in dogs, **although little investigation into this treatment modality has been undertaken.**
   3. Treatment with **doxorubicin or cisplatin** has resulted in a response in approximately 40–50% of cases, but survival has been much shorter than with other treatment modalities.
I. **Hypothyroidism** can be a complication of most of the treatments, so levothyroxine supplementation should be instituted if clinical signs and thyroid function tests confirm its presence.

VII. Prognosis
A. **Smaller and freely moveable tumors carry a better prognosis** than those that are fixed to surrounding tissue or larger. The **incidence of metastasis is increased when the tumor diameter exceeds 5 cm or when both lobes of the thyroid gland are affected.**
B. **Without treatment,** median survival of dogs with thyroid carcinoma has been reported to be 3 months, but dogs with slow-growing carcinomas may live over one year.
C. Dogs with **mobile thyroid carcinomas treated by surgical excision** have a median survival time of over 3 years.
D. Dogs treated with **radioiodine** have a median survival of 27–30 months, although dogs with metastatic disease have a shorter survival (12–19 months).
E. **External beam radiation therapy** of dogs with fixed, invasive carcinomas results in median survival of 2–4 years or longer; even dogs with extensive metastasis can have prolonged survival.

VIII. Prevention
No known prevention.

References and Further Readings

Feldman EC, Nelson RW. Canine thyroid tumors and hyperthyroidism. In: Feldman EC, Nelson RW, eds. *Canine and Feline Endocrinology and Reproduction*, 3rd edn. Philadelphia: Saunders, 2004, pp. 219–249.
Liptak JM. Canine thyroid carcinoma. *Clin Tech Small Anim Pract* 2007;22:75–81.
Theon AP, Marks SL, Feldman ES, Griffey S. Prognostic factors and patterns of treatment failure in dogs with unresectable differentiated thyroid carcinomas treated with megavoltage irradiation. *J Am Vet Med Assoc* 2000;216:1775–1779.
Worth AJ, Zuber RM, Hockin M. Radioiodide (^{131}I) therapy for the treatment of canine thyroid carcinoma. *Aust Vet J* 2005;83:208–214.

CHAPTER 29

Hyperthyroidism in Cats

Mark E. Peterson

Pathogenesis

- Hyperthyroidism occurs as a result of an increase in the circulating concentrations of the thyroid hormones, thyroxine (T_4), and triiodothyronine (T_3).
- Benign thyroid adenoma (adenomatous hyperplasia) affecting one (30%) or both lobes (70%) of the thyroid gland is the most common cause.

Classical Signs

- Most cats are >10 years of age, with a median age of 13 years.
- Weight loss despite an increased appetite.
- Hyperactivity and vomiting common.
- Palpable thyroid nodule in most cats.

Diagnosis

- High serum concentrations of total T_4 confirms diagnosis in most cats.

Treatment

- Antithyroid drugs (methimazole, carbimazole).
- Surgical thyroidectomy.
- Radioactive iodine (radioiodine; ^{131}I).
- Nutritional therapy (low-iodine diet).

I. Pathogenesis

A. **Hyperthyroidism (thyrotoxicosis)** is a multisystemic disorder resulting from excessive circulating concentrations of the active thyroid hormones T_3 and T_4.

B. Benign **adenomatous hyperplasia (adenoma)** of one (30%) or both (70%) thyroid lobes is the most common pathological abnormality associated with hyperthyroidism in cats, occurring in 96–98% of cases.

C. **Thyroid carcinoma** is a rare cause of hyperthyroidism in cats, accounting for approximately 2–4% of cats.

Clinical Endocrinology of Companion Animals, First Edition. Edited by Jacquie Rand.
© 2013 John Wiley & Sons, Inc. Published 2013 by John Wiley & Sons, Inc.

D. To date, the **underlying etiology** responsible for the thyroid changes remains obscure and is probably multifactorial. However, studies have indicated numerous environmental and nutritional factors, which may play a role in the pathogenesis of this disorder.

E. Possible **risk factors:**

1. Diet composed entirely or primarily of canned cat food.
2. Certain varieties of canned cat food (fish, liver, or giblet flavor).
3. Cans with plastic linings and pop-top lids may pose a greater risk than sachets or cans which require a can opener to open them. This is potentially due to the release of chemicals such as bisphenol-A and bisphenol-F from the lacquer linings of the pop-top cans.
4. Diets containing either excess *or* deficient amounts of iodine have been implicated.
5. Regular use of insecticidal products (flea products) on the cat or fly sprays within the household.
6. Exposure to herbicides and fertilizers.
7. Exposure to flame-retardant chemical contaminants including polybrominated diphenyl ethers (PBDEs). Excessive PBDEs have been identified in household dust from contaminated carpet padding, polyurethane foams, furniture, and mattresses.

II. Signalment

A. Hyperthyroidism most commonly occurs in middle-aged to older cats with a median **age** of 12–13 years.

B. Only 5% of hyperthyroid cats are <10 years of age.

C. There is no obvious **breed** susceptibility. Two genetically related breeds (Siamese and Himalayan [Colourpoint Persian]) and purebred cats have been reported to be at *decreased* risk of developing hyperthyroidism.

D. Male and female cats are affected equally.

III. Clinical Signs

A. The typical historical findings and clinical signs of hyperthyroidism are listed in Table 29.1.

B. **Weight loss** is the most commonly recognized sign of hyperthyroidism in cats. Hyperthyroidism is so common that it should always be considered in cats that have lost weight, whether supporting signs such as tachycardia are present or not.

C. The weight loss seen in cats with hyperthyroidism is often associated with an **increased appetite.** However, some cats maintain a normal appetite or even develop a reduced appetite.

D. **Hyperactivity,** exhibited particularly as **nervousness, restlessness, and aggressive behavior,** may be apparent in some hyperthyroid cats. These signs may be more obvious when attempts are made to restrain the cat and are therefore often more noticeable to veterinarians than to owners themselves.

E. **Anxiety and restlessness** can be obvious to owners if the cat yowls. **Aimless pacing** and easily **interrupted sleep** patterns have been described and this presumably reflects a state of confusion, anxiety, and nervousness.

F. Skin changes that often develop in hyperthyroid cats include a **dull or matted hair coat.** Some hyperthyroid cats can groom obsessively resulting in **alopecia** and even **miliary dermatitis.**

G. **Gastrointestinal signs** including vomiting or diarrhea are not uncommon in cats with hyperthyroidism:

1. **Vomiting** may be associated with rapid overeating; **diarrhea** is most likely due to intestinal hypermotility although malabsorption is also a factor.

H. **Polyuria and polydipsia (PU/PD)** occur in about half of hyperthyroid cats, but PU/PD can be marked in some cats:

1. Various mechanisms may be responsible, including concurrent primary renal dysfunction, renal medullary washout because of increased renal blood flow, and primary polydipsia because of a hypothalamic disturbance.

I. **Heart murmur and other cardiac signs** are common and frequently the most significant findings on initial physical examination:

1. **Tachycardia** (rate >240 beats per minute) is found in about half the hyperthyroid cats.
2. A powerful apex beat and systolic murmurs are also commonly encountered. Such murmurs are frequently associated with dynamic right and left ventricular outflow obstruction rather than primary mitral or tricuspid regurgitation. Hyperthyroidism is probably the single most important factor for the development of murmurs in older cats.

Table 29.1   Clinical findings in cats with hyperthyroidism.

Finding	Percentage of cats
Historic owner complaints	
Weight loss	85–95%
Polyphagia	60–75%
Polyuria/polydipsia	45–60%
Increased activity, anxiety	30–55%
Vomiting	30–45%
Dyspnea, tachypnea, or panting	20–35%
Diarrhea	15–20%
Large fecal volume	10–20%
Decreased appetite	5–10%
Decreased activity	5–10%
Weakness	5–10%
Physical examination findings	
Large thyroid gland	80–95%
Thin (low body condition score)	60–70%
Hyperkinesis	50–65%
Tachycardia	50–60%
Heart murmur	35–55%
Unkempt hair coat, matting, alopecia	15–30%
Gallop rhythm	15–25%
Aggressive	10–15%
Hypertension	10–15%
Increased nail growth	5–10%
Congestive heart failure	1–2%

3. Gallop rhythms attributed to rapid ventricular filling can also occur.

4. Occasionally **arrhythmias** are found, particularly **ectopic atrial and ventricular arrhythmias**.

J.   Mild to moderate **hypertension** was previously considered important in hyperthyroid cats. However, these cats are typically only mildly hypertensive and, when present, may simply reflect the reduced tolerance of hyperthyroid cats to stressful situations such as the veterinary examination ("white-coat" phenomenon).

K.   **Palpable goiter** is present in most, if not all, cats with hyperthyroidism. Thyroid lobes are not normally palpable. In hyperthyroid cats, either **unilateral or bilateral thyroid enlargement** (goiter) is invariably present since all hyperthyroid cats have either adenomas or carcinomas as the underlying cause of the disease:

1. There are two general techniques used to palpate the thyroid gland in cats:

a. With the **classic palpation technique**: the cat is restrained in sitting position and the front legs held still. The neck of the cat is extended, and the clinicians' thumb and index finger are placed on each side of the trachea and swept downwards from the larynx to the sternal manubrium. Palpation of a mobile subcutaneous nodule or a "blip" that slips under the fingertips determines the presence of a goiter.

Table 29.2 Common hematological and biochemical abnormalities associated with hyperthyroidism in cats.

Percentage of cats	
Complete blood count	
Erythrocytosis	30–55%
Anemia	1–5%
Lymphopenia	15–40%
Eosinopenia	15–35%
Leukocytosis	15–20%
Serum chemistry profile	
High alanine aminotransferase (ALT)	80–90%
High alkaline phosphatase (ALP)	60–75%
High aspartate aminotransferase (AST)	30–45%
Azotemia	20–25%
Hyperglycemia	15–20%
Hyperphosphatemia	10–20%
Hyperbilirubinemia	3–4%
Complete urinalysis	
Specific gravity >1.040	40–60%
Specific gravity <1.015	3–6%
Proteinuria (high protein:creatinine>0.4)	30–70%

  b. With the alternative **Norsworthy technique,** the clinician is positioned directly behind the standing cat. The head of the cat is raised and turned (45°) alternatively to the right or left, away from the side that is assessed (i.e., to palpate the right thyroid lobe, turn the cat's head to the left). The tip of the clinician's index finger is placed in the groove formed by the trachea and sternothyroid muscle just below the larynx and then moved downwards in the groove to the thoracic inlet). If the thyroid lobe is enlarged, a characteristic "blip" is felt as the index finger passes the goiter.
L. Rarely cats develop **apathetic hyperthyroidism** and present with **apathy, depression, weakness, and anorexia:**
  1. Although weight loss is present in these cats, it is accompanied by anorexia, instead of increased appetite. Most cats with apathetic hyperthyroidism have **concurrent severe nonthyroidal illness** such as renal failure, cardiac disease, or neoplasia.

IV. Diagnosis
A. A variety of procedures, including a **complete blood count, serum chemistry analysis,** and **complete urinalysis,** are recommended in the workup of all cats with suspected hyperthyroidism (Table 29.2). Often this database simply lends support to the diagnosis, but these screening tests are most useful if concurrent disorders are present and an accurate prognosis is required. Specific **thyroid function tests,** especially a **total serum T_4 determination,** are necessary to confirm a diagnosis.
B. **Hematological findings** are usually nonspecific and mostly not clinically important (Table 29.1). **Anemia,** when present, is almost never caused by the hyperthyroid state and a search for another cause should be undertaken.
C. **Serum biochemistry abnormalities** are common in cats with hyperthyroidism (Table 29.1):
  1. **Mild to marked increases in the serum activities of many liver enzymes,** including **alanine aminotransferase (ALT)** and **alkaline phosphatase (ALP)** are the most common and striking biochemical abnormalities

of feline hyperthyroidism. These liver enzymes changes and T_4 concentrations are related, with liver enzyme abnormalities being more common in cats with severe hyperthyroidism. These high liver enzymes return to normal upon successful treatment of hyperthyroidism.

2. Before treatment, mild to moderate **increases in serum concentrations of urea and creatinine** may be found in just over 20% of hyperthyroid cats. Such a prevalence of concurrent renal dysfunction or **chronic kidney disease (CKD)** is not unexpected in a group of older or aged cats:

    a. These abnormalities, particularly the high urea concentration, may be exacerbated by the increased protein intake and protein catabolism of hyperthyroidism.

    b. On the other hand, in hyperthyroid cats **without concurrent CKD or azotemia, circulating creatinine concentrations are lowered,** which may be related in part to a loss of muscle mass.

    c. However, this lowering of serum creatinine (and urea in some cats) is primarily the result of the increase in glomerular filtration rate (GFR) that occurs in hyperthyroid cats. These effects have implications in assessing the presence of primary renal dysfunction in hyperthyroid cats (see below).

D. **Urinalysis** is generally unremarkable but is useful in differentiating other diseases with similar clinical signs such as diabetes mellitus:

    1. The **urine-specific gravity** is variable, but concurrent (masked) renal disease should be considered in all cats that have values <1.040. Cats with concurrent CKD can occasionally have values >1.040 but most cats have less concentrated urine.

    2. Mild **proteinuria** is commonly observed and may reflect glomerular hypertension and hyperfiltration or differences in tubular handling of protein. Proteinuria found on routine urinalysis should be confirmed by measuring the **urine protein:creatinine (UPC) ratio:**

        a. Normal cats have a UPC ratio of <0.2, where many hyperthyroid cats have borderline high (0.2–0.4) or overt proteinuria (>0.4).

        b. Such proteinuria resolves upon successful treatment of hyperthyroidism.

E. On **thoracic radiography,** mild to severe cardiac enlargement is evident in about half of hyperthyroid cats:

    1. In the vast majority of cats, this **cardiomegaly** is reversible with correction of the hyperthyroid state.

    2. With severe hyperthyroidism, cats may develop congestive heart failure, as evidenced by **pleural effusion and pulmonary edema** on thoracic radiography.

F. The most common **echocardiographic findings** in hyperthyroid cats include left ventricular hypertrophy, left atrial and ventricular dilation, and interventricular septum hypertrophy:

    1. However, most of these changes are subtle and are of little clinical relevance.

    2. Increased fractional shortening (reflecting increased cardiac contractility) is common and invariably normalizes upon successful treatment of the hyperthyroidism.

G. **Confirming the diagnosis of hyperthyroidism** requires use of one of more **thyroid function tests** to demonstrate increased production of circulating thyroid hormones, suppressed pituitary thyroid-stimulating hormone (TSH) secretion, or increased thyroidal radioisotope uptake:

    1. **Elevated circulating thyroid hormone concentrations** (T_4 and T_3) are the biochemical hallmarks of hyperthyroidism and are extremely specific for its diagnosis with very few false positive results reported. Methods for their measurement are readily accessible, relatively cheap, and do not involve specific sampling requirements:

        a. Serum total T_4 is preferable as a screening test for hyperthyroidism with a test sensitivity of over 90% (Figure 29.1). However, approximately 10% of all hyperthyroid cats have serum total T_4 concentration within the reference range limits. Such T_4 values are usually within the mid to high end of the reference range. Thus, while a high total T_4 value is indicative of hyperthyroidism, finding a single reference range T_4 value does not preclude such a diagnosis:

            1) In early or mildly affected cases, **serum total T_4 concentrations can fluctuate** in and out of the reference range. Such fluctuation occurs in all hyperthyroid cats but the degree of fluctuation is of little diagnostic significance in cats with markedly elevated T_4 concentrations.

            2) **Severe nonthyroidal illness** is capable of **suppressing serum total T_4 concentrations** to below the reference range in euthyroid cats. Similarly, marginally elevated serum total T_4 concentrations may be suppressed to the mid to high end of the reference range in cats with mild hyperthyroidism and concurrent moderate to severe nonthyroidal disease.

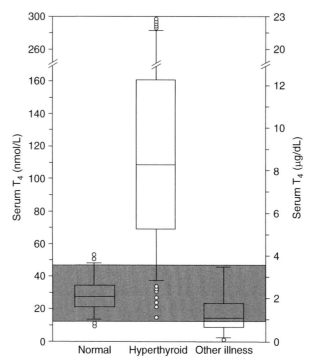

Figure 29.1 Box plots of the serum concentrations of total T_4 concentrations tests in 172 clinically normal cats, 917 cats with untreated hyperthyroidism, and 221 cats with nonthyroidal disease. For each box plot, the T-bars represent the main body of data, which in most instances is equal to the range. The box represents the interquartile range (i.e., the 25th percentile to 75th percentile range or the middle half of the data). The horizontal bar in the box is the median. Outlying data points are represented by open circles. The shaded area indicates the reference interval, which was established by use of the nonparametric method of percentile estimates with confidence intervals to determine the 2.5th percentile to 97.5th percentile range for results from the clinically normal cats (From Peterson ME, Melian C, Nichols R. Measurement of serum concentrations of free thyroxine, total thyroxine, and total triiodothyronine in cats with hyperthyroidism and cats with nonthyroidal disease. *J Am Vet Med Assoc* 2001;218:529–336, with permission).

3) In early or mildly hyperthyroid cats (with no concurrent illnesses), **serum total T_4** concentrations will **eventually increase** into the diagnostic thyrotoxic range upon retesting a few weeks later.

4) Concurrent hyperthyroidism should always be suspected in severely ill cats with mid to high reference range serum total T_4 concentrations.

5) Alternatively, other diagnostic tests may provide a means of diagnosing hyperthyroidism in these cats (see below).

b. **Serum total T_3** is less useful than T_4 as a diagnostic test, since over 30% of hyperthyroid cats have normal circulating T_3 concentration. The majority of hyperthyroid cats with normal T_3 concentrations are early or mildly affected. Measurement of total T_3 is **not recommended** for investigation of hyperthyroidism in cats.

c. Determination of **serum free T_4** concentrations, as measured by equilibrium dialysis, is a **more sensitive diagnostic test** than total T_4 in cats with hyperthyroidism (Figure 29.2):

1) Up to 98% of hyperthyroid cats will have a high free T_4 value, compared to 90% of cats with high total T_4 values.

2) Free T_4 cannot, however, be used as a routine screening test since **nonthyroidal disease can cause falsely high free T_4 values** in up to 12% of nonhyperthyroid cats (Figure 29.2). These cats generally have corresponding total T_4 values in the lower half or below the reference range.

3) Caution is therefore advised in using serum-free T_4 measurements by equilibrium dialysis as the sole diagnostic test for hyperthyroidism. It is more reliable if interpreted with a corresponding total T_4 value. High-normal total and free T_4 concentrations are consistent with hyperthyroidism, whereas a low total T_4 together with a high free T_4 is usually associated with nonthyroidal illness.

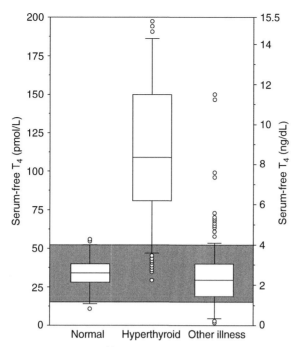

Figure 29.2 Box plots of the serum concentrations of free T_4 concentrations tests in 172 clinically normal cats, 917 cats with untreated hyperthyroidism, and 221 cats with nonthyroidal disease. See Figure 29.1 for key (From Peterson ME, Melian C, Nichols R. Measurement of serum concentrations of free thyroxine, total thyroxine, and total triiodothyronine in cats with hyperthyroidism and cats with nonthyroidal disease. *J Am Vet Med Assoc* 2001;218:529–336, with permission).

2. In human patients, measurement of circulating **TSH** concentration is usually used as a first-line discriminatory test of thyroid function:

   a. A species-specific feline TSH assay has not yet been developed; however, assays for measuring canine TSH (cTSH) are widely available, and it has been suggested that TSH measurement using this test may provide some diagnostic information in cats with suspected hyperthyroidism.

   b. Theoretically, as in people, it could be expected that **TSH levels should be low** in early stages of hyperthyroidism before the T_4 is elevated.

   c. **Caution is advised in interpreting TSH values in cats.** The current canine assays only detect approximately 35% of recombinant feline TSH, making it difficult to distinguish normal values from the suppressed values expected in cats with hyperthyroidism.

   d. Perhaps the only use for such TSH measurement would be to exclude hyperthyroidism, that is, finding a normal rather than suppressed cTSH value.

3. With **thyroid imaging (scintigraphy)**, hyperthyroid cats usually exhibit **increased thyroidal uptake of radioisotope**: radioactive iodine (^{123}I or ^{131}I) or technetium-99 M as pertechnetate (^{99m}TcO$_4^-$):

   a. Percentage uptake or increased **thyroid:salivary ratio** may be calculated and both are strongly correlated with circulating thyroid hormone concentration and provide a sensitive means of diagnosing hyperthyroidism (Figures 29.3–29.5).

   b. Thyroid imaging may be useful in assessment of thyroid involvement prior to surgical thyroidectomy.

   c. However, apart from expense and the difficulties in dealing with radioisotopes, few veterinarians have access to the nuclear medicine equipment needed to obtain thyroid images or perform thyroid uptake determinations.

4. In cats with suspected hyperthyroidism but normal serum T_4 concentrations, **dynamic thyroid function testing** (e.g., **T_4 suppression test** or the **TRH stimulation test**) can be used to help in diagnosis. However, in the majority of hyperthyroid cats found to have a normal T_4 concentration, identification of

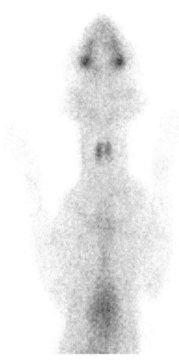

Figure 29.3 Normal thyroid image (scintigraphy) performed using 99 m-TcO4⁻ in a 16-year-old neutered male DSH cat with a history of weight loss and chronic gastrointestinal symptoms. The serum T₄ within the reference range, but the free T₄ was high. This study was performed to investigate the potential for early hyperthyroidism but was interpreted as normal. Note the bilateral symmetry of the thyroid lobes as well as the normal size and normal thyroid:salivary uptake ratio of <1.0. This cat was subsequently diagnosed with alimentary lymphosarcoma based on endoscopically acquired intestinal biopsies.

concurrent disease, repeat total T_4 values, or simultaneous measurement of free T_4 concentrations allows confirmation of the diagnosis. Further diagnostic tests are rarely required:

    a. Protocols and interpretive advice for these tests are outlined in Table 29.3.

    b. Nowadays such dynamic tests should only be considered in cats with clinical signs suggestive of hyperthyroidism when repeated total T4 concentration remains within reference range or free T4 analysis and thyroid imaging is unavailable or diagnostically unhelpful.

V. Differential Diagnoses

A. Because the clinical signs of hyperthyroidism in cats can be so variable and generally affect many body systems, a number of differential diagnoses must be considered in cats having a possible diagnosis of hyperthyroidism. These diseases include **diabetes mellitus, CKD, hepatic disease, gastrointestinal disease, and neoplasia.**

B. Similarly, because heart murmurs and cardiomegaly are so common in hyperthyroid cats, **primary cardiac disease** (cardiomyopathy) must also be considered, as should cardiac disease secondary of other conditions, for example, hypertension, acromegaly, etc.

C. Finally, **anxiety-related misbehavior** must also be included in the differential list.

VI. Treatment

A. General principles:

    1. Hyperthyroidism can be treated in four ways: **medical management** with methimazole or carbimazole, **surgical thyroidectomy, radioactive iodine (¹³¹I) and nutritional therapy.**

    2. Each form of treatment has advantages and disadvantages that should be considered when formulating a treatment plan for the individual hyperthyroid cat.

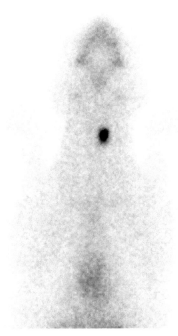

Figure 29.4 Thyroid scintigraphy performed using 99 m-TcO4⁻ on a 9-year-old spayed female DLH cat with a history of weight loss, recent onset of gastrointestinal symptoms, polydipsia, and polyuria. This cat's T$_4$ was within the reference range and the free T$_4$ was elevated. This patient has a small unilateral, left-sided thyroid adenoma. Note the increased radionuclide uptake (thyroid:salivary uptake ratio >1.0) in a mildly enlarged left thyroid lobe combined with the absence of visualization of the right thyroid lobe secondary to feedback suppression.

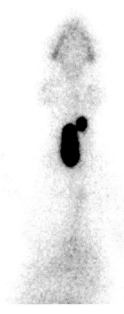

Figure 29.5 Thyroid scintigraphy performed on a 14-year-old spayed female DLH cat with a history of weight loss and increased appetite and elevated T$_4$ level. Note the bilateral asymmetric increase in radionuclide uptake in both enlarged thyroid lobes.

Table 29.3 Commonly used protocols for dynamic function tests for the diagnosis of hyperthyroidism in cats.

	T_3 suppression	TRH stimulation	TSH stimulation	
Drug	Liothyronine (Cytomel)	TRH	Bovine TSH	Human TSH
Dose	25 µg 8 hourly for 7 doses	0.1 mg/kg	0.5 IU/kg	0.025–0.20 mg/cat
Route	Oral	Intravenous	Intravenous	Intravenous
Sampling times	0 and 2–4 h after last dose	0 and 4 h	0 and 6 h	1 and 6–8 h
Assay	Total T_4 Total T_3	Total T_4	Total T_4	Total T_4
Interpretation				
Euthyroidism	>50% suppression	>60% increase	>100% increase	>100% increase
Hyperthyroidism	<35% suppression	<50% increase	Minimal/no increase	Not determined

T_4, thyroxine; T_3, triiodothyronine; TRH, thyrotropin-releasing hormone; TSH, thyroid-stimulating hormone.

3. Medical management and nutritional therapy are considered "reversible," whereas surgical thyroidectomy and ^{131}I are "permanent" treatments.

4. The major advantages and disadvantages of the main forms of therapy are outlined in **Table 29.4.**

B. **Treatment considerations:**

1. **Concurrent conditions (nonthyroidal disorders):**

a. **CKD** is very common in older cats so it is not surprising that CKD is commonly found concurrent with hyperthyroidism. The increased GFR and reduced muscle mass induced by hyperthyroidism can mask underlying CKD:

1) Because it is not always possible to predict which hyperthyroid cats have underlying CKD, a **treatment trial with methimazole, carbimazole** or, possibly, nutritional therapy should be considered in all cats in which CKD is suspected.

2) Immediate **permanent therapy** (^{131}I **or surgical thyroidectomy**) without a methimazole/carbimazole trial is only appropriate for relatively young cats with completely normal serum urea and creatinine concentration, and urine specific gravity of >1.040.

3) The **serum T_4 and renal parameters should be rechecked after 30 days methimazole/carbimazole administration.** If renal parameters remain normal after euthyroidism is restored, it is safe to proceed with **permanent therapy such as thyroidectomy or radioactive iodine.**

4) Mild to moderate kidney disease should not preclude permanent treatment of hyperthyroidism. Recent research provides evidence that **hyperthyroidism may contribute to the development or progression of CKD** in cats, suggesting that leaving a hyperthyroid cat untreated (or poorly regulated with methimazole) may be detrimental to long-term kidney function. Treating and curing hyperthyroidism may help to both reverse renal damage and preserve the remaining kidney function.

b. **Cardiac disease** associated with hyperthyroidism is mild and reversible in most cats with hyperthyroidism. Murmurs and tachycardia are common but often do not result in clinical signs. On the occasions when cats show more severe cardiac changes such as **congestive heart failure** or **aortic thromboembolism,** these should be stabilized before a cat undergoes thyroidectomy or radioiodine therapy.

c. Mild to moderate **hypertension** develops in approximately 10–15% of untreated hyperthyroid cats and is generally reversible upon induction of euthyroidism. Conversely, some cats are normotensive when hyperthyroidism is diagnosed but may become hypertensive after becoming euthyroid. Most of these cats, however, have some degree of **concurrent renal disease.** If hypertension is severe or persists after treatment of hyperthyroidism, these cats should be managed with **amlodipine.**

d. **Hepatic disease** is often suspected in cats with untreated hyperthyroidism because of their **high liver enzymes (serum ALT and ALP).** At the time of diagnosis, it is not always possible to know if increased liver enzymes are due to hepatic disease unrelated to hyperthyroidism or merely a

Table 29.4   Advantages and disadvantages of treatment modalities for cats with hyperthyroidism.

	Methimazole or carbimazole	Surgery	Radioiodine
Availability of treatment	Readily available	Skilled surgeon needed	Radiation license needed
Ease of treatment	Intermediate	Most difficult	Simple
Hospitalization time	None	1–7 days	1–4 weeks
Anesthesia required	No	Yes	No
Time until euthyroid	1–3 weeks	1–2 days	1–12 weeks
Persistent hyperthyroidism	Low (Dose-related)	Rare (usually ectopic tissue)	Low (Dose-related)
Reversible or permanent	Reversible	Permanent	Permanent
Cures disease	No (tumor continues to grow)	Yes	Yes
Relapse/ recurrence	High	Intermediate	Low
Lifelong medication	Yes	No	No
Cost	Variable (inexpensive in short-term)	Intermediate to high	Generally highest
Complications			
Hypoparathyroidism	Never	Common	Never
Permanent hypothyroidism	Never	Intermediate	Rare (Dose-related)
Anorexia, vomiting	Common	Rare	Never
Hematologic effects	Rare (thrombocytopenia, agranulocytosis, serum ANA)	Never	Rare (Only with very high doses)
Neurologic Damage	Never	Rare (vocal cord paralysis, Horner's syndrome)	Never

manifestation of hyperthyroidism. If underlying primary liver disease is expected, especially if the cat is showing signs of **apathetic hyperthyroidism** (e.g., anorexia, depression, etc.), a **treatment trial with methimazole or carbimazole** should be considered.

    e. Client circumstances such as cost of therapy is a major consideration in many instances. Medical therapy costs far less initially. However, the cost of ongoing monitoring can exceed that of thyroidectomy or ^{131}I therapy over a period of many months to years.

C. **Medical therapy:**

    1. Chronic management with antithyroid drugs is a practical treatment option for many cats. Medical management requires **no special facilities** and is readily available. **Anesthesia is avoided,** as are the surgical complications associated with thyroidectomy (Table 29.4).

    2. However, medical management has many disadvantages. This form of treatment is **not curative,** is highly **dependent on owner and cat compliance** and requires **regular biochemical monitoring** to ensure the efficacy of treatment. Most importantly, the thyroid tumor continues to grow and, after many months, may **transform from adenoma to thyroid carcinoma** in some cats.

    3. Long-term medical management is best reserved for cats of advanced age or for those with concurrent diseases, and for when owners refuse either surgery or radioactive iodine.

    4. In addition to long-term treatment, medical management is also necessary **prior to surgical thyroidectomy** to decrease the metabolic and cardiac complications associated with hyperthyroidism. Short-term medical management is often recommended as **trial therapy prior to** ^{131}**I therapy** to determine the effect of restoring euthyroidism on renal function.

5. **Methimazole and carbimazole** are antithyroid drugs used in cats:

   a. **Methimazole** is specifically licensed for treatment of feline hyperthyroidism both in Europe and USA as 2.5- and 5-mg tablets (**Felimazole**, Dechra Veterinary Products):

      1) For most hyperthyroid cats, a starting dose of 2.5 mg methimazole is administered once to twice daily as recommended.

   b. **Carbimazole** is available for human use in many European countries (NeoMercazole, Amdipharm), Australia, and Japan. It exerts its antithyroid effect through immediate conversion to methimazole when administered orally:

      1) For most hyperthyroid cats, a starting dose of regular carbimazole of 5 mg twice daily is effective in restoring euthyroidism.

   c. **Carbimazole**, as a novel **once daily controlled-release formulation** (10- or 15-mg tablets) was recently licensed for cats in Europe (**Vidalta**, Intervet Schering-Plough). Administration of this drug with food significantly enhances its absorption:

      1) The starting dose for controlled release carbimazole is 15 mg administered once daily. In cats with mild hyperthyroidism (total T_4 concentration <100 nmol/L), a 10 mg once daily is recommended.

   d. **Carbimazole and methimazole** can be reformulated in a pluronic lecithin organogel (PLO) for **transdermal administration**:

      1) Both antithyroid drugs are generally effective in cats when administered at a dose of 2.5 mg twice daily transdermally. The gel is applied in a thin layer to the nonhaired portion of the pinnae.

      2) Transdermal administration is associated with fewer gastrointestinal side effects than the oral route, but some cats resent manipulation of their ears and crusting can occur between doses leading to erythema.

      3) Such custom formulation increases expense of therapy and the stability of the product is not guaranteed.

      4) Owners need to be cautioned to use gloves for application; allergic skin reactions have occurred in owners.

   e. **Monitoring** of cats on antithyroid drugs is extremely important:

      1) **Initially**, cats should be reassessed after **2–3 weeks** and a serum total T_4 concentration measured. If euthyroidism has not been achieved, the dose of methimazole or carbimazole can be increased in 2.5–5 mg increments, reassessing the cat again in 2–3 weeks. Lack of owner or cat compliance should first be eliminated as a reason for a failure of therapy.

      2) When monitoring, **time of serum T_4 sampling** in relation to the administration of the antithyroid drug is not important.

      3) The goal of medical therapy is to maintain total T_4 concentrations within the **lower half of the reference range**.

      4) For **long-term management** (once euthyroidism has been achieved), the daily antithyroid drug dosage is adjusted to the lowest possible dose that effectively maintains euthyroidism. Once the dosage has stabilized, the cat should be monitored every 3–6 months and as needed clinically.

   f. Because antithyroid medications have no effect on the underlying lesion, the **thyroid nodules continue to grow** larger and larger over time. This may necessitate an increased daily dose with time.

   g. Most **clinical adverse reactions** occur within the first 3 months of therapy:

      1) Mild clinical side effects of **vomiting, anorexia, or depression** occur in approximately 10–15% of cats, usually within the first 3 weeks of therapy. In most cats, these reactions are transient and do not require permanent drug withdrawal.

      2) Early in the course of therapy, mild and transient **hematological abnormalities,** including lymphocytosis, eosinophilia, or leucopenia, develop in up to 15% of cats without any apparent clinical effect. More serious hematological complications occur in <5% of cats and include agranulocytosis and thrombocytopenia.

      3) Self-induced **excoriations of the head and neck** occasionally develop, usually within the first 6 weeks of therapy.

      4) **Hepatopathy** characterized by marked increases in liver enzymes and bilirubin concentration occurs in <2% of cats. Withdrawal of the medication and symptomatic therapy is required.

5) Other rarely reported side effects include a bleeding tendency without thrombocytopenia, prolongation of clotting times, and acquired myasthenia gravis.

6) **All of the adverse effects are reversible** upon discontinuation of the medication.

D. **Surgical thyroidectomy:**

1. Thyroidectomy is a **highly curative treatment** for hyperthyroidism. However, thyroidectomy can be associated with significant morbidity and mortality, especially in cats with severe hyperthyroidism (Table 29.4).

2. Ideally, the cat would be **managed preoperatively** with antithyroid drugs. After **methimazole or carbimazole** treatment has maintained euthyroidism for 1–3 weeks, anesthetic and surgical complications will be greatly minimized. The last dose of methimazole or carbimazole should be given on the morning of surgery.

3. In cats that cannot tolerate antithyroid drug treatment, alternate preoperative preparation with **β-adrenoceptor-blocking drugs** (e.g., propranolol or atenolol) should be used, or nutritional therapy could be considered.

4. **Surgery** entails either unilateral or bilateral thyroidectomy. Because most cats have involvement of both thyroid lobes, bilateral thyroidectomy is indicated in most cats.

5. The two major techniques for bilateral thyroidectomy include the **intracapsular and extracapsular methods.** The aim of both techniques is to remove the adenomatous thyroid tissue while preserving parathyroid function:

   a. The major problem with the **intracapsular technique for thyroidectomy** is that it can be difficult to remove the entire thyroid capsule (and therefore all abnormal thyroid tissue) while concurrently preserving parathyroid function. Small remnants of thyroid tissue that remain attached to the capsule may regenerate and produce recurrent hyperthyroidism.

   b. The main advantage of the **extracapsular technique** is that the incidence of relapse is much less than that of the intracapsular technique because the entire thyroid capsule is removed together with the thyroid lobe.

6. Many **potential complications** are associated with thyroidectomy, including **hypoparathyroidism,** laryngeal nerve damage (most commonly associated with voice change), and Horner's syndrome (Table 29.4):

   a. The most serious complication is **hypocalcemia,** which develops after the parathyroid glands are injured or inadvertently removed. Since only one parathyroid gland is required for maintenance of normocalcemia, hypoparathyroidism develops **only in cats treated with bilateral thyroidectomy.**

   b. If the surgeon recognizes that all parathyroid glands have been inadvertently removed, they can **autotransplant parathyroid tissue** into a muscular pouch in the neck where revascularization and return of function may occur.

   c. After bilateral thyroidectomy, it is important to **monitor serum calcium concentration daily** until it has stabilized within the normal range.

   d. In most cats with **iatrogenic hypoparathyroidism,** clinical signs associated with **hypocalcemia** will develop within **1–3 days of surgery.**

   e. Although mild hypocalcemia (6.5–7.5 mg/dL; 1.6–1.9 mmol/L) is common during this immediate postoperative period, laboratory evidence of hypocalcemia alone does not require treatment. However, if accompanying signs of **muscle tremors, tetany, or convulsions develop,** therapy with vitamin D and calcium is strongly indicated.

   f. Although hypoparathyroidism may be permanent in some cats, **spontaneous recovery of parathyroid function** may occur weeks to months after surgery.

7. Temporary **hypothyroidism** develops in most cats after unilateral or bilateral thyroidectomy, with serum T_4 concentrations falling to subnormal levels for 2–3 months. However, clinical signs of hypothyroidism are rare and oral levothyroxine (L-T_4) supplementation is rarely required (Table 29.4):

   a. If signs of postoperative hypothyroidism do develop (e.g., severe lethargy), L-T_4 (0.1 to 0.2 mg/day) can be given, but this supplementation can generally be stopped after 2–3 months.

   b. Serum T_4 concentrations almost always spontaneously return to reference range limits within a few weeks to months in cats treated with thyroidectomy.

8. Because of the potential for **recurrence of hyperthyroidism,** all cats should have serum T_4 concentration monitored once or twice a year (Table 29.4):

    a. If hyperthyroidism recurs after bilateral thyroidectomy, treatment with either antithyroid drugs or radioiodine is favored over reoperation; the incidence of surgical complications (especially hypoparathyroidism) is considerably higher in subsequent operations.

E. **Radioactive iodine therapy:**

  1. Radioactive iodine (**radioiodine**; ^{131}I) provides a simple, effective, and safe treatment for cats with hyperthyroidism and is regarded by most veterinarians to be the **treatment of choice** for cats with hyperthyroidism.

  2. Treatment with radioiodine has **many advantages** over other treatment methods:

    a. It avoids inconvenience of daily oral administration of antithyroid drugs as well as the side effects commonly associated with these drugs.

    b. Radioiodine also eliminates the risks and perioperative complications associated with anesthesia and surgical thyroidectomy (Table 29.4).

    c. A single administration of radioiodine restores euthyroidism in most (95%) hyperthyroid cats. The therapy is simple and relatively stress free for most cats.

  3. There are some **downsides** of radioiodine treatment, however:

    a. Its use requires **special radioactive licensing** and hospitalization facilities, and extensive compliance with local and state radiation safety laws.

    b. Major drawback for most owners is that their cat must be kept **hospitalized for a certain period of time** (5–10 days in most treatment centers; but up to a month in some places) and visiting is not allowed.

  4. The **principle behind this treatment** is that thyrocytes concentrate iodine but do not differentiate between stable and radioactive iodine:

    a. In cats with hyperthyroidism, radioiodine is concentrated primarily in the hyperplastic or neoplastic thyroid cells, where it irradiates and destroys the hyperfunctioning tissue.

    b. In hyperthyroid cats, any normal thyroid tissue tends to be protected from the effects of radioiodine, because the uninvolved thyroid tissue is suppressed and receives only a small dose of radiation.

  5. The **goal of treatment** is to administer a dose of radioiodine that will restore euthyroidism while avoiding iatrogenic hypothyroidism. Unfortunately, there is no definitive method to determine the best dose of ^{131}I for cats:

    a. **Fixed doses** are **not recommended** as they can provide too low a ^{131}I dose and not cure the disease. More commonly, fixed dose methods give too high a ^{131}I dose, resulting in hypothyroidism.

    b. More precise, variable ^{131}I doses can be estimated by use of a **scoring system** that takes into consideration the severity of clinical signs, the size of the cat's thyroid gland, and the serum T_4 concentration. Yet more precision can be gained with thyroid imaging (scintigraphy) since it can also be used to estimate thyroid tumor volume and identify ectopic (intrathoracic) thyroid tissue.

  6. Most hyperthyroid cats treated with radioactive iodine are **cured by a single dose** (Figure 29.6). Approximately 5% of cats, however, fail to respond completely and remain hyperthyroid after treatment with radioiodine:

    a. In **cats that remain hyperthyroid** 3 months after initial ^{131}I treatment, retreatment is generally recommended because virtually all cats with **persistent hyperthyroidism** after the first treatment can be cured by a second treatment.

  7. A proportion of cats treated with radioiodine will develop **permanent hypothyroidism**, with clinical signs developing 2–6 months after treatment:

    a. Clinical signs associated with iatrogenic hypothyroidism may include **lethargy, nonpruritic seborrhea sicca, matting of hair, and marked weight gain**; bilateral symmetric alopecia does not develop.

    b. Diagnosis of **hypothyroidism** is based upon clinical sign, subnormal serum total T_4 and free T_4 concentrations, high serum cTSH values, and the response to replacement L-T_4 therapy).

    c. **Lifelong L-T_4 supplementation** is needed (i.e., 0.1–0.2 mg L-thyroxine per day).

  8. **Relapse after** ^{131}I is possible but rare. When it does occur, relapse generally develops between 2 or more years after treatment. Because of this possibility, rechecking serum total T_4 annually is recommended.

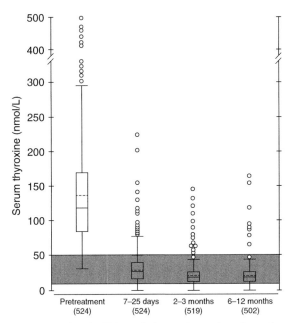

Figure 29.6 Box plots of serum T_4 concentrations in 524 cats before and at various times after administration of radioiodine for treatment of hyperthyroidism. See Figure 29.1 for key. Shaded area indicates normal ranges for T_4 concentration for cats. (From Peterson ME, Becker DV. Radioiodine treatment of 524 cats with hyperthyroidism. *J Am Vet Med Assoc* 1995;207: 1422–1428, with permission).

9. In cats with **thyroid carcinoma** (incidence <2–4% of all hyperthyroid cats), radioiodine offers the best chance for successful cure of the tumor because it concentrates in all hyperactive thyroid cells, that is, carcinomatous tissue, as well as metastasis:

   a. Thyroid carcinomas are more resistant to the effect of ^{131}I than thyroid adenomas (adenomatous hyperplasia) and the size of thyroid carcinomas is usually much larger.

   b. Therefore, **extremely high doses of radioiodine** (1110 mBq) are almost always needed for destruction of all malignant tissue.

   c. A combination of **surgical debulking** followed by high-dose ^{131}I is also useful in treating cats with thyroid carcinoma.

   d. Longer periods of hospitalization will be required with use of such high-dose ^{131}I administration because of the prolonged radioiodine excretion.

F. Nutritional therapy (iodine-deficient diet):

   1. Recent studies have indicated that use of a diet with restricted iodine levels (Hill's Prescription Diet y/d Feline –Thyroid Health) can result in normalization of T_4 levels in hyperthyroid cats and provide a further option for medical management of this disease. The basis for using this diet is that iodine is an essential component of both T4 and T3; without suffcient iodine, the thyroid cannot produce excess thyroid hormones. This is an iodine-deficient diet, containing levels below the minimum daily requirement for adult cats.

   2. By 4 weeks, about 70% of hyperthyroid cats exclusively eating y/d will be euthyroid. By 8 weeks, about 90% of cats will be euthyroid. By 12 weeks, almost all cats should have normal T_4 values. This therapy appears to be more effective in cats with only moderate elevations of T_4 than cats with severe hyperthyroidism.

   3. A major indication for the use of this y/d diet for management of feline hyperthyroidism is in cats that are not candidates for definitive treatment of the underlying thyroid tumor(s) with surgery or radioiodine, which remains the treatments of choice. In addition, nutritional management with y/d food (canned rather than the dry y/d) could be considered in cats whose owners are not able to give oral medication or in cats that develop side effects from methimazole/carbimazole.

4. Despite some advantages, nutritional management has many disadvantages:

   a. First of all, feeding this diet cannot cure hyperthyroidism. Rather, feeding y/d just offers control (withholding fuel for thyroid tumor). The thyroid tumor remains and will continue to grow larger. As now documented in cats with long-standing hyperthyroidism, transformation of adenoma to thyroid carcinoma can occur unless definitive treatment (surgery or radioiodine treatment) is used to cure the disease.

   b. The cats fed this diet must not eat any other cat diet, table food, or treats because even tiny amounts of iodine may lead to failure of this diet to effectively control hyperthyroidism.

   c. If the diet is stopped, relapse will develop; the cat must eat only this diet for rest of his/her lifetime.

   d. The long-term consequences of this iodine deficient diet are not known, especially in normal cats in households that are also fed this diet. For this reason, y/d should not be the only diet fed to normal cats, which can be an issue for owners with multiple cats in the same household.

   e. The composition (protein/fat/carbohydrate breakdown) of y/d reveals that it is a high-carbohydrate, relatively low-protein diet. Feeding y/d for long periods is less than an "ideal" diet for an obligate carnivore, especially in an older hyperthyroid cat with severe muscle wasting.

VII. Prognosis

A. With proper treatment, the prognosis of most cats with hyperthyroidism is **good to excellent**.

B. The specific prognosis for each individual cat depends on the cat's age and condition at the time of diagnosis, duration of the disease, and the presence of concurrent diseases (e.g., CKD).

C. Like most other diseases, hyperthyroidism is best diagnosed and treated in its early rather than the advanced stages. The prognosis also depends on the treatment type as well as the cat's response to treatment.

VIII. Prevention

A. Unfortunately, there is no known way to prevent the development of hyperthyroidism in cats.

References and Further Readings

Birchard SJ. Thyroidectomy in the cat. Clin Tech Small Anim Pract 2006;21:29–33.

Frenais R, Rosenberg D, Burgaud S, Horspool LJ. Clinical efficacy and safety of a once-daily formulation of carbimazole in cats with hyperthyroidism. *J Small Anim Pract* 2009;50:510–515.

Hibbert A, Gruffydd-Jones T, Barrett EL, et al. Feline thyroid carcinoma: Diagnosis and response to high-dose radioactive iodine treatment. *J Feline Med Surg* 2009;11:116–124.

Langston CE, Reine NJ. Hyperthyroidism and the kidney. *Clin Tech Small Anim Pract* 2006:21:17–21.

Melendez LM, Yamka RM, Forrester SD et al. Titration of dietary iodine for reducing serum thyroxine concentrations in newly diagnosed hyperthyroid cats [abstract]. *J Vet Intern Med* 2011;25:683.

Peterson ME. Diagnostic tests for hyperthyroidism in cats. *Clin Tech Small Anim Pract* 2006;21(1):2–9.

Peterson ME, Becker DV. Radioiodine treatment of 524 cats with hyperthyroidism. *J Am Vet Med Assoc* 1995;207: 1422–1428.

Peterson ME, Kintzer PP, Hurvitz AI. Methimazole treatment of 262 cats with hyperthyroidism. *J Vet Intern Med* 1988;2: 150–157.

Peterson ME, Melian C, Nichols R. Measurement of serum concentrations of free thyroxine, total thyroxine, and total triiodothyronine in cats with hyperthyroidism and cats with nonthyroidal disease. *J Am Vet Med Assoc* 2001;218:529–536.

Peterson ME, Ward CR. Etiopathologic findings of hyperthyroidism in cats. *Vet Clin North Am Small Anim Pract* 2007;37:633–645.

Trepanier LA. Pharmacologic management of feline hyperthyroidism *Vet Clin North Am Small Anim Pract* 2007;37:775–788.

Wakeling J, Moore K, Elliott J, et al. Diagnosis of hyperthyroidism in cats with mild chronic kidney disease. *J Small Anim Pract* 2008;49:287–294.

Yu S, Wedekind KJ, Burris PA et al. Controlled level of dietary iodine normalizes serum total thyroxine in cats with naturally occurring hyperthyroidism [abstract]. *J Vet Intern Med* 2011;25:683.

CHAPTER 30

Hyperthyroidism/Thyroid Neoplasia in Other Species

Michelle L. Campbell-Ward

Pathogenesis

- Clinical hyperthyroidism is rare in horses, small exotic mammals, birds, and reptiles: few documented cases exist.
- Thyroid neoplasia is more common but is rarely associated with overt clinical disease.

Classical Signs

- Often none.
- Palpable ventral cervical mass in the case of neoplasia.
- Weight loss, excitability, polyphagia, and tachycardia in clinical cases.

Diagnosis

- Demonstration of increased circulating concentrations of free fractions of thyroid hormones.
- Complicated by lack of validated assays for many species.
- Suspected neoplasms can be biopsied.

Treatment

- May not be required depending on clinical signs.
- Thyroidectomy/surgical excision of neoplasms.

I. Pathogenesis

A. Hyperthyroidism is defined as a **pathologic and sustained state of hypermetabolism caused by elevated concentrations of thyroid hormones** (thyroxine [T4] and triiodothyronine [T3]) in the circulation.

B. In general terms, causes of hyperthyroidism include hyperfunctioning thyroid nodules, thyroid neoplasia, oversupplementation of exogenous thyroid hormone and pituitary dysfunction leading to increased thyroid-stimulating hormone secretion which results in increased T4 production.

Clinical Endocrinology of Companion Animals, First Edition. Edited by Jacquie Rand.
© 2013 John Wiley & Sons, Inc. Published 2013 by John Wiley & Sons, Inc.

C.   High thyroid hormone concentrations are a feature of certain **physiological states and thyroid hormone levels may vary due to external influences**. These factors should be considered when interpreting hormone levels for a particular individual:

1.   In horses, high thyroid hormone levels are seen during pregnancy in mares, in fetuses in late pregnancy, and in foals in the first few weeks of life.

2.   Thyroid hormone concentrations in birds and reptiles are influenced by ambient temperature, photoperiod, food intake, and dietary composition. As such thyroid size can vary seasonally. In relation to avian hatchlings, thyroid function varies widely between species (it is well developed in precocial species compared to altricial species).

3.   Thyroid hormone metabolism plays an important role in molting (birds) and ecdysis/shedding (reptiles).

D.   **Clinical hyperthyroidism is rare in horses, small exotic mammals, birds, and reptiles:** few documented cases exist. Although hyperthyroidism due to thyroid neoplasia has been occasionally reported, most cases of neoplasia of this gland are not associated with thyroid dysfunction:

1.   Horses are at risk of accelerated thyroid hormone production when exposed to increased quantities of iodine-containing compounds such as expectorants, counterirritants, some drugs (e.g., sodium iodide, potassium iodine, and iodinated glycerol), contrast media, leg paints, and povidone-based shampoos.

2.   There are no reports of hyperthyroidism in the horse associated with an autoimmune condition.

E.   **Thyroid neoplasia has been reported in many species** and may originate from undifferentiated cells, parafollicular cells, and follicular epithelial cells. (Note that birds do not have parafollicular cells in their thyroid glands.) However, **overt clinical disease is rarely described in cases of thyroid neoplasia:**

1.   Thyroid gland neoplasia is not uncommon in horses. **Benign microfollicular adenoma is the most commonly diagnosed type.** The vast majority of cases are euthyroid, but both hypothyroidism and hyperthyroidism have been reported in association with thyroid adenocarcinoma. Multiple endocrine neoplasia (MEN) has also been described in horses in which multiple endocrine gland neoplasms occur, including thyroid involvement.

2.   Thyroid neoplasia, including adenoma and adenocarcinoma is frequently reported in psittacine birds. The tumors are not usually functionally secreting.

3.   A single case report of hyperthyroidism in a green iguana attributed the condition to a thyroid follicular adenoma. Thyroid gland adenomas and carcinomas have been reported in chelonians.

II.   Signalment

A.   **Horses:**

1.   Thyroid neoplasia tends to occur more frequently in **lightweight breeds** than in draft breed horses.

2.   Thyroid neoplasia is more common in **older horses** (>16 years):

a.   A survey of aged horses revealed thyroid tumors in 30% of the animals; with no tumors in horses <18 months old.

B.   **Birds:**

1.   **Budgerigars and cockatiels** appear to be overrepresented in cases of avian thyroid neoplasia.

III.   Clinical Signs

A.   Regardless of the species involved, **many thyroid neoplasms produce no clinical signs** and the disease is diagnosed as an incidental finding at necropsy.

B.   **Horses:**

1.   Weight loss, cachexia, tremors, excitability, tachycardia, tachypnoea, polyphagia, and sweating have been described in suspect hyperthyroid cases.

2.   Constant swallowing or changes in respiration may occur as a result of the space-occupying nature of large thyroid neoplasms.

C.   **Birds:**

1.   Palpable mass in the neck.

2.   Respiratory signs referable to the mass placing pressure on the trachea.

3.   Signs of crop dysfunction (e.g., regurgitation, dysphagia).

D. **Reptiles:**
    1. Palpable mass in the ventral cervical region near the thoracic inlet.
    2. Weight loss, polyphagia, hyperactivity, increased aggression, loss of dorsal spines (iguanas), and tachycardia may be seen.
    3. Hyperthyroidism has been suspected in snakes that undergo frequent ecdysis.

IV. Diagnosis
A. Demonstration of **increased circulating concentrations of free fractions of thyroid hormones**. Note that validated assays to test samples from many species have not been reported. In such cases, it may be useful to test a number of clinically normal age-matched controls for comparison:
    For example, in the case report describing hyperthyroidism in an iguana, the measured T4 level (30 nmol/L [2.33 µg/dL]) in the patient was found to be significantly higher than the level measured in clinically healthy adult iguanas (3.81±0.84 nmol/L [0.30±0.07 µg/dL]).
B. One case report describes a T3 suppression test in which T4 concentrations did not decrease in an affected horse compared with controls.
C. Thyroid neoplasia can be confirmed by cytology of fine needle aspirate samples or preferably **histopathological examination of biopsy samples**. Immunohistochemistry or electron microscopy may be necessary to distinguish between some types of thyroid neoplasia.

V. Differential Diagnoses
A. Cervical masses may be caused by goiter, neoplasia associated with other cervical structures, abscesses, granulomas, or crop impactions.
B. Weight loss accompanied by neurological and/or cardiovascular disturbances may be due to a wide variety of systemic diseases, many of which are more common than thyroid disease. A thorough history and clinical examination is warranted in all cases regardless of species.

VI. Treatment
A. Horses:
    1. Antithyroid therapy has been used in the form of potassium iodide at a dose of 1 g per horse q 24 h per os.
    2. **Thyroidectomy** may be necessary but has variable success.
    3. In cases of thyrotoxicosis due to exposure to iodine-containing compounds, administration of glucocorticoids may alleviate the signs.
B. **Clinically silent thyroid neoplasms do not usually warrant treatment**, although **surgical excision is recommended for large masses**. Potential complications of surgery include infection, hemorrhage, and in horses laryngeal hemiplegia. Given that the parathyroid glands of some species (e.g., horses, reptiles) are not connected to the thyroid itself, hypocalcemia is not always considered a complication. Once the thyroid gland has been removed, thyroid hormone supplementation may be required to maintain concentrations of thyroid hormones within the normal reference range. Patients that have undergone unilateral/partial thyroidectomy or tumor debulking do not usually require thyroid hormone supplementation:
    1. Thyroidectomy in an iguana case proved to be curative; with T4 levels comparable to clinically healthy adults 173 days post surgery.
C. A snake with excessively frequent ecdysis (every 2 weeks) responded to methimazole (1 mg/kg q 24 h) by returning to a more regular ecdysis cycle. However, it is worth noting that hyperthyroidism in this case was not confirmed by measurement of thyroid hormone levels.
D. Radiotherapy has not been reported to date in these species for the treatment of thyroid neoplasia.

VII. Prognosis
A. Most thyroid tumors are benign and are not associated with thyroid dysfunction. The prognosis is therefore **good** in the majority of cases.

VIII. Prevention
A. There are no specific preventative measures.

References and Further Readings

Breuhaus BA. Thyroid glands. In: Smith BP, ed. *Large Animal Internal Medicine*, 4th edn. St Louis, MO: Mosby Elsevier, 2009, pp. 1347–1351.

Frye FL. *Biomedical and Surgical Aspects of Captive Reptile Husbandry*, 2nd edn. Malabar: Krieger Publishing, 1991.

Garner MM. Overview of biopsy and necropsy techniques. In: Mader DR, ed. *Reptile Medicine and Surgery*, 2nd edn. St Louis, MO: Saunders Elsevier, 2006, pp. 569–580.

Hernandez-Divers SJ, Knott C, MacDonald J. Diagnosis and surgical treatment of thyroid adenoma-induced hyperthyroidism in a green iguana (*Iguana iguana*). *J Zoo Wildl Med* 2001;32(4):465–475.

Leach MW. A survey of neoplasia in pet birds. *Semin Avian Exot Pet Med* 1992;1:52–64.

Lightfoot TL. Overview of tumours: Section I—Clinical avian neoplasia and oncology. In: Harrison GJ, Lightfoot TL, eds. *Clinical Avian Medicine*, Vol. 2. Palm Beach, FL: Spix Publishing, 2006, pp. 560–565.

Percy DH, Barthold SW. *Pathology of Laboratory Rodents and Rabbits*, 3rd edn. Ames, IO: Blackwell Publishing, 2007.

Rae M. Endocrine diseases in pet birds. *Semin Avian Exot Pet Med* 1995;4:32–38.

Ramirez S, McClure JJ, Moore RM, et al. Hyperthyroidism associated with a thyroid adenocarcinoma in a 21-year old gelding. *J Vet Intern Med* 1998;12:475–477.

Reavill DR. Neoplasia. In: Girling SJ, Raiti P, eds. *BSAVA Manual of Reptiles*, 2nd edn. Gloucester: British Small Animal Veterinary Association, 2004, pp. 309–318.

Schmidt RE, Reavill DR. The avian thyroid gland. *Vet Clin North Am Exot Anim Pract* 2008;11:15–23.

Toribio RE. Thyroid gland. In: Reed SM, Bayly WM, Sellon DC, eds. *Equine Internal Medicine*, 3rd edn. St Louis, MO: Saunders Elsevier, 2010, pp. 1251–1260.

CHAPTER 31

Hypocalcemia in Dogs

Patricia A. Schenck and Dennis Chew

Pathogenesis

- Clinical signs only result when ionized calcium (iCa) falls below a critical level.
- Causes of hypocalcemia can be parathyroid independent or parathyroid dependent.
- The most common cause of chronic hypocalcemia is primary hypoparathyroidism.
- The most common cause of acute hypocalcemia in combination with clinical signs related to hypocalcemia is periparturient tetany (eclampsia).
- Hypocalcemia is usually underestimated in dogs when serum total calcium (tCa) is used.
- Hypocalcemia based on low serum tCa concentration is commonly seen with hypoalbuminemia; however, low iCa concentration may or may not be present.

Classical Signs

- The most common clinical signs associated with hypocalcemia are muscle tremors and fasciculations, facial rubbing, muscle cramping, stiff gait, seizures, restlessness, aggression, disorientation, and cutaneous hypersensitivity.
- Acute development of hypocalcemia is typically associated with severe clinical signs; there may be few clinical signs of hypocalcemia if the underlying problem is chronic.

Diagnosis

- Hypocalcemia is defined as a tCa concentration <8.0 mg/dL (2.0 mmol/L) or iCa concentration <5.0 mg/dL (1.25 mmol/L).
- Parathyroid hormone (PTH) should be measured in conjunction with iCa to determine whether PTH production is appropriate; measurement of serum 25-hydroxyvitamin D may be helpful to identify cases in which decreased intake of vitamin D is the cause of hypocalcemia.

Clinical Endocrinology of Companion Animals, First Edition. Edited by Jacquie Rand.
© 2013 John Wiley & Sons, Inc. Published 2013 by John Wiley & Sons, Inc.

Treatment

- Specific therapy depends on the cause of hypocalcemia.
- Acute symptomatic hypocalcemia requires treatment with IV calcium salts to effect.
- Symptomatic subacute and chronic hypocalcemia require treatment with oral calcium salts and/or active vitamin D compounds.

Prognosis

- Prognosis depends on the underlying cause of hypocalcemia.
- Prognosis is excellent for properly treated eclampsia and good to excellent for primary hypoparathyroidism.

I. Pathogenesis

A. Serum tCa is composed of protein-bound calcium (pCa), complexed calcium (cCa), and iCa. The **iCa fraction is the biologically active fraction.**

B. Hypocalcemia develops when there is a decrease in bone mobilization of calcium, an increase in loss of calcium in urine or milk, a decrease in gastrointestinal calcium absorption, calcium translocation intracellularly, or a combination of these mechanisms:

1. A **decrease in serum iCa typically stimulates the synthesis and release of PTH** from the parathyroid glands.

2. **PTH** causes a **decrease in urinary calcium excretion,** and an **increase in bone resorption.**

3. PTH also stimulates production of calcitriol (1,25-dihydroxyvitamin D), the active form of Vitamin D, from 25-hydroxyvitamin D by upregulation of the renal enzyme 1α-hydroxylase.

4. Calcitriol causes an increase in calcium absorption in the gut and also increases bone resorption.

5. Increased PTH production continues if a continued decrease in iCa concentration exists or there is persisting hyperphosphatemia. This creates a secondary hyperparathyroidism in which PTH is elevated, and serum iCa concentration is within the reference range or low.

C. Causes of hypocalcemia are listed in Table 31.1.

D. Mechanisms for hypocalcemia in **eclampsia** include a poor dietary calcium source, calcium loss during lactation, and/or abnormal parathyroid gland function.

E. **Primary hypoparathyroidism** is **usually idiopathic,** though immune mechanisms are thought to be important (Figure 31.1). **Other causes** of hypoparathyroidism include **postoperative** (after neck surgery that disrupts the blood supply to the parathyroid glands), spontaneous **infarction** of a parathyroid gland tumor, and both **acute hypermagnesemia** or **severe magnesium depletion.**

Table 31.1   Causes of hypocalcemia in dogs.

Most common	Occasional	Uncommon
Hypoalbuminemia	Soft tissue trauma or rhabdomyolysis	Lab error
Azotemic chronic kidney disease	Hypoparathyroidism	Improper anticoagulant (EDTA)
Puerperal tetany (eclampsia)	Ethylene glycol intoxication	Infarction of parathyroid gland adenoma
Acute renal failure	Phosphate enema	Intestinal malabsorption or severe
Acute pancreatitis	Post-NaHCO$_3$ administration	starvation
Cause not identified (often trivial	Emergency and critical care (sepsis,	Hypovitaminosis D
magnitude and transient)	SIRS)	Diabetes mellitus
		Rapid infusion of phosphate
		Vitamin D-resistant rickets
		Drug administration
		Blood transfusion with citrated
		anticoagulant

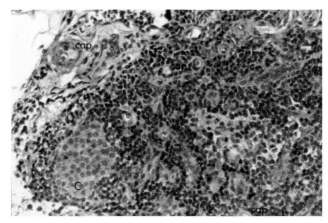

Figure 31.1 Lymphocytic-plasmacytic parathyroiditis as the cause for primary hypoparathyroidism in a Schnauzer dog. Note infiltration of lymphocytes and plasma cells surrounding chief cells (C) of the parathyroid gland in what is thought to be an immune reaction that destroys functioning parathyroid gland tissue. cap – capillary (Courtesy of Dr. Robert G. Sherding, The Ohio State University College of Veterinary Medicine).

F. Mechanisms of low iCa in **pancreatitis** include sequestration of calcium into peripancreatic fat (saponification), increased circulating free fatty acids, increased calcitonin secretion, and PTH resistance or deficit resulting from hypomagnesemia.
G. Decreased calcitriol synthesis and mass law interactions of calcium with increased serum phosphorus concentration are probable causes of hypocalcemia **in chronic renal failure**.
H. **Nutritional secondary hyperparathyroidism** is associated with lack of sufficient dietary vitamin D intake or low calcium/high phosphorus concentrations in the diet.
I. With **rhabdomyolysis**, hypocalcemia usually occurs as a consequence of calcium translocation into damaged muscles.
J. One possible mechanism of hypocalcemia **in small intestinal disease** is an increase in calcium/fatty acid complexes in the intestinal lumen that decrease intestinal calcium absorption. Also, malabsorption of vitamin D can lead to hypovitaminosis D and decreased intestinal calcium absorption.
K. **Bicarbonate administration** IV results in increased protein binding of calcium, thereby decreasing the iCa fraction.
L. After **acute reversal of chronic hypercalcemia**, hypocalcemia, if it occurs, is the result of parathyroid gland atrophy and inadequate ability to synthesize and secrete PTH. This happens most frequently following the removal of a parathyroid adenoma that has caused primary hyperparathyroidism.
M. **Tumor lysis syndrome** occurs when there is rapid destruction of tumor cells following chemotherapy which can result in hyperphosphatemia. Hypocalcemia develops when calcium precipitates with phosphate and the salts are deposited into soft tissues.
N. **Phosphate enemas** result in hypocalcemia after rapid absorption of phosphate and subsequent mass law interaction with serum calcium.
O. Oxalate metabolites that result from **ethylene glycol toxicity** can chelate calcium and become deposited in soft tissues, resulting in hypocalcemia.
P. **Vitamin D-Resistant Rickets (VDRR)**: VDRR type 2 is a genetic condition associated with downregulation of the function or numbers of vitamin D receptors in target tissues. Circulating calcitriol concentrations will be elevated. VDRR type 1 is associated with a genetic defect in the metabolic activation of 25-hydroxy-vitamin D to the most active vitamin D metabolite 1,25-dihydroxyvitamin D (calcitriol). Circulating calcitriol concentrations are, therefore, low.
Q. After its **rapid infusion, phosphate** complexes with circulating calcium and promotes deposition of calcium phosphate salts into soft tissues due to mass law interactions.
R. The cause of hypocalcemia in **emergency and critical care patients** is largely unknown and likely to be multifactorial.

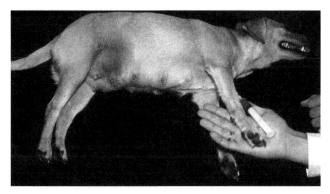

Figure 31.2 Eclampsia in a bitch shortly after parturition. Note rigor in between seizures. IV needle has been placed for the administration of calcium salts. (Courtesy of Dr. Charles Capen, The Ohio State University College of Veterinary Medicine).

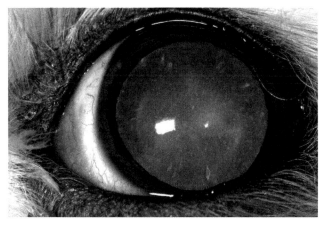

Figure 31.3 Multiple punctate cortical ("snowflake") cataracts may occur in dogs with hypocalcemia secondary to primary hypoparathyroidism. (Courtesy of Dr. Anne Gemensky Metzler, The Ohio State University College of Veterinary Medicine).

S. **Diabetes mellitus**—cause of hypocalcemia is unknown.

T. Drug administration: **Enrofloxacin**—cause unknown; **mithramycin**—decreased osteoclastic bone resorption; **bisphosphonates**—decreased osteoclastic bone resorption.

II. Signalment

A. **Eclampsia** usually occurs in females of small breeds that have recently whelped a litter of puppies. It is **more common in those with large litters.**

B. Breeds at higher risk for **primary hypoparathyroidism** include **miniature schnauzers, standard schnauzers, Scottish terriers, West Highland white terriers, and dachshunds. Mean age of occurrence is 6 years; females** are more commonly affected.

C. There does not appear to be any age-, sex-, or breed-related predispositions for the other causes of hypocalcemia.

III. Clinical Signs

A. Decreased serum iCa concentration **increases excitability of neuromuscular tissue,** which accounts for many of the clinical signs of hypocalcemia:

    1. The **most common clinical signs** associated with hypocalcemia are **muscle tremors and fasciculations, facial rubbing, muscle cramping, stiff gait, seizures, restlessness, aggression, disorientation, and hypersensitivity** (Figure 31.2).

    2. Clinical signs of hypocalcemia that **may occur** include **panting, pyrexia, lethargy, depression, anorexia, tachycardia, and posterior lenticular cataracts** (Figure 31.3).

3. **Uncommon clinical signs** of hypocalcemia include polyuria, polydipsia, hypotension, respiratory arrest, or death.

B. Clinical signs **usually do not occur until serum tCa is <6.5 mg/dL (1.6 mmol/L)**. Some dogs (especially those in chronic renal failure) may not show clinical signs of hypocalcemia until serum tCa concentration is <5.0 mg/dL (1.2 mmol/L):

1. **Acute development** of hypocalcemia is typically associated with **severe clinical signs**.

2. If the underlying problem has been chronic and there has been sufficient time for physiologic adaptation, then few clinical signs of hypocalcemia may be present.

3. Clinical signs of hypocalcemia are **uncommon** when hypocalcemia occurs in association **with secondary hyperparathyroidism and chronic renal failure**.

C. **Electrolyte and acid-base abnormalities can impact hypocalcemia**:

1. **Exercise or excitement** leading to respiratory alkalosis may cause or exacerbate the degree of hypocalcemia following increased binding of iCa to protein sites.

2. **Rapid infusion of alkali** to correct metabolic acidosis can cause seizures in those with marginal hypocalcemia.

IV. Diagnosis

A. **Definition of hypocalcemia**:

1. Using serum tCa, hypocalcemia is usually defined as a concentration <8.0 mg/dL (2.00 mmol/L) (Figure 31.4).

2. Using serum iCa, hypocalcemia is usually defined as a concentration <5.0 mg/dL (1.25 mmol/L).

3. There can be **unpredictable discordance between serum tCa and serum iCa measurements**. In one study, 27% of sick dogs were classified as hypocalcemic by tCa, but when iCa was measured, 31% were hypocalcemic. **Hypocalcemia is usually underestimated in dogs when serum tCa is used**.

4. Hypocalcemia based on serum tCa is relatively common in sick dogs.

B. Measurement of calcium:

1. **Trivial decreases in serum tCa are common and may not be persistent. Pursuit of a specific diagnosis in these instances is not warranted**.

2. **Serum iCa concentration should be measured any time that a persistent decrease in serum tCa is detected. Serum iCa should especially be measured in all cases of chronic renal failure** since the diagnostic error in using **tCa** to predict iCa increases greatly with this disorder.

3. **Do not use adjustment formulas** to correct the tCa to serum total protein or albumin concentration as the formulas do not accurately predict the serum iCa concentration.

4. Do not directly compare serum iCa results to those obtained from heparinized plasma or whole blood (from a blood gas analyzer or point-of-care analyzer). The **iCa concentration is lower in heparinized plasma or whole blood than in serum**.

5. **Do not use EDTA plasma** for collection of blood for iCa measurement. EDTA chelates calcium, and EDTA plasma will yield falsely low iCa results.

6. In dogs, serum tCa is normally 9.0–11.5 mg/dL (2.2–3.8 mmol/L) and serum iCa is normally 5.0–6.0 mg/dL (1.2–1.5 mmol/L).

7. To convert mmol/L to mg/dL, multiply mmol/L by 4.

C. **PTH should be measured** in conjunction with iCa measurement to determine whether PTH production is appropriate:

1. **Patients** with low iCa and low PTH concentrations have absolute hypoparathyroidism. If serum iCa is low and PTH is within the reference range, the PTH response is inappropriate, as PTH is expected to be elevated with low iCa.

2. Hypocalcemia associated with increased serum PTH is classified as **parathyroid-independent hypocalcemia**. In these cases, hypocalcemia exists from redistribution of calcium into other body spaces, excess phosphorus effects, or from deficiencies of vitamin D or dietary calcium.

D. Measurement of serum 25-hydroxyvitamin D may be helpful to identify cases in which decreased intake of vitamin D is the cause of hypocalcemia.

E. Calcitriol measurement may be useful to differentiate VDRR from those with renal disease in patients with normal serum 25-hydroxyvitamin D concentration. Calcitriol concentrations are increased in those with type 2 VDRR and decreased in those with type 1.

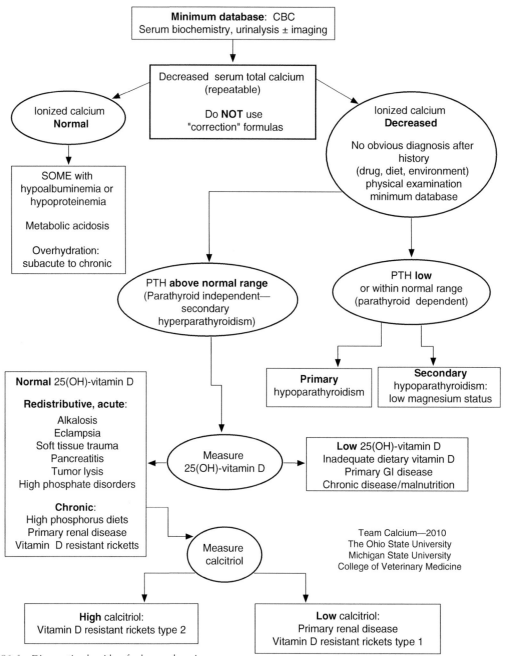

Figure 31.4 Diagnostic algorithm for hypocalcemia.

F. **Causes of hypocalcemia are listed in Table 31.1.** Identification of the underlying cause of hypocalcemia requires appropriate diagnostic testing. Most cases of hypocalcemia are parathyroid independent, that is, PTH concentration is appropriately increased.

G. **Hypoalbuminemia** is the most common condition observed with hypocalcemia based on serum tCa measurement but the least important:

1. Hypocalcemia is usually mild, and there are no clinical signs of hypocalcemia.

2. **Do not use correction formulas** to adjust serum tCa to serum total protein or albumin. These correction formulas do not improve the prediction of actual iCa concentration.

H. **Renal failure is the second most common disorder associated with hypocalcemia:**

   1. Most dogs with azotemic chronic kidney disease (CKD) and decreased serum iCa concentration do not show clinical signs directly related to hypocalcemia.

   2. Decreased serum iCa concentration is seen in approximately 30–40% of dogs with CRF.

   3. Acute renal failure and postrenal failure results in hypocalcemia that is more likely to be symptomatic.

I. **Emergency and critical care:**

   1. Low serum iCa concentration is **common in the intensive care setting** and is **more common in septic patients.**

   2. **Sepsis, systemic inflammatory response syndrome, hypomagnesemia, and blood transfusions** have been associated with hypocalcemia. **Cardiopulmonary resuscitation** may also result in hypocalcemia.

J. **Acute pancreatitis** may be associated with hypocalcemia.

K. Dogs with **diabetes mellitus** may exhibit hypocalcemia:

   1. In one study, approximately 47% of dogs with nonketotic diabetes had hypocalcemia; in another study, 52% of dogs with diabetic ketoacidosis had ionized hypocalcemia.

   2. In the second study, survival was correlated to degree of anemia, hypocalcemia, and acidosis.

L. **Puerperal (periparturient) tetany (eclampsia)** usually occurs about 1–3 weeks postpartum in females of small breeds, especially those with a small body weight to litter number ratio:

   1. iCa is <3.2 mg/dL (0.8 mmol/L) in nearly all dogs with clinical signs.

   2. Some dogs have iCa <3.2 mg/dL (0.8 mmol/L) but do not display classic signs of hypocalcemia.

M. **Rhabdomyolysis** may be associated with hypocalcemia, but clinical signs directly referable to hypocalcemia are uncommon.

N. **Small intestinal disease,** especially lymphangiectasia, may be associated with hypocalcemia:

   1. **Protein-losing enteropathy** is also associated with low serum iCa and ionized magnesium concentrations.

   2. Serum PTH is typically elevated, and serum 25-hydroxyvitamin D is low (due to its loss in nonabsorbed fat through the stool).

O. **Alkali (sodium bicarbonate) administration** can result in serum total and ionized hypocalcemia.

P. **Acute reversal of chronic hypercalcemia.**

Q. **Tumor lysis syndrome.**

R. **Nutritional secondary hyperparathyroidism** is associated with diets providing excess phosphate, insufficient calcium, or both:

   1. Serum iCa concentration typically is low, with an elevation in PTH concentration. iCa can be restored to normal due to the correcting effects of increased PTH in some cases.

   2. Nutritional secondary hyperparathyroidism tends to cause **osteopenia of the long bones and vertebrae.** A stiff gait, bone pain, and multiple bone fractures are common. This is a syndrome that occurs mostly in **young growing dogs fed a predominantly meat-based diet.**

   3. With the feeding of a BARF (biologically appropriate raw food or bones and raw food) or other unbalanced homemade diets, the occurrence of nutritional secondary hyperparathyroidism is more likely.

   4. Calcitriol concentration is typically increased in those with VDRR type 2 and decreased with type 1; it is normal to low in nutritional secondary hyperparathyroidism.

S. **Drug administration:**

   1. Drugs that can induce hypocalcemia include **enrofloxacin, mithramycin, bisphosphonates, and phosphate enemas.**

   2. **Phosphate enemas should not be used in small dogs or debilitated patients of any size.** Clinically occult hyperphosphatemia and hypocalcemia were reported in dogs in which a sodium phosphate enema was used as a bowel prep prior to colonoscopy, but they resolved within 24 h.

T. **Primary hypoparathyroidism** is an absolute or relative deficiency of PTH secretion that may be **permanent or transient:**

   1. Since magnesium status can impact PTH secretion, **measurement of ionized magnesium is recommended** in cases of hypoparathyroidism. A large percentage of dogs with primary hypoparathyroidism (58%) also exhibit low or marginal ionized magnesium concentration.

    2. Serum tCa concentration is usually <6.5 mg/dL (**1.6 mmol/L**), and **most have hyperphosphatemia.** Mean serum iCa concentration in hypoparathyroid dogs was 3.16 mg/dL (0.79 mmol/L) in one study (reference range 5.0–5.8 mg/dL; 1.25–1.45 mmol/L).

    3. Most dogs have episodes of tetany or seizures.

    4. Primary hypoparathyroidism is **characterized by low serum iCa concentration with an inappropriately low PTH concentration.**

U. Following **ethylene glycol ingestion,** seizures may be noted within hours of ingestion.

V. Differential Diagnosis

A. **Other causes of neuromuscular clinical signs similar to those produced by hypocalcemia** include primary brain disease (epilepsy, brain tumors, encephalitis, etc.), glycogen storage disorders, hepatic encephalopathy, toxins (strychnine, metaldehyde, etc.), and musculoskeletal disorders (myopathies, arthritis, hip dysplasia, etc.).

VI. Treatment

A. General treatment for hypocalcemia is listed in Table 31.2.

B. **Treatment must be individualized** based on the severity of clinical signs, magnitude of hypocalcemia, rapidity of development of hypocalcemia, the trend of serial serum calcium measurements, and the underlying disease:

    1. **Puerperal tetany is the condition that most often requires acute correction of hypocalcemia:**

        a. After treatment with intravenous calcium gluconate, iCa is normal within 25 min in most dogs.

        b. Nearly all dogs are discharged within several hours of treatment.

        c. Puppies <4 weeks old should be removed for 24 h and fed a canine milk replacer. Those older than 4 weeks can be weaned.

        d. Calcium carbonate 50 mg/kg q 12 h with meals for remainder of lactation period. Vitamin D may also be required.

    2. **Primary hypoparathyroidism is the only condition requiring both acute and chronic therapy.** Both calcium and vitamin D supplementation are usually necessary. **Magnesium supplementation may also be beneficial** if serum ionized magnesium concentration was initially marginal or low.

    3. Hypocalcemia should be anticipated in **dogs undergoing parathyroidectomy for treatment of parathyroid adenoma:**

        a. Therapy should be **initiated before the development of clinical signs of hypocalcemia.**

        b. Supplementation with active vitamin D metabolites should be started prior to surgery in patients with severe hypercalcemia, traditionally defined as having a serum tCa concentration of 14.0 mg/dL (3.5 mmol/L) or greater.

        c. Supplementation with active vitamin D metabolites will be necessary in those in which postsurgical calcium concentration rapidly declines to below the reference range.

C. The goal of therapy is to increase serum iCa concentration to alleviate clinical signs of hypocalcemia and to minimize the likelihood of developing hypercalcemia. The target serum iCa concentration is just below or in the lower part of the reference range.

D. **Acute management** of hypocalcemia includes treatment with **intravenously administered calcium salts:**

    1. Calcium gluconate is the calcium salt of choice because it is nonirritating if injected perivascularly.

    2. The **heart rate and electrocardiogram should be monitored during infusion of calcium salts.** Bradycardia may signal the onset of cardiotoxicity from rapid infusion of calcium.

E. Subacute management of hypocalcemia:

    1. The **initial calcium injection will decrease signs of hypocalcemia for 1–12 h.**

    2. **Vitamin D metabolites such as calcitriol should be administered as soon as possible if hypocalcemia is expected to be protracted** (e.g., primary hypoparathyroidism, parathyroid gland atrophy from longstanding hypercalcemia). Calcitriol will exert initial effects on the intestine within 3–4 h but **maximal effects to enhance intestinal absorption of calcium will take several days.**

    3. **Continuous intravenous calcium infusion is recommended** until oral medications provide control of serum calcium concentration.

    4. **Subcutaneous administration of calcium salts should not be given, even if diluted.** Some dogs exhibit severe reactions to the subcutaneous administration of calcium salts, resulting in euthanasia.

Table 31.2 Treatment of hypocalcemia.

Drug	Preparation	Calcium content	Dose	Comment
Parenteral calcium*				
Calcium gluconate	10% solution	9.3 mg of Ca/mL	a. Slow IV to effect (0.5–1.5 mL/kg IV)	For acute treatment to stop clinical signs of hypocalcemia; stop if bradycardia or shortened QT interval occurs
			b. 5–15 mg/kg/h IV	Infusion to maintain normal Ca
				SQ calcium salts—can cause severe skin necrosis/mineralization even when diluted. It is best NOT to give any calcium salts SQ
Calcium chloride	10% solution	27.2 mg of Ca/mL	5–15 mg/kg/h IV	Only given IV as extremely caustic perivascularly
Oral calcium**				
Calcium carbonate	Many sizes	40% tablet	25–50 mg/kg/day	Most common calcium supplement
Calcium lactate	325, 650 mg tablets	13% tablet		Higher doses (e.g., 100 mg/kg/day) divided with meals may be required for lactating bitches following recovery from clinical eclampsia
Calcium chloride	Powder	27.2%		May cause gastric irritation
Calcium gluconate	Many sizes	10%		
Vitamin D				Time for maximal effect to occur	Time for toxicity effect to resolve
Vitamin D_2 (ergocalciferol)***			Initial: 4000–6000 U/kg/day; maintenance: 1000–2000 U/kg once daily to once weekly	5–21 days	1–18 weeks. Although less expensive then calcitriol, it has longer time to effect and greater risk of hypercalcemia
1,25-$(OH)_2$ D_3 (calcitriol)***			Initial: 20–30 ng/kg/day for 3–4 days; maintenance: 5–15 ng/kg/day	1–4 days	2–14 days Supplement of choice

*Do not mix calcium solution with bicarbonate-containing fluids as precipitation may occur.
**Calculate dose on elemental calcium content.
***For treatment of hypoparathyroidism.

F.   **Chronic management** of hypocalcemia:
1.   **Supplemental calcium is administered orally. Calcium carbonate** is most commonly used.
2.   **Vitamin D metabolite supplementation** is necessary for patients with primary hypoparathyroidism or postoperative hypocalcemia that fails to resolve spontaneously:
   a.   **Ergocalciferol** is inexpensive, but high doses are necessary, and **time to effect is long.** Hypercalcemia frequently develops during its use, due to its high lipid solubility and time required to saturate fat stores, and is prolonged even after discontinuation of supplementation.
   b.   **Calcitriol** is the active vitamin D metabolite and the **supplement of choice.** Calcitriol has a short half-life with a rapid onset of action. If hypercalcemia occurs due to overdose, the hypercalcemia quickly subsides after withdrawal of calcitriol.
   c.   **The goal for optimal concentration of circulating calcium is to be slightly lower than the normal range:**
      1)   This helps protect the kidneys.
      2)   PTH normally removes calcium from renal tubular fluid.
      3)   At higher circulating calcium concentrations, more calcium is filtered at any level of glomerular filtration rate (GFR), providing more tubular exposure to calcium and the calcium is not removed in the absence of PTH.
      4)   Hypercalciuria poses a risk for development of renal dysfunction and CKD as well as urinary stone formation.
G.   **Periods of hypocalcemia and hypercalcemia often occur sporadically during initial management** of those with chronic hypocalcemia, as dose adjustments are made in an attempt to achieve optimal circulating calcium concentrations:
1.   **Daily measurement of circulating calcium concentration is necessary** during initial stabilization. iCa **measurements are preferred** over tCa during acute management.
2.   **Weekly serum calcium measurement is sufficient during maintenance therapy until the target serum calcium concentration has been maintained.** Use of serum tCa is often adequate to make clinical decisions during this time, especially if serum ionized and tCa concentrations have paralleled each other during earlier treatments.
3.   **Serum calcium concentration should be measured every 3 months in patients with hypoparathyroidism.** Some patients are sufficiently stable that twice yearly evaluations will suffice.
H.   **Hypercalcemia is a serious adverse side effect** of treatment that can result in renal damage or death. Owners should be aware of clinical signs of hypercalcemia (e.g., polydipsia, polyuria, anorexia, vomiting, and lethargy) and should be instructed to seek veterinary care if they occur.
I.   Patients that can maintain serum iCa concentration within the target range **can be managed successfully for years.** Calcitriol maintains serum iCa concentration in the target zone better than other vitamin D supplements.
J.   Vitamin D metabolite treatment is **gradually tapered and discontinued in dogs with postsurgical hypoparathyroidism** because the hypocalcemia is usually transient:
1.   Vitamin D compounds are typically tapered first by about 25% to see if circulating iCa remains at the desired level. If reasonable levels are maintained, a further taper of 25% is attempted.
2.   Calcium compounds are usually tapered after the decrement in vitamin D treatments have resulted in a stable level of calcemia, usually by 25% at each interval.
3.   Dogs with hypocalcemia typically require treatment for 6–12 weeks after removal of a parathyroid gland.
4.   Permanent hypoparathyroidism is likely if there is failure to maintain acceptable serum iCa concentration after the reduction of vitamin D metabolite dose at 3 months.

VII.   Prognosis
A.   **Chronic kidney disease:** The prognosis overall is guarded and dependent on appropriate therapy and response to treatment. Improvement in iCa status often accompanies optimal serum phosphorus control and supplementation with active vitamin D compounds.
B.   **Emergency and critical care:** The prognosis is dependent on treatment and response to therapy for sepsis and critical illness.

C.   **Acute pancreatitis:** The prognosis overall is dependent on the response to therapy. Hypocalcemia typically resolves as does the pancreatitis.

D.   **Diabetes mellitus:** The prognosis for resolution of hypocalcemia is unknown.

E.   **Eclampsia:** The prognosis for resolution of hypocalcemia is excellent following appropriate therapy.

F.   **Rhabdomyolysis:** Hypocalcemia typically resolves as the underlying muscle injury improves.

G.   **Small intestinal disease:** Improvement in calcium status depends on the underlying disease and response to treatment. Prognosis could be guarded to excellent depending on the underlying cause.

H.   **Alkali administration:** Prognosis for restoration of normal serum calcium is excellent following cessation of alkali treatment.

I.   **Acute reversal of chronic hypercalcemia:** The prognosis is guarded for restoration of normocalcemia without calcium-specific treatments. With appropriate therapy, prognosis is good to excellent.

J.   **Tumor lysis syndrome:** Prognosis is poor to grave due to the underlying malignancy.

K.   **Nutritional secondary hyperparathyroidism:** Prognosis is excellent if a proper diet is provided.

L.   **Drug administration:** Prognosis for restoration of normocalcemia is variable depending on the type of drug. The prognosis for survival following phosphate enema administration can be poor (depending on the magnitude of hyperphosphatemia, hypocalcemia, and renal failure).

M.   **Primary hypoparathyroidism:** Prognosis for normocalcemia and overall survival is good to excellent with appropriate therapy. Prognosis for long-term survival is lower in those that develop hypercalcemia in response to therapy with ergocalciferol (due to duration of effect of this vitamin D compound).

N.   **Ethylene glycol toxicity:** Prognosis is grave.

VIII. Prevention

A.   Feed a nutritionally complete and balanced diet to prevent the occurrence of nutritional secondary hyperparathyroidism.

B.   Limit exposure to drugs or compounds that can cause hypocalcemia (e.g., ethylene glycol, mithramycin, phosphate enemas, etc.).

C.   Ensure that females of small dog breeds with large litters receive an adequate diet with adequate calories and calcium to prevent eclampsia.

D.   Initiate vitamin D supplementation prior to parathyroid gland removal in patients with severe hypercalcemia due to parathyroid gland disease, for example, adenoma.

E.   Provide optimal serum phosphorus control in patients with chronic renal failure; calcitriol therapy for prevention/control of renal secondary hyperparathyroidism may help maintain serum iCa.

References and Further Readings

Drobatz KJ, Casey KK. Eclampsia in dogs: 31 cases (1995–1998). *J Am Vet Med Assoc* 2000;217(2):216–219.

Hess RS, Saunders HM, Van Winkle TJ, Ward CR. Concurrent disorders in dogs with diabetes mellitus: 221 cases (1993–1998). *J Am Vet Med Assoc* 2000;217(8):1166–1173.

Holowaychuk MK, Hansen BD, DeFrancesco TC, Marks SL. Ionized hypocalcemia in critically ill dogs. *J Vet Intern Med* 2009;23(3):509–513.

Hume DZ, Drobatz KJ, Hess RS. Outcome of dogs with diabetic ketoacidosis: 127 dogs (1993–2003). *J Vet Intern Med* 2006;20(3):547–555.

Russell NJ, Bond KA, Robertson ID, Parry BW, Irwin PJ. Primary hypoparathyroidism in dogs: A retrospective study of 17 cases. *Aust Vet J* 2006;84(8):285–290.

Schenck PA. Serum ionized magnesium concentrations in association with canine calcium metabolic disorders. *J Vet Intern Med* 2008;22(3):796–797.

Schenck PA and Chew DJ. Prediction of serum ionized calcium concentration by use of serum total calcium concentration in dogs. *Am J Vet Res* 2005;66(8):1330–1336.

Schenck PA and Chew DJ. Calcium: Total or ionized? *Vet Clin North Am Small Anim Pract* 2008;38(3):497–502.

Schenck PA, Chew DJ, Nagode LA, Rosol TJ. Disorders of calcium: Hypercalcemia and hypocalcemia. In: Dibartola S, ed. *Fluid Therapy in Small Animal Practice*, 3rd edn. St. Louis: Elsevier, 2006, p. 122–194.

CHAPTER 32

Hypocalcemia in Cats

Patricia A. Schenck and Dennis Chew

Pathogenesis

- Clinical signs only result when ionized calcium (iCa) falls below a critical level.
- Causes of hypocalcemia can be parathyroid independent or parathyroid dependent.
- The most common cause of chronic hypocalcemia is primary hypoparathyroidism.
- The most common cause of acute hypocalcemia in combination with clinical signs related to hypocalcemia is periparturient tetany (eclampsia).

Classical Signs

- The most common clinical signs associated with hypocalcemia are muscle tremors and fasciculations, facial rubbing, muscle cramping, stiff gait, seizures, restlessness, aggression, disorientation, and hypersensitivity.
- Anorexia and lethargy are common signs of hypocalcemia in the cat and prolapse of the third eyelid is occasionally observed with acute hypocalcemia.
- *Acute development of hypocalcemia is typically associated with severe clinical signs; there may be few clinical signs if the underlying problem is chronic.*

Diagnosis

- *Hypocalcemia is defined as a total calcium (tCa) concentration <7.0 mg/dL (1.75 mmol/L) or iCa concentration <4.5 mg/dL (1.1 mmol/L).*
- Parathyroid hormone (PTH) should be measured in conjunction with iCa measurement to determine whether PTH production is appropriate; measurement of serum 25-hydroxyvitamin D may be helpful to identify cases in which decreased intake of vitamin D is the cause of hypocalcemia.

Clinical Endocrinology of Companion Animals, First Edition. Edited by Jacquie Rand.
© 2013 John Wiley & Sons, Inc. Published 2013 by John Wiley & Sons, Inc.

Treatment

- Specific therapy depends on the cause of hypocalcemia.
- Acute symptomatic hypocalcemia requires treatment with intravenous (IV) calcium salts, to effect.
- Symptomatic subacute and chronic hypocalcemia require treatment with oral calcium salts and/or active vitamin D compounds.

Prognosis

- Prognosis depends on the underlying cause of hypocalcemia.
- Prognosis is excellent for properly treated eclampsia and good to excellent for primary hypoparathyroidism.

I. Pathogenesis
A. Serum tCa is composed of protein-bound calcium (pCa), complexed calcium (cCa), and iCa. The iCa fraction is the biologically active fraction.
B. **Hypocalcemia develops when** there is a decrease in bone mobilization of calcium, an increase in loss of calcium via urine or milk, a decrease in gastrointestinal absorption of calcium, translocation of calcium intracellularly, or a combination of these mechanisms:
    1. A decrease in serum iCa typically stimulates the synthesis and release of PTH from the parathyroid gland.
    2. PTH causes a **decrease in urinary calcium excretion** and an **increase in bone resorption.**
    3. PTH also stimulates the production of calcitriol (1,25-dihydroxyvitamin D) from 25-hydroxyvitamin D (produced in liver from vitamin D) by up-regulation of 1α-hydroxylase.
    4. Calcitriol causes an increase in vitamin D absorption in the gut and also increases bone resorption.
    5. Increased production of PTH continues if there is a continued decrease in iCa concentration or persisting hyperphosphatemia. This creates a secondary hyperparathyroidism in which PTH is elevated and serum iCa concentration is within the reference range or low.
C. **Causes of hypocalcemia** are listed in Table 32.1.
D. **Hypoalbuminemia is the most common condition associated with hypocalcemia,** but the least important. Hypocalcemia is usually mild, and there are no clinical signs of hypocalcemia.
E. **Azotemic chronic kidney disease** (CKD): Decreased calcitriol synthesis and mass law interactions of calcium with increased serum phosphorus concentration are probable causes of hypocalcemia.
F. **Emergency and critical care cases:**
    1. Low serum iCa concentration is common in the intensive care setting and is more common in septic patients.
    2. Urethral obstruction, eclampsia, sepsis, systemic inflammatory response syndrome, hypomagnesemia, and blood transfusions have been associated with hypocalcemia. Cardiopulmonary resuscitation may also result in hypocalcemia.
G. **Pancreatitis:** Mechanisms of low iCa include sequestration of calcium into peripancreatic fat (saponification), increased free fatty acids, increased calcitonin, and PTH resistance or deficit resulting from hypomagnesemia.
H. **Eclampsia:** Mechanisms for hypocalcemia include a poor dietary source of calcium, loss of calcium during lactation, and/or abnormal parathyroid gland function.
I. **Urethral obstruction:** Low serum iCa concentration is not a consequence of deficient secretion of PTH, nor does it appear related to serum concentrations of 25-hydroxycholecalciferol. It likely is a consequence of increased serum phosphorus concentration.
J. **Rhabdomyolysis or soft tissue trauma:** Hypocalcemia usually occurs as a consequence of translocation of calcium into damaged muscles.
K. **Severe small intestinal disease:** Mechanisms of hypocalcemia include calcium/fatty acid complexes in the intestinal lumen that decrease intestinal calcium absorption. Malabsorption of vitamin D can also lead to hypovitaminosis D and decreased intestinal calcium absorption.

Table 32.1 Causes of hypocalcemia in the cat.

Most common	Occasional	Uncommon
Hypoalbuminemia	Soft tissue trauma or rhabdomyolysis	Lab error
Chronic renal failure	Hypoparathyroidism	Improper anticoagulant (EDTA)
Puerperal tetany (eclampsia)	Ethylene glycol intoxication	Infarction of parathyroid gland
Acute kidney failure	Phosphate enema	adenoma
Acute pancreatitis	Post-NaHCO$_3$ administration	Rapid infusion of phosphate
Undefined		Intestinal malabsorption or severe starvation
		Hypovitaminosis D
		Blood transfusion with citrated anticoagulant

L. **Alkali administration:** Results in increased protein binding of calcium, thereby decreasing the iCa fraction.
M. **Acute reversal of chronic hypercalcemia:** This happens most frequently following removal of a parathyroid adenoma that has caused primary hyperparathyroidism and atrophy of nontumorous parathyroid tissue.
N. **Tumor lysis syndrome:** Occurs when there is rapid destruction of tumor cells following chemotherapy. Hypocalcemia develops when calcium-phosphate salts are deposited into soft tissues.
O. **Drug administration can cause hypocalcemia:**
   1. Drugs that can induce hypocalcemia include enrofloxacin, mithramycin, bisphosphonates, and phosphate enemas.
P. **Phosphate enemas:** Result in hypocalcemia after rapid absorption of phosphate and subsequent mass law interaction with serum calcium. They should not be used in cats as they are too dangerous, especially if they are sick before the enema.
Q. **Ethylene glycol toxicity:** Oxalate metabolites can chelate calcium and become deposited in soft tissues, resulting in hypocalcemia.
R. **Nutritional secondary hyperparathyroidism:** Associated with lack of sufficient dietary vitamin D or low calcium/high phosphorus concentrations in the diet. This most commonly occurs in cats fed mainly meat diets (cow's milk provides insufficient calcium to correct imbalance).
S. **Primary hypoparathyroidism:** Surgical removal or injury to the parathyroid glands during thyroidectomy to correct hyperthyroidism is the most common cause in cats. Idiopathic chronic inflammation of parathyroid tissue occurs sporadically.
T. **Vitamin D–dependant rickets:** Type 2 is a genetic condition associated with down-regulation of the function or numbers of vitamin D receptors in the target tissues (resulting in high circulating calcitriol). Type 1 is associated with a genetic defect in the metabolic activation of 25(OH) vitamin to the most active vitamin D metabolite 1,25-dihydroxyvitamin D, resulting in low circulating calcitriol.

II. Signalment
A. **Primary hypoparathyroidism:** Occurs more often in male cats. Siamese cats may be overrepresented.
B. Other causes of hypocalcemia: There does not appear to be any age-, sex-, or breed-related predispositions for these disorders.

III. Clinical Signs
A. **Decreased serum iCa concentration increases excitability of neuromuscular tissue, which accounts for many of the clinical signs of hypocalcemia:**
   1. The most common clinical signs associated with hypocalcemia are **muscle tremors and fasciculations,** facial rubbing, muscle cramping, stiff gait, seizures, restlessness, aggression, disorientation, and hypersensitivity:
      a. Neuromuscular signs in cats with **primary hypoparathyroidism** are similar to those in dogs. **Anorexia and lethargy** are more common in cats than in dogs, but seizures have not been reported to be induced by excitement, as occurs in dogs.

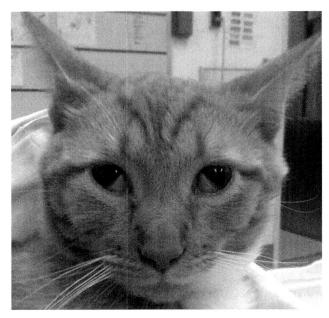

Figure 32.1 Bilateral prolapse of the nictitans often occurs during the development of acute hypocalcemia in the cat. (Courtesy of Dr. Philip Lerche, The Ohio State University College of Veterinary Medicine.)

2. Other clinical signs of hypocalcemia may include **panting, pyrexia, lethargy,** depression, anorexia, tachycardia, and posterior lenticular cataracts. In contrast to dogs, **prolapse of the third eyelid** is occasionally observed in cats with acute hypocalcemia, but is not usually seen with chronic hypocalcemia (Figure 32.1).

3. Uncommon clinical signs of hypocalcemia include polyuria, polydipsia, hypotension, respiratory arrest, or death.

4. Clinical signs of acute postoperative hypocalcemia following thyroidectomy are similar in dogs and cats:

    a. Tetany or facial twitching has not been observed in cats after thyroidectomy until serum tCa concentration is <6.9 mg/dL (1.7 mmol/L).

B. **Clinical signs usually do not occur until serum tCa is <6.5 mg/dL (1.62 mmol/L).** Some patients (especially those in CKD) may not show clinical signs of hypocalcemia until serum tCa concentration is <5.0 mg/dL (1.25 mmol/L), likely a consequence of CKD-associated acidosis that shifts calcium from protein bound stores so that more exists in the ionized form:

1. Acute development of hypocalcemia is typically associated with severe clinical signs.

2. If the underlying problem has been chronic and there has been sufficient time for physiologic adaptation, then there may be few clinical signs of hypocalcemia.

3. Clinical signs of hypocalcemia are uncommon when hypocalcemia occurs in association with renal secondary hyperparathyroidism.

C. Electrolyte and acid-base abnormalities can impact hypocalcemia:

1. Exercise or excitement associated with respiratory alkalosis may cause hypocalcemia.

2. Rapid infusion of alkali to correct metabolic acidosis can cause seizures in those with marginal hypocalcemia due to increased binding of calcium at the expense of iCa.

3. Correction of hypokalemia in cats with concurrent hypocalcemia can precipitate the onset of clinical signs of hypocalcemia.

IV. Diagnosis (see Figure 31.4, Diagnostic algorithm for hypocalcemia)

A. **Definition of hypocalcemia:**

1. Using serum **tCa,** hypocalcemia in cats is usually defined as a concentration <7.0 mg/dL (1.75 mmol/L).

2. Using serum iCa, hypocalcemia is usually defined as a concentration <4.5 mg/dL (1.1 mmol/L).

3. There can be unpredictable discordance between serum tCa and serum iCa measurements. In one study, 49% of sick cats were classified as hypocalcemic based on serum tCa concentration. When iCa was measured, only 27% were hypocalcemic. **Hypocalcemia is usually overestimated in cats when serum tCa is used.**

4. Hypocalcemia based on serum iCa is relatively common and was observed in 27% of sick cats in one study.

B. **Measurement of calcium:**

1. Trivial decreases in serum tCa are common and may not be persistent. Pursuit of a specific diagnosis in these instances is not warranted.

2. Serum iCa concentration should be measured when a decrease in serum tCa is persistent. Ideally, serum iCa should also be measured in all cases of azotemic CKD. It is debatable if iCa should be determined in patients with mild decreases in total serum calcium associated with hypoalbuminemia.

3. Do not directly compare serum iCa results to those obtained from heparinized plasma or whole blood (when using a blood gas analyzer or point-of-care analyzer). The iCa concentration is lower in heparinized plasma or whole blood than in serum.

4. **Do not use EDTA plasma for collection of blood for iCa measurement.** EDTA chelates calcium, and EDTA plasma will yield falsely low iCa results.

5. In cats, serum tCa is normally 8.0–10.5 mg/dL (2.0–2.6 mmol/L), and serum iCa is normally 4.5–5.5 mg/dL (1.1–1.4 mmol/L).

6. If serum tCa is <6.0 mg/dL (1.5 mmol/L) or iCa is <3.2 mg/dL (0.8 mmol/L), clinical signs are usually present.

7. To convert mmol/L to mg/dL, multiply mmol/L by 4.

C. **PTH should be measured** in conjunction with iCa measurement in patients with chronically low tCa concentrations to determine whether PTH production is appropriate:

1. **Patients with low iCa and low PTH concentrations have absolute hypoparathyroidism.** If serum iCa is low and PTH is within the reference range, the PTH response is inappropriate (sometimes referred to as "relative hypoparathyroidism"), as PTH is expected to be elevated with low iCa.

2. **Hypocalcemia associated with increased serum PTH is classified as parathyroid-independent hypocalcemia.** In these cases, hypocalcemia exists from redistribution of calcium into other body spaces, excess phosphorus effects, or from deficiencies of vitamin D or dietary calcium.

D. **Measurement of serum 25-hydroxyvitamin D** may be helpful to identify cases in which decreased intake or malabsorption of vitamin D is the cause of hypocalcemia.

E. **Calcitriol measurement** may be useful to differentiate vitamin D resistant rickets from those with azotemia CKD in patients with normal serum 25-hydroxyvitamin D concentration:

1. Vitamin D–dependent rickets type 2 is characterized by hypocalcemia, secondary hyperparathyroidism, normal 25-hydroxyvitamin D, high plasma calcitriol concentrations, and clinical signs of rickets.

2. Type 1 rickets is characterized by similar findings except that there are low concentrations of calcitriol indicative of an activation defect involving renal 1-alpha-hydroxylase that normally facilitates conversion of 25-hydroxyvitamin D to 1,25-dihydroxyvitamin D.

F. Causes of hypocalcemia are listed in Table 32.1. Identification of the underlying cause of hypocalcemia requires appropriate diagnostic testing. Most cases of hypocalcemia are parathyroid independent, that is, PTH concentration is appropriately increased.

G. **Hypoalbuminemia is the most common cause of hypocalcemia,** but is usually mild and not associated with clinical signs of hypocalcemia.

H. **Azotemic kidney disease is associated with hypocalcemia:**

1. Most cats with azotemic CKD and decreased serum iCa concentration do not show clinical signs of hypocalcemia.

2. In cats with azotemic CKD, about 15% were hypocalcemic based on serum tCa concentration. Based on iCa concentration, 14% of cats with moderate azotemic CKD and 56% with advanced azotemic CKD had hypocalcemia. Hypocalcemia is underappreciated when based on results of tCa measurement, especially with advancing azotemia.

3. Acute renal failure and postrenal failure results in hypocalcemia that is more likely to be symptomatic. It is difficult in these clinical settings to determine with certainty which signs are specifically due to hypocalcemia, as other electrolyte and acid-base disturbances often occur concomitantly.

I. **Emergency and critical care cases:**
   1. Low serum iCa concentration is common in severely ill cats, especially septic patients, or cats with urethral obstruction, eclampsia, sepsis, systemic inflammatory response syndrome, and hypomagnesemia, or following blood transfusions or cardiopulmonary resuscitation.

J. **Acute pancreatitis** may be associated with hypocalcemia:
   1. In cats with acute pancreatitis, iCa was low in 61% of cats in one study.
   2. Pansteatitis has been reported to create severe hypocalcemia in a cat from similar mechanisms.

K. **Puerperal (periparturient) tetany (eclampsia)** is rare in cats which more commonly exhibit signs during the last 3 weeks of pregnancy:
   1. Signs of **depression, weakness, tachypnea,** and **mild muscle tremors** are most common; vomiting and anorexia are less common, and prolapse of the third eyelid occurs in some cats. Hypothermia (instead of hyperthermia as seen in dogs) is observed.

L. **Urethral obstruction:** Hypocalcemia was present in **34% of cats** with urethral obstruction in one study:
   1. Serum iCa was >3.2 but <4.0 mg/dL (>0.8 but <1.0 mmol/L) in 14% and ≤3.2 mg/dL (≤0.8 mmol/L) in 6% of cats with urethral obstruction in one study.
   2. Hypocalcemia is likely to develop in cats that have hyperkalemia and metabolic acidosis.
   3. Alkalinizing infusions to correct metabolic acidosis are often considered for treatment of cats with urethral obstruction, but these can decrease both tCa and iCa concentrations which can be dangerous as tetany can develop, as well as increasing risk for respiratory and cardiac collapse in those with marginal iCa at presentation.

M. **Rhabdomyolysis** may be associated with hypocalcemia, but clinical signs are uncommon.

N. **Small intestinal disease** may be associated with hypocalcemia:
   1. Protein-losing enteropathy is also associated with low iCa and low ionized magnesium.
   2. Serum PTH is typically elevated in these cases, and serum 25-hydroxyvitamin D is low.

O. **Alkali (sodium bicarbonate) administration** can result in hypocalcemia:
   1. Twitching has been observed on rare occasion during infusion of sodium bicarbonate solutions to cats with urethral obstruction.

P. **Acute reversal of chronic hypercalcemia.**

Q. **Tumor lysis syndrome.**

R. **Drug administration can cause hypocalcemia including** enrofloxacin, mithramycin, and bisphosphonates.

S. **Phosphate enemas** can cause rapid onset of hypocalcemia associated with rapid absorption of phosphorus, especially if the cat is dehydrated before the enema.

T. Following **ethylene glycol ingestion,** seizures may be noted within hours of ingestion.

U. **Nutritional secondary hyperparathyroidism is associated with diets providing excess phosphate, insufficient calcium or both:**
   1. Serum iCa concentration typically is low, with an elevation in PTH concentration.
   2. Nutritional secondary hyperparathyroidism tends to cause osteopenia of the long bones and vertebrae. A stiff gait, bone pain, and multiple bone fractures are common.
   3. History of feeding of BARF (biologically appropriate raw food or bones and raw food) and other unbalanced homemade diets, which makes the occurrence of nutritional secondary hyperparathyroidism more likely.
   4. In six young cats with nutritional secondary hyperparathyroidism, serum iCa and phosphorus concentrations were low. Calcitriol concentration was increased in most, and serum 25-hydroxyvitamin D concentration was low. PTH concentration was increased in all cats. These cats had been fed either meat only, meat combined with vegetables, or vegetables only. Dietary calcium intake was less than one-tenth of the minimal nutritional requirement. An unfavorable calcium to phosphorus ratio existed for all diets.

V. **Primary hypoparathyroidism** is an absolute or relative deficiency of PTH secretion that may be permanent or transient. Hypoparathyroidism is rare in cats:

   1. Since magnesium status can impact PTH secretion, measurement of ionized magnesium is recommended in cases of hypoparathyroidism. A large percentage of cats with primary hypoparathyroidism (52%) exhibit low or marginal ionized magnesium concentration.
   2. Serum tCa concentration is usually <6.5 mg/dL (1.62 mmol/L) and most have hyperphosphatemia. Mean serum iCa concentration in hypoparathyroid cats was 2.9 mg/dL (0.72 mmol/L) in one study (reference range 4–5.6 mg/dL; 1.0–1.4 mmol/L).
   3. Primary hypoparathyroidism is characterized by low serum iCa concentration with an inappropriately low PTH concentration.
   4. Primary hypoparathyroidism requires lifelong treatment with calcium and vitamin D supplementation.

V. Differential Diagnosis

A. **Other causes of neuromuscular clinical signs** similar to those produced by hypocalcemia include primary brain disease (epilepsy, brain tumors, encephalitis, etc.), glycogen storage disorders, hepatic encephalopathy, toxins (strychnine, metaldehyde, etc.), musculoskeletal disorders (myopathies, arthritis, hip dysplasia, etc.).

VI. Treatment

A. For general treatment for hypocalcemia including doses of drugs, please refer to Table 31.2, Treatment of hypocalcemia.

B. **Treatment must be individualized based on the severity of clinical signs, magnitude of hypocalcemia, rapidity of development of hypocalcemia, and the trend of serial serum calcium measurements:**

   1. **Puerperal tetany** is the condition that most often requires acute correction of hypocalcemia.
   2. Cats respond to parenteral calcium gluconate initially and to oral calcium supplementation throughout gestation and lactation.
   3. **Primary hypoparathyroidism** is the only condition requiring both acute and long-term therapy. Both calcium and vitamin D supplementation are usually necessary. Magnesium supplementation may also be beneficial if serum ionized magnesium concentration was initially low.
   4. Hypocalcemia should be anticipated in cats undergoing **parathyroidectomy for treatment of parathyroid adenoma:**
      a. Therapy should be initiated before the development of clinical signs of hypocalcemia.
      b. Supplementation with active vitamin D metabolites should be started prior to surgery in patients with severe hypercalcemia (see Table 31.2, page 324 for dose).

C. The goal of therapy is to increase serum calcium concentration to alleviate clinical signs of hypocalcemia and to minimize the likelihood of developing hypercalcemia.

D. **Acute management of hypocalcemia includes treatment with intravenously administered calcium salts** (see Table 31.2, page 324 for dose):

   1. Calcium gluconate is the calcium salt of choice because it is nonirritating if injected perivascularly.
   2. **Subcutaneous administration of calcium salts should not be given,** even if diluted, as reactions severe enough to cause death or warrant euthanasia are known to occur in dogs and severe calcinosis has been described in one cat.
   3. The heart rate and electrocardiogram should be monitored during infusion of calcium salts. Bradycardia may signal the onset of cardiotoxicity from rapid infusion of calcium.

E. **Subacute management of hypocalcemia:**

   1. The initial injection of calcium will decrease signs of hypocalcemia for 1–12 h.
   2. Vitamin D metabolites such as calcitriol should be administered as soon as possible (see Table 31.2). Calcitriol will exert initial effects on the intestine within 3–4 h but maximal effects of enhanced calcium absorption may be exerted within 1–4 days.
   3. Continuous IV infusion of calcium is recommended until oral medications provide control of serum calcium concentration.

F. **Chronic management of hypocalcemia:**

   1. Supplemental calcium is administered orally. Calcium carbonate is most commonly used (see Table 31.2, Treatment of hypocalcemia, for doses of calcium products).

2. Vitamin D supplementation is necessary for patients with primary hypoparathyroidism or postoperative hypocalcemia that fails to resolve spontaneously (see Table 31.2, Treatment of hypocalcemia, for doses of vitamin D products):

    a. Ergocalciferol is inexpensive, but high doses are necessary, and time to effect is long. Ergocalciferol is highly lipid soluble and undergoes extensive storage in fat. Once fat is saturated with this compound, the risk of the development of hypercalcemia greatly increases if the clinician becomes impatient and continues to escalate the dose because of suboptimal levels of circulating calcium. If overdosed, hypercalcemia is often prolonged (weeks to months).

    b. Calcitriol is the active vitamin D metabolite and the supplement of choice. Calcitriol has a short half-life in the circulation with a rapid onset of action. If hypercalcemia occurs due to overdose, the hypercalcemia quickly subsides after withdrawal of calcitriol since its biological effect half life is several days.

G. Periods of hypocalcemia and hypercalcemia occur sporadically during initial management of hypocalcemia:

    1. **Daily measurement of serum tCa concentration during stabilization is necessary**; weekly serum calcium measurement is sufficient during maintenance therapy until the target serum calcium concentration has been maintained. Serum calcium concentration should be measured every 3 months in patients with hypoparathyroidism.

H. Hypercalcemia is a serious adverse side effect of treatment that can result in renal damage or death. Owners should be aware of clinical signs of hypercalcemia (anorexia, vomiting, lethargy, polydipsia, polyuria).

I. Patients that can maintain serum iCa concentration within the target range can be managed successfully for years:

    1. Management with calcitriol is more successful in maintaining serum iCa concentration in the target zone than are other vitamin D supplements.

J. Vitamin D metabolite treatment is gradually tapered and discontinued in cats with postsurgical hypoparathyroidism because the hypocalcemia is usually transient:

    1. Most cats are able to maintain normal serum iCa concentrations 2 weeks after thyroidectomy, although some may take as long as 3 months.

    2. Permanent hypoparathyroidism is likely if there is failure to maintain acceptable serum iCa concentration after the reduction of vitamin D metabolite dose at 3 months.

VII. Prognosis

A. **Chronic kidney disease:** The prognosis overall is guarded and dependent on appropriate therapy and response to treatment. Improvement in iCa status often accompanies optimal serum phosphorus control and supplementation with active vitamin D compounds.

B. **Emergency and critical care cases:** The prognosis is dependent on treatment and response to therapy for sepsis and critical illness.

C. **Acute pancreatitis:** The prognosis overall is dependent on the response to therapy. Hypocalcemia typically resolves as the pancreatitis resolves.

D. **Urethral obstruction:** Most cats survive with appropriate therapy for urethral obstruction.

E. **Eclampsia:** The prognosis for resolution of hypocalcemia is excellent following appropriate therapy.

F. **Rhabdomyolysis:** Hypocalcemia typically resolves as the underlying muscle injury improves.

G. **Small intestinal disease:** Improvement in calcium status depends on the underlying disease and response to treatment. Prognosis could be guarded to excellent depending on the underlying cause.

H. **Alkali administration:** Prognosis for restoration of normal serum calcium is excellent following cessation of alkali treatment.

I. **Acute reversal of chronic hypercalcemia:** The prognosis is guarded for restoration of normocalcemia without calcium-specific treatments. With appropriate therapy, prognosis is good to excellent.

J. **Tumor lysis syndrome:** Prognosis is poor to grave due to the underlying malignancy.

K. **Nutritional secondary hyperparathyroidism:** Prognosis is excellent if a proper diet is provided, although skeletal deformity may persist and predispose to constipation.

L. **Drug administration:** Prognosis for restoration of normocalcemia is variable depending on the type of drug. The prognosis following phosphate enema administration can be poor.

M.   **Primary hypoparathyroidism:** Prognosis for normocalcemia is good to excellent with appropriate therapy. Prognosis is lower in those that develop hypercalcemia in response to therapy with ergocalciferol.

N.   **Ethylene glycol toxicity:** Prognosis is grave.

VIII. Prevention

A.   Feed a nutritionally complete and balanced diet to prevent the occurrence of nutritional secondary hyperparathyroidism.

B.   Limit exposure to drugs or compounds that can cause hypocalcemia (ethylene glycol, mithramycin, phosphate enemas, etc.).

C.   Make sure that female cats receive a balanced diet with adequate calories and calcium during the last 3 weeks of pregnancy to prevent eclampsia.

D.   Initiate vitamin D supplementation prior to parathyroid gland removal in those patients with severe hypercalcemia to prevent development of hypocalcemia after removal of a parathyroid adenoma.

E.   Provide optimal serum phosphorus control in patients with azotemic CKD; calcitriol therapy for prevention/control of renal secondary hyperparathyroidism may help maintain serum iCa.

References and Further Readings

Drobatz KJ, Hughes D. Concentration of ionized calcium in plasma from cats with urethral obstruction. *J Am Vet Med Assoc* 1997;211(11):1392–1395.

Drobatz KJ, Ward C, Graham P, Hughes D. Serum concentrations of parathyroid hormone and 25-OH vitamin D_3 in cats with urethral obstruction. *J Vet Emerg Crit Care* 2005;15(3):179–184.

Fascetti AJ, Hickman MA. Preparturient hypocalcemia in four cats. *J Am Vet Med Assoc* 1999;215(8):1127–1129.

Kimmel SE, Washabau RJ, Drobatz KJ. Incidence and prognostic value of low plasma ionized calcium concentration in cats with acute pancreatitis: 46 cases (1996–1998). *J Am Vet Med Assoc* 2001;219(8):1105–1109.

Naan EC, Kirpensteijn J, Kooistra HS, Peeters ME. Results of thyroidectomy in 101 cats with hyperthyroidism. *Vet Surg* 2006;35(3):287–293.

Schenck PA. Serum ionized magnesium concentrations in association with feline calcium metabolic disorders. *J Vet Intern Med* 2008;22(3):797.

Schenck PA and Chew DJ. Calcium: Total or ionized? *Vet Clin North Am Small Anim Pract* 2008;38(3):497–502.

Schenck PA and Chew DJ. Prediction of serum ionized calcium concentration by serum total calcium concentration in cats. *Can J Vet Res* 2010;74 (3):209–213.

Schenck PA, Chew DJ, and Behrend EN. Updates on hypercalcemic disorders. In: August J, ed. *Consultations in Feline Internal Medicine*, St. Louis: Elsevier. 2005, pp. 157–168.

Schenck PA, Chew DJ, Nagode LA, Rosol TJ. Disorders of calcium: Hypercalcemia and hypocalcemia. In: Dibartola S, ed. *Fluid Therapy in Small Animal Practice*, 3rd edn. St. Louis: Elsevier. 2006, pp. 122–194.

Tomsa K, Glaus T, Hauser B, Fluckiger M, Arnold P, Wess G, Reusch C. Nutritional secondary hyperparathyroidism in six cats. *J Small Anim Pract* 1999;40(11):533–539.

Zini E, Hauser B, Ossent P, Dennler R, Glaus TM. Pansteatitis and severe hypocalcaemia in a cat. *J Feline Med Surg* 2007;9(2):168–171.

CHAPTER 33

Hypocalcemia in Other Species

Michael Stanford, John Keen and Michelle L. Campbell-Ward

Hypocalcemia in Horses

Pathogenesis

- Signs of hypocalcemia are due to derangements in the ionized fraction of total plasma calcium.
- Parathyroid hormone (PTH) is the most important hormone regulating calcium levels.
- The most common causes of hypocalcemia are lactation, gastrointestinal disease, and strenuous exercise.

Classical Signs

- Muscle fasciculations and/or muscle stiffness/tetany.
- Synchronous diaphragmatic flutter/thumps.
- Smooth muscle dysfunction (e.g., gastrointestinal ileus).
- Seizures or coma if severe and prolonged.

Diagnosis

- Clinical signs.
- Low plasma ionized calcium (<1.5 mmol/L) or total calcium (<2.6 mmol/L).

Treatment

- Intravenous calcium borogluconate to effect.
- Oral calcium supplementation long term.

I. Pathogenesis
A. Calcium distribution and control mechanisms:
   1. **Intracompartmental distribution.**
   Only **0.1% of total body calcium** is in **extracellular fluid**. The rest is found in the **skeleton (99%)** or intracellular compartments (0.9%). Of the calcium portion in plasma, approximately **40–45% is bound**

Clinical Endocrinology of Companion Animals, First Edition. Edited by Jacquie Rand.
© 2013 John Wiley & Sons, Inc. Published 2013 by John Wiley & Sons, Inc.

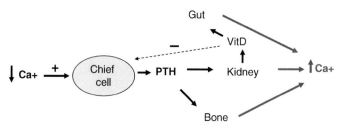

Figure 33.1 Diagram showing the crucial role of parathyroid hormone (PTH) in the face of hypocalcemia in the horse. Calcium sensors in the chief cells of the parathyroid gland sense low ionized calcium levels thereby increasing PTH secretion. PTH effect is mainly not only on the kidney to increase calcium absorption but also on bone to effect release of calcium and on the gut (via increased activation of Vitamin D) to effect increased absorption.

to anionic proteins (mainly albumin), **5% is complexed with small anions** (e.g., lactate), and **55–60% is ionized.** The ionized form is the biologically active form therefore it is **derangements to ionized calcium levels rather than the total plasma calcium that lead to clinical signs of hypocalcemia.**

2. Control of calcium levels.

As in other species, calcium is controlled by three hormones: **PTH** and **vitamin D** which aim to increase ionized calcium levels (Figure 33.1) and **calcitonin** which aims to lower calcium levels. In **horses, PTH is of primary importance** and consequently most is known about this hormone. Vitamin D is thought to have minor importance in the horse while little is known about calcitonin. Key features of calcium homeostasis in the horse are:

    a. The kidney is the major site for control of calcium and phosphorous levels and the site of vitamin D activation. Large amounts of calcium are excreted through the urinary tract in normal horses. **PTH increases calcium resorption** and **decreases phosphate resorption.**

    b. **Calcium extraction from the diet,** which occurs mainly in the proximal small intestine, is **very efficient** in horses.

    c. **Vitamin D** appears to have **minimal regulatory effect** on calcium absorption from the gut in the horse.

    d. Dietary constituents such as phosphorous and oxalate can affect calcium balance long term by impairing gut absorption.

B. **Causes of hypocalcemia:**

There are many causes of hypocalcemia in the horse including:

    1. **Prolonged exercise**—low calcium may be due to losses in sweat or due to respiratory and/or metabolic alkalosis:

        a. These conditions are most likely to occur in endurance type events or following exertion during warm weather conditions.

    2. **Lactation:** due to calcium sequestration in the milk.

    3. **Gastrointestinal diseases** including colitis:

        a. Hypocalcemia is probably due to a combination of electrolyte losses in the gastrointestinal tract along with the effect of sepsis and endotoxemia.

    4. **Sepsis/systemic inflammatory response syndrome/endotoxemia:**

        a. The pathophysiological mechanisms causing hypocalcemia with this syndrome are largely obscure, but are possibly due to interstitial/intracellular sequestration of calcium or derangements in the hormones controlling calcium (e.g., impaired PTH secretion).

    5. **Post transport:** the pathophysiology of hypocalcemia under these circumstances is obscure.

    6. **Hypoparathyroidism**—PTH is an important hormone governing acute calcium balance:

        a. Lack of PTH activity reduces calcium resorption from the renal tubules, reduces bone mobilization, and affects gut uptake of calcium via vitamin D. The net result is low ionized calcium.

        b. This condition may be a **primary parathyroid problem** or secondary to **low plasma magnesium.**

    7. **Severe rhabdomyolysis:** may cause calcium sequestration into degenerating cells, reducing plasma ionized calcium levels.

8. **Any condition causing alkalosis:** this increases calcium binding to anionic proteins, causing a reduction in ionized calcium.

9. **High dietary phosphorous or oxalates:** these may antagonize calcium uptake from the gastrointestinal tract.

10. **Low serum albumin** reduces the total calcium (40–45% of total calcium is bound to albumin) but **does not affect the ionized level** unless there are other processes concurrently affecting ionized levels.

C. **Effects of hypocalcemia:**

Extracellular ionized calcium is important for **stabilizing cell membranes of excitable cells such as nerve and skeletal or cardiac muscle;** the effects of acute **hypocalcemia** are therefore **increased excitability/activity** in such tissues. In contrast, extracellular calcium is essential for **contraction of smooth muscle;** therefore, hypocalcemia leads to **impaired smooth muscle contractility.** Chronic calcium deficiency, a much rarer condition in the horse, leads to abnormalities in bone and cartilage.

D. Pathogenesis of **synchronous diaphragmatic flutter/"thumps":** calcium, along with other cations, antagonize sodium permeability through cell membrane ion channels. Therefore in **hypocalcemia,** cell membranes, including those of **neurons, become hyperexcitable.** Since the phrenic nerve courses over the right atrium, **contraction of the heart leads to rhythmic stimulation of the phrenic nerve** and therefore diaphragm twitching in synchrony with the heart beat. Other ion (e.g., magnesium) and fluid deficits may contribute to this effect. Clinically, there is twitching of the flank and often a sound is audible (hence the term "thumps").

II. Signalment

There is no known breed or age predisposition for hypocalcemia. The disorder is seen more frequently however in **lactating mares.**

III. Clinical Signs

A. **Acute hypocalcemia:**

Clinical signs of acute hypocalcemia are **very varied** and depend on the degree of hypocalcemia as well as the chronicity. They include effects on the following:

1. **Skeletal muscle:**
   a. Increased muscle tone including **trismus** (spasm of masticatory muscles—"lockjaw").
   b. **Gait abnormalities:**
      1) **Stiff, stilted,** sometimes hypermetric gait.
      2) Hind limb ataxia.
   c. **Muscle fasciculations** (especially the temporal, masseter, and triceps muscles).
2. **Cardiac muscle:**
   a. Tachycardia.
   b. Cardiac arrhythmias.
3. **Neurological system:**
   a. Synchronous diaphragmatic flutter (="thumps").
   b. Convulsions/seizures.
   c. Coma.
4. **Smooth muscle:**
   a. Dysphagia.
   b. Ileus.
5. **Other:**
   a. Salivation.
   b. Anxiety.
   c. Profuse sweating.
   d. Elevated body temperature.
   e. Death.

B. **Chronic hypocalcemia/calcium deficiency:**

Clinical signs of chronic calcium deficiency are considerably rarer and comprise **skeletal abnormalities** such as **lameness** and increased predisposition to **fracture.** Note that calcium levels measured in the blood may

Table 33.1 Likely degree of hypocalcemia in the horse based on the severity of clinical signs (Ca$_{tot}$ = total calcium; Ca$_i$ = ionized calcium).

Ca$_{tot}$ (mmol/L)	Ca$_i$ (mmol/L)	Severity of clinical signs
2–2.6	1.1–1.5	MILD: increased excitability
1.25–2	0.7–1.1	MODERATE: tetanic spasms and incoordination
<1.25	<0.7	SEVERE: recumbency and stupor

be within normal reference ranges or only marginally low. PTH levels are usually high. Therefore, clinical signs of acute hypocalcemia noted above may not be readily evident.

IV. Diagnosis

A. **Signalment**, in particular lactating mares.

B. History and clinical signs.

C. **Low serum calcium levels.** Ideally, the **ionized fraction should be measured** although this may not always be possible. If only total calcium can be measured, then the ionized fraction may be estimated. A useful guide to the degree of hypocalcemia based on clinical severity is shown in Table 33.1.

D. **Magnesium is often low** (<0.6 mmol/L [1.5 mg/dL]) in cases of hypocalcemia and may contribute to the clinical signs; therefore, this should also be **measured concurrently**.

E. Evaluating cases with recurrent hypocalcemia or possible chronic calcium deficiency:

1. **PTH is low** (<0.25 pmol/L) in hypoparathyroidism leading to hypocalcemia and hyperphosphatemia (>1.8 mmol/L [5.6 mg/dL]). Magnesium may also be low, as a consequence of or perhaps contributing to the disorder.

2. Vitamin D appears to have limited importance in the horse with regard to calcium metabolism. Deficiencies have not been reported in the literature.

3. **Evaluating the oxalate content of the diet** may be useful, although signs of chronic deficiency are more common than overt hypocalcemia in these cases.

V. Differential Diagnoses

A. Tetanus.

B. Laminitis.

C. Acute rhabdomyolysis.

D. Equine grass sickness.

VI. Treatment

A. Some horses may not require treatment. For example, **racehorses** after racing may develop a **self-resolving hypocalcemia** due to a mild respiratory or metabolic alkalosis. If in doubt, treatment should be initiated before signs progress.

B. **Intravenous** administration of **calcium-containing solutions** is very effective:

1. In the UK, available preparations of calcium borogluconate (20 and 40%) provide approximately 6 and 12 g of calcium per 400 mL, respectively.

2. As an approximation, an ionized blood calcium level of 1.2 mmol/L (4.81 mg/dL) with a total calcium of 2.5 mmol/L (10.02 mg/dL) corresponds to a 6–7 g deficit of calcium in a 500-kg horse.

3. As a rule of thumb therefore, with moderate signs of hypocalcemia, 400–600 mL of 20% calcium borogluconate diluted at least 1 in 4 with saline, Hartmann's solution, or dextrose saline is effective.

4. Administration should be slow (over at least 15 min) and clinical monitoring is essential during administration in case of cardiac arrhythmias. The infusion should be stopped if there is an alteration in cardiac rate or rhythm.

C. Relapses can occur; therefore some cases may require repeated or continued treatment. Reanalysis of calcium levels on a regular basis is essential.

D. **Oral supplementation of calcium carbonate: 20 g/day** is the basic equine requirement for calcium in a 500-kg horse. In times of high demand such as pregnancy, lactation, growth, or intense exercise, 40–80 g/day may be more appropriate.

E. In **endurance events**, horses may benefit from **preemptive electrolyte supplementation.**

VII. Prognosis

A. **Good** with appropriate therapy in cases of acute hypocalcemia.

VIII. Prevention

A. Ensure **calcium intake is sufficient,** especially in high risk individuals, for example, lactating mares and endurance horses.

B. Avoid dietary items high in oxalates.

Hypocalcemia in Ferrets, Rabbits, and Rodents

Pathogenesis

- Low ionized calcium levels.
- May occur due to increased calcium demands in the periparturient period or during lactation; dietary factors are likely to contribute.

Classical Signs

- Neurological signs ranging from ataxia or tremors through to coma.

Diagnosis

- Based on signalment, history, clinical signs, and blood biochemistry.

Treatment

- Calcium administration; dietary correction.

I. Pathogenesis

A. **Hypocalcemia** may develop during **late gestation, the periparturient period or lactation** in breeding animals as a result of increased calcium demand. It may be associated with pregnancy toxemia.

B. Low dietary calcium and high dietary phosphorus are predisposing factors.

C. Rabbits have an unusual calcium metabolism resulting in a 30–50% higher normal serum calcium concentration than other mammals (Table 33.2):

1. Rabbit serum calcium concentrations vary widely and **reflect dietary intake.**
2. **Fractional urinary excretion** of calcium is approximately **44% in the rabbit,** compared to <2% in most mammals.
3. Passive absorption of dietary calcium from the gastrointestinal tract is very efficient and does not require vitamin D if dietary levels of calcium are adequate.
4. Rabbits consuming a **low-calcium, high-phosphorus diet** (e.g., a diet of exclusively **commercial cereal/legume mixes**) may develop **nutritional secondary hyperparathyroidism** characterized by increased serum PTH, hyperphosphatemia, hypovitaminosis D, and decreased bone mass. When alveolar bone is lost, the bone of the mandible may be most affected and acquired dental disease may be the end result.

II. Signalment

Obese multiparous females with **large litters** may be more at risk of developing hypocalcemia.

III. Clinical Signs

A. **Neurological signs** which may include ataxia, posterior paresis/paralysis, tremors, convulsions, or coma.

Table 33.2 Reference ranges for normal total calcium levels in rabbits, ferrets, and selected rodent species.

Species	Total calcium (mmol/L)	Total calcium (mg/dL)
Rat	1.9–3.2	7.6–12.8
Mouse	1.1–2.4	4.4–9.6
Gerbil	0.9–1.5	3.6–6.0
Hamster	2.1–3.1	8.4–12.4
Guinea pig	2.4–3.1	9.6–12.4
Chinchilla	1.4–3.0	5.6–12.0
Rabbit	3.0–4.2	12.0–16.8
Ferret	1.9–2.4	7.6–9.6

B. Generalized weakness, depression.
C. Anorexia.
D. Collapse.
E. Clear, acidic urine in the herbivorous species which tend to have calcium crystalluria and as such cloudy urine in health.

IV. Diagnosis
A. Based on review of reproductive status and diet along with clinical signs.
B. Demonstration of a **low serum calcium level, preferably** the **ionized** fraction.

V. Differential Diagnoses
A. Pregnancy toxemia.
B. Viral, protozoal, or bacterial meningitis/encephalitis (e.g., lymphocytic choriomeningitis virus, toxoplasmosis, listeriosis, encephalitozoonosis, rabies).
C. Trauma (e.g., head or spinal).
D. Central nervous system neoplasia.
E. Heat stress.
F. *Baylisascaris* infection.
G. Toxicity (e.g., heavy metals, botulism).
H. Epilepsy.
I. *Trixacarus caviae* infection (guinea pigs).
J. Insulinoma (ferrets) (see Chapter 23).

VI. Treatment
A. For immediate treatment, 100 mg/kg **calcium gluconate** can be given im, ip, or sc. This may be diluted with warmed isotonic fluids prior to administration.
B. If a dietary deficiency is suspected, the inclusion of **calcium rich foods or oral supplementation** should be considered.

VII. Prognosis
A. Fair to good if the diagnosis is reached promptly and appropriate treatment provided without delay.

VIII. Prevention
A. Ensure the diet of breeding females is sufficiently high in calcium. Supplementation should be considered where dietary levels are considered inadequate.

Hypocalcemia in Pet Birds

Pathogenesis

- Hypocalcemia occurs when there is a low serum ionized calcium concentration.
- Most cases in captive birds are acknowledged to be associated with nutritional secondary hyperparathyroidism associated with feeding a diet with inadequate calcium and/or vitamin D content.

Classical Signs

- Seizures in adult birds.
- Juvenile osteodystrophy in growing birds.

Diagnosis

- Measurement of low serum ionized calcium concentration.

Treatment

- Calcium supplementation.
- Vitamin D supplementation and provision of UV-b radiation to stimulate endogenous Vitamin D synthesis.

I. Pathogenesis
A. **Control of calcium metabolism in birds:**
  1. Calcium is the most prevalent mineral in the adult bird constituting over **30% of the total mineral content**. It exists as three fractions in avian serum: an ionized salt, calcium bound to proteins, and complex calcium bound to a variety of anions (citrate, bicarbonate, and phosphate).
  2. Calcium has two important physiological roles in the bird providing structural strength for the avian skeleton and playing a vital role in many biochemical reactions within the body via its concentration as the ionized salt in tissue fluids.
  3. **Ionized calcium**, the **physiologically active fraction** of serum calcium, is essential for bone homeostasis, muscle and nerve conduction, blood coagulation, and the control of hormone secretion, **particularly vitamin D$_3$ and PTH**.
  4. The control of calcium metabolism in birds has developed into a highly efficient homeostatic system able to respond quickly to sudden demands for calcium. This is required for the **production of hard-shelled eggs** and the **rapid growth rate in young birds**.
  5. Calcium is controlled mainly by **PTH, metabolites of vitamin D$_3$**, and **calcitonin** that act on the target organs (liver, kidney, gastrointestinal tract, and bone) in direct response to changes in serum ionized calcium concentrations.
  6. **Estrogen and prostaglandins** also have a role in calcium regulation in the bird.
  7. There are **distinct differences between the mammalian and avian system.** The most dramatic difference between the two phylogenetic groups **is in the rate of skeletal metabolism in birds at times of demand.** Domestic **chickens** will **correct hypocalcemic** challenges **within minutes**, whereas similarly challenged mammals respond over a period of 24 h.
  8. Egg-laying hens require **10% of the total body calcium reserves for egg production in a 24 h period**. The calcium required for eggshell production is obtained by **increased intestinal absorption** and from the highly labile reservoir found in the **medullary bone**, normally visible radiographically in sexually mature female birds (Figure 33.2).
  9. In the normal bird, serum ionized calcium concentration is kept within a tight range by the controlling influence of PTH.
  10. The parathyroid glands, found at the thoracic inlet of the bird, normally respond to hypocalcemia by increasing their rate of secretion of PTH from the chief cells.

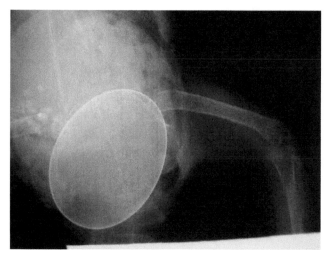

Figure 33.2   A dorsal-ventral radiograph of an egg bound Blue-Fronted Amazon parrot. The film demonstrates the presence of medullary bone in mature female birds. The characteristic fluffy appearance of medullary bone can be visualized in the medullary cavity of the femur. The bird was diagnosed with egg peritonitis and a salpingohysterectomy was performed to remove the egg.

11. **Hypocalcemia occurs** when there is **a failure** of the **parathyroid controlled homeostatic mechanisms** that normally protect against falling blood calcium concentrations.

B. **Nutrition of cage and aviary birds:**

1. **Chronic malnutrition** is a common clinical presentation in captive parrots characterized by multiple nutrient deficiencies or excesses rather than problems with a single dietary component, usually associated with **feeding seed-based diets.** The calcium content of seeds traditionally fed to psittacine birds is low (**<0.1%**):

   a. It has been shown that parrots fed diets consisting of **<50% balanced formulated food** risk deficiency of several vitamins and minerals, particularly **vitamin A, vitamin E, and calcium.**

2. **Raptors** fed an unsupplemented **all meat diet** are susceptible to disorders of calcium metabolism. They should always receive **whole prey** in their diet.

3. The absorption and excretion of phosphate and calcium is interdependent. The dietary calcium to phosphate ratio is therefore important and **calcium to phosphate ratio of 2:1 (as in bone) is considered optimal for birds:**

   a. Many **seed diets** contain **suboptimal ratios** often as high as 1:37. This is certainly considered to be a factor in the development of nutritional secondary hyperparathyroidism.

4. The nutritional requirements of birds vary with their physiological state:

   a. At maintenance only small amounts of dietary calcium are required to replace losses through urine and feces. This is thought to be **<0.2–0.5% in adult nonlaying chickens.**

   b. The calcium requirement increases **in the egg laying bird:**

      1) During the breeding season, many species in the wild **supplement their diet with insects** in order to increase their dietary calcium and protein.

      2) The increased calcium requirement **depends on clutch size and frequency** in addition to the amount of calcium deposited in the shell.

      3) **Small birds** have a **higher calcium requirement** as they lay proportionately larger eggs than bigger birds.

      4) **Precocial species** have a **higher** calcium requirement than altricial birds due to producing larger eggs.

      5) The increase in calcium requirement in laying pet birds is less than in production poultry. The **calcium requirement** of **a laying hen is between 2.25% and 3.25% for continuous egg production,** but cockatiels will produce well-shelled eggs on 0.85% dry matter calcium.

      6) The **majority of the calcium for the shell** is obtained from **medullary bone formed in the weeks before egg production** so any increase in calcium requirement is spread over a period of time.

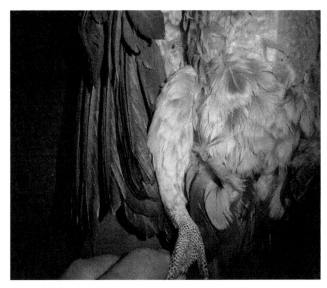

Figure 33.3   Juvenile osteodystrophy in a 12-week-old hand-reared grey parrot. There is severe bowing of the tibiotarsus.

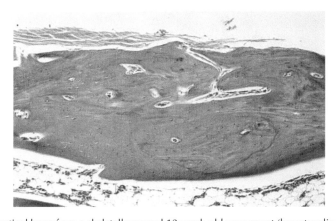

Figure 33.4   Section of cortical bone from a skeletally normal 12-week-old grey parrot (hematoxylin and eosin 200×).

   c. The calcium requirement **is high in the growing chick:**
     1) During growth, the **requirement** for calcium is **highest** at the **start of life** decreasing as full adult size is reached.
     2) The calcium requirement of chickens is significantly affected by the growth rate of the birds.
     3) Psittacine chicks (altricial birds) experience rapid skeletal growth and would be expected to have greater requirements than precocial birds due to greater growth rates and poor calcification of the skeleton at hatching, but surprisingly, this increase is not excessive (**1% dry matter of diet appears sufficient**).
     4) The **correct vitamin D₃ content**, however, is **essential** and failure to provide sufficient would be expected to cause **osteodystrophy** in **young psittacine chicks** (Figures 33.3–33.5).
5. **Vitamin D:**
   a. Vitamin D₃ was traditionally classed as a fat-soluble vitamin. It is now **classified** as a **steroid hormone.**
   b. It is supplied via the **diet** or by **endogenous synthesis** from vitamin D₃ precursors requiring **exposure to UV-b light.** There is some evidence that **vitamin D₃ metabolism varies between avian species** but **vitamin D₃ deficiency is a relatively common problem in companion birds:**

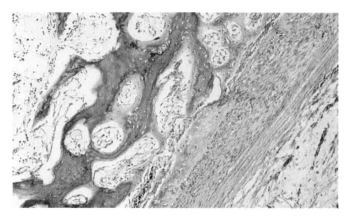

Figure 33.5   Section of cortical bone from a grey parrot with juvenile osteodystrophy. There is a loss of normal osteoid and replacement with fibrous tissue especially in the periosteal region (hematoxylin and eosin, 200×).

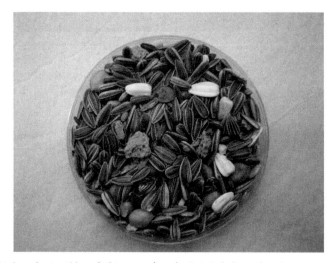

Figure 33.6   Traditional bird seed mix. Although this type of seed mix is imbalanced and encourages selective feeding, it is still the most common diet used by aviculturists for captive psittacine birds.

    1) **Poultry** do not have a dietary requirement for vitamin D_3 if they receive adequate radiation in the **285–315 nm spectra.**

    2) In poultry, endogenous vitamin D_3 **synthesis occurs** on the **featherless areas** of the legs and face.

    3) The ultraviolet light required for endogenous vitamin D_3 synthesis can either be supplied naturally from full spectrum sunlight or using artificial lamps manufactured to provide UV-b radiation. **Exposure to direct unfiltered sunlight is the optimal way to provide UV-b light.**

    4) As most domestic poultry and captive parrots are kept indoors, they are prone to **vitamin D deficiencies unless** fed a **diet with adequate vitamin D_3 or supplied artificial UV-b light.**

    5) UV-b lamp technology is constantly changing but a useful source of up-to-date information is available via http://www.uvguide.co.uk.

6. **Nutritional secondary hyperparathyroidism** is a sequel to a nutritional imbalance characterized by an increase in PTH secretion in response to a disturbance in mineral homeostasis. It is the **most common cause of hypocalcemia in pet birds:**

    a. **Nutritional secondary hyperparathyroidism in captive cage and aviary birds and poultry has traditionally been attributed to feeding cereal/seed-based diets with a low vitamin D_3 and calcium content** (Figure 33.6).

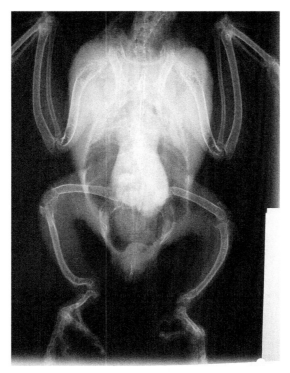

Figure 33.7 A dorsal-ventral radiograph of an 8-month-old captive grey parrot. The radiograph indicates evidence of juvenile osteodystrophy with bowing in both tibiotarsi. There is also obvious distortion in both wings. The radiographs were taken as part of a postpurchase examination and the bird was otherwise healthy.

    b. **These diets are also typically high in phosphate,** which forms **phytate complexes with** the **calcium** reducing bioavailabilty of the mineral.

    c. **Nutritional secondary hyperparathyroidism** in carnivore avian species, including **raptors,** is associated with feeding unsupplemented **all meat diets** with an inappropriate calcium:phosphate ratio.

7. **Metabolic bone disease** is a nonspecific term used to describe morphological defects that can occur during bone growth or remodeling of the adult skeleton:

    a. Metabolic bone disease is usually due to **primary nutritional deficiencies.**

    b. Osteodystrophy is defined as the failure of normal bone development.

    c. Clinically, osteodystrophy presents as **distortion of bone,** with associated increased susceptibility to **pathological fractures** and **abnormalities** of both **gait** and **posture.**

    d. Osteodystrophy has been demonstrated in many species of birds radiographically (Figures 33.7 and 33.8):

        1) Feeding a **diet** with **inadequate calcium** and **vitamin D₃** is responsible for the development of osteodystrophy.

        2) It has been postulated that the **hand rearing of young psittacine birds** may predispose to osteodystrophy **due to increased activity and lack of sibling support.**

II. Signalment

A. **Adult grey parrots** more frequently present with **hypocalcemic seizures** compared with other psittacine birds fed similar diets.

B. Juvenile grey parrots more frequently present with **juvenile osteodystrophy** compared with other psittacine birds fed similar diets (Figure 33.9).

C. **Goshawks** are more susceptible to **hypocalcemic seizures** compared with other raptor species.

D. All raptor chicks fed unsupplemented all meat diets are susceptible to **osteodystrophy.**

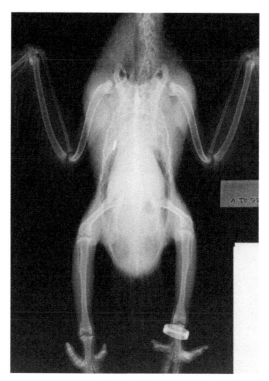

Figure 33.8 A typical ventral dorsal radiograph from a 12-week-old grey parrot fed a formulated diet demonstrating normal skeletal growth in the species.

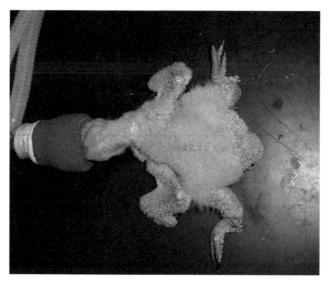

Figure 33.9 A 6-week-old captive bred hand-reared grey parrot with severe juvenile osteodystrophy. There is obvious bilateral bowing of the tibiotarsus. Radiography revealed evidence of osteodystrophy in wings, legs, and spine with numerous pathological fractures. The bird was euthanized on humane grounds. The bird had been hand reared on a cereal diet with no additional calcium or vitamin D_3 supplementation.

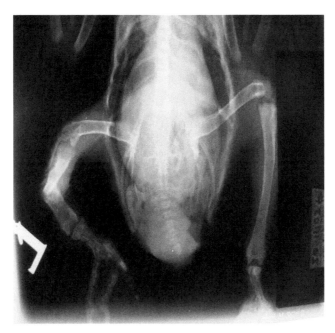

Figure 33.10 Radiograph of a Harris Hawk chick fed an unsupplemented all meat diet. There is a pathological fracture of the left tibiotarsus. The bird was euthanized due to the severity of the condition.

E. **Poultry** kept **indoors** and fed **diets** containing **inadequate calcium** and/or **vitamin D** are susceptible to osteodystrophy during growth or **cage layer paralysis** as adults (neurological symptoms associated with low blood ionized calcium concentrations).

III. Clinical Signs

A. Signs in adult birds are similar to those for acute hypocalcemia in other species resulting from **enhanced neuromuscular irritability.**

B. Range from **slight ataxia** and **head twitching** to **full seizures.**

C. The **wings** are usually **extended** with severe loss of coordination and the birds may exhibit **nystagmus** with pronounced facial twitching.

D. The birds show irritable and abnormal behavior.

E. Hypocalcemic females, particularly poultry species, can present with **egg binding** although this is more usually due to oversized, overproduced, or malpositioned eggs rather than an absolute calcium deficiency.

F. Birds can produce **poor quality egg shells** or deformed eggs when fed a diet containing low calcium or vitamin D_3.

G. **Hypocalcemia** in captive **hand-reared parrot and raptor chicks** presents as a metabolic bone disease (specifically juvenile osteodystrophy) with **deformity of the long bones and pathological fractures** identified radiographically (Figure 33.10).

H. Osteodystrophy can occur in growing poultry denied access to adequate calcium, vitamin D, or UV-b radiation.

IV. Diagnosis

A. The measurement of **serum ionized calcium**, rather than serum total calcium, provides a more precise estimate of an individual's calcium status especially in the diseased avian patient (Table 33.3). A laboratory reference range for **ionized calcium** in healthy grey parrots was found to be **0.96–1.22 mmol/L** (3.85–4.89 mg/dL) and this appears **consistent for most bird species:**

    1. The majority of veterinary pathology laboratories only report a **total calcium** value, which reflects the total combined levels of **ionized calcium, protein-bound calcium, and complexed calcium.**

Table 33.3 Normal ranges for calcium metabolism in birds.

Parameter	Reference range
Ionized calcium (mmol/L)	0.96–1.22
Total calcium (mmol/L)	2.00–3.00
Inorganic phosphate (mmol/L)	1.00–3.40
25-hydroxycholecalciferol (nmol/L)	7.20–380.00
Parathyroid hormone (pg/mL)	<7.00*
1,25-dihydroxycholecalciferol (nmol/L)	<10.00*
Magnesium (mmol/L)	0.88–1.28

*For poultry as no published reference range for psittacine birds.

2.   This can lead to misinterpretation of calcium results in birds, as any change in **protein-bound calcium is not thought to have any pathophysiological significance.**

3.   In **laying female birds, serum albumin** levels may **rise** by up to **100%** to provide albumin for yolk and albumen production. A blood sample analyzed at this time shows **inflated total calcium** concentrations due to an increased protein-bound calcium fraction while the ionized calcium level is not affected.

4.   The binding reaction between the calcium ion and albumin is strongly pH dependent so **acid base imbalances** will **also affect ionized calcium levels.**

5.   **Blood** samples for ionized calcium assays should be **analyzed as soon as possible** after venipuncture as changes in the pH of the sample will affect the accuracy of the ionized calcium levels.

6.   It is important to **chill the samples** immediately to **reduce glycolysis** by the red blood cells which continue to produce lactic acid as a by-product **reducing the pH** of the sample.

7.   **The sample will lose carbon dioxide if it is exposed to room air, increasing the pH of the sample and subsequently reducing the ionized calcium measured.**

8.   In grey parrots, delaying sample analysis for up to 72 h has not been found to significantly affect ionized calcium assays.

9.   **Heparin binds calcium.** This is a potential problem with analyzing bird samples, as heparin is the normal anticoagulant used. Each unit of heparin has been demonstrated to bind 0.001 mmol/L of ionized calcium. It is therefore **important to achieve the correct ratio of heparin** anticoagulant to blood volume by filling the blood sample tubes with the required amount.

10.   **The thick-billed parrot** has **lower ionized calcium** concentrations than those reported for other birds (0.82–1.13 mmol/L [3.29–4.53 mg/dL]).

B. In normocalcemic birds the concentration of **25-hydroxycholecalciferol** is not expected to fall below 26 nmol/L (10.4 ng/mL) and would normally be expected to be above 50 nmol/L (20.0 ng/mL):

1.   The concentration of **25-hydroxycholecalciferol correlates** well with **dietary vitamin D₃** intake or **exposure to UV-b** light.

2.   **The measurement of 25-hydroxycholecalciferol is considered the best assessment of vitamin D₃** status in an individual as it has a longer half-life than other vitamin D₃ metabolites.

3.   **Sample handling** for vitamin D₃ assays is **not critical** and assays are available for both plasma and serum samples. There is no requirement for freezing samples prior to analysis, as the vitamin is **stable at room temperature.** Repeated freeze–thaw cycles of the sample should be avoided, however, as the hormone will denature.

4.   Vitamin D₃ results need to be **interpreted in context of the diet and the levels of UV-b light** received by the individual.

C. Nutritional secondary hyperparathyroidism can be diagnosed by direct measurement of PTH:

1.   Most human assays concentrate on the mid and terminal segments of the PTH molecule due to the very short half-life **of the biologically active 1–34 N sections.**

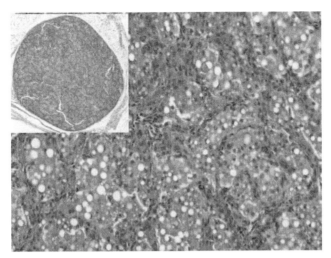

Figure 33.11   Parathyroid gland from a juvenile peregrine falcon (*Falco peregrinus*) with nutritional secondary hyperparathyroidism. The bird presented with bilateral pathological fractures of the tibiotarsi. The gland demonstrates hypertrophy of the chief cells with evidence of vacuolation throughout the gland (hematoxylin and eosin, 20× magnification main images, insert 2× magnification).

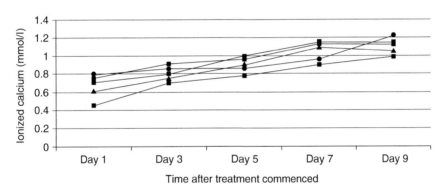

Figure 33.12   Response of plasma ionized calcium concentrations in birds following treatment for hypocalcemia.

2. Unfortunately correlation in structure between the poultry and mammalian PTH molecule is very poor in the middle and terminal sections so PTH assays have traditionally been difficult in birds.

3. The avian and mammalian PTH molecule has greatest homology in the biologically active 1–34 N regions. **Only assays measuring the 1–34 N section are relevant in birds,** and these are increasingly commercially available.

4. PTH is extremely labile and any assay requires exacting sample handling to produce good results.

5. The hormone is labile at >20 °C (68 °F) so it should be **analyzed immediately** following venipuncture or the sample **rapidly frozen** to −70 °C (−94 °F). Repeated freeze–thaw cycles will also denature the hormone.

6. Proteolytic enzymes present in serum and plasma affect PTH and it is apparently more stable if blood is taken into **sample tubes containing EDTA** or protease inhibitors such as aprotinin.

7. Histological examination of the parathyroid gland of birds suffering from nutritional secondary hyperparathyroidism **show hypertrophic chief cells and considerable vacuolation** (Figure 33.11).

V. Differential Diagnoses

A. Neurological signs may be attributable to:

   1. Hepatic encephalopathy.

   2. Hypoglycemia.

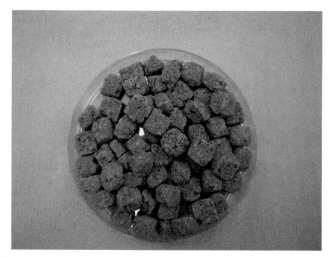

Figure 33.13 The use of formulated pellet diets has been demonstrated to prevent disorders of calcium metabolism (Harrison's High Potency Course™ diet).

    3. Toxicity (e.g., heavy metals, pesticides, plants, drugs).
    4. Infectious central nervous system disease (bacterial, fungal, parasitic, viral).
    5. Epilepsy.
    6. Trauma.
B.   **Fractures/bone deformities** in young birds may be traumatic in origin.

VI.   Treatment
A.   **Calcium gluconate** (10%) 10–50 mg/kg intramuscularly (IM) q 12 h.
B.   **Vitamin D$_3$** 3300 IU/kg IM.
C.   Provision of **UV-b radiation**.
D.   It can take up to **7 days** for ionized calcium concentrations to **normalize** (Figure 33.12).
E.   Consider **surgery** to repair pathological fractures or corrective surgery in severe cases of juvenile osteodystrophy.
F.   Correct husbandry by providing a **balanced diet** containing adequate vitamin D and calcium. Ensure birds receive **UV-b radiation** either through **natural sunlight** or **artificial lamps**.

VII. Prognosis
A.   **Excellent in adults** after acute signs subside and husbandry has been corrected.
B.   **Good in chicks** suffering from juvenile osteodystrophy although chronic orthopedic disease may be a problem.

VIII. Prevention
A.   Provide **diet with adequate vitamin D$_3$ and calcium content:**
    1. Formulated diets are recognized to prevent nutritional problems in cage and aviary birds.
    2. The use of vitamin supplementation to prevent nutritional disease though widespread is associated with problems as intake cannot be effectively monitored. Additionally, the provision of a formulated diet has been demonstrated to be more successful in preventing nutritional problems in birds as it eliminates selective feeding (Figure 33.13).
    3. Raptors should be fed **whole adult prey** items at least once per week to prevent disorders of calcium metabolism.
    4. Provision of soluble **limestone grit** is a useful source of calcium for poultry.
B.   Consider **UV-b provision:**
    1. **Poultry only require 30 min UV-b radiation per 24 h** for adequate vitamin D synthesis.

2. Natural **unfiltered** sunlight is the best form of UV-b radiation but artificial lights can be used for birds kept indoors.

C. Prevent **excessive movement** in young hand-reared chicks by creating nests or rearing birds in small groups.

Hypocalcemia in Pet Reptiles

Pathogenesis

- Usually secondary to nutritional or renal secondary hyperparathyroidism.

Classical Signs

- Muscle tremors or fasciculations.

Diagnosis

- Based on history, signalment, clinical signs, and serum ionized calcium levels.

Treatment

- Calcium administration and husbandry correction.

I. Pathogenesis
A. Hypocalcemia in reptiles is most commonly seen **in animals with nutritional secondary hyperparathyroidism** (see Chapter 37).
B. **Vitamin D$_3$ deficiency** and **improper dietary calcium:phosphorus ratio** are implicated (e.g., feeding a carnivore an exclusively red meat diet).
C. Hypocalcemia may also occur as a consequence of **renal secondary hyperparathyroidism.**

II. Signalment
A. Among the reptile groups, **lizards** seem especially prone to hypocalcemia, **particularly oviparous females.**

III. Clinical Signs
A. **Muscle tremors** and fasciculations; tetany. The initial signs may be unilateral or bilateral **twitching of the digits** which progresses to generalized **tetanic spasms.**
B. **Flaccid paralysis.**
C. Death can occur due to heart failure.

IV. Diagnosis
A. History.
B. Clinical examination.
C. **Radiography** to identify hypomineralized bone if prolonged hypocalcemia is suspected.
D. **Serum calcium levels;** as total blood calcium levels may be normal or subnormal, it is preferable to measure **ionized calcium.**
E. Serum phosphorus levels are usually elevated.

V. Differential Diagnoses
A. Septicemia/toxemia.
B. Bacterial, fungal, viral, or parasitic meningitis/encephalitis.
C. **Trauma.**
D. **Toxicity.**
E. **Hepatic or renal disease.**
F. Hypoglycemia.

G.   Central nervous system neoplasia.

H.   Other nutritional deficiencies (e.g., thiamine, biotin, vitamin E/selenium).

VI.   Treatment

A.   Administration of **parenteral calcium** (10–200 mg/kg **calcium gluconate** subcutaneously, intramuscularly, intracelomically or intravenously) q 6–8 h as required for immediate therapy of reptiles with **neurological signs.**

B.   Once stabilized, parenteral calcium may be discontinued and oral **calcium glubionate/borogluconate** (10 mg/kg q 12–24 h) or **calcium carbonate powder** used as a supplement while efforts are made to correct any underlying causes.

VII.   Prognosis

A.   **Fair if** identified in the **early stages,** and rapid treatment/husbandry correction is possible.

B.   **Poor if** hypocalcemia is **prolonged** and associated with severe clinical signs.

VIII.   Prevention

A.   Providing the appropriate husbandry (including nutrition and environmental conditions) for the species concerned is of paramount importance.

References and Further Readings

Aguilera-Tejero E, Estepa JC, López I, et al. Polycystic kidneys as a cause of secondary hypoparathyroidism in a horse. *Equine Veterinary Journal* 2000;32(2):167–169.

Antillon A, Scott ML, Krook L, et al. Metabolic response of laying hens to different dietary levels of calcium, phosphorus and vitamin D. *The Cornell Veterinarian* 1977;167:413–444.

Arnold SA, Kram MA, Hintz HF, et al. Nutritional secondary hyperparathyroidism in the parakeet. *The Cornell Veterinarian* 1973;64(1):37–46.

Baker DH, Biehl RR, Emmert JL. Vitamin D₃ requirement of young chicks receiving diets varying in calcium and available phosphorus. *British Poultry Science* 1998;39(3):413–417.

Bannister DW, Candlish JK. The collagenolytic activity of avian medullary bone: Effect of laying status and parathyroid extract. *British Poultry Science* 1973;14:121–125.

Bar A, Rosenberg J, Perlman R, et al. Field rickets in turkeys; relationship to vitamin D. *Poultry Science* 1987;66:68–72.

Bar A, Sharvit M, Noff D, et al. Absorption and excretion of cholecalciferol and of 25 hydroxycholecalciferol and metabolites in birds. *J Nutr* 1980;110(10):1930–1934.

Bar A, Vax E, Striem S. Relationship among age, eggshell thickness and vitamin D metabolism and its expression in the laying hen. *Comparative Biochemistry and Physiology. Part A, Molecular & Integrative Physiology* 1999;123(2):147–154.

Barber PJ, Elliot J, Torrance AG. Measurement of feline intact parathyroid hormone: Assay validation and sample handling studies. *The Journal of Small Animal Practice* 1993;34:614–619.

Barlet JP. Plasma calcium, inorganic phosphorus and magnesium levels in pregnant and lactating rabbits. *Reprod Nutr Dev* 1980;20:647–651.

Bennett RA, Mehler SJ. Neurology. In: Mader DR, ed. *Reptile Medicine and Surgery*, 2nd edn. St Louis: Saunders Elsevier, 2006, pp. 239–250.

Bentley PJ, ed. Calcium metabolism. In: *Comparative Vertebrate Endocrinology*. Cambridge: Cambridge University Press, 1998, pp. 269–301.

Blind E, Gagel RF. Assay methods: Parathyroid hormone, parathyroid hormone-related protein and calcitonin. In: Favus MJ, ed. *Primer on the Metabolic Bone Disease and Disorders of Bone Metabolism*, 5th edn. Philadelphia: Lippincott, Williams and Wilkins, 1999, pp. 119–128.

Blunt JW, Deluca HF, Schnoes HK. 25 hydroxycholecalciferol: A biologically active metabolite of vitamin D₃. *Biochemistry* 1968;7:3317–3322.

Brue RN. Nutrition. In: Ritchie RW, Harrison GJ, Harrison LR, eds. *Avian Medicine: Principals and Applications*. Lake Worth, Florida: Wingers Publishing, 1994, pp. 63–95.

Burgos-Trinidad M, Brown AJ, DeLuca HF. A rapid assay for 25-hydroxyvitamin D and 1,25-dihydroxyvitamin D hydroxylase. *Analytical Biochemistry* 1990;190(1):102–107.

Bush BM. In: *Interpretation of Laboratory Results for Small Animal Clinicians*. Oxford: Blackwell Scientific, 1991, pp. 367–368.

Candlish JK, Taylor TG. The response time to the parathyroid hormone in the laying fowl. *J Endocrinol* 1970;48:143–144.

Carpenter JW. *Exotic Animal Formulary*, 3rd edn. St Louis: Elsevier Saunders, 2005.

Carrier D, Auriemma J. A developmental constraint in fledging time in birds. *Biological Journal of the Linnean Society* 1992;47:61–77.

Carrier D, Leon LR. Skeletal growth and function in the Californian Gull (*Larus californicus*). *J Zool Soc Lond* 1990;222:375–389.

Castillo L, Tanaka Y, Wineland MJ, et al. Production of 1,25-dihydroxyvitamin D3 and formation of medullary bone in the egg-laying hen. *Endocrinology* 1979;104(6):1598–1601.

Classen HL. Management factors in leg disorders. In: Whitehead CC, ed. *Bone Biology and Skeletal Disorders in Poultry. Poultry Science Symposium Number Twenty-three*. Oxford: Carfax Publishing Company, 1992, pp. 201–203.

Couëtil LL, Sojka JE, Nachreiner RF. Primary hypoparathyroidism in a horse. *Journal of Veterinary Internal Medicine* 1998;12:45–49.

Dacke CG. Calcium homeostasis. In: Whittow GC, ed. *Sturkie's Avian Physiology*, 5th edn. London: Academic Press, 2000, pp. 472–485.

Deftos LJ, Roos BA, Oates EL. Calcitonin. In: Favus MJ, ed. *Primer on the Metabolic Bone Disease and Disorders of Bone Metabolism*, 5th edn. Philadelphia: Lippencott, Williams and Wilkins, 1999, pp. 99–104.

Earle KE, Clarke NR. The nutrition of the budgerigar (*Melopsittacus undulatus*). *J Nutr* 1991;121:186–192.

Eckermann-Ross C. Hormonal regulation and calcium metabolism in the rabbit. *The Veterinary Clinics of North America. Exotic Animal Practice* 2008;11:139–152.

Edwards HM Jr. Nutritional factors and leg disorders. In: Whitehead CC, ed. *Bone Biology and Skeletal Disorders in Poultry. Poultry Science Symposium Number Twenty-three*. Carfax Publishing Company, Oxford, 1992, pp. 167–195.

Edwards HM Jr. Nutrition and skeletal problems in poultry. *Poultry Science* 2000;79(7):1018–1023.

Edwards HM Jr. Effects of UVB irradiation of very young chickens on growth and bone development. *Br J Nutr* 2003;90(1):151–160.

Edwards HM Jr, Elliot MA, Soonchareryning S. Effect of dietary calcium on tibial dyschondroplasia. Interaction with light, cholecalciferol, 1,25-dihydroxycholecalciferol, protein and synthetic zeolite. *Poultry Science* 1992;71(12):2041–2055.

Etches RJ. Calcium logistics in the laying hen. *J Nutr* 1987;117:619–628.

Fowler ME. Metabolic bone disease. In: Fowler ME, ed. *Zoo and Wild Animal Medicine*, 3rd edn. Philadelphia: WB Saunders, 1986, pp. 63–82.

Freedman MT, Bush M, Novak GR. Nutritional and metabolic bone disease in a zoological collection: A review of radiographic findings. *Skeletal Radiology* 1976;1:87–96.

Gilardi JD, Duffy SS, Munn CA, et al. Biochemical functions of geophagy in parrots: Detoxification of dietary toxins and cytoprotective effects. *J Chem Ecol* 1999;25(4):897–922.

Gilsanz V, Roe TF, Antunes J, et al. Effect of dietary calcium on bone density in growing rabbits. *Am J Physiol* 1991;260(23):E471–E476.

Graveland J. Avian eggshell formation in calcium rich and calcium poor habitats—Importance of snail shells and anthropogenic calcium sources. *Canadian Journal of Zoology* 1996;74:1035–1044.

Graveland J, Van Gijzen T. Arthropods and seeds are not sufficient as calcium sources for shell formation and skeletal growth in passerines. *Ardea* 1994;82:299–314.

Harcourt-Brown F. Textbook of rabbit medicine. Edinburgh: Butterworth Heinemann, 2002.

Harcourt-Brown NH. Incidence of juvenile osteodystrophy in hand reared parrots (*Psittacus e psittacus*). *Vet Rec* 2003;152:438–439.

Harcourt-Brown NH. Development of the skeleton and feathers of dusky parrots (*Pionus fuscus*) in relationship to their behaviour. *Vet Rec* 2004;154:42–48.

Hess L, Mauldin G, Rosenthal K. Estimated nutrient content of diets commonly fed to pet birds. *Vet Rec* 2002;150:399–403.

Hochleithner M. Convulsions in African Grey parrots in connection with hypocalcaemia: Five selected cases. *Proceedings 2nd European Symposium Avian Medicine and Surgery*, 1989, pp. 44–52.

Hochleithner M, Hochleithner C, Harrison GL. Evidence of hypoparathyroidism in hypocalcaemic African Grey Parrots. *The Avian Examiner*, special supplement spring. HBD International Ltd., Brentwood, 1997.

Holick MF, Adams JS, Clemens TL. Photoendocrinology of vitamin D_3: the past, present and future. In: Norman AW, Schaefer K, Herrath DV, eds. *Vitamin D, Chemical, Biochemical and Clinical Endocrinology of Calcium Metabolism*. Berlin: Walter de Gruyter, 1982, pp. 1151–1156.

Hollamby S. Rodents: Neurological and musculoskeletal disorders. In: Keeble E, Meredith A, eds. *BSAVA Manual of Rodents and Ferrets*. Gloucester: British Small Animal Veterinary Association, 2009, pp. 161–168.

Hollis BW, Clemens TL, Adams JS. Vitamin D_3 metabolites. In: Flavus MJ, ed. *Primer on the Metabolic Bone Diseases and Disorders of Mineral Metabolism*, 3rd edn. Philadelphia: Lippincott, Williams and Wilkins, 1999, pp. 124–128.

Howard LL, Kass PH, Lamberski N, et al. Serum concentrations of ionized calcium, vitamin D_3 and parathyroid hormone in captive thick billed parrots (*Rhynchopsitta pachyrhyncha*). *Journal of Zoo and Wildlife Medicine* 2004;35(2):147–153.

Hudson NP, Church DB, Trevena J, et al. Primary hypoparathyroidism in two horses. *Australian Veterinary Journal* 1999;77:504–508.

Hurwitz S. Calcium homeostasis in birds. *Vitamins and Hormones* 1989;45:173–221.

Hurwitz S, Pines M. Regulation of bone growth. In: Pang PKT, Schreibman M, eds. *Vertebrate Endocrinology: Fundamentals and Biochemical Implications*. New York: Academic Press, 1991, pp. 229–235.

Ibanez R. Bone mineral density measurement techniques. *Anales del Sistema Sanitario de Navarra* 2003;**26:19–27.**

Johnson MS, Ivey ES. Parathyroid and ultimobranchial glands: Calcium metabolism in birds. In: Fudge AM, Antinoff N, eds. *Semin Avian Exot Pet Med* 2002;11(2):84–94.

Jose-Cunilleras E. Abnormalities of body fluids and electrolytes in athletic horses. In: Hinchcliff KW, Kaneps AJ Geor RJ, eds. *Equine Sports Medicine and Surgery*, Philadelphia: WB Saunders, 2004, pp. 899–918.

Keeble E. Neurology. In: Girling SJ, Raiti P, eds. *BSAVA Manual of Reptiles*, 2nd edn. Gloucester: British Small Animal Veterinary Association, 2004, pp. 273–288.

Kenny AD. Parathyroid and ultimobranchial glands. In: Sturkie PD, ed. *Avian Physiology*, 4th edn. New York: Springer-Verlag, 1986, pp. 466–478.

Kirkwood JE, Duignan PJ, Kemper NF, et al. The growth rate of the tarsometatarsus of birds. *J Zool Soc Lond* 1989;217: 403–416.

Klasing KC. Minerals. In: Klasing KC, ed. *Comparative Avian Nutrition*. New York: CAB International, 1998, pp. 290–295.

Kostka V, Krautwald ME, Tellhelm B, et al. A contribution to radiological examination of bone alterations in psittacines, birds of prey and pigeons. *Proceedings of the Association of Avian Veterinarians*. Lake Worth, USA, 1988, pp. 37–59.

Koutsos EA, Matson KD, Klasing KC. Nutrition of birds in the order Psittaciformes. *Journal of Avian Medicine and Surgery* 2001;15:257–275.

Koutsos EA, Tell LA, Woods LW, et al. Adult cockatiels (*Nymphicus hollandicus*) at maintenance are more sensitive to diets containing excess vitamin A than to vitamin A-deficient diets. *J Nutr* 2003;113(6):1898–1902.

Kratser FH, Vohra P. *Chelates in animal nutrition*. Boca Raton: CRC Press, 1986.

Lewis PD, Perry GC, Morris TR. Ultraviolet radiation and laying pullets. *British Poultry Science* 2000;41(2):131–135.

Lim SK, Gardella T, Thompson A, et al. Full length chicken parathyroid hormone: Biosynthesis in *Escherichia coli* and analysis of biological activity. *J Biol Chem* 1991;266:3709–3714.

Loveridge N, Thomson BM, Farquharson C. Bone growth and turnover. In: Whitehead CC, ed. *Bone Biology and Skeletal Disorders in Poultry. Poultry Science Symposium Number Twenty-three*. Oxford: Carfax Publishing Company, 1992, pp. 3–11.

Lumeij JT. Relationship of plasma calcium to total protein and albumin in grey (*Psittacus erithacus*) and Amazon (*Amazona spp.*) parrots. *Avian Pathology* 1990;19:661–667.

Lumeij JT, Remple JD, Riddle KE. Relationship of plasma total protein and albumin to total calcium in peregrine falcons (*Falco peregrinus*). *Avian Pathology* 1993;22:183–188.

MacWhirter P. Malnutrition. In: Ritchie BW, Harrison GJ, Harrison LR, eds. *Avian Medicine: Principles and Application*. Lake Worth, Florida: Wingers Publishing, 1994, pp. 842–861.

Mattila P, Lehikoinen K, Kiiskinen T, et al. Cholecalciferol and 25-hydroxycholecalciferol content of chicken egg yolk as affected by the cholecalciferol content of feed. *Journal of Agricultural and Food Chemistry* 1999;47(10):4089–4092.

McDonald LJ. Hypocalcemic seizures in an African Grey parrot. *Can Vet J* 1988;29:928–930.

Mehotra M, Gupta SK, Kumar K, et al. Calcium deficiency-induced secondary hyperparathyroidism and osteopenia are rapidly reversible with calcium supplementation in growing rabbit pups. *Br J Nutr* 2006;95:582–590.

Meredith A. General biology and husbandry. In: Meredith A, Flecknell P, eds. *BSAVA Manual of Rabbit Medicine and Surgery*, 2nd edn. Gloucester: British Small Animal Veterinary Association, 2006, pp. 1–17.

Meredith A, Johnson-Delaney C, eds. *BSAVA Manual of Exotic Pets*, 5th edn. Gloucester: British Small Animal Veterinary Association, 2010.

Morrissey RL, Cohn RM, Empson RN Jr, et al. Relative toxicity and metabolic effects of cholecalciferol and 25 hydroxycholecalciferol in chicks. *J Nutr* 1977;107(6);1027–1034.

National Research Council Nutrient Requirements of Poultry. Washington, DC: National Academy Press, 1994.

Norman AW. The avian as an animal model for the study of the vitamin D endocrine system. *The Journal of Experimental Zoology* 1990;4(Suppl):37–45.

Norris SA, Pettifor JM, Gray DA, et al. Calcium metabolism and bone mass in female rabbits during skeletal maturation: effects of dietary calcium intake. *Bone* 2001;29(1):62–69.

Paré JA, Paul-Murphy J. Disorders of the reproductive and urinary systems. In: Quesenberry KE, Carpenter JW, eds. *Ferrets, Rabbits and Rodents—Clinical Medicine and Surgery*, 2nd edn. Philadelphia: WB Saunders, 2004, pp. 183–193.

Pines M, Bar A, Hurwitz S. Isolation and purification of avian parathyroid hormone using a high performance liquid chromatography, and some of its properties. *General and Comparative Endocrinology* 1984;53(2):224–231.

Randell MG. Nutritionally induced hypocalcemic tetany in an Amazon parrot. *Journal of the American Veterinary Medical Association* 1981;179(111):1277–1278.

Richardson PRK, Mundy PJ, Plug I. Bone crushing carnivores and their significance to osteodystrophy in griffon vulture chicks. *Journal of Zoology* 1986;210:23–43.

Robben JH, Lumeij JT. A comparison of parrot food commercially available in the Netherlands. *Tijdschrift Voor Diergeneeskunde* 1989;114(1):19–25.

Rosskopf WJ, Woerpel RW. Egg binding in caged and aviary birds. *Modern Veterinary Practice* 1984;65(6):437–440.

Rosskopf WJ, Woerpel RW, Lane RA. The hypocalcaemic syndrome in African Greys: An updated clinical viewpoint. *Proceedings Association of Avian Veterinarians*, 1985, pp. 129–132.

Roudybush TE. Nutrition. In: Rosskopf W, Worpel R, eds. *Diseases of Cage and Aviary Birds*. Baltimore: Williams and Wilkins, 1996, pp. 218–234.

Roudybush TE. Psittacine nutrition. *The Veterinary Clinics of North America. Exotic Animal Practice* 1999;2(1):111–125.

Schoemaker NJ, Lumeij JT, Dorrestein GM, et al. Nutrition-related problems in pet birds. *Tijdschrift Voor Diergeneeskunde* 1999;124(2):39–43.

Stanford MD. The measurement of ionised calcium in grey parrots. In: *Proceedings of the British Veterinary Zoological Society Autumn meeting, Royal Veterinary College, Potters Bar,* 10–11 November, 2001, pp. 21–24.

Stanford MD. Development of a parathyroid hormone assay in grey parrots. In: *Proceedings of the British Veterinary Zoological Society Spring meeting Chester,* 11–12 May, 2002a, pp. 37.

Stanford, M.D. Determination of 25-hydroxyvitamin D in seed fed grey parrots. *Proceedings of Joint Nutritional Symposium, Antwerp, Belgium, 21–25 August,* 2002b pp. 142–141.

Stanford MD. Cage and aviary birds. In: Meredith A, Redrobe S, eds. *BSAVA Manual of Exotic Pets.* Gloucester: British Small Animal Veterinary Association, 2002c, p. 161.

Stanford MD. Measurement of ionised calcium in grey parrots (*Psittacus e. erithacus*): The effect of diet. *Proceedings of the European Association of Avian Veterinarians 7th European meeting, Tenerife, Spain,* April 22–26, 2003a, pp. 269–275.

Stanford MD. Measurement of 25-hydroxycholecalciferol in captive grey parrots (*Psittacus e erithacus*). *Vet Rec* 2003b;153:58–59.

Stanford MD. Clinical pathology of hypocalcaemia in grey parrots. *Proceedings of the International Conference on Exotics 2005, Fort Lauderdale, Florida, US.* 2005a, 7.2 Supplement, pp. 28–34.

Stanford MD. Nutrition and nutritional disease. In: Harcourt-Brown NH, Chitty J, eds. *BSAVA Manual of Psittacine Birds,* 2nd edn. Gloucester: British Small Animal Veterinary Association, 2005b, pp. 136–155.

Stark JM, Ricklefs RE. The development of the skeleton. In: Stark JM, Ricklefs RE, eds. *Avian Growth and Development Evolution within the Altricial-Precocial Spectrum.* Oxford: Oxford University Press, 1998, pp. 64–74.

Taylor TG, Dacke CG. Calcium metabolism and its regulation. In: Freeman BM, ed. *Physiology and Biochemistry of the Domestic Fowl,* Vol. 5. London: Academic Press, 1984, pp. 125–170.

Thorp BH. Abnormalities in the growth of leg bones. In: Whitehead CC, ed. *Bone Biology and Skeletal Disorders in Poultry. Poultry Science Symposium Number Twenty-three.* Oxford: Carfax Publishing Company, 1992, pp. 147–167.

Tian XQ, Chen TC, Lu Z, et al. Characterization of the translocation process of vitamin D3 from the skin into the circulation. *Endocrinology* 1994;135(2):655–661.

Toribio RE. Calcium disorders. In: Reed SM, Bayly WM, Sellon DC, eds. *Equine Internal Medicine,* 2nd edn. Philadelphia: WB Saunders, 2004, pp. 1295–1327.

Ullrey DE, Allen ME, Baer DJ. Formulated diets versus seed mixtures for psittacines. *J Nutr* 1991;121(11 Suppl):S193–S205.

Ullrey DE, Bernard JB. Vitamin D Metabolism, sources, unique problems in zoo animals, meeting needs. In: Fowler ME, Miller RE, eds. *Zoo and Wild Animal Medicine Current Therapy,* 4th edn. Philadelphia: WB Saunders, 1999, pp. 63–78.

Williams TD, Reed WL, Walzem RL. Egg size variation: Mechanisms and hormonal control. In:. Dawson A, Chaturvedi CM, eds. *Avian Endocrinology.* Pangbourne: Alpha Science International Ltd., 2001, pp. 205–213.

Wilson S, Duff SR. Effects of vitamin or mineral deficiency on the morphology of medullary bone in laying hens. *Research in Veterinary Science* 1991;50(2):216–221.

Yarger JG, Saunders CA, McNaughton JL, et al. Comparison of dietary 25-hydroxycholcalciferol and cholecalciferol in broiler chickens. *Poultry Science* 1995;74(7):1159–1167.

CHAPTER 34

Hypercalcemia in Dogs

Patricia A. Schenck and Dennis Chew

Pathogenesis

- Clinical signs occur when serum ionized calcium (iCa) rises above a critical level.
- Causes of hypercalcemia can be parathyroid independent or parathyroid dependent (primary hyperparathyroidism).
- The most common cause of hypercalcemia in dogs is malignancy.

Classical Signs

- The most common clinical signs associated with hypercalcemia include polyuria, polydipsia, anorexia, lethargy, and weakness.
- Clinical signs are most severe when hypercalcemia develops rapidly.
- If iCa concentration is >1.75 mmol/L (7.0 mg/dL), clinical signs are usually present.

Diagnosis

- Hypercalcemia is defined as a total calcium (tCa) concentration >12.0 mg/dL (3.0 mmol/L) or iCa concentration >6.0 mg/dL (1.50 mmol/L).
- Hypercalcemia is usually overestimated when serum tCa concentration is used.
- Parathyroid hormone (PTH) concentration should be measured in conjunction with iCa measurement to determine whether PTH production is appropriate.
- Measurement of PTH-related protein (PTHrP) concentration may be helpful in cases of suspected malignancy.
- Measurement of serum 25-hydroxyvitamin D may be helpful to identify cases of vitamin D toxicity.

Treatment

- Specific therapy depends on the cause of hypercalcemia.
- If serum tCa is >16 mg/dL (4 mmol/L), aggressive therapy is usually warranted.
- General therapy includes the administration of fluids, diuretics, glucocorticoids, and/or bisphosphonates.

Clinical Endocrinology of Companion Animals, First Edition. Edited by Jacquie Rand.
© 2013 John Wiley & Sons, Inc. Published 2013 by John Wiley & Sons, Inc.

Prognosis

- Prognosis is dependent on the underlying cause of hypercalcemia.
- Prognosis is good for most cases of primary hyperparathyroidism, hypoadrenocorticism, and hypervitaminosis D if treatment is adequate.

I. Pathogenesis
A. Serum tCa is composed of protein-bound calcium (pCa; 34%), complexed calcium (cCa; 10%), and iCa (56%). The **iCa fraction is the biologically active fraction**.
B. Development of hypercalcemia:
   1. Normal hormonal action:
      a. **PTH** secretion from the parathyroid glands is **responsible for the minute-to-minute control of circulating calcium concentration** through rapid effects on bone mobilization; it works to increase serum calcium concentration. In the kidney, PTH increases calcium reabsorption and promotes phosphorus excretion.
      b. **Calcitriol, that is, active vitamin D** secretion from normal kidneys manages the **day-to-day control of calcium,** largely through effects on intestinal calcium absorption; it works to increase serum calcium concentration.
      c. **Calcitonin** secreted from the thyroidal parafollicular cells serves to minimize postprandial hypercalcemia; its **effect on overall calcium metabolism is minor.**
   2. **Hypercalcemia develops primarily when there is an increase in bone mobilization of calcium or a decrease in urinary calcium loss:**
      a. An increase in serum iCa concentration decreases PTH secretion, increases intracellular degradation of PTH by chief cells, and decreases PTH synthesis from normal parathyroid glands.
      b. Calcitonin secretion is stimulated in an attempt to minimize the magnitude of hypercalcemia.
      c. Calcitriol synthesis is decreased both through direct inhibition by iCa and by decreased stimulation because of decreased PTH concentration.
      d. The outcome of the above response is to increase urinary calcium excretion and to decrease the degree of bone mobilization of calcium as countervailing mechanisms to limit the degree of hypercalcemia.
   3. In **primary hyperparathyroidism,** the abnormal parathyroid gland(s) (parathyroid adenoma, carcinoma, or hyperplasia) **continues to secrete PTH even though hypercalcemia is present** and is termed a "parathyroid-dependent" hypercalcemia. There is an increased serum iCa concentration with an inappropriately high PTH secretion.
   4. In **"parathyroid-independent" causes** of hypercalcemia, hypercalcemia **occurs due to many processes** including elaboration of other secretory factors (such as PTHrP, interleukins, or tumor necrosis factor) or as a result of excessive vitamin D ingestion:
      a. In these instances, the parathyroid gland responds in a normal fashion to hypercalcemia, and PTH secretion is very low.
      b. Thus, in parathyroid-independent hypercalcemia, serum iCa concentration is elevated and PTH shows appropriate suppression (below normal or in the lower third of the reference range).
C. Causes of hypercalcemia are listed in Table 34.1.
D. Transient hypercalcemia:
   1. **Dehydration** is occasionally associated with serum tCa concentrations of 12.0–13.5 mg/dL (3.0–3.4 mmol/L).
   2. **Increased serum albumin or total protein** can result in an increased serum tCa concentration as more calcium binds to protein.
E. Hypoadrenocorticism:
   1. Approximately half the cases have an elevation of serum tCa, but only about 25% have a mild elevation of serum iCa.
   2. The pathogenesis of hypercalcemia in hypoadrenocorticism is not fully understood.

Table 34.1 Differential diagnosis for hypercalcemia.

Nonpathologic causes	Transient causes
Nonfasting (minimal increase)	Hemoconcentration
Physiologic growth of the young	Hyperproteinemia
Lab error	Severe environmental hypothermia (rare)
Spurious	
Hyperlipidemia	

Pathologic or consequential—persistent causes

Parathyroid dependent: primary hyperparathyroidism
Parathyroid independent:
  Malignancy associated (most common cause of hypercalcemia in dogs)
    Lymphoma (common)
    Anal sac apocrine gland adenocarcinoma (common)
    Multiple myeloma
    Metastatic bone tumors (rare)
    Miscellaneous tumors (lymphocytic leukemia, mammary carcinoma, fibrosarcoma, pancreatic
      adenocarcinoma, testicular interstitial cell tumor, lung carcinoma, squamous cell carcinoma, thyroid
      adenocarcinoma, clitoral adenocarcinoma, and osteosarcoma)
  Idiopathic hypercalcemia (most common association in cats; very uncommon in dogs)
  Hypoadrenocorticism
  Renal failure
  Hypervitaminosis D
    Iatrogenic
    House plants (calcitriol glycosides; *Cestrum diurnum* or day-blooming jessamine)
    Rodenticide (cholecalciferol)
    Antipsoriasis creams (calcipotriol or calcipotriene containing)
  Granulomatous disease
    Blastomycosis, schistosomiasis, histoplasmosis, coccidioidomycosis, panniculitis, injection granuloma, and
      sterile dermatitis
  Skeletal lesions (nonmalignant; uncommon)
    Osteomyelitis (bacterial or mycotic)
    Hypertrophic osteodystrophy
    Craniomandibular osteopathy
    Disuse osteoporosis (immobilization)
  Ingestion of excessive calcium-containing intestinal phosphate binders
  Ingestion of excessive calcium supplementation (calcium carbonate)
  Raisin/grape toxicity
  DMSO administration to treat calcinosis cutis
  Hypervitaminosis A
  Aluminum exposure (intestinal phosphate binders)
  Acromegaly

Modified from Schenck PA, Chew DJ. Hypercalcemia: A quick reference. *Vet Clin North Am Small Anim Pract* 2008;38:449–453.

    3. Some of the increase in tCa can be accounted for by hemoconcentration.

F. In azotemic chronic kidney disease (CKD), **serum tCa concentration may be elevated, but serum iCa is uncommonly so:**

    1. In most cases, the increase in serum tCa is due to an increase in the cCa fraction.
    2. **Iatrogenic factors may play a role:**
      a. Excessive calcitriol supplementation to treat secondary hyperparathyroidism can cause hypercalcemia.
      b. The use of calcium carbonate-containing intestinal phosphate binders may cause hypercalcemia.

3. **Tertiary hyperparathyroidism:**
   a. The **iCa fraction increases due to a change in the set point for iCa.**
   b. Tertiary hyperparathyroidism involves a subset of patients with azotemic CKD that develop elevated iCa concentration and excessive PTH secretion that is not inhibited by high serum iCa concentration.
   c. It is likely that such patients had high PTH concentrations in association with normal or low serum iCa concentration (i.e., renal secondary hyperparathyroidism) earlier in the clinical course of azotemic CKD.
   d. Autonomous PTH secretion from the parathyroid glands is unlikely, but the set point for PTH secretion may be altered in chronic renal failure (CRF) such that higher iCa concentrations are necessary to inhibit PTH secretion:
      1) Decreases in serum calcitriol concentration, the number of calcitriol receptors in the parathyroid glands, and calcitriol–vitamin D receptor interactions caused by uremic toxins may contribute to the increased set point.
      2) Decreased calcium receptor number, which both establishes the set point and depends on calcitriol functionality for synthesis of its mRNA from parathyroid cell DNA, may also contribute to the altered set-point.
   e. Dogs with elevated iCa concentration and marked hyperparathyroidism may have greater calcitriol receptor deficits in their parathyroid cells, which leads to poorly controlled PTH synthesis and parathyroid gland hyperplasia.
   f. Deficient calcitriol functionality caused by vitamin D receptor deficits may also lead to calcium receptor deficits and the set point elevations involved in tertiary hyperparathyroidism.
G. **Cancer-associated hypercalcemia:**
   1. Types include humoral hypercalcemia of malignancy and local osteolytic hypercalcemia induced by metastases to bone or malignancies in the bone marrow.
   2. **Humoral hypercalcemia of malignancy:**
      a. Mechanisms:
         1) **Excessive PTHrP secretion** plays a role in the pathogenesis of hypercalcemia in most cases.
         2) PTHrP binds PTH receptors and causes the same effects with regard to calcium.
         3) Cytokines such as IL-1, TNF-α, and TGF-α may also cause humoral hypercalcemia of malignancy.
      b. **Lymphoma:**
         1) Associated with humoral hypercalcemia.
         2) Hypercalcemia is found in 20–40% of cases.
         3) Lymphomas associated with hypercalcemia are usually **T cell**, and approximately 30% of lymphomas are T cell.
      c. **Adenocarcinoma of the apocrine glands of the anal sac:**
         1) Associated with humoral hypercalcemia.
         2) Hypercalcemia is noted in approximately 50% of cases.
      d. **Other neoplasms that can cause humoral hypercalcemia of malignancy** are thymoma, myeloma, melanoma, or carcinomas originating in the lungs, pancreas, thyroid gland, skin, mammary gland, nasal cavity, and adrenal medulla.
   3. Local osteolytic hypercalcemia:
      a. Due to **metastatic bone disease or hematologic malignancies** in the bone marrow.
      b. Hypercalcemia is due to induction of local bone resorption.
      c. **Carcinomas of the mammary gland, prostate, liver, and lung most frequently metastasize to bones** in dogs; and the humerus, femur, and vertebrae are the most common sites of metastasis.
      d. Hematologic malignancies that can cause hypercalcemia are most commonly **multiple myeloma and lymphoma:**
         1) Thus, lymphoma can cause hypercalcemia by two mechanisms—humoral and local osteolysis.
         2) Hypercalcemia has been reported in 17% of dogs with multiple myeloma.
      e. **Primary bone tumors are not often associated with hypercalcemia.**

H. Primary hyperparathyroidism:

1. In Keeshonden, the gene associated with the development of primary hyperparathyroidism has been identified.

2. **A single parathyroid gland adenoma is the underlying lesion in most dogs,** regardless of breed.

3. Multiple adenomas may be found in a small percentage.

4. Parathyroid gland carcinoma is rare and parathyroid gland hyperplasia an uncommon lesion causing primary hyperparathyroidism.

I. Hypervitaminosis D:

1. Causes:

a. **Excessive dietary supplementation** of vitamin D (cholecalciferol or ergocalciferol).

b. **Overdose of calcitriol** (1-25 dihydroxyvitamin D), dihydrotachysterol cholecalciferol (vitamin D_3), or ergocalciferol (vitamin D_2) during treatment of hypoparathyroidism or overdose of calcitriol for renal secondary hyperparathyroidism.

c. Ingestion of plants containing glycosides of calcitriol (i.e., ***Cestrum diurnum* or day-blooming jessamine,** not to be confused with jasmine).

d. Ingestion of a **cholecalciferol-containing rodenticide.**

e. Ingestion of **topical ointments containing vitamin D analogues (calcipotriene) for treatment of human psoriasis:**

1) The minimal lethal dose of calcipotriene is 65 µg/kg in dogs.

2) There is rapid onset of hypercalcemia and hyperphosphatemia, with rapid catabolism of calcipotriene.

3) Hypercalcemia decreases after several days.

2. Hypercalcemia results primarily from increased intestinal absorption of calcium, but increased osteoclastic bone resorption and calcium reabsorption from renal tubules also contribute.

J. Granulomatous disease:

1. Hypercalcemia results from calcitriol synthesis by activated macrophages within granulomatous inflammation.

2. Granulomatous diseases associated with hypercalcemia include **blastomycosis, histoplasmosis, coccidioidomycosis, schistosomiasis, panniculitis, injection-site granuloma, and dermatitis.**

K. Other uncommon or rare causes of hypercalcemia:

1. Acute intrinsic renal failure:

a. Occasionally associated with mild hypercalcemia, especially during the diuretic phase of recovery.

b. Mechanism unknown.

2. Nonmalignant skeletal lesions:

a. Hypercalcemia due to local osteolysis.

b. Causes include bacterial and fungal osteomyelitis, hypertrophic osteodystrophy, and craniomandibular osteopathy.

3. Disuse osteoporosis after prolonged immobilization due to loss of bone mineral.

4. Overuse of calcium-containing intestinal phosphate binders can cause hypercalcemia due to simple oversupplementation.

5. Overdose of calcium-containing compounds:

a. Can occur during treatment of hypocalcemia.

b. Hypercalcemia due to spontaneous ingestion of rocks containing calcium carbonates has been described in a dog.

6. Grape or raisin toxicity:

a. In some cases of grape or raisin ingestion associated with acute intrinsic renal failure, mild to severe total hypercalcemia develops, but iCa status has not been reported.

b. The pathogenesis of nephrotoxicity associated with grape or raisin ingestion is unknown, but ochratoxin may be a toxic component.

c. Ingestion can be as little as 0.41–1.1 oz of grapes or raisins per kilogram body weight.

II. Signalment

A. **Hypoadre-nocorticism:**

1. More common in **younger dogs** (median age 4 years); female dogs are more likely to be affected than males.

2. Breeds at higher risk of hypoadrenocorticism include Great Danes, Portuguese water dogs, Great Pyrenees, Rottweilers, standard Poodles, West Highland white terriers, soft-coated Wheaten terriers, bearded collies, Nova Scotia duck-tolling retrievers, and Chinese cresteds.

3. A **genetic basis** has been proven in standard poodles, bearded collies, and Nova Scotia duck-tolling retrievers.

B. **Primary hyperparathyroidism:**

1. The mean age of affected dogs is 10.5 years.

2. **Breeds with an increased risk** include the Keeshond, Briard, American Eskimo, English setter, Siberian husky, Rhodesian ridgeback, Norwegian elkhound, Irish setter, wirehaired fox terrier, English Springer spaniel, Australian shepherd, Dachshund, Lhasa Apso, Shih Tzu, and golden retriever.

3. A **genetic basis** has been proven in Keeshonden.

4. **Dogs with a decreased risk** include the cocker spaniel, German shepherd dog, Shetland sheepdog, Labrador retriever, and miniature schnauzer.

C. Various age, breed, or sex predispositions exist for other causes of hypercalcemia; the reader is referred to specific texts on those topics.

III. Clinical Signs

A. **Polyuria, polydipsia, anorexia, lethargy, and weakness are the most common** clinical signs of hypercalcemia in dogs:

1. **Vomi**ting, depression, weakness, and constipation can occur.

2. Uncommon signs include cardiac arrhythmias, seizures, muscle twitching, and death.

B. Clinical signs are **most severe when hypercalcemia develops rapidly.**

C. The **magnitude of the hypercalcemia is also important:**

1. If serum tCa is >15.0 mg/dL (3.7 mmol/L) or iCa is >7.2 mg/dL (1.8 mmol/L), clinical signs are usually present.

2. If serum tCa is >18.0 mg/dL (4.5 mmol/L) or iCa is >8.8 mg/dL (2.2 mmol/L), the patient is usually critically ill.

D. **Interaction with phosphorus is important.** If serum tCa (mg/dL) multiplied by the serum phosphorus (mg/dL) concentration is >70, tissue mineralization is likely.

E. **Clinical signs due to the disease causing the hypercalcemia may also be present:**

1. Hypoadrenocorticism should be considered as a differential diagnosis in any case of hypercalcemia, as the clinical signs of ionized hypercalcemia of any cause are similar to those of hypoadrenocorticism.

2. With primary hyperparathyroidism, clinical signs related to hypercalcemia are either mild (e.g., polydipsia, polyuria, lethargy, and weakness) or absent in many affected dogs:

a. In a review of 210 dogs with primary hyperparathyroidism, no clinical signs were noted in 71% of dogs. The most common clinical signs were related to urinary tract infection or urolithiasis.

b. Urinary tract infection was present in 29% of dogs with primary hyperparathyroidism, and urolithiasis was reported in 31%.

IV. Diagnosis

A. **Definition of hypercalcemia** (Figure 34.1):

1. Using serum tCa, hypercalcemia is usually defined as a concentration >12.0 mg/dL (3.0 mmol/L).

2. Using serum iCa, hypercalcemia is usually defined as a concentration >6.0 mg/dL (1.50 mmol/L).

3. **Unpredictable discordance between serum tCa and serum iCa measurements often exists**, especially in dogs with CRF:

a. In one study, 21% of dogs with azotemic CKD were classified as hypercalcemic based on serum tCa, but when iCa was measured, only 8% were hypercalcemic.

b. Hypercalcemia is usually overestimated in dogs when serum tCa concentration is used.

4. Hypercalcemia based on serum iCa is relatively common and was observed in 19% of sick dogs in one study.

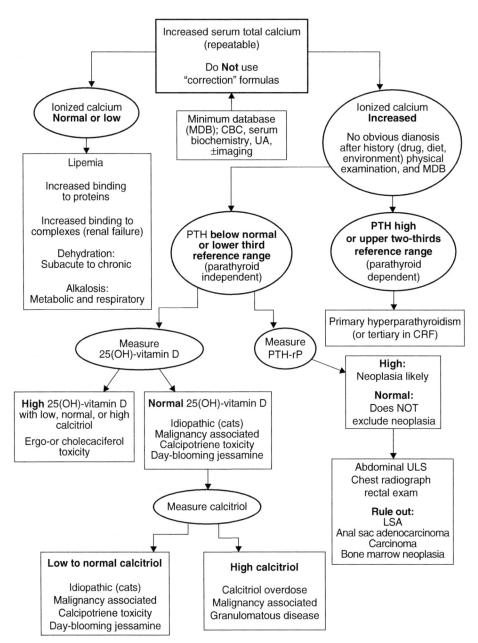

Figure 34.1 Algorithm for approach to definitive diagnosis for hypercalcemia. (Modified from Schenck PA, Chew DJ. Hypercalcemia: A quick reference. *Vet Clin North Am Small Anim Pract* 2008;38:449 453). MDB—minimum data base, ULS—ultrasound, LSA—lymphosarcoma.

B. Measurement of calcium:
   1. **Serum iCa concentration should be measured any time that an increase in serum tCa is detected.** Serum iCa should also be measured in **all cases of CRF.**
   2. **Do not use adjustment formulas to correct the tCa to serum total protein or albumin concentration** as these formulas do not accurately predict the serum iCa concentration.
   3. Do not directly compare serum iCa results to those obtained from heparinized plasma or whole blood (from a blood gas analyzer or point-of-care analyzer). The **iCa concentration is lower in heparinized plasma or whole blood than in serum.**

4. **Do not use EDTA plasma** for collection of blood for calcium measurement. EDTA chelates calcium, and EDTA plasma will yield falsely low results.

5. In dogs, serum tCa is normally 9.0–11.5 mg/dL (2.2–2.9 mmol/L) and serum iCa is normally 5.0–6.0 mg/dL (1.2–1.5 mmol/L).

6. To convert mmol/L to mg/dL, multiply mmol/L by 4.

C. **PTH concentration should be measured in conjunction with iCa measurement** to determine whether PTH production is appropriate:

1. **Patients with elevated iCa and inappropriately high PTH concentrations typically have primary hyperparathyroidism.** If serum iCa is elevated and PTH is within the upper two-thirds of the reference range or elevated, the PTH response is inappropriate, as PTH is expected to be low (below normal or in the lower third of the reference range) with elevated iCa.

2. Hypercalcemia associated with low serum PTH is classified as parathyroid-independent hypercalcemia.

3. Of hypercalcemic canine samples submitted for hormone analysis to specialist endocrinology laboratories, approximately 40% have primary hyperparathyroidism and 50% have parathyroid-independent hypercalcemia. However, because of sample bias, primary hyperparathyroidism is overrepresented compared to that reported from referral clinics for hypercalcemic dogs in general.

D. **Measurement of serum 25-hydroxyvitamin D concentration** may be helpful to identify cases in which increased vitamin D intake is the cause of hypercalcemia.

E. **Calcitriol concentration measurement** may be helpful in patients with normal serum 25-hydroxyvitamin D concentration.

F. Other tests may be indicated depending on the suspected underlying cause.

V. Differential Diagnoses

A. Potential causes of hypercalcemia are listed in Table 34.1.

B. In dogs, **neoplasia is the most common cause of hypercalcemia, followed by hypoadrenocorticism, primary hyperparathyroidism, and renal failure (elevation of serum tCa but not iCa).**

C. **Transient** hypercalcemia:

1. Should be suspected if dehydration is present and serum tCa concentrations are mildly elevated (12.0–13.5 mg/dL or 3.0–3.4 mmol/L) or serum albumin or protein concentrations are increased.

2. In addition, serum calcium concentration will rapidly return to normal when dehydration has been corrected.

D. **Hypoadrenocorticism:**

1. The hypercalcemia is typically mild.

2. The magnitude of hypercalcemia is greater in more severely affected dogs.

3. Serum tCa concentration returns to normal after 1–2 days of hormone replacement therapy.

4. Some combinations of hyperkalemia, hyponatremia, and decreased sodium:potassium ratio suggest the diagnosis.

5. **Hypercalcemia due to hypoadrenocorticism in the absence of altered sodium and potassium concentrations, though possible, is rare.**

E. Azotemic CKD:

1. The finding of hypercalcemia with primary renal azotemia poses a diagnostic problem since hypercalcemia can cause renal failure or can develop as a consequence of renal failure.

2. **Serum iCa concentration is usually normal to low in patients with azotemic CKD.**

3. **Measurement of serum iCa concentration to assess calcium status is critical** in azotemic CKD:

   a. **Serum tCa measurement incorrectly assesses iCa status in about 36% of dogs with azotemic CKD.**

   b. Adjustment formulas should not be used, as they do not accurately determine iCa status in approximately 53% of dogs with azotemic CKD.

   c. **Serum tCa measurement or adjusted tCa measurement overestimates hypercalcemia and underestimates hypocalcemia in dogs with azotemic CKD.**

4. The incidence of elevated tCa in azotemic CKD is about 14%, and increases with the severity of azotemia. Fewer than 10% of dogs with azotemic CKD have increased serum iCa concentrations.

5. In tertiary hyperparathyroidism, azotemic CKD patients have increased iCa with excessive PTH secretion.

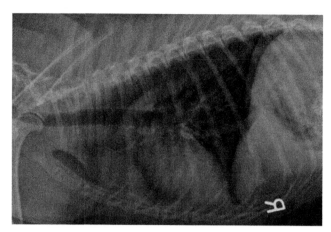

Figure 34.2   Mediastinal lymphosarcoma associated with hypercalcemia in a dog. Note mass cranial to the heart on this lateral radiograph of the thorax. (Courtesy of Dr. Felipe Galvao, The Ohio State University College of Veterinary Medicine and the Radiology Section).

F.   **Cancer-associated** hypercalcemia:
1. This is the most common cause of hypercalcemia in dogs.
2. Since malignancy causes **parathyroid-independent** hypercalcemia, it **should be suspected when serum iCa concentration is increased, PTH is suppressed** (below normal or in the lower third of the reference range) **and PTHrP is increased. Hypophosphatemia is often present** if kidney function is normal.
3. In dogs, malignancies commonly associated with hypercalcemia include **T-cell lymphoma** (**Figure 34.2**) and **adenocarcinoma of the apocrine glands of the anal sacs.**
4. If hypercalcemia due to malignancy is suspected:
   a. A complete physical exam should be repeated paying particular attention to lymph nodes. A thorough rectal exam should be done with careful palpation of the anal sacs and sublumbar lymph nodes.
   b. Any enlarged lymph nodes should be aspirated and cytology performed.
   c. Three-view thoracic radiographs should always be done:
      1) The mediastinum should be evaluated for the presence of a mass.
      2) Metastatic disease from the tumor causing the hypercalcemia may be present.
   d. Abdominal ultrasound may be helpful:
      1) May identify a tumor anywhere.
      2) Particular attention should be paid to the liver, spleen, and lymph nodes for the presence of lymphoma.
   e. Other tests to consider to screen for lymphoma:
      1) Aspirate and cytology of lymph nodes that palpate normally.
      2) Bone marrow aspirate and cytology.
5. **Tumors of the apocrine gland of the anal sacs:**
   a. **Should not be confused with the common perianal adenoma** that is not associated with hypercalcemia.
   b. On occasion, both anal sacs may feel normal but metastases are detected in the regional lymph nodes. Repeated palpation of the anal sac often discloses the primary nodule that was missed.
   c. **Circulating PTHrP concentrations are highest in dogs with apocrine adenocarcinomas of the anal sac** and sporadic carcinomas associated with humoral hypercalcemia of malignancy.
6. Hematologic malignancies:
   a. **Hematologic malignancies that cause hypercalcemia are typically multiple myeloma and lymphoma** (**Figure 34.3**).
   b. With multiple myeloma:
      1) Bone marrow aspirate and cytology should be performed.

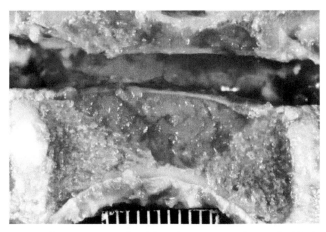

Figure 34.3 Local osteolytic hypercalcemia associated with lymphosarcoma in the vertebral body of a dog. This lesion was present in other vertebrae and some internal organs also. The finding of obvious bone loss at necropsy or on radiographs usually excludes humoral hypercalcemia of malignancy. Hypercalcemia is largely the result of activated osteoclastic bone resorption from the local lesion. (Courtesy of Dr. Donald Meuten North Carolina State Univeristy and Dr. Dennis Chew The Ohio State University).

      2) Osteolytic disease may be present on radiographs.

      3) Hyperglobulinemia due to a monoclonal gammopathy may be present.

      4) Urine should be screened for the presence of Bence-Jones proteinuria.

  7. Tumors metastatic to bone:

    a. Solid tumors that metastasize to bone rarely produce hypercalcemia.

    b. Carcinomas of the mammary gland, prostate, liver, and lung most frequently metastasize to bones in dogs, with the humerus, femur, and vertebrae being the most common sites.

    c. Primary bone tumors are not often associated with hypercalcemia.

    d. Areas of osseous pain should be radiographed; radiographic lesions should be aspirated and/or biopsied with appropriate evaluation (e.g., cytology and/or histopathology, culture, etc.).

G. **Primary hyperparathyroidism:**

  1. Primary hyperparathyroidism is **uncommon**. In about 90% of dogs with primary hyperparathyroidism, it is caused by a single parathyroid adenoma (**Figure 34.4**).

  2. In primary hyperparathyroidism, **serum iCa concentration is elevated and PTH is inappropriately high for the level of hypercalcemia:**

    a. In a review of 210 dogs with primary hyperparathyroidism, all had hypercalcemia and 65% had hypophosphatemia.

    b. Serum PTH concentration was within the reference range in 73% of dogs and above the reference range in the rest.

  3. A parathyroid mass is rarely if ever palpable in dogs.

  4. **Ultrasonography of the neck can be helpful** in the diagnosis, but it **requires operator experience and an ultrasound unit with a high-frequency transducer** to achieve good resolution (**Figure 34.5**).

H. **Hypervitaminosis D:**

  1. Clinical signs are those encountered with development of ionized hypercalcemia, though often they are more severe due to rapid and severe increases. Soft tissue mineralization is more severe with hypervitaminosis D; tongue necrosis may be a more specific lesion in dogs.

  2. Should be suspected with history of access to rodenticides, plants that cause hypercalcemia (i.e., *Cestrum diurnum* or day blooming jessamine, not to be confused with jasmine), or antipsoriasis creams as well as in dogs that are treated with any form of Vitamin D and/or oral calcium supplements.

  3. Hypercalcemia usually develops within 24 h after ingestion and is often severe.

  4. **Hyperphosphatemia is often noted, and azotemia is initially absent but can subsequently develop.**

(b)

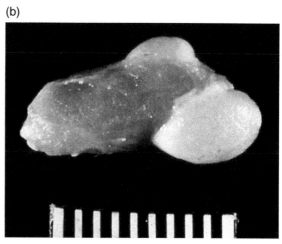

(a)

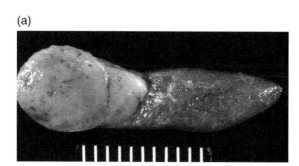

Figure 34.4   (a) Single large parathyroid adenoma (left) in sagittal section, embedded in thyroid tissue of a dog with hypercalcemia due to primary hyperparathyroidism. (Courtesy of Dr. Charles Capen, The Ohio State University College of Veterinary Medicine). (b) Multiple parathyroid adenomas in a dog with primary hyperparathyroidism. Though this is less common than the finding of a single adenoma, as many as four adenomas can be encountered. It is difficult to make the histopathologic distinction between multiple adenomas and parathyroid gland hyperplasia. (Courtesy of Dr. Larry Nagode, The Ohio State University College of Veterinary Medicine, Department of Veterinary Biosciences).

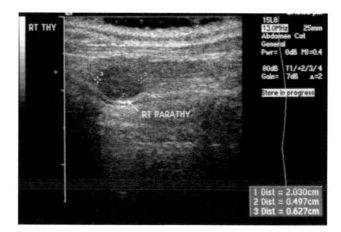

Figure 34.5   Ultrasonography of a single large parathyroid gland adenoma associated with hypercalcemia in a dog. If a parathyroid gland nodule >2 mm is found, surgery is usually recommended. A parathyroid nodule of 2–4 mm is consistent with hyperplasia and >4 mm that of adenoma. (Courtesy of the Radiology Section Center for Veterinary Medicine, The Ohio State University).

5. PTH concentration is suppressed.
6. Vitamin D metabolite concentrations:
    a. **Serum concentration of 25-hydroxyvitamin D will be elevated in cases of treatment overdose, cholecalciferol rodenticide ingestion, or excessive dietary supplementation of vitamin D.**
    b. **Concentration of 25-hydroxyvitamin D may be normal in cases of plant or antipsoriasis ointment ingestion.**
I. Granulomatous disease:
    1. **Clinical signs of the underlying disease** (e.g., blastomycosis, histoplasmosis, coccidioidomycosis, and schistosomiasis) **may predominate** and can include uveitis, bone pain, cutaneous masses and/or draining tracts, respiratory difficulty, cough, large bowel diarrhea, and weight loss depending on the specific disease.

2. Serum iCa concentration is increased, and PTH is suppressed; PTHrP should be normal to undetectable.

3. **Serum calcitriol concentrations are increased.** Decreasing levels of calcitriol accompany successful treatment that restores normocalcemia.

4. Specific tests may be indicated depending on the suspected disease, for example, serum fungal titers, PCR, or urine antigen testing.

J. **Acute intrinsic renal failure** can be diagnosed based on acute onset of renal disease and ruling out other causes.

K. **Nonmalignant skeletal lesions:**

1. **Radiographs** of the affected bone will be necessary for diagnosis.

2. **Bone biopsy** may be required:

   a. **Histopathology** should be performed.

   b. **Bacterial and fungal cultures** should be submitted if indicated.

   c. **Fungal titers** may be of use if fungal disease is suspected.

L. Disuse osteoporosis after prolonged immobilization can be diagnosed based on history.

M. Overuse of calcium-containing intestinal phosphate binders should be suspected based on history of administration.

N. Hypercalcemia from spontaneous ingestion of rocks should be suspected based on history.

O. Grape or raisin toxicity should be suspected based on history of ingestion.

VI. Treatment

A. An overview of treatment of hypercalcemia is provided in Table 34.2.

B. The magnitude of hypercalcemia, rate of development, whether the calcium concentration is continuing to increase, and modifying effects of other electrolytes and acid-base disturbances should all be considered when deciding on a treatment plan:

1. Serum tCa concentration of 16 mg/dL (4 mmol/L) or greater usually warrants aggressive therapy. Serum tCa concentration approaching 20 mg/dL (5 mmol/L) merits crisis management if clinical signs are severe.

2. Depending on the degree of neurologic, cardiac, and renal dysfunction induced by the hypercalcemia and concurrent deleterious factors, animals with serum tCa <16 mg/dL (4 mmol/L) may also require aggressive treatment.

3. Acidosis magnifies the effects of hypercalcemia by shifting more calcium to the ionized fraction.

4. Serum phosphorus concentration is important in decision making because soft tissue mineralization is potentiated by hyperphosphatemia when the product of multiplying calcium concentration by phosphorus concentration, both in mg/dL, is >70.

5. Animals with rapid and progressive development of hypercalcemia usually display severe clinical signs and require aggressive therapy.

C. **Removal of the underlying cause** of the hypercalcemia is the definitive treatment.

D. **Supportive therapy is often needed** to decrease serum calcium concentration to a less toxic level while waiting for a definitive diagnosis to be established.

E. Parenteral fluids, furosemide, sodium bicarbonate, glucocorticoids, or combinations of these treatments reduce serum calcium concentrations in most animals:

1. **Fluid therapy:**

   a. The **first goal of fluid therapy is to correct dehydration** because hemoconcentration contributes to hypercalcemia.

   b. **Dehydration should be corrected within 4–6 h** of presentation in animals with severe clinical signs of hypercalcemia. Normocalcemia may be restored by fluid therapy alone if the hypercalcemia was initially mild.

   c. **Physiologic saline** (0.9% NaCl) is the solution of choice. It is preferred to lactated Ringer's solution since it contains no calcium and more sodium than lactated Ringer's solution.

   d. The **intravenous (IV) route is always needed for treatment of ionized hypercalcemia in animals with severe clinical signs.** Subcutaneous fluids are not helpful initially but could be useful when weaning off IV fluids or in those dogs with minimal hypercalcemia.

Table 34.2   Treatment of hypercalcemia.

Treatment	Dose	Indications	Comments
Volume expansion			
SQ Saline (0.9%)	75–100 mL/kg/day	Mild hypercalcemia	Contraindicated if peripheral edema is present
IV saline (0.9%)	100–125 mL/kg/day	Moderate to severe hypercalcemia	Contraindicated if congestive heart failure and/or hypertension present
Diuretics			
Furosemide	1–4 mg/kg q 8–12 h IV, SQ, PO; constant rate infusion 0.2–1 mg/kg/h	Moderate to severe hypercalcemia	Volume expansion is necessary prior to use of this drug
Glucocorticoids			
Prednisone	1–2.2 mg/kg BID PO, SQ, IV	Moderate to severe hypercalcemia	Use of these drugs prior to identification of etiology of hypercalcemia may make definitive diagnosis difficult
Prednisolone	5–20 mg/cat/day PO	Feline idiopathic hypercalcemia	Follow by 6 mL tap water and "buttering" of nose
Dexamethasone	0.1–0.22 mg/kg BID IV, SQ		
Inhibition of bone resorption			
Calcitonin	4–6 IU/kg SQ BID to TID	Hypervitaminosis D toxicity	Response may be short lived. Vomiting may occur
Bisphosphonates		Moderate to severe chronic hypercalcemia	Expensive Large and rapid doses IV associated with acute renal failure
Etidronate	5–15 mg/kg Daily to BID		
Clodronate	20–25 mg/kg in a 4-h IV infusion		Approved in Europe; availability in USA limited
Pamidronate	1.3–2.0 mg/kg in 150 mL 0.9% saline in a 2-h IV infusion; can repeat in 1–3 weeks	Hypervitaminosis D	Well studied in dogs
Alendronate	1–4 mg/kg, q 48–72 h PO; 10–30 mg/cat once weekly followed by 6 mL PO tap water and "buttering" of lips	Adjunctive therapy for malignancy-associated hypercalcemia or primary hyperparathyroidism Feline idiopathic hypercalcemia	
Shifting of ionized calcium to other fractions			
Sodium bicarbonate	1 mEq/kg slow IV bolus (may give up to 4 mEq/kg total dose)	Severe, life-threatening hypercalcemia	Requires close monitoring. Rapid onset of action

2. Diuretics:
   a. **Furosemide** is important for treatment of persistent hypercalcemia.
   b. Furosemide promotes enhanced urinary calcium loss.
   c. **Thiazides should not be used** since they may result in hypocalciuria and may aggravate hypercalcemia.
   d. **Adequate hydration before initiation of and during furosemide administration is essential.**
3. Sodium bicarbonate:
   a. Serum iCa concentration is reduced with sodium bicarbonate infusion as the serum pH becomes more alkalotic, calcium binding to serum proteins increases.
   b. Infusion of sodium bicarbonate is most often used **in the presence of severe metabolic acidosis or in those with severe hypercalcemic crisis** (e.g., collapse, encephalopathy, and cardiac arrhythmia).
   c. Reduction in total serum calcium concentration is slight after sodium bicarbonate administration alone.
   d. Sodium bicarbonate infusion is **most likely to be helpful in combination with other treatments.**
4. Glucocorticoids:
   a. Glucocorticoids can significantly reduce serum iCa concentration in patients with hypercalcemia, especially those with lymphoma, apocrine gland adenocarcinoma of the anal sacs, multiple myeloma, thymoma, hypoadrenocorticism, hypervitaminosis D, hypervitaminosis A, or granulomatous disease.
   b. **When possible, glucocorticoids should be withheld from animals for which a diagnosis of the underlying disease has not been established:**
      1) Lymphocytolysis **can make a cytologic or histopathologic diagnosis of lymphoma much more difficult or impossible.** Effects of glucocorticoids may similarly make it difficult to definitively diagnose leukemias or multiple myeloma as the cause for hypercalcemia.
      2) Treatment with glucocorticoids alone before initiation of a traditional combination chemotherapy protocol for lymphoma **can potentially decrease survival duration by 50%.**
5. Calcitonin:
   a. Treatment with calcitonin **may be useful in those with severe hypercalcemia.** It is almost always used in combination with other treatments and is **not considered effective alone.**
   b. Calcitonin treatment is **expensive,** its effect is **unpredictable,** effects are **short lived,** and resistance often develops after a few days.
   c. Vomiting and anorexia are common side effects in dogs.
6. Bisphosphonates:
   a. Bisphosphonates inhibit bone resorption by decreasing osteoclast activity and function.
   b. Bisphosphonates are **given when the underlying disease causing the hypercalcemia cannot be completely or quickly treated (especially in those with severe hypercalcemia), as occurs in hypervitaminosis D (cholecalciferol) or from malignancy that is nonresectable and not responding to chemotherapy.**
   c. **Dehydration should be corrected** before bisphosphonate use to lessen the chance of renal injury.
   d. IV infusion of pamidronate has been used to treat hypercalcemia. Clodronate has also been used clinically to treat hypercalcemia.

F. **Specific treatment for hypoadrenocorticism:**
   1. Treatment of dehydration and hormone deficiencies is key (see Chapter 2).
   2. Hypercalcemia usually resolves with specific treatment for hypoadrenocorticism and does not require further therapy.
G. **Specific treatment for azotemic CKD:**
   1. A complete description is beyond the scope of the book and the reader is referred elsewhere.
   2. Treatment with low-dose calcitriol therapy to reduce PTH synthesis improves quality of life, reduces progression of chronic renal disease, and prolongs life.
   3. Low-dose calcitriol therapy is considered after dietary phosphate restriction and use of intestinal phosphate binders to control serum phosphorus levels to <5.5 mg/dL (1.8 mmol/L), preferably to levels <4.5 mg/dL (1.45 mmol/L).

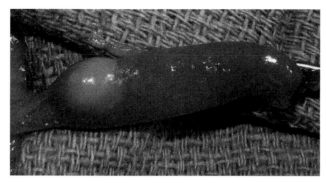

Figure 34.6   Obvious parathyroid gland mass at surgery in a dog with primary hyperparathyroidism. Note polar mass embedded in the thyroid gland that is nearing complete excision. (Courtesy of Dr. Stephen Birchard, The Ohio State University College of Veterinary Medicine).

    4. Ideally, PTH concentrations are monitored during treatment with calcitriol to ensure it either decreases or stays within the reference range.

    5. Hypercalcemia is very uncommon in dogs treated with lower dosages of calcitriol (2.5–4.0 ng/kg/day). Even so, it is **important to monitor circulating calcium status** at least with tCa, though measurement of iCa provides more useful information especially for those with azotemic CKD. Calcium should be measured at 1 and 4 weeks after initiating therapy and then every 4 months thereafter to ensure that hypercalcemia does not develop.

H. Specific treatment for hypervitaminosis D:

    1. When associated with **cholecalciferol intoxication, treatment of hypercalcemia may be necessary for several weeks** because of the long half-lives of cholecalciferol (29 days in dogs) and vitamin D metabolites:

        a. **Aggressive therapy for 1 week** or more may be required.

        b. **Maintenance therapy** with prednisone and furosemide should be continued **for 1 month.**

        c. A **low-calcium diet is important** to reduce intestinal calcium absorption.

    2. **Noncalcium-containing intestinal phosphorus binders** (e.g., aluminum hydroxide, sevelamer hydrochloride, and lanthanum carbonate):

        a. May be beneficial in addition to a phosphorus-restricted diet to minimize the degree of hyperphosphatemia, hopefully restoring serum phosphorus concentration to within the reference range.

        b. Doses are usually from 30 to 100 mg/kg divided in meals and adjusted based on the serum phosphorus concentration achieved.

    3. **IV pamidronate protocols** are very useful during treatment of hypervitaminosis D (Table 34.2). Since this compound **may take up to 72 h to achieve salutary effects,** other treatments to control hypercalcemia must be initially given until this effect is achieved.

I. Specific treatment for primary hyperparathyroidism:

    1. **Surgery to remove the parathyroid adenoma is the treatment of choice (Figure 34.6).** Occasionally, more than one parathyroid gland mass is visible which should also be removed:

        a. In 47 dogs undergoing surgery to remove a parathyroid mass, 94% resulted in control of hypercalcemia.

        b. Hypercalcemia resolved in 1–6 days.

        c. **Hypocalcemia may occur postoperatively,** especially if the serum tCa is >14 mg/dL (3.5 mmol/L) before surgery:

            1) **Hypocalcemia without clinical signs usually does not require treatment unless the serum tCa is <6 mg/dL (1.5 mmol/L).**

            2) Treatment with supplemental calcium or vitamin D metabolites is required if tCa is <6 mg/dL (1.5 mmol/L) or clinical signs of hypocalcemia are present (see Chapter 31).

            3) If the patient is treated with oral calcitriol (7.5 ng/kg/BID) for 7–10 days prior to surgery, hypocalcemia in the postsurgical period can be minimized.

    d. If the patient is unstable, bisphosphonate therapy for 1–2 months prior to surgery may decrease the serum calcium concentration, increase the chance for renal repair, and increase the recovery of the atrophied parathyroid glands.

  2. **Ultrasound-guided ethanol ablation** is an alternative to surgery:

    a. In a review of 110 dogs with primary hyperparathyroidism, 72% of ethanol ablation procedures resulted in resolution of hypercalcemia within 1–4 days.

    b. Requires extensive technical expertise.

  3. **Ultrasound-guided radiofrequency heat ablation** of the parathyroid mass is also used as a treatment:

    a. In 49 dogs treated with heat ablation, 90% experienced control of their disease with resolution of the hypercalcemia within 1–6 days.

    b. Requires extensive technical expertise and the equipment is expensive.

    c. If multiple masses present, surgery may be preferred.

VII. Prognosis

A. **Prognosis is dependent on the underlying cause** of hypercalcemia.

B. **Hypoadrenocorticism:** Excellent following fluid repletion and replacement hormone therapy; with spontaneous disease, lifelong therapy is required.

C. **Renal failure:**

    a. Usually tCa, not iCa, is increased in azotemic CKD so calcium-specific treatment is not indicated.

    b. An increased tCa concentration is not known to be associated with pathology in the face of a normal iCa.

D. **Humoral hypercalcemia of malignancy and malignant local osteolytic hypercalcemia:** Good to excellent for the initial response of hypercalcemia to treatment and poor for long-term survival due to the underlying malignancy.

E. **Primary hyperparathyroidism:**

  1. **In cases of parathyroid gland adenoma, the prognosis is excellent following surgical removal.**

  2. **In cases of parathyroid adenocarcinoma, prognosis is guarded** depending on the ability to remove the entire tumor. Following surgery, 94% of dogs had control of hypercalcemia for a median of 581 days.

F. **Hypervitaminosis D:** Good to excellent if hypercalcemia is identified and adequate treatment started early enough.

G. **Granulomatous disease:**

    a. Good to excellent if the cause is fungal and the organisms can be eradicated.

    b. Good to excellent for control of sterile dermatitis and panniculitis while on glucocorticoids.

    c. Good to excellent if sterile granulomatous masses can be completely excised.

H. **Grape or raisin ingestion:** Guarded to fair. About 50% survive with intensive supportive care.

I. **Nonmalignant skeletal disease:** Good if the underlying lesion such as hypertrophic osteodystrophy or craniomandibular osteopathy resolve.

VIII. Prevention

A. Prevent exposure to excessive vitamin D.

B. Prevent exposure to grapes and raisins.

C. Prevent ingestion of excessive calcium supplementation or calcium carbonate-containing rocks.

References and Further Readings

Adamantos S, Boag A. Total and ionised calcium concentrations in dogs with hypoadrenocorticism. *Vet Rec* 2008; 163(1):25–26.

Eubig PA, Brady MS, Gwaltney-Brant SM, Khan SA, Mazzaferro EM, Morrow CMK. Acute renal failure in dogs after the ingestion of grapes or raisins: A retrospective evaluation of 43 dogs (1992–2002). *J Vet Intern Med* 2005;19(5):663–674.

Feldman EC, Hoar B, Pollard R, Nelson RW. Pretreatment clinical and laboratory findings in dogs with primary hyperparathyroidism: 210 cases (1987–2004). *J Am Vet Med Assoc* 2005;227(5):756–761.

Gow AG, Gow DJ, Bell R, Simpson JW, Chandler ML, Evans H, Berry JL, Herrtage ME, Mellanby RJ. Calcium metabolism in eight dogs with hypoadrenocorticism. *J Small Anim Pract* 2009;50(8):426–430.

Hare WR, Dobbs CE, Slayman KA, et al. Calcipotriene poisoning in dogs. *Vet Med* 2000;95:770–778.

Hostutler RA, Chew DJ, Jaeger JQ, et al. Uses and effectiveness of pamidronate disodium for treatment of dogs and cats with hypercalcemia. *J Vet Intern Med* 2005;19:29–33.

Messinger JS, Windham WR, Ward CR. Ionized hypercalcemia in dogs: A retrospective study of 109 cases (1998–2003). *J Vet Intern Med* 2009;23(3):514–519.

Morrow CMK, Valli VE, Volmer PA, et al. Canine renal pathology associated with grape or raisin ingestion: 10 cases. *J Vet Diagn Invest* 2005;17:223–231.

Rasor L, Pollard R, Feldman EC. Retrospective evaluation of three treatment methods for primary hyperparathyroidism in dogs. *J Am Anim Hosp Assoc* 2007;43(2):70–77.

Rosol TJ, Nagode LA, Couto CG, et al. Parathyroid hormone (PTH)-related protein, PTH, and 1,25-dihydroxyvitamin D in dogs with cancer-associated hypercalcemia. *Endocrinology* 1992;131:1157–1164.

Rumbeiha WK, Fitzgerald SD, Kruger JM, et al. Use of pamidronate disodium to reduce cholecalciferol-induced toxicosis in dogs. *Am J Vet Res* 2000;61:9–13.

Rumbeiha WK, Kruger JM, Fitzgerald SF, et al. Use of pamidronate to reverse vitamin D3-induced toxicosis in dogs. *Am J Vet Res* 1999;60:1092–1097.

Schenck PA, Chew DJ. Prediction of serum ionized calcium concentration by use of serum total calcium concentration in dogs. *Am J Vet Res* 2005;66(8):1330–1336.

Schenck PA, Chew DJ. Calcium: Total or ionized? *Vet Clin North Am Small Anim Pract* 2008;38(3):497–502.

Schenck PA, Chew DJ, Nagode LA, Rosol TJ. Disorders of calcium: hypercalcemia and hypocalcemia. In: Dibartola S, Ed. *Fluid Therapy in Small Animal Practice*, 3rd edn. St. Louis: Elsevier, 2006, pp. 122–194.

Williams LE, Gliatto JM, Dodge RK, et al. Carcinoma of the apocrine glands of the anal sac in dogs: 113 cases (1985–1995). *J Am Vet Med Assoc* 2003;223:825–831.

CHAPTER 35

Hypercalcemia in Cats

Dennis Chew and Patricia A. Schenck

Pathogenesis

- Clinical signs occur when serum ionized calcium (iCa) rises above a critical level.
- Causes of hypercalcemia can be parathyroid independent or parathyroid dependent (primary hyperparathyroidism).
- The most common causes of hypercalcemia in cats are idiopathic hypercalcemia, chronic renal failure (total calcium [tCa]), and malignancy.
- Hypercalcemia is usually underestimated when serum tCa is used.

Classical Signs

- The most common clinical sign associated with hypercalcemia is anorexia; other common signs include vomiting, depression, weakness, and constipation. Polyuria and polydipsia are much less commonly reported than in dogs.
- Clinical signs are most severe when hypercalcemia develops rapidly.
- Cats with idiopathic hypercalcemia may have no clinical signs, or transient signs thought to be insignificant.

Diagnosis

- Hypercalcemia is defined as a tCa concentration >11.0 mg/dL (2.75 mmol/L) or iCa concentration >5.7 mg/dL (1.40 mmol/L).
- Parathyroid hormone (PTH) should be measured in conjunction with iCa measurement to determine whether PTH production is appropriate.
- Measurement of PTH-related protein (PTHrP) may be helpful in cases of suspected malignancy; measurement of serum 25-hydroxyvitamin D may be helpful to identify cases of vitamin D toxicity.

Treatment

- Specific therapy depends on the cause.
- General therapy includes the administration of fluids, diuretics, glucocorticoids, and/or bisphosphonates.

Clinical Endocrinology of Companion Animals, First Edition. Edited by Jacquie Rand.
© 2013 John Wiley & Sons, Inc. Published 2013 by John Wiley & Sons, Inc.

Prognosis

- Prognosis is dependent on the underlying cause.
- Prognosis is good for most cases of idiopathic hypercalcemia, vitamin D toxicity, primary hyperparathyroidism, and hypoadrenocorticism if treatment is adequate.

I. Pathogenesis
A. Serum tCa is composed of protein-bound calcium (pCa), complexed calcium (cCa), and iCa. The iCa fraction is the biologically active fraction.
B. Development of hypercalcemia:
  1. Hypercalcemia develops primarily when there is an increase in bone mobilization of calcium, an increase in intestinal calcium absorption, or a decrease in urinary loss of calcium (decreased glomerular filtration rate [GFR] or increased tubular reabsorption of calcium). Hypercalcemia based on measurement of tCa but not iCa can occur with increases in circulating complexes (as can happen in azotemic chronic kidney disease [CKD]):
    a. An increase in serum iCa concentration decreases PTH secretion if the parathyroid gland is healthy, increases intracellular degradation of PTH in parathyroid gland chief cells, and decreases PTH synthesis.
    b. Increased calcitonin secretion is stimulated in an attempt to minimize the magnitude of hypercalcemia.
    c. Calcitriol synthesis in the kidney is decreased both through direct inhibition by iCa and by decreased stimulation because of decreased PTH concentration.
    d. The overall outcome is to increase urinary excretion of calcium and to decrease the bone mobilization of calcium in an effort to limit the degree of hypercalcemia.
  2. In **primary hyperparathyroidism**, the parathyroid adenoma continues to secrete PTH even though hypercalcemia is present. This is termed a **"parathyroid-dependent"** hypercalcemia. With primary hyperparathyroidism, there is an increased serum iCa concentration, with an inappropriate PTH secretion. Most cases in cats are caused by a single parathyroid adenoma.
  3. In **"parathyroid-independent"** causes of hypercalcemia, hypercalcemia occurs due to other secretory factors (such as PTHrP, interleukin, or tumor necrosis factor) or as a result of excessive vitamin D ingestion. In these instances, the parathyroid gland responds in a normal fashion to the hypercalcemia and PTH secretion is very low. Thus in parathyroid-independent hypercalcemias, serum iCa concentration is elevated and PTH shows appropriate suppression in response to the hypercalcemia.
C. Causes of hypercalcemia are listed in Table 35.1.
D. Transient hypercalcemia:
  1. Dehydration is occasionally associated with mild increases in serum tCa concentrations that rapidly return to normal when dehydration has been corrected.
  2. Increased serum albumin or total protein can result in an increased serum tCa concentration as more calcium binds to protein.
E. **Idiopathic hypercalcemia** has been recognized in the last 20 years in cats. It now appears to be **the most common cause of hypercalcemia in cats in the USA.** The pathogenesis of idiopathic hypercalcemia is unknown. It does not appear to be due to excessive serum vitamin D or calcitriol concentrations, though some cats could be especially sensitive to "normal" concentrations of these vitamin D metabolites. Specific nutrients in the diet may play a role, but this has not been proven. A role for acquired dysfunction of the calcium-sensing receptor is possible but has not been investigated.
F. **Cancer-associated hypercalcemia:** Mechanisms of hypercalcemia include humoral hypercalcemia of malignancy, and local osteolytic hypercalcemia induced by metastases to bone, and malignancies in the bone marrow.
G. **Humoral hypercalcemia of malignancy:** Excessive secretion of PTHrP plays a role in the pathogenesis of hypercalcemia in some cases, but cytokines such as IL-1, TNF-α, and TGF-α may also cause hypercalcemia:
  1. **Metastatic tumors and hematologic malignancies:** Hypercalcemia is due to the induction of local bone resorption.

Table 35.1   Causes of hypercalcemia in cats.

Nonpathologic	Transient or inconsequential
Nonfasting (minimal increase)	Hemoconcentration
Growth in young cats	Hyperproteinemia
Laboratory error	Hypoadrenocorticism
Spurious (lipemia, detergent contamination of sample)	Severe environmental hypothermia

Pathologic or consequential (persistent)

Parathyroid dependent: primary hyperparathyroidism

Parathyroid independent:

  Idiopathic hypercalcemia

  Malignancy associated

    Humoral hypercalcemia of malignancy (lymphoma, squamous cell carcinoma [head and neck], and other carcinomas)

    Hematologic malignancies (lymphoma, multiple myeloma, myeloproliferative disease, leukemia)

    Metastatic or primary bone neoplasia—not reported in cats

Chronic renal failure (elevation of tCa)

Hypervitaminosis D (iatrogenic, plants, rodenticide, antipsoriasis creams)

Granulomatous disease (blastomycosis, mycobacteriosis, dermatitis, panniculitis, injection reaction)

Acute renal failure (diuretic phase)

Nonmalignant skeletal lesions (osteomyelitis, hypertrophic osteodystrophy)

Excessive calcium-containing intestinal phosphate binders

Excessive calcium supplementation

Hypervitaminosis A

Acromegaly

Thyrotoxicosis

Aluminum exposure (intestinal phosphate binders)

H. **CKD (IRIS stages 2–4)**—Serum tCa may be elevated, but serum iCa is uncommonly elevated:
   1. The increase in serum tCa may be due to an increase in the cCa fraction as in dogs, but this has not been proven in cats.
   2. Excessive supplementation with calcitriol can cause hypercalcemia.
   3. The use of calcium carbonate intestinal phosphate binders may cause hypercalcemia.
   4. Tertiary hyperparathyroidism occurs in some CRF patients with long-standing secondary hyperparathyroidism. The iCa fraction increases due to a change in the set point for iCa.
I. **Tertiary hyperparathyroidism** refers to the condition in a small subset of CKD patients with CKD who develop increased iCa with excessive PTH secretion. It is likely that these patients had renal secondary hyperparathyroidism earlier in the clinical course of CKD. Downregulation of the vitamin D receptor in the parathyroid glands plays a pivotal role in this and occurs secondary to calcitriol deficits encountered during azotemic CKD.
J. **Primary hyperparathyroidism** is rare and most cases in cats are caused by a single parathyroid adenoma.
K. **Hypoadrenocorticism** is a rare cause of hypercalcemia in cats.

L. **Hypervitaminosis D**: Toxicity results from excess cholecalciferol, ergocalciferol, 25-hydroxyvitamin D, calcitriol, or analogues of calcitriol. Hypercalcemia results from increased intestinal absorption of calcium, but increased osteoclastic bone resorption and calcium reabsorption from renal tubules also contribute:

    1. Vitamin D toxicity in cats is uncommonly reported due to the fact that cats appear to be somewhat resistant to cholecalciferol toxicity when the diet is otherwise complete and balanced.

    2. Causes of hypervitaminosis D:

        a. **Excessive dietary supplementation of vitamin D**. Hypervitaminosis D with hypercalcemia, azotemia, high concentrations of 25-hydroxyvitamin D, and/or renal calcification has been described in cats fed a commercial cat food in which the cholecalciferol content of the diet greatly exceeded the dietary requirements of vitamin D.

        b. **Overdose during treatment of hypoparathyroidism**.

        c. **Ingestion of plants** containing glycosides of calcitriol (*Cestrum diurnum*, *Solanum malacoxylon*, and *Trisetum flavescens*).

        d. **Ingestion of cholecalciferol-containing rodenticide**.

        e. **Ingestion of topical ointments containing vitamin D analogues** (calcipotriene) for the treatment of human psoriasis is possible but not specifically reported in cats. Anecdotal reports of this ingestion exist for cats following licking of ointment off humans, unlike dogs that usually ingest the tube. It would be anticipated that toxicity would be far less severe with gradual ingestion of these small amounts from licking.

M. **Granulomatous disease**—Hypercalcemia results from calcitriol synthesis by activated macrophages in granulomatous inflammation:

    1. Granulomatous disease associated with hypercalcemia includes histoplasmosis, *Nocardia*, and mycobacterial infection. Cats with blastomycosis, cryptococcosis, actinomyces, and injection-site granulomas have been observed to have hypercalcemia, possibly due to enhanced synthesis of calcitriol.

II. Signalment

A. **Idiopathic hypercalcemia**:

    1. Cats with idiopathic hypercalcemia range from 0.5 to 20 years old (mean 9.8 years).

    2. There is no sex predilection, but long-haired cats are overrepresented.

B. **Primary hyperparathyroidism**:

    1. Primary hyperparathyroidism is rare in cats.

    2. The mean age of affected cats is approximately 13 years.

    3. There is no sex predilection, but Siamese cats appear to be predisposed.

C. **Other causes of hypercalcemia**: There does not appear to be any age-, breed-, or sex-related predispositions for the other causes of hypercalcemia.

III. Clinical Signs

A. **Anorexia is the most common clinical sign of hypercalcemia** in cats:

    1. Vomiting, depression, weakness, constipation, polyuria, and polydipsia may occur.

    2. Uncommon signs include cardiac arrhythmias, seizures, muscle twitching, and death.

B. **Clinical signs are most severe when hypercalcemia develops rapidly.**

C. The magnitude of the hypercalcemia is also important:

    1. If serum tCa is >15.0 mg/dL (3.75 mmol/L) or iCa is >7.2 mg/dL (1.8 mmol/L), clinical signs are usually present.

    2. If serum tCa is >18.0 mg/dL (4.5 mmol/L) or iCa is >8.8 mg/dL (2.2 mmol/L), the patient is usually critically ill.

D. **Interaction with phosphorus is important.** If serum tCa (mg/dL)×phosphorus concentration is >70, tissue mineralization is likely.

E. **Cats with idiopathic hypercalcemia may have no clinical signs.** In one study, 46% of cats with **idiopathic hypercalcemia** had no clinical signs, 18% had mild weight loss with no other clinical signs, 6% had inflammatory bowel disease, 5% had chronic constipation, 4% were vomiting, and 1% were anorectic. Uroliths or renoliths were observed in 15% and calcium oxalate stones were specifically noted in 10% of cases. Cats with **idiopathic hypercalcemia** do not commonly exhibit polyuria and polydipsia.

F. Clinical signs are **vague in cats with Vitamin D excess,** and include anorexia, lethargy, vomiting, tremors, constipation, and polyuria (especially if renal damage has been sustained).

G. Hypercalcemia usually develops within 24 h after ingestion of **rat-bait poison containing cholecalciferol,** and is often severe. Hyperphosphatemia is often noted, and azotemia is initially absent but can subsequently develop. PTH concentration is suppressed by the hypercalcemia (a parathyroid-independent hypercalcemia).

H. In **primary hyperparathyroidism,** clinical signs related to hypercalcemia are either mild (anorexia, polydipsia, polyuria, lethargy, and weakness) or absent in many affected cats. Calcium-containing uroliths may occur. **A mass associated with the parathyroid gland is palpable in about 50% of cats with primary hyperparathyroidism.** This mass lesion is sometimes confused with an enlargement of the thyroid gland.

IV. Diagnosis

A. **Definition of hypercalcemia:**
1. Using serum tCa, hypercalcemia is usually defined as a concentration >11.0 mg/dL (2.75 mmol/L), though many labs list an upper reference range closer to 10.0 mg/dL (2.5 mmol/L).
2. Using serum iCa, hypercalcemia is usually defined as a concentration >5.7 mg/dL (1.40 mmol/L).
3. **There is often an unpredictable discordance between serum tCa and serum iCa measurements.** In one study, 7% of cats were classified as hypercalcemic based on serum tCa, but when iCa was measured, 17% were hypercalcemic. **Hypercalcemia is usually underestimated in cats when serum tCa concentration is used.**
4. **Hypercalcemia based on serum iCa is relatively common and was observed in 17% of sick cats in one study.**

B. **Measurement of calcium:**
1. **Serum iCa concentration should be measured any time that an increase in serum tCa is detected.** Serum iCa should also be measured in all cases of azotemic CKD.
2. Do not directly compare *serum* iCa results to those obtained from heparinized plasma or whole blood (when using a blood gas analyzer or point-of-care analyzer). The iCa concentration is lower in heparinized plasma and whole blood than in serum.
3. **Do not use EDTA plasma for collection of blood for iCa measurement.** EDTA chelates calcium, and EDTA plasma will yield falsely low iCa results.
4. In cats, serum tCa is normally 8.0–10.5 mg/dL (2.0–2.6 mmol/L) and serum iCa is normally 4.5–5.5 mg/dL (1.1–1.4 mmol/L).
5. To convert mmol/L to mg/dL, multiply mmol/L by 4.

C. **PTH should be measured in conjunction with iCa measurement,** to determine whether PTH production is appropriate:
1. Patients with elevated iCa and inappropriately high or "normal" PTH concentrations have primary hyperparathyroidism. If serum iCa is elevated and PTH is within the upper reference range or elevated, the PTH response may be inappropriate, as PTH is expected to be suppressed with elevated iCa. **About 10% of hypercalcemic cats have primary hyperparathyroidism** based on analysis of samples submitted to veterinary endocrine labs.
2. Hypercalcemia associated with low serum PTH is classified as parathyroid-independent hypercalcemia. **About 80% of hypercalcemic cats have parathyroid-independent hypercalcemia.**

D. **Measurement of serum 25-hydroxyvitamin D** may be helpful to identify cases in which increased intake of vitamin D is the cause of hypercalcemia.

E. **Calcitriol measurement** may be helpful in patients with normal serum 25-hydroxyvitamin D concentration.

V. Differential Diagnoses

A. Potential causes of hypercalcemia are listed in **Table 35.1.** An algorithm for the diagnostic approach for definitive diagnosis of hypercalcemia is identical for dogs and cats and is listed in **Figure 34.1.**

B. In cats from North America, **idiopathic hypercalcemia** is the most common cause of hypercalcemia although surveys for the causes of hypercalcemia have not been reported in cats since 2000; CKD (elevation of tCa but not iCa) and neoplasia are listed as the most common causes of hypercalcemia in the literature.

C. **Transient hypercalcemia:**
1. **Dehydration** resulting in increased serum albumin or total protein is occasionally associated with mild increases in serum tCa concentrations that rapidly return to normal when dehydration has been corrected.

D. **Idiopathic hypercalcemia:**
1. **Idiopathic hypercalcemia** appears to be **the most common cause of hypercalcemia in cats in the USA.**
2. **No clinical signs are observed in half the cases.** Remaining cats had signs associated with hypercalcemia including mild weight loss, chronic constipation, vomiting, and anorexia. Uroliths or renoliths were observed in 15%.
3. Hypercalcemia is often discovered during review of results from routine serum biochemistry (preanesthesia, wellness exams, and minor GI signs).
4. **Increased serum iCa, suppressed PTH (parathyroid-independent hypercalcemia), normal range 25-hydroxyvitamin D, and negative PTHrP are expected findings in cats with idiopathic hypercalcemia:**
   a. Serum phosphorus is usually in the normal range unless it is increased due to concurrent CRF.
   b. Mean urinary specific gravity was 1.036 in one study; cats with hypercalcemia often maintain the ability to concentrate urine to >1.030 if they do not have concurrent CKD.
5. The diagnosis of **idiopathic hypercalcemia** is largely one of exclusion.
E. **Cancer-associated hypercalcemia:**
1. **This is one of the most common causes of hypercalcemia in cats.**
2. **Humoral hypercalcemia of malignancy:**
   a. Malignancy causes a parathyroid-independent hypercalcemia, where serum iCa concentration is increased and PTH is suppressed. Hypophosphatemia can be present due to effects of PTHrP to occupy the PTH/PTHrP receptor on the renal tubules which results in phosphaturia.
   b. In the cat, malignancies commonly associated with hypercalcemia include lymphoma, multiple myeloma, squamous cell carcinoma, bronchogenic carcinoma/adenocarcinoma, osteosarcoma, fibrosarcoma, undifferentiated sarcoma, undifferentiated renal carcinoma, anaplastic carcinoma of the lung and diaphragm, and thyroid carcinoma. **Approximately one-third of tumors associated with hypercalcemia in cats are lymphoma, another one-third are squamous cell carcinoma, and the remaining one-third from other carcinomas.** Lymphomas are less common in cats with hypercalcemia than dogs with hypercalcemia.
   c. With lymphoma, involvement has been renal, generalized, gastrointestinal, mediastinal, laryngeal, nasal, or cutaneous.
   d. Squamous cell carcinoma has been found in mandibular, maxillary, pulmonary, and ear canal locations.
   e. Excessive secretion of PTHrP plays a role in the pathogenesis of hypercalcemia in some cases, but cytokines such as IL-1, TNF-α, and TGF-α may also cause or contribute to the development and maintenance of hypercalcemia.
3. **Tumors metastatic to bone:**
   a. Solid tumors that metastasize to bone produce hypercalcemia by the induction of local bone resorption associated with tumor growth, but this is not a common occurrence.
   b. Primary bone tumors are not often associated with hypercalcemia.
4. **Hematologic malignancies:** These malignancies are typically multiple myeloma and lymphoma.
F. **CKD:**
1. **Finding hypercalcemia in a cat with primary renal azotemia poses a diagnostic problem since hypercalcemia can cause renal failure or can develop as a consequence of renal failure.**
2. **Serum tCa is elevated in 11.5–58% of cats with azotemic CKD,** and the incidence of elevated tCa increases with severity of azotemia.
3. Serum iCa concentration is usually normal to low in cats with CRF:
   a. Cats with **azotemic CKD** have a higher incidence of ionized hypercalcemia as compared to dogs; in 102 cats with **azotemic CKD,** 29% were hypercalcemic, 61% were normocalcemic, and 10% were hypocalcemic based on serum iCa concentration.
4. **Measurement of serum iCa concentration to assess calcium status is critical in azotemic CKD:**
   a. Serum tCa measurement incorrectly assesses iCa status in about 33% of cats with **azotemic CKD.**
   b. Serum tCa measurement underestimates hypercalcemia and overestimates normocalcemia in cats with **azotemic CKD.**

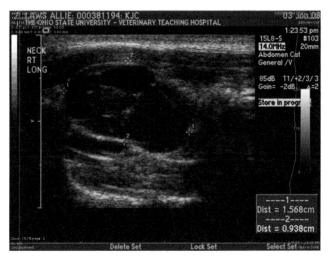

Figure 35.1   Cystic changes associated with a parathyroid gland carcinoma in a cat. (Courtesy of Dr. Kelly Cairns and the Radiology Section Center for Veterinary Medicine, The Ohio State University.)

5. **Causes of increased calcium in azotemic CKD:**
   a. The cCa fraction may be increased, causing an increase in the tCa fraction; iCa concentrations are normal in these instances.
   b. An increase in iCa may be associated with the use of calcium carbonate intestinal phosphate binders. Serum iCa will rapidly return to normal after discontinuation of treatment.
   c. Ionized hypercalcemia may occur in patients who receive excessive doses of calcitriol. Hypercalcemia is very uncommon in patients treated with lower dosages of calcitriol (2.5–4.0 ng/kg/day).
G. **Tertiary hyperparathyroidism** occurs in a small subset of CRF patients with CKD who develop increased iCa with excessive PTH secretion. It is likely that these patients had renal secondary hyperparathyroidism earlier in the clinical course of CKD:
   1. Azotemic CKD and the presence of ionized hypercalcemia occur in some cats with idiopathic hypercalcemia (PTH is generally increased in those with azotemic CKD and is low in **idiopathic hypercalcemia**).
H. **Primary hyperparathyroidism:**
   1. Clinical signs related to hypercalcemia are either mild or absent in many affected cats. **A cystic mass associated with the parathyroid gland is palpable in about 50% of cats with primary hyperparathyroidism.**
   2. Serum iCa concentration is elevated, and PTH is inappropriately high for the level of hypercalcemia (either elevated or in the upper part of the reference range).
   3. **Ultrasonography of the neck can be helpful in the diagnosis,** but it requires an ultrasound unit with a high-frequency transducer to achieve good resolution. Identification of an enlarged parathyroid gland(s) >4 mm provides support for this diagnosis. Some cats have cystic changes around the parathyroid tumor **(Figure 35.1)**.
I. **Hypoadrenocorticism:**
   1. Hypoadrenocorticism is rare in cats, and hypercalcemia is noted in only about 8% of them based on tCa.
   2. Serum tCa concentration returns to normal after 1–2 days of steroid replacement therapy.
J. **Hypervitaminosis D:**
   1. Toxicity results from excess cholecalciferol, ergocalciferol, 25-hydroxyvitamin D, calcitriol, or analogues of calcitriol.
   2. Serum concentration of 25-hydroxyvitamin D will be elevated in cases of treatment overdose, cholecalciferol-rodenticide ingestion, or excessive dietary supplementation of vitamin D. Concentration of 25-hydroxyvitamin D may be normal in cases of plant or psoriasis ointment ingestion.

Table 35.2   Treatment of hypercalcemia.

Treatment	Dose	Indications	Comments
Volume expansion			
SQ saline (0.9%)	75–100 mL/kg/day	Mild hypercalcemia	Contraindicated if peripheral edema is present
IV saline (0.9%)	100–125 mL/kg/day	Moderate to severe hypercalcemia	Contraindicated in congestive heart failure and hypertension
Diuretics			
Furosemide	1–4 mg/kg q 12 h–q 8 h IV, SQ, PO	Moderate to severe hypercalcemia	Volume expansion is necessary prior to use of this drug
Glucocorticoids			
Prednisone	1–2.2 mg/kg q 12 h PO, SQ, IV	Moderate to severe hypercalcemia	Use of these drugs prior to identification of etiology may make definitive diagnosis difficult
Dexamethasone	0.1–0.22 mg/kg q 12 h IV, SQ		
Inhibition of bone resorption			
Calcitonin	4–6 IU/kg SQ q 12 h to q 8 h	Hypervitaminosis D toxicity	Response may be short lived. Vomiting may occur.
Bisphosphonates			
Etidronate (EHDP)	5–15 mg/kg daily to q 12 h	Moderate to severe chronic hypercalcemia	Expensive
Clodronate	20–25 mg/kg in a 4-h IV infusion		Approved in Europe; availability in USA limited
Pamidronate	1.3–2.0 mg/kg in 150 mL 0.9% saline a 2-h IV infusion; can repeat in 1–3 weeks	Well studied in hypervitaminosis D in dogs	
Alendronate	1–4 mg/kg q 48–72 h PO	Malignancy associated hypercalcemia adjunctive; primary hyperparathyroidism adjunctive	
	10–30 mg/cat once weekly followed by 6 mL PO tap water and "buttering" of lips	Idiopathic hypercalcemia—cats	

K. **Granulomatous disease:**

   1. Hypercalcemia in the presence of granulomatous disease is rare but occurs associated with histoplasmosis, *Nocardia*, and mycobacterial infection, blastomycosis, cryptococcosis, actinomyces, and injection-site granulomas.

   2. Serum iCa concentration is increased and PTH is suppressed (a parathyroid-independent hypercalcemia).

VI. Treatment

A. For an overview of treatment, see **Table 35.2**.

B. As in dogs, the magnitude of hypercalcemia, rate of development, whether the calcium concentration is continuing to increase, and modifying effects of other electrolytes and acid-base disturbances should all be considered when deciding on a treatment plan:

   1. The degree of neurologic, cardiac, and renal dysfunction induced by the hypercalcemia and other concurrent deleterious factors dictate the need for aggressive treatment.

2. Acidosis magnifies the effects of hypercalcemia by shifting more calcium to the ionized fraction.
3. Serum phosphorus concentration is important in decision making because soft tissue mineralization is potentiated by hyperphosphatemia.
4. Cats with rapid and progressive development of hypercalcemia usually display serious clinical signs and require aggressive therapy.

C. **Removal of the underlying cause of the hypercalcemia is the definitive treatment.**

D. **Supportive therapy** is often needed to decrease serum calcium concentration to a less toxic level while waiting for a definitive diagnosis to be established.

E. Parenteral fluids, furosemide, sodium bicarbonate, glucocorticoids, or combinations of these treatments reduce serum calcium concentrations in most animals that are severely affected (acutely ill):

1. **Fluid therapy:**
   a. The first goal of fluid therapy is to correct dehydration because hemoconcentration contributes to hypercalcemia.
   b. Dehydration should be corrected within 4–6 h of presentation in animals with severe hypercalcemia. Normocalcemia may be restored by fluid therapy alone if the hypercalcemia is initially mild.
   c. Physiologic saline (0.9% NaCl) is the solution of choice for correction of dehydration and hypercalcemia. This solution is preferred to lactated Ringer's solution since physiologic saline does not contain any calcium and contains more sodium that lactated Ringer's solution, which promotes renal loss of calcium.

2. **Diuretics:**
   a. **Furosemide** is important for treatment of persistent hypercalcemia.
   b. Furosemide promotes enhanced urinary calcium loss.
   c. Thiazides should not be used since they may result in hypocalciuria and may aggravate hypercalcemia.
   d. Adequate hydration during furosemide administration is essential.

3. **Sodium bicarbonate:**
   a. Infusion of sodium bicarbonate has been studied in cats at 1–4 mEq/kg as a bolus infusion.
   b. This treatment is most often used in the presence of metabolic acidosis or in those cats with a severe hypercalcemic crisis (collapse, encephalopathy, and cardiac arrhythmia).
   c. Sodium bicarbonate infusion is most likely to be helpful in combination with other treatments.
   d. Serum iCa concentration is reduced with sodium bicarbonate infusion because the pH becomes more alkalotic, and there is increased binding of calcium to serum proteins.

4. **Glucocorticoids:**
   a. Glucocorticoids can significantly reduce serum iCa concentration in patients with hypercalcemia, especially in those with lymphoma, multiple myeloma, thymoma, hypoadrenocorticism, hypervitaminosis D, hypervitaminosis A, or granulomatous disease.
   b. When possible, corticosteroids should be withheld from animals for which a diagnosis has not been established because lymphocytolysis can make a histopathologic diagnosis of lymphoma much more difficult or impossible.

5. **Calcitonin:**
   a. Treatment with calcitonin may be useful in those with severe hypercalcemia.
   b. Calcitonin treatment is expensive, its effect is unpredictable, effects are short lived, and resistance often develops after a few days.
   c. Vomiting and anorexia are common side effects in dogs.

6. **Bisphosphonates:**
   a. Bisphosphonates inhibit bone resorption by decreasing osteoclast activity and function.
   b. Dehydration should be corrected before bisphosphonate use to lessen the chance of renal injury.
   c. Intravenous infusions of pamidronate and clodronate have been used to treat hypercalcemia in a few cats.
   d. Oral alendronate has been used in a limited number of cats with **idiopathic hypercalcemia** with apparent safety and efficacy. Oral alendronate at 3 mg/kg once weekly for 22 weeks followed by 9 mg/kg twice weekly for an additional 27 weeks was well tolerated in a small number of cats treated for odontoclastic resorptive tooth lesions. The usual starting dose for treatment of **idiopathic hypercalcemia**

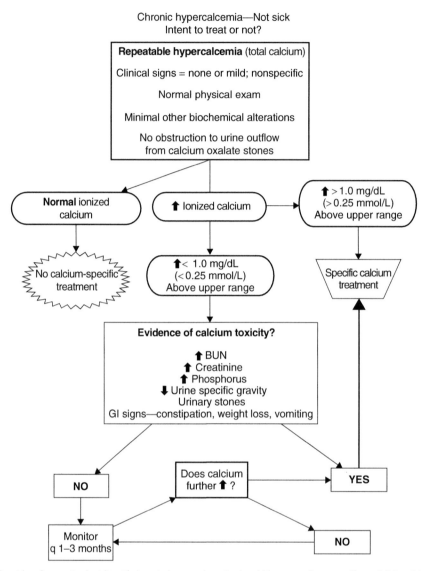

Figure 35.2 Algorithm for use in deciding if chronic hypercalcemia should be treated now or if watchful waiting could be safe.

using alendronate is 10 mg/cat/week. Based on the response in iCa, the dose is adjusted to a final dose of 5–30 mg/cat/week (**Figure 35.3**) It is important to give alendronate on an empty stomach. Bisphosphonates are poorly absorbed in general and this absorption approaches 0% with food in the stomach so we recommend a 12-h fast followed by pilling. Alendronate administered in tuna water was significantly less bioavailable than alendronate delivered in water in one study. Due to concerns about esophagitis, we recommend following the pill by 6 mL tap water and "buttering" of the nose to enhance salivation and speed the transit of the medication to the stomach.

F. **Specific therapy for idiopathic hypercalcemia** (**Figures 35.2 and 35.3** provide algorithms to help in deciding if treatment is needed now or not, and what treatment path may be chosen):

    1. The feeding of increased dietary fiber decreases serum iCa in some cats but not others. The beneficial effect of a higher fiber diet may be through decreasing the intestinal absorption of calcium.

    2. The feeding of a renal veterinary diet sometimes decreases serum iCa in some cats but not others. The beneficial effect may be through less acidification or other unknown nutrient interactions of these diets.

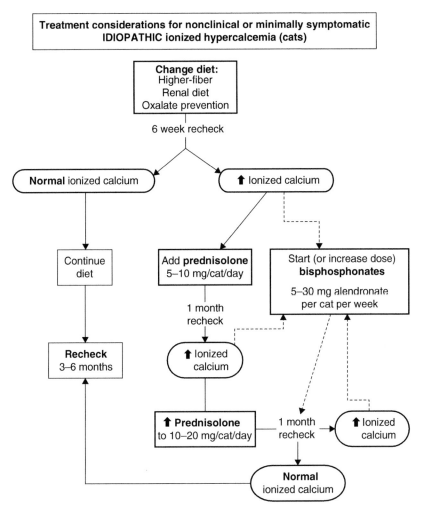

Figure 35.3 Treatment paths for consideration for cats with idiopathic hypercalcemia. Though prednisolone has been chosen historically after diet modification has failed to control circulating calcium, bisphosphonates appear to be emerging as the preferred second choice of treatment.

3. Prednisolone therapy may result in long-term decrease in iCa concentration. The effects may last for months to years in some cats at doses of 5–20 mg prednisone per cat per day.

4. When dietary modification and prednisolone fail to decrease serum iCa concentration, bisphosphonate treatment can be considered.

5. The impetus to prescribe therapy for cats with **idiopathic hypercalcemia** is more pressing when the magnitude of ionized hypercalcemia continues to increase or clinical signs become more obvious:

    a. Aggressive treatment to decrease serum calcium is warranted in cats with CRF or those with calcium-containing urinary stones.

6. Specific treatment for **idiopathic hypercalcemia** is impossible because the pathogenesis remains unknown. Due to efficacy and apparent safety, alendronate has become the second choice for treatment of IHC after or in addition to dietary modification in our hospital. Reports of the efficacy of alendronate in restoration of normocalcemia have yet to be published in a series of cats.

G. **Specific therapy for primary hyperparathyroidism:** Surgery to remove the parathyroid adenoma is the treatment of choice:

1. Hypocalcemia postsurgery may occur as in the dog. Treatment with supplemental calcium or vitamin D metabolites may be required. Hypocalcemia without clinical signs usually does not require treatment unless the serum tCa is <6 mg/dL (1.5 mmol/L).

2. We have less experience in cats using a preemptive protocol with calcitriol treatment to minimize postsurgical hypocalcemia.

H. **Specific treatment for secondary hyperparathyroidism:** Treatment with low-dose calcitriol therapy to reduce PTH synthesis conceivably improves quality of life, reduces progression of renal disease, and prolongs life, but evidence-based medicine for this is not as established as that for the dog. **There is generally no rationale for prescribing calcitriol treatment for hypercalcemia found in CRF**, unless it is an ionized hypercalcemia attributed to the development of tertiary hyperparathyroidism.

I. **Treatment of vitamin D toxicity** should be aggressive and may need to be prolonged. Greater survival has been reported in cats than in dogs following ingestion of rat bait containing cholecalciferol.

VII. Prognosis

A. **Prognosis is dependent on the underlying cause.**

B. **Idiopathic hypercalcemia:** Prognosis is good to excellent for initial restoration of normocalcemia with treatment.

C. **Malignancy-associated hypercalcemia:** Prognosis is good for initial restoration of normocalcemia following treatment of the underlying malignancy. Prognosis is poor to grave for long-term survival from the malignancy.

D. **Hypervitaminosis D:** Prognosis is good for resolution of hypercalcemia.

VIII. Prevention

A. Prevent exposure to excessive vitamin D in rodenticides, houseplants, and antipsoriasis creams.

References and Further Readings

Barber PJ, Elliott J. Feline chronic renal failure: calcium homeostasis in 80 cases diagnosed between 1992 and 1995. *J Small Anim Pract* 1998;39:108–116.

Bolliger AP, Graham PA, Richard V, et al. Detection of parathyroid hormone-related protein in cats with humoral hypercalcemia of malignancy. *Vet Clin Pathol* 2002;31:3–8.

Chew DJ, Leonard M, Muir W 3rd. Effect of sodium bicarbonate infusions on ionized calcium and total calcium concentrations in serum of clinically normal cats. *Am J Vet Res* 1989;50:145–150.

Chew DJ, Schenck PA. Advances in the treatment of hypercalcemia—The veterinary perspective. *Proceedings from the American College of Veterinary Internal Medicine Meeting*, Anaheim, CA, 2010.

Hostutler RA, Chew DJ, Jaeger JQ, et al. Uses and effectiveness of pamidronate disodium for treatment of dogs and cats with hypercalcemia. *J Vet Intern Med* 2005;19:29–33.

Midkiff AM, Chew DJ, Randolph JF, et al. Idiopathic hypercalcemia in cats. *J Vet Intern Med* 2000;14:619–626.

Mohn KL, Jacks TM, Schleim KD, et al. Alendronate binds to tooth root surfaces and inhibits progression of feline tooth root resorption: A pilot proof-of-concept study. *J Vet Dent* 2009;26(2):74–81.

Patel RT, Caceres A, French AF, McManus PM. Multiple myeloma in 16 cats: a retrospective study. *Vet Clin Pathol* 2005;34(4):341–352.

Peterson ME, Greco DS, Orth DN. Primary hypoadrenocorticism in ten cats. *J Vet Intern Med* 1989:3:55–58.

Savary KC, Price GS, Vaden SL. Hypercalcemia in cats: A retrospective study of 71 cases (1991–1997). *J Vet Intern Med* 2000;14:184–189.

Schenck PA. Serum ionized magnesium concentrations in dogs and cats with hypoparathyroidism. *J Vet Intern Med* 2005;19(3):462.

Schenck PA, Chew DJ. Calcium: Total or ionized? *Vet Clin North Am Small Anim Pract* 2008;38(3):497–502.

Schenck PA, Chew DJ. Prediction of serum ionized calcium concentration by serum total calcium concentration in cats. *Can J Vet Res* 2010;74(3):209–213.

Schenck PA, Chew DJ, Behrend EN. Updates on hypercalcemic disorders. In: August J, ed. *Consultations in Feline Internal Medicine*. St. Louis: Elsevier, 2005, pp. 157–168.

Schenck PA, Chew DJ, Nagode LA, Rosol TJ. Disorders of calcium: Hypercalcemia and hypocalcemia. In: Dibartola S, ed. *Fluid Therapy in Small Animal Practice*, 3rd edn. St. Louis: Elsevier, 2006, pp. 122–194.

Schenck PA, Chew DJ, Refsal K, et al. Calcium metabolic hormones in feline idiopathic hypercalcemia. *J Vet Intern Med* 2004;18:442.

CHAPTER 36

Hypercalcemia in Other Species
Michelle L. Campbell-Ward

Hypercalcemia in Horses

Pathogenesis

- Multiple causes including renal failure, hypervitaminosis D, neoplasia, hyperparathyroidism, and granulomatous disease.
- Can lead to cardiac rate and rhythm abnormalities and soft tissue mineralization of vital organs.

Classical Signs

- Anorexia, lethargy, weight loss, poor performance, depression, polyuria/polydipsia, and other signs dependent upon underlying cause.

Diagnosis

- Serum biochemistry.

Treatment

- Fluid therapy, furosemide diuresis, glucocorticoids, or surgery, for example, for neoplasia.

I. Pathogenesis
A. Hypercalcemia is defined as an **elevated serum calcium level** (i.e., >3.4 mmol/L [13.5 mg/dL]).
B. **Parathyroid hormone (PTH), calcitonin, and vitamin D** act in conjunction with the **intestine, bone, kidneys, and parathyroid glands** to **maintain calcium homeostasis**. Disturbances in calcium homeostasis resulting in hypercalcemia occur with organ dysfunction, abnormalities in hormonal balance or production of a PTH analogue. Regardless of the underlying pathology, hypercalcemia **can lead to cardiac rate and rhythm abnormalities and soft tissue mineralization of vital organs**.
C. Hypercalcemic disorders in the horse can be divided into two broad groups:
   1. **Parathyroid-dependent** hypercalcemia/primary hyperparathyroidism.

Clinical Endocrinology of Companion Animals, First Edition. Edited by Jacquie Rand.
© 2013 John Wiley & Sons, Inc. Published 2013 by John Wiley & Sons, Inc.

2. **Hypercalcemia independent of parathyroid gland function** (i.e., hypercalcemia develops despite parathyroid gland suppression). This may be seen in a variety of conditions (e.g., renal failure, vitamin D intoxication, secondary hyperparathyroidism, and neoplasia).

D. Parathyroid-dependent hypercalcemia:

1. **Primary hyperparathyroidism** results from parathyroid **hyperplasia** or parathyroid **adenoma** formation. It is rare in horses.

2. In this condition, the chief cells of the parathyroid gland secrete excessive and autonomous amounts of PTH and do not respond to the negative feedback of calcium. **Elevated PTH concentrations** in turn lead to **increased renal calcium reabsorption** (hypocalciuria), **decreased phosphorus reabsorption** (hyperphosphaturia), **increased bone resorption**, and **increased 1,25 (OH)$_2$ D$_3$ synthesis.**

3. The end result is loss of cortical bone and the development of a condition termed **osteodystrophia fibrosa**, in which there is an excessive accumulation of subperiosteal unmineralized connective tissue.

E. Hypercalcemia independent of parathyroid gland function:

1. Renal secondary hyperparathyroidism/renal failure:

a. Renal secondary hyperparathyroidism is not a well recognized condition in the horse.

b. **Horses with chronic renal failure tend to be hypercalcemic** but this is thought to be **due to an inability of the kidneys to eliminate calcium** rather than an elevated PTH level. In fact, **serum PTH concentrations** in horses with chronic renal failure and hypercalcemia are often in the **low to normal range.** Serum phosphorus concentrations are variable and unlike in other species with renal disease, may be low.

2. Nutritional secondary hyperparathyroidism:

a. Nutritional secondary hyperparathyroidism is associated with **diets** with one or more of the following features:

1) **Low in calcium and/or high in phosphorus.**

2) **High in oxalates.**

3) With a phosphorus:calcium ratio of 3:1 or higher.

b. Such diets are associated with hyperphosphatemia and the **induction of parathyroid cell hyperplasia.** Although some horses with this condition are hypercalcemic, the majority are normocalcemic or slightly hypocalcemic.

3. Hypervitaminosis D:

a. Hypervitaminosis D is a **potentially fatal condition** that **can occur due to intoxication with either ergocalciferol (vitamin D$_2$) or cholecalciferol (vitamin D$_3$).**

b. In addition to oversupplementation, it may also occur due to the ingestion of plants **containing vitamin D analogues** such as *Solanum glaucophyllum* (*S. malacoxylon*) in South America, *S. sodomaeum* in Hawaii, day blooming jasmine (*Cestrum diurnum*) in the southern United States, and *Trisetum flavescens* in Europe.

c. Hypervitaminosis D increases the **intestinal absorption** and **renal reabsorption of calcium and phosphorus.**

d. As vitamin D is an important negative regulator of parathyroid cell proliferation, **hypervitaminosis D** causes **parathyroid cell atrophy** and decreased PTH secretion. In addition, the associated hypercalcemia contributes to decreased PTH secretion, lowering bone turnover.

4. Humoral hypercalcemia of malignancy (HHM):

a. HHM, also referred to as **pseudohyperparathyroidism**, refers to a paraneoplastic condition of horses with certain types of neoplasia. In fact, **hypercalcemia is the most common paraneoplastic finding in horses.** The development of hypercalcemia in these cases is thought to be due to **secretion of PTH-related protein (PTHrP)** by the neoplastic cells.

b. **PTHrP interacts with PTH receptors** to increase renal reabsorption of calcium, renal elimination of phosphorus, and bone resorption.

c. In horses, HHM has been demonstrated in cases of gastric, vulvar, and preputial **squamous cell carcinoma, adrenocortical carcinoma, multiple myeloma, lymphosarcoma, and ameloblastoma.**

5. **Neonatal hypercalcemia and asphyxia:**
   a. Some authors have reported hypercalcemia in neonatal foals that does not appear to be associated with renal failure, excessive PTH secretion, or excessive calcium administration. A consistent feature of these cases is **peripartum asphyxia.** Many of these foals have severe hypotension, somnolence, and often die of asphyxia. The pathogenesis is unclear but placental insufficiency and excessive production of PTHrP are thought to play a role.
6. **Idiopathic systemic granulomatous disease:**
   a. This is a **rare immune disease** of horses and ponies characterized by granuloma formation in several organs including the skin.
   b. Increased **expression of PTHrP** by the **macrophages** of granulomas has been found in a pony with this condition and may explain the hypercalcemia that is seen in some cases.

II. Signalment
A. Varies with the underlying condition, for example:
   1. Chronic renal failure is more common in middle-aged to older horses (>15 years).
   2. Some types of neoplasia that are associated with hypercalcemia are more common in certain groups. For example, cutaneous squamous cell carcinoma tends to occur in **middle-aged** to **older horses** with **unpigmented areas of skin.**

III. Clinical Signs
A. Hypercalcemia, regardless of etiology, can cause a **variety of nonspecific clinical signs:**
   1. **Polyuria/polydipsia and/or dehydration** (due to the direct effects of calcium on renal function and/or secondary to renal mineralization).
   2. Lethargy/depression.
   3. **Cardiac dysrhythmias** (due to reduced membrane excitability).
   4. **Gastrointestinal signs,** for example, colic, choke, or constipation.
   5. **Weight loss**/poor body condition and inappetence.
   6. Poor performance.
B. Depending on the underlying disease process, other clinical signs may be noted:
   1. **Enlargement of the facial bones** (primary hyperparathyroidism or nutritional secondary hyperparathyroidism).
   2. **Lameness, stiffness,** or reluctance to move (hypervitaminosis D, bone neoplasia, primary hyperparathyroidism, or nutritional secondary hyperparathyroidism).
   3. **Fractures** (bone neoplasia, primary hyperparathyroidism, or nutritional secondary hyperparathyroidism).
   4. **Crusting skin lesions** often affecting mucocutaneous junctions and coronary bands (systemic granulomatous disease).
   5. Enlarged lymph nodes (lymphoma).
   6. **Palpable mass** (neoplasia or granuloma).
   7. Renal pain (chronic renal failure).
   8. Dysuria (chronic renal failure).
   9. Sudden death (due to cardiovascular mineralization) (hypervitaminosis D).

IV. Diagnosis
A. **Measurement of serum total calcium** is required for diagnosis. Values >3.4 mmol/L (13.5 mg/dL) are consistent with hypercalcemia in horses.
B. A detailed **history** must be obtained and **other diagnostic tests will be necessary to identify the underlying etiology** (and thereby determine prognosis and optimal treatment protocols) (Tables 36.1 and 36.2).
C. Given the relative incidence of the causative diseases, it is suggested that:
   1. **Initial efforts concentrate on assessing renal function and the possibility of hypervitaminosis D.**
   2. If neither renal failure nor vitamin D intoxication seems likely and hypercalcemia persists, attempt to **exclude neoplasia.**

	Diagnostic test	Expected/suggestive results
Common causes		
Chronic renal failure	Transrectal examination of the urinary tract	Palpable renal abnormalities (firm, irregular surface); renal pain; palpable (enlarged) ureters; occasionally palpable ureteroliths
	Hematology and serum biochemistry	Azotemia; mild anemia; hypoalbuminemia; hypophosphatemia; electrolyte aberrations
	Urinalysis	Isosthenuria (u.s.g = 1.008–1.012); moderate to marked proteinuria may be seen depending on the etiology of the renal dysfunction
	Renal ultrasonography	Small renal size, abnormal renal architecture, and/or variably increased echogenicity suggestive of fibrosis
	Ultrasound guided renal biopsy	Histopathological evidence of renal pathology
Hypervitaminosis D	History	Oversupplementation with vitamin D or ingestion of plants containing vitamin D analogues
	Serum biochemistry	Azotemia; hypochloremia; hyperphosphatemia
	Measurement of serum levels of vitamin D metabolites	Elevated
	Urinalysis	Often hyposthenuria or isosthenuria
	Radiography	Increased bone density; decreased size of medullary cavity; calcification of soft tissues
	Necropsy	Mineralization of kidneys, liver, lymph nodes, lungs, ligaments, tendons, large vessels, and/or endocardium; osteopetrosis of long bones; parathyroid gland atrophy— although this can be challenging to assess as the glands are small and vary in location
Uncommon causes		
Neoplasia (humoral hypercalcemia of malignancy)	Biochemistry	Hypophosphatemia
	PTH assay	Low to normal
	PTHrP assay	Elevated
	Urinalysis	Hypocalciuria; hyperphosphaturia
	FNA and/or biopsy of any mass or masses; collection of abdominal or thoracic fluid where indicated	Presence of neoplastic cells on cytology and/or histopathology
Hyperparathyroidism	Serum biochemistry	Hypophosphatemia (primary hyperparathyroidism) or hyperphosphatemia (nutritional secondary hyperparathyroidism)
	Measurement of serum levels of vitamin D metabolites	Low to normal
	PTH assay	High
	Urinalysis	Hypocalciuria; hyperphosphaturia
	Radiography	Decreased facial and long bone density; fibrous proliferation of the maxilla and mandible; resorption of the dental alveolar sockets; loss of the lamina dura surrounding the molars
	Nasal endoscopy	Stenosis of the nasal passages
	Necropsy	Enlargement of the maxilla and mandible; accumulation of fibrous tissue around the facial bones; stenosis of the nasal passages; loose cheek teeth; increased bone fragility; parathyroid gland hyperplasia

PTH = parathyroid hormone; PTHrP = parathyroid hormone–related protein; FNA = fine needle aspirate; u.s.g = urine specific gravity.

Table 36.2   Equine reference values for total calcium, phosphorus, parathyroid hormone (PTH), and parathyroid hormone–related protein (PTHrP).

Parameter	Normal range
Total calcium	2.8–3.4 mmol/L (11.1–13.5 mg/dL)
Phosphorus	0.39–1.6 mmol/L (1.2–4.8 mg/dL)
PTH	1–4 pmol/L (9.5–38 pg/mL)
PTHrP	<1 pmol/L (<10 pg/mL)

3. Finally if all the previous work-up has failed to identify a cause, rarer hypercalcemic syndromes should be considered, for example, hyperparathyroidism and systemic granulomatous disease.

D. Note that blood samples collected in **standard EDTA** tubes **may clot** if the serum calcium concentration is markedly elevated. This occurs when there is insufficient EDTA to bind all the calcium, leaving some available to complete the clotting process.

V. Differential Diagnoses

A. Given that a proportion of the extracellular calcium is protein bound, **total calcium results should be interpreted in light of total protein and albumin concentrations.** Total serum calcium may be falsely elevated if the horse is hyperalbuminemic; equally hypoalbuminemia may obscure true hypercalcemia.

B. **Hemolysis and lipemia** may **falsely elevate total calcium** results.

C. Other conditions that may present with **similar nonspecific clinical signs:**
1. **Renal disease without hypercalcemia.**
2. **Hepatic disease.**
3. **Diabetes mellitus** (see Chapter 17).
4. **Cardiac disease.**
5. **Hypoadrenocorticism** (see Chapter 3).
6. Any disease that results in anemia.

VI. Treatment

A. Hypercalcemia rarely presents as an equine emergency.

B. If total calcium levels are markedly elevated, the following medical treatment may be indicated:
1. **Intravenous fluid therapy** with **0.9% saline solution.**
2. The administration of loop diuretics. **Furosemide** is the diuretic of choice because it inhibits the sodium/potassium/chloride cotransporter in the distal tubules, thereby increasing the urinary excretion of calcium. **Thiazide diuretics are contraindicated** because they stimulate calcium reabsorption.

C. Other therapeutic measures should be directed toward **addressing the underlying disease process:**
1. **Chronic renal failure:**
   a. Intravenous or oral **fluid therapy** will promote dieresis.
   b. Antibiotics may be indicated if secondary infection is present.
   c. **Dietary management** should focus on **low-calcium, limited-protein (<10%)** rations and free access to water, electrolytes, and carbohydrates.
   d. Vitamin B and anabolic steroids may be helpful to stimulate appetite.
   e. Any nephrotoxic medications must be discontinued.
   f. Electrohydraulic or laser lithotripsy via an endoscope inserted into the ureter is the recommended approach to the treatment of the rare cases with obstructive nephrolithiasis or ureterolithiasis.
2. **Vitamin D intoxication:**
   a. **Discontinue supplementation/eliminate access to causative plants.**
   b. **Glucocorticoids** may be helpful because in horses they decrease intestinal absorption of calcium, increase urinary excretion of calcium, and decrease bone resorption.
   c. Dietary calcium and phosphate levels should be decreased.

    d. The use of **calcium binding agents** such as sodium phytate which is high in many cereals has been proposed as an adjunctive measure.

   3. Neoplasia:

    a. Surgical excision, radiotherapy, or cryosurgery may be options for localized tumors resulting in HHM.

    b. Some horses with lymphoma may improve with chemotherapy.

   4. Primary hyperparathyroidism:

    a. Theoretically, parathyroidectomy is the treatment of choice, although this is often impractical for several reasons (e.g., localizing the pathologic gland is challenging, cost).

VII. Prognosis

A. The prognosis for horses with hypercalcemia is variable depending on the underlying disease, but in general is **guarded to poor** as persistent untreated hypercalcemia may lead to renal failure and organ mineralization.

VIII. Prevention

A. **Avoid oversupplementation** with vitamin D.

B. **Eliminate access to plants that contain vitamin D analogues.**

C. Provide appropriate treatment for renal disease and neoplasia in the earliest stages when possible.

Hypercalcemia in Rabbits

Pathogenesis

- May develop secondary to high dietary calcium intake, chronic renal failure, hypervitaminosis D, and a variety of other diseases.
- Sequelae include renal calcification and arteriosclerosis.

Classical Signs

- Anorexia, weakness, weight loss, polyuria/polydipsia, and other signs dependent upon underlying cause.

Diagnosis

- Serum biochemistry.

Treatment

- Dietary correction, fluid therapy, supportive care, and treatment of any underlying disease process.

I. Pathogenesis

A. **Rabbits have an unusual calcium metabolism** resulting in a **30–50% higher normal serum total calcium concentration** than other mammals (Table 33.2). The ionized fraction of calcium, however, is comparable to that of other mammals:

   1. Rabbit serum calcium concentrations vary widely and **reflect dietary intake.**

   2. Fractional urinary excretion of calcium is approximately 44% in the rabbit, compared to <2% in most mammals.

   3. Passive absorption of dietary calcium from the gastrointestinal tract is very efficient and does not require vitamin D if dietary levels of calcium are adequate.

B. Total blood calcium levels may be affected by age and reproductive status.

C. Compared to other mammalian species, a reduction in PTH concentration occurs at relatively high levels of blood calcium.

D. **Causes of hypercalcemia** in the rabbit include:
    1. **High dietary calcium intake.**
    2. **Chronic renal failure** (impaired calcium excretion).
    3. **Primary or secondary hyperparathyroidism.** Development of secondary hyperparathyroidism as a complication of chronic renal failure depends on the mineral content of the diet. Rabbits fed a normal diet of ~1.2% calcium and 0.6% phosphorus have been shown to develop hypercalcemia, hypophosphatemia, and low PTH levels in the course of chronic renal failure, therefore suggesting that rabbits are resistant to renal secondary hyperparathyroidism. However, **hyperparathyroidism can develop** if **uremic rabbits** are fed a **low-calcium, high-phosphorus diet.**
    4. **Paraneoplastic syndrome** (e.g., secondary to lymphoma, thymoma, or primary/metastatic osteolytic bone neoplasia).
    5. **Osteomyelitis or diffuse osteoporosis.**
    6. **Granulomatous disease.**
    7. **Severe hypothermia.**
    8. **Hypervitaminosis D** (via rodenticide or plant ingestion or excessive supplementation) which results in metastatic calcification of soft tissues, including the kidney, liver, arterial walls, and muscle.
E. **Rabbits are especially predisposed to the renal consequences of hypercalcemia** (impaired renal function; calcification) as the urinary system is the main route for calcium excretion. Initially, renal compromise will be subclinical but progressive mineralization of the kidney causes nephron damage and chronic renal failure.
F. Spontaneous **aortic arteriosclerosis** has been reported in hypercalcemic rabbits and in rabbits fed a diet high in calcium and vitamin D.

II. Signalment
A. There are no reported sex or breed predispositions.

III. Clinical Signs
A. Clinical signs tend to be **nonspecific and vary depending on the underlying etiology:**
    1. Weight loss/poor body condition.
    2. Weakness.
    3. Polyuria/polydipsia.
    4. Dysuria/hematuria.
    5. Anorexia.
    6. Gastrointestinal ileus or diarrhea.
    7. Decreased appetite.
    8. Palpably small and irregular kidneys.
    9. Ataxia or paralysis.
    10. Death.

IV. Diagnosis
A. **Measurement of serum total calcium** is required for diagnosis. Values >**4.2 mmol/L** (16.8 mg/dL) are consistent with hypercalcemia in rabbits. Ideally, ionized calcium should also be measured.
B. A nonregenerative anemia may be detected on hematology if renal compromise is a feature.
C. Radiography may reveal **calcification of soft tissues,** including the renal vessels and the aorta.
D. **Renal function should be assessed** (serum biochemistry, urinalysis, and renal ultrasonography).

V. Differential Diagnoses
A. **An erroneous diagnosis** of hypercalcemia is frequently made by clinicians unfamiliar with the high normal total serum calcium levels of rabbits compared to other mammals.
B. **Lipemia** may artifactually elevate total calcium values.

VI. Treatment
A. **Dietary correction** is indicated if calcium and/or vitamin D levels are considered excessive.
B. **Fluid therapy** (0.9% sodium chloride) is indicated if renal function is compromised.
C. Treat any identified underlying disease process and provide general supportive care.

VII. Prognosis

A.   **Good** if hypercalcemia simply **reflects a high dietary calcium** intake, and soft tissue calcification and renal failure have not yet developed.

B.   **Guarded to poor** if hypercalcemia is secondary to an **underlying disease** process.

VIII. Prevention

A.   Avoid excessive dietary levels of calcium and vitamin D.

B.   Avoid access to rodenticides that contain vitamin D.

Hypercalcemia in Pet Birds and Reptiles

Pathogenesis

- May be physiological (most common) or pathological in origin.

Classical Signs

- Physiological: none.
- Pathological: anorexia, polyuria/polydipsia, depression, muscle weakness, and painful joints.

Diagnosis

- Measurement of total (and ideally ionized) calcium in the blood.

Treatment

- Physiological: none required.
- Pathological: fluid therapy and dietary correction.

I.   Pathogenesis

A.   **Physiological hypercalcemia:**

1. Hypercalcemia in birds and reptiles is most often physiological in origin and **associated with increased estrogen secretion, production of calcium-binding proteins** (e.g., albumin), **calcium mobilization from medullary bone, and lipemic interference.**

2. In oviparous species, **increased phosphorus and calcium concentrations are observed during egg formation** in females. Generally, these occur together and the calcium:phosphorus ratio stays above 1 in healthy individuals. If the calcium:phosphorus ratio is <1, renal disease should be investigated.

3. In **laying female birds**, the serum albumin level may rise by up to 100% and total calcium can be as high as **10 mmol/L (40 mg/dL) without clinical complications.**

B.   Pathological hypercalcemia:

1. Pathological hypercalcemia in birds and reptiles occurs most commonly due to **long-term provision of a diet with excessive calcium and/or vitamin D_3 levels.** This is usually associated with overzealous use of vitamin and/or mineral supplements. The feeding of plants containing vitamin D analogues may also result in hypercalcemia. Vitamin D_3 oversupplementation is exacerbated by high dietary levels of calcium or phosphorus. Hyperparathyroidism, neoplasia, osteomyelitis, and granulomatous disease are other possible causes of hypercalcemia but their association with calcium derangements remains largely undescribed in these taxonomic groups.

2. Little information is available regarding the required and toxic levels of vitamin D for most avian and reptilian species.

3. Long-term consumption of high levels of calcium may interfere with magnesium, manganese, and zinc absorption causing secondary deficiencies.

4. The end result of oversupplementation is **hypercalcinosis** characterized by **calcification of soft tissues** (including arterial walls and kidneys), **visceral gout, urate nephrosis,** and/or demineralization of bone.

II. Signalment

A. **Entire female birds and reptiles are predisposed to physiological hypercalcemia.**

B. Macaws, cockatiels, and African grey parrots appear to be particularly sensitive to vitamin D toxicity.

C. Budgerigars appear to be sensitive to hypercalcemia associated with high dietary calcium levels.

III. Clinical Signs

A. **Physiological hypercalcemia:**
   1. **None** other than normal reproductive activity, for example, egg laying.

B. **Pathological hypercalcemia:**
   1. Poor weight gain in growing animals.
   2. Increased embryo mortality/poor hatchability (toxic levels of calcium and vitamin D_3 are transferred to the embryo).
   3. Depression.
   4. Anorexia.
   5. Nausea.
   6. Polyuria/polydipsia.
   7. Painful joints.
   8. Muscle weakness.
   9. Disorientation.

IV. Diagnosis

A. Hypercalcemia is diagnosed on the basis of **biochemistry confirming high blood calcium levels. Ideally, both total and ionized calcium should be measured.** Where available, species specific reference ranges should be sought for comparison.

B. If hypercalcemia is confirmed and not likely to be associated with normal physiological processes, the following diagnostic approach may be helpful:
   1. **A thorough dietary history** should be obtained.
   2. **Radiography** is useful to assess bone density, renal size, and to detect mineralization of tissues.
   3. **Assessment of uric acid** levels in blood: hyperuricemia frequently accompanies pathological hypercalcemia.
   4. Measurement of vitamin D3 metabolites in the blood may aid the diagnostic process although for the majority of species more research is required to validate these tests and define reference ranges.

V. Differential Diagnoses

A. As is the case in mammals, it appears that correlations between calcium, total protein, and albumin exist in birds and reptiles. However, the specific relationship differs markedly between species. **Total calcium values should not be interpreted without consideration of the total protein and albumin concentration.**

B. **Hemolysis, lipemia, and bacterial contamination** of the sample may falsely elevate total calcium results.

VI. Treatment

A. **Physiological hypercalcemia does not require treatment.**

B. **Pathological hypercalcemia** is treated by **diuresis with a calcium-deficient crystalloid,** for example, 0.9% sodium chloride, and **dietary correction:**
   1. Furosemide treatment may be helpful if hypercalcemia persists despite fluid therapy.
   2. Cortisol has been suggested as an adjunctive measure for the treatment of vitamin D toxicity in reptiles.

VII. Prognosis

A. Poor in the case of pathological hypercalcemia if tissue calcification and visceral or articular gout are present.

VIII. Prevention

A. Feed a balanced diet appropriate for the species concerned, ensuring dietary levels of calcium and vitamin D are not excessive.

References and Further Readings

Bas S, Bas A, Estepa JC, et al. Parathyroid gland function in the uremic rabbit. *Domest Anim Endocrinol* 2004;26:99–110.

Boland RL. *Solanum malacoxylon*: A toxic plant which affects animal calcium metabolism. *Biomed Environ Sci* 1988;1:414–423.

Calvert I. Nutritional problems. In: Girling SJ, Raiti P, eds. *BSAVA Manual of Reptiles*, 2nd edn. Gloucester: British Small Animal Veterinary Association, 2004, pp. 289–308.

Campbell TW. Clinical pathology of reptiles. In: Mader DR, ed. *Reptile Medicine and Surgery*, 2nd edn. St Louis: Saunders Elsevier, 2006, pp. 453–470.

Dorrestein GM, de Wit M. Clinical pathology and necropsy. In: Harcourt-Brown N, Chitty J, eds. *BSAVA Manual of Psittacine Birds*, 2nd edn. Gloucester: British Small Animal Veterinary Association, 2005, pp. 60–86.

Echols MS. Evaluating and treating the kidney. In: Harrison GJ, Lightfoot TL, eds. *Clinical Avian Medicine*, Vol. 2. Palm Beach: Spix Publishing, 2006, pp. 451–491.

Eckermann-Ross C. Hormonal regulation and calcium metabolism in the rabbit. *Vet Clin North Am Exot Anim Pract* 2008;11:139–152.

Frank N, Hawkins JF, Couetil LL, et al. Primary hyperparathyroidism with osteodystrophia fibrosa of the facial bones in a pony. *J Am Vet Med Assoc* 1998;212:84–86.

Garibaldi BA, Pecquet Goad ME. Hypercalcemia with secondary nephrolithiasis in a rabbit. *Lab Anim Sci* 1988;38(3):331–333.

Harcourt-Brown F. *Textbook of Rabbit Medicine*. Edinburgh: Butterworth Heinemann, 2002.

Harr KE. Diagnostic value of biochemistry. In: Harrison GJ, Lightfoot TL, eds. *Clinical Avian Medicine*, Vol. 2. Palm Beach: Spix Publishing, 2006, pp. 611–629.

Harrington DD. Acute vitamin D2 (ergocalciferol) toxicosis in horses: Case report and experimental studies. *J Am Vet Med Assoc* 1982;180:867–873.

Harrington DD, Page EH. Acute vitamin D3 toxicosis in horses: Case reports and experimental studies of the comparative toxicity of vitamins D2 and D3. *J Am Vet Med Assoc* 1983;182:1358–1369.

Jenkins JR. Clinical pathology. In: Meredith A, Flecknell P, eds. *BSAVA Manual of Rabbit Medicine and Surgery*, 2nd edn. Gloucester: British Small Animal Veterinary Association, 2006:pp. 45–51.

Johnston MS, Ivey ES. Parathyroid and ultimobranchial glands: Calcium metabolism in birds. *Semin Avian and Exot Pet Med* 2002;11(2):84–93.

Lavoie J-P, Hinchcliff, KW. *Blackwell's Five-Minute Veterinary Consult: Equine*, 2nd edn. Ames: Lippincott Williams and Wilkins, 2008.

Lumeij JT. Relationship of plasma calcium to total protein and albumin in grey (*Psittacus erithacus*) and Amazon (*Amazona spp.*) parrots. *Avian Pathol* 1990;19:661–667.

Lumeij JT, Remple JD, Riddle KE. Relationship of plasma total protein and albumin to total calcium in peregrine falcons (*Falco peregrinus*). *Avian Pathol* 1993;22:183–188.

Macwhirter P. Malnutrition. In: Ritchie BW, Harrison GJ, Harrison LR, eds. *Avian Medicine—Principles and Application*. Lake Worth: Wingers, 1994, pp. 842–861.

Marr CM, Love S, Pirie HM. Clinical, ultrasonographic and pathological findings in a horse with splenic lymphosarcoma and pseudohyperparathyroidism. *Equine Vet J* 1989;21:221–226.

de Matos R. Calcium metabolism in birds. *Vet Clin North Am Exot Anim Pract* 2008;11:59–82.

Oglesbee BL. *The 5-Minute Veterinary Consult: Ferret and Rabbit*. Ames: Blackwell Publishing, 2006.

Orcutt CJ. Cardiovascular disorders. In: Meredith A, Flecknell P, eds. *BSAVA Manual of Rabbit Medicine and Surgery*, 2nd edn. Gloucester: British Small Animal Veterinary Association, 2006, pp. 96–102.

Peauroi JR, Fisher DJ, Mohr FC, et al. Primary hyperparathyroidism caused by a functional parathyroid adenoma in a horse. *J Am Vet Med Assoc* 1998;212:1915–1918.

Reusch B. Urogenital system and disorders. In: Meredith A, Flecknell P, eds. *BSAVA Manual of Rabbit Medicine and Surgery*, 2nd edn. Gloucester: British Small Animal Veterinary Association, 2006, pp. 85–95.

Rosol TJ, Nagode LA, Robertson JT, et al. Humoral hypercalcemia of malignancy associated with ameloblastoma in a horse. *J Am Vet Med Assoc* 1994;204:1930–1933.

Roudybush T. Nutritional disorders. In: Rosskopf WJ, Woerpel RW, eds. *Diseases of Cage and Aviary Birds*. Baltimore: Williams and Wilkins, 1996, pp. 490–500.

Schoemaker NJ, Lumeij JT, Beynen AC. Polyuria and polydipsia due to vitamin and mineral oversupplementation of the diet of a salmon crested cockatoo (*Cacatua moluccensis*) and blue and gold macaw (*Ara ararauna*). *Avian Pathol* 1997;26:201–209.

Schott HC II. Chronic renal failure in horses. *Vet Clin North Am Equine Pract* 2007;23:593–612.

Sellers RS, Toribio RE, Blomme EA. Idiopathic systemic granulomatous disease and macrophage expression of PTHrP in a miniature pony. *J Comp Pathol* 2001;125:214–218.

Shell LG, Saunders G. Arteriosclerosis in a rabbit. *J Am Vet Med Assoc* 1989;194(5):679–680.

Stanford M. Calcium metabolism. In: Harrison GJ, Lightfoot TL, eds. *Clinical Avian Medicine*, Vol. 1. Palm Beach: Spix Publishing, 2006, pp. 141–151.

Suva LJ, Winslow GA, Wettenhall RE, et al. A parathyroid hormone-related protein implicated in malignant hypercalcemia: Cloning and expression. *Science* 1987;237:893–896.

Toribio RE. Parathyroid gland and calcium dysregulation. In: Smith BP, ed. *Large Animal Internal Medicine*, 4th edn. St Louis: Mosby Elsevier, 2009, pp. 1355–1363.

Toribio RE. Disorders of calcium and phosphorus. In: Reed SM, Bayly WM, Sellon DC, eds. *Equine Internal Medicine*, 3rd edn. St Louis: Saunders Elsevier, 2010, pp. 1277–1291.

Toribio RE. Disorders of calcium and phosphate metabolism in horses. *Vet Clin North Am Equine Pract* 2011;27:129–147.

Vernau KM, Grahn BH, Clarke-Scott HA, et al. Thymoma in a geriatric rabbit with hypercalcemia and periodic exophthalmos. *J Am Vet Med Assoc* 1995;206(6):820–822.

Warren HB, Lausen NC, Segre GV, et al. Regulation of calciotropic hormones in vivo in the New Zealand white rabbit. *Endocrinology* 1989;125:2683–2690.

Zimmerman JE, Guddens WT, DiGiaborno RF, et al. Soft tissue mineralization in rabbits fed a diet containing excess vitamin D. *Lab Anim Sci* 1990;40(2):212–215.

CHAPTER 37

Nutritional Secondary Hyperparathyroidism in Reptiles

Kevin Eatwell

Pathogenesis

- Hyperparathyroidism occurs as a result of a deficiency (relative or absolute) of calcium.
- Most cases in reptiles are due to a lack of dietary calcium in combination with insufficient ultraviolet (UV)-b radiation.
- Other factors can be involved such as high phosphorus diets, suboptimal temperatures, or increased demand for calcium.
- Snakes fed whole mammal prey are not reported to suffer from this condition.

Classical Signs

- Skeletal deformity and compressible face or shell (chelonians).
- Lack of truncal lifting.
- Tetany and seizures (lizards) or flaccid paralysis (chelonians).
- Prolapse of cloacal organs.

Diagnosis

- Clinical history.
- Low blood ionized calcium.
- Radiographic or CT evidence of pathological fractures and low bone density.

Treatment

- Calcium and vitamin D therapy.
- Phosphate binders and calcitonin may be indicated.
- Supportive care and stabilization.
- Treatment of secondary complications and/or underlying disease states.
- Husbandry improvement including UV-b provision.
- Dietary correction.

Clinical Endocrinology of Companion Animals, First Edition. Edited by Jacquie Rand.
© 2013 John Wiley & Sons, Inc. Published 2013 by John Wiley & Sons, Inc.

I. Pathogenesis

A. **A reduction in the ionized calcium level** in the circulation leads to the **release of parathyroid hormone (PTH)** from the parathyroid gland. This acts on the osteoclasts of the reptile to **liberate calcium and other products from the bony cortices,** which provide the structural framework and strength of the skeleton, and to increase renal tubular reabsorption of calcium while simultaneously increasing phosphorus excretion in the urine. PTH also acts on the kidney to stimulate the **release of 1,25-dihydroxycholecalciferol** (active vitamin D). Vitamin D then acts on the intestine to increase uptake of calcium and on the skeleton to liberate even more calcium from the bone stores. Low blood ionized calcium leads to **increased nerve excitability and reduced motor end plate function:**

  1. In chronic cases, a compensatory parathyroid hypertrophy results. Importantly, the negative feedback mechanism that normally operates may fail, such that increasing serum calcium no longer suppresses the production of PTH from a now overactive parathyroid gland.

B. In clinical cases, problems are usually caused by one or more of the following factors: **dietary calcium deficiency, imbalances in the dietary calcium to phosphorus ratio, and hypo- or hypervitaminosis D.** A lack of vitamin D (cholecalciferol) can be due to either dietary deficiency or **failure to provide adequate UV-b radiation** (naturally or artificially).

C. **The ultimate result is:**

  1. **A reduction in blood ionized calcium** levels leading to **tetany and flaccid paralysis** (when there is a sudden demand for calcium or the case has become severe).

  2. And/or a **reduction in the skeletal calcium content** and hence structural strength, leading to soft malleable bones, when the deficiency has been medium to long term. This represents the most common form of **metabolic bone disease** in reptiles.

D. **Common husbandry errors** increasing the risk of nutritional secondary hyperparathyroidism (NSHP) include:

  1. **Suboptimal environmental temperatures.** Production of vitamin D_3 in the skin is crucially temperature dependent.

  2. **No artificial UV-b light provided and/or insufficient exposure to natural sunlight,** especially for diurnal species.

  3. **UV-b light bulb in need of replacement.**

  4. **UV-b light placed too far away from the reptile.**

  5. **Artificial UV-b source placed too far away from the basking site.**

  6. **Diet with an inverted calcium to phosphorus ratio.**

  7. **Lack of appropriate dusting of herbivorous food with a calcium and vitamin D supplement.**

  8. **Lack of appropriate dusting and gut loading of invertebrate prey with a calcium and vitamin D supplement.**

  9. **Overfeeding leading to excessive growth rate.**

  10. **Lack of exercise.**

E. **Animal risk factors** include:

  1. **Hepatic disease.**

  2. **Renal disease.**

  3. **Skin disease.**

  4. **Reproductive activity.**

II. Signalment

A. **Juvenile** or rapidly growing lizards and chelonians are more commonly affected by the depletion of bone stores.

B. **Reproductively active female** lizards and chelonians are more prone to hypocalcemia.

C. **Most cases present with a history of poor husbandry and diet.**

D. **Snakes fed whole mammal prey are not reported to suffer from this condition.**

III. Clinical Signs

A. **Deformity of the skeletal elements** leading to distorted shape (vertebral column and long bones of the limbs) and compressible skull (Figure 37.1). Stunted growth may be a feature in young animals. The lay term "rubber jaw" is often used by owners to describe facial deformities that result.

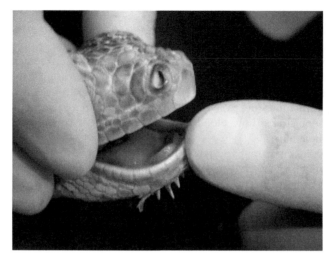

Figure 37.1   A green iguana (*Iguana iguana*) demonstrating a classical sign of nutritional secondary hyperparathyroidism: the skull and jaw bones are easily compressible.

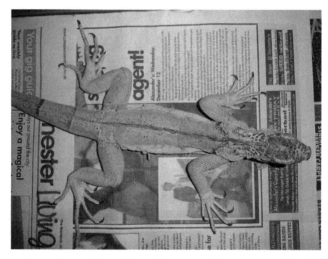

Figure 37.2   This green iguana (*Iguana iguana*) is unable to lift its body off the ground and is suffering from dysecdysis (abnormal skin sloughing).

B. **Lack of truncal lifting** (Figure 37.2).

C. **Pathological fractures** of the limbs.

D. **Shell deformities** and softening of the carapace and plastron in chelonians (Figure 37.3).

E. **Dermal hemorrhages** between the epidermal scutes and the dermal bone in chelonians.

F. **Cloacal prolapse** of the hemipenis, cloaca, colon, bladder, or oviducts are all possible (Figure 37.4).

G. **Hypocalcemic tetany** in lizards; only anecdotally reported in chelonians. Muscle fasciculations and hyperreflexia may also be seen.

H. Hypocalcemia causing **flaccid paralysis** in lizards and chelonians.

I. **Dysecdysis (abnormal sloughing) and general debility** due to chronicity of the disease process.

J. **Secondary renal disease** contributing to collapse.

IV. Diagnosis

A. **Clinical history in combination with typical clinical signs is indicative of NSHP.**

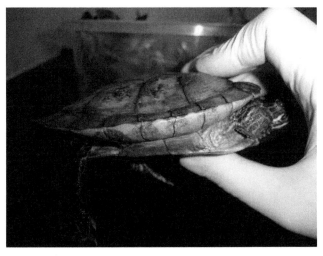

Figure 37.3   This yellow bellied terrapin (*Trachemys scripta scripta*) has a compressible shell.

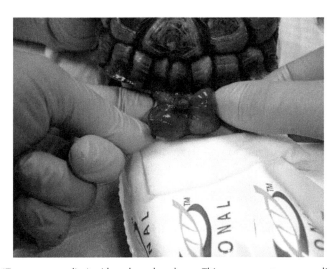

Figure 37.4   A box turtle (*Terrapene carolina*) with a cloacal prolapse. This can present as a complication of hypocalcemia in both lizards and chelonians.

B. A significant amount of the body's circulating calcium may be protein bound but the proportion bound is highly variable and as such **total calcium values are not helpful in the diagnosis of NSHP.**
C. Ionized calcium will be reduced (typically <2.4 mg/dL [0.6 mmol/L]) in cases of hypocalcemic tetany or paralysis.
D. **25-hydroxycholecalciferol levels may be reduced.** However, there are only a few reports of normal values in reptiles which can make interpretation of results challenging.
E. **Radiography or CT examination may demonstrate reduced bone density,** bone deviations, fibrous osteodystrophy, or pathological fractures. In older animals, bone deviations with acceptable bone density or healed fractures can indicate historic NSHP.
F. **Reproductive activity** should also be critically assessed using radiography, ultrasound, or celioscopy, as concurrent reproductive disease may require medical or surgical treatment as part of the therapy for NSHP (Figure 37.5).

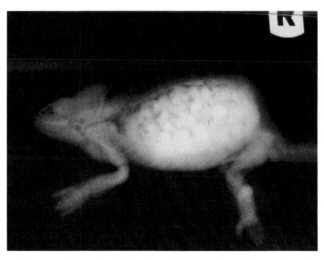

Figure 37.5 A lateral horizontal beam radiograph of a female veiled chameleon (*Chamaeleo calyptratus*). Bone density is poor and the animal is gravid with multiple follicles filling the entire coelomic cavity.

V. Differential Diagnoses

A. **Renal secondary hyperparathyroidism.** Severe renal disease can lead to reduced active vitamin D production and lead to similar clinical signs. Equally concurrent renal disease in patients with NSHP is possible as excessively elevated PTH levels have been shown to be nephrotoxic. It is important to thoroughly evaluate the patient for renal disease and this may include blood biochemistry, assessment of the glomerular filtration rate, or renal biopsy for histopathological examination. In many cases, **hyperphosphatemia may complicate therapy.**

B. **Other bone disorders** such as spinal osteomyelitis (bacterial or fungal) can be seen in aged lizards. Hypertrophic osteopathy, osteopetrosis, and Paget's disease (osteitis deformans) have also been reported in reptiles.

C. **Cloacal prolapses** can also occur due to trauma of the local tissues, excessive straining due to cloacoliths, egg production, foreign body ingestion, and parasitism. Radiography, fecal parasitology, and cloacal endoscopy may be required to rule out these conditions.

D. If **neurological signs** are present with ionized calcium levels over 2.4 mg/dL (0.6 mmol/L), the clinician should look towards other differentials such as trauma, infectious agents, xanthomatosis, hypoglycemia, or toxins.

E. **Trauma** leading to fractures of the limbs in lizards. In these cases, the bone density will be assessed as normal on radiography or CT examination.

VI. Treatment

A. **General principles:**
   1. The **primary goals** of therapy are:
      a. **To achieve eucalcemia.**
      b. To provide **supportive care.**
      c. To **control and correct secondary complications** such as cloacal prolapses.
      d. To **identify any underlying predisposing disease states** and manage these.
      e. To provide **dietary and husbandry correction** long term. Considerations include appropriate supplementation of dietary items, aiming for a dietary calcium to phosphorus ratio of >2:1, ensuring background and basking temperatures are suitable for the species, and providing access to natural sunlight and/or an appropriate artificial UV-b source.
   2. A suggested protocol is outlined in Table 37.1 but is subject to much variation depending on the severity of the case.

B. **Thermal therapy:**
   1. All reptiles should be **warmed to their optimal temperatures** prior to the administration of therapeutics. These are species specific and ranges should be sought from reference material:

Table 37.1　Suggested treatment protocol for collapsed hypocalcemic reptiles.

Day 1	Diagnostic procedures	Radiography and blood profile (including ionized calcium, uric acid, and phosphorus levels) to evaluate disease status
	Treatment	Warm the reptile to its optimal temperature Provide fluid therapy at 30 mL/kg, by parenteral routes Provide a UV light source Start parenteral calcium gluconate therapy at 100–200 mg/kg q 6 h (give slowly and dilute with fluids if using intravenous or intraosseous routes) Consider treatment with 1,25-dihydroxycholecalciferol at 1 ng/kg PO q 12 h Treat any secondary complications and underlying conditions accordingly
Day 2	Diagnostic procedures	Consider reevaluating ionized calcium levels to determine when parenteral calcium therapy can be stopped
	Treatment	Start supportive nutrition if urinated Provide oral 25-hydroxycholecalciferol or cholecalciferol and calcium therapy
Day 3	Treatment	Stop oral 1,25-dihydroxycholecalciferol therapy Continue supportive care and oral calcium and vitamin D therapy Place an esophagostomy tube if required Send home once stable with ongoing medication
Day 7	Diagnostic procedures	Reevaluate ionized calcium levels
	Treatment	Consider salmon calcitonin at this point

Note: The protocol used may need to be modified depending on the species presented, the severity and chronicity of nutritional secondary hyperparathyroidism, and any concurrent disease problems identified.

　　a. **An even background temperature** should be provided for collapsed reptiles (as they are unable to move about freely to thermoregulate).

　　b. In reptiles capable of thermoregulation, a **basking site** should be provided.

C. Calcium therapy:

　1. Even in animals with acceptable levels of ionized calcium, calcium therapy is indicated. This provides a source for not only stabilizing the blood levels but also integration into the bone matrix. Caution is to be advised in those animals suffering from hyperphosphatemia as calcium therapy can lead to further elevations in phosphorus by decreasing glomerular filtration rate, renal blood flow, and leading to the release of phosphorus from cells. Phosphorus binders can be used alongside diuresis to reduce phosphorus levels:

　　a. **Parenteral calcium gluconate** can be used in severe cases and is given by any parenteral route. For intravenous or intraosseous use, it is best diluted with fluids and administered slowly. Dosages commonly employed are 100–200 mg/kg, every 6 h. Ideally, treatment should be based on serial ionized calcium concentrations and the clinical response to therapy.

　　b. **Oral calcium supplementation** should be provided in those animals with an acceptable ionized calcium level that are well enough to tolerate oral therapy. This can be provided either in a liquid format, such as **calcium borogluconate**, or as **calcium carbonate** powder. Levels provided are arbitrary but dosing regimens are often provided on commercial products.

D. UV light:

　1. This should be provided to all reptiles suffering from NSHP, specifically **UV-b light (wavelength 290–320 nm)**. Some species have a greater ability to utilize UV light than others for the production of vitamin D:

a. An **artificial light source** should be used. Many designs are commercially available for reptiles and include metal halide and mercury vapor lamps (which also act as heat sources), compact bulbs, or fluorescent tubes. The output of these sources should be verified at the reptile's level with a UV meter. Exposure levels required vary among reptile species.

b. **Solar radiation** should also be provided when weather conditions allow exposure to direct unfiltered sunlight. The reptile must be warmed to its optimal temperature to benefit from UV light sources.

E. **Vitamin D therapy:**

1. Vitamin D can be given in any of three formulations: oral cholecalciferol, 25–hydroxycholecalciferol, or 1,25-dihydroxycholecalciferol. Many oral formulations contain cholecalciferol in combination with calcium. Ideally, measurement of the blood 25-hydroxycholecalciferol should be performed to avoid toxicity. Nephrocalcinosis is a potential complication of therapy. It should be noted that the ability of all species of reptile to utilize oral vitamin D is questionable:

a. **1,25-dihydroxycholecalciferol** is available as oral capsules containing 0.25 or 0.5 µg. The capsule contents can be mixed with olive oil to increase absorption. It is generally only used in the initial phase of treatment, where immediate effectiveness is required. The recommended dose is based on anecdotal reports: 1 ng/kg is given orally q 12 h.

b. **25-hydroxycholecalciferol or cholecalciferol** can be provided at the same time and can be continued over the first few weeks.

F. **Supportive care:**

1. It is highly likely that reptiles suffering from NSHP will have had reduced access to food and water prior to presentation:

a. **Fluid therapy** should be administered by parenteral or enteral routes depending on the severity of the case. This is of particular importance for phosphate diuresis when reptiles are suffering from hyperphosphatemia.

b. **Nutritional support** is of secondary importance after the animal has been successfully rehydrated and any electrolyte imbalances corrected. If the reptile is anorexic, as is often the case, nutritional support can be achieved using a number of commercially available products. Liquidized food can be provided via tube/gavage feeding; for longer term support, the placement of an esophagostomy tube should be considered. The metabolic rate of reptiles is much lower than mammals and the level of nutritional support is adjusted accordingly.

G. **Providing exercise:**

1. Exercise is vital in order to stimulate normal bone growth due to mechanical loading and this is often overlooked. Caution is advised though as those reptiles considered at risk of pathological fractures will require their activity to be initially curtailed:

a. Getting tortoises or large lizards **outside in a run** is probably one of the best options both for the physiological and psychological well being of the reptile.

b. Allowing **exercise indoors** is more appropriate for smaller reptiles and the time spent out of their enclosure should be based on the relative size of the reptile and the room temperature. The reptile should be returned to its enclosure prior to excessive cooling.

H. **Phosphorus binders:**

1. Where phosphorus has been elevated, phosphorus binders may be used to reduce the risk of mineralization of tissues, prior to calcium supplementation. Phosphate binders only act on intestinal phosphorus:

a. **Aluminum hydroxide** can be given orally at a dose rate of 50 mg/kg q 12 h. Care has to be taken with commercial antacids as some can contain magnesium at excessive levels for reptiles.

b. **Calcium acetate, citrate, or carbonate** also act to bind phosphorus and can be given orally.

c. **Fluid diuresis** will also reduce plasma phosphorus levels.

I. **Calcitonin therapy:**

1. There have been some studies on the effects of serial injections of calcitonin in reptiles. Calcitonin acts to reduce bone liberation of calcium. However, some studies have shown calcitonin to have limited effects even with daily administration in reptiles. It is best used in combination with serial monitoring of blood ionized calcium levels to reduce the risk of hypocalcemia and to permit evaluation of its effectiveness:

a. **Salmon calcitonin** (a synthetic calcitonin) is available commercially and has been used at a dose of 50 IU/kg in lizards after a week of initial therapy and stabilization. This treatment can be repeated after a further week. In chelonians, a dose of 1.5 IU/kg has been recommended as a one-off treatment.

J. **PTH therapy:**

1. In humans, PTH is used to treat osteopenia as it has an anabolic effect on bone. There have been no such effects reported in reptiles.

K. **Treatment of underlying predisposing factors or secondary complications:**

1. This is an important aspect of therapy and may influence prognosis. The reader is directed to more detailed texts on the management of related conditions:

a. Underlying conditions such as **reproductive disease** should be diagnosed and managed appropriately.

b. Secondary complications such as **cloacal prolapse** will require specific treatment.

c. **Renal function** should be evaluated in every patient and if renal disease is diagnosed, it must be treated accordingly.

d. External coaptation, such as lightweight splints, should be used to stabilize pathological fractures. Internal fixation implants are not appropriate.

VII. Prognosis

A. Prognosis depends on the severity of the case presented and can vary from good to grave. Severe cases with significant debility or cases presented by owners who are resistant to implementing husbandry changes should be euthanized on humane grounds. Milder cases will respond to therapy and husbandry changes although anatomical distortions will remain long term. Many reptiles can lead acceptable lives despite this, provided that mobility and respiration are not overly impaired. Some chelonians will require modification of the carapace to allow free limb and head movement.

VIII. Prevention

A. Providing the **appropriate husbandry** (including nutrition and environmental conditions) for the species concerned is of paramount importance. Identifying animals in greater need of calcium and vitamin D is important (such as growing juveniles or reproductively active females) as their environment and diet will need to be modified accordingly.

References and Further Readings

Bentley PJ. Hormones and calcium metabolism. In: Bentley PJ, ed. *Comparative Vertebrate Endocrinology*. Cambridge: Cambridge University Press, 1976, pp. 218–241.

Burgmann PM, Mcfarlen J, Thiesenhausen K. Causes of hypocalcaemia and metabolic bone disease in *Iguana iguana. J Small Exot Anim Med* 1993;2(2):63–68.

Calvert I. Nutritional problems. In: Girling S, ed. *BSAVA Manual of Reptiles*, 2nd edn. Cheltenham: British Small Animal Veterinary Association, 2004, pp. 289–308.

Gibbons PM. Comparative vertebrate calcium metabolism and regulation. *Proc Assoc Reptil Amphib Vet* 2001;267–276.

Klaphake E. A review of phosphorous for the reptile practitioner. *Proc Assoc Reptil Amphib Vet* 2001;281–286.

Kline LW. A hypocalcaemic response to synthetic salmon calcitonin in the green iguana *Iguana iguana. Gen Comp Endocrinol* 1981;44:476–479.

Mader DR. Metabolic bone diseases. In: Mader DR, ed. *Reptile Medicine and Surgery*, 2nd edn. St Louis: Saunders, 2006, pp. 841–851.

Mader DR, Garner MM. Metabolic bone disease in reptiles. *Proc Assoc Reptil Amphib Vet* 2001;287–289.

McArthur S, Wilkinson RJ, Barrows MG. Tortoises and turtles. In: Meredith A, Redrobe S, eds. *BSAVA Manual of Exotic pets*, 4th edn. Gloucester: British Small Animal Veterinary Association, 2002, pp. 208–222.

Rosol TJ, Taylor JL, Fischbach DG, et al. Effects of daily administration of human parathyroid hormone (1–34) or salmon calcitonin in green iguanas, *Iguana iguana*. In: Danes J, Dacke C, Filk C, Gay C, eds. *Calcium Metabolism: Comparative Endocrinology*. Bradley Stoke, Bristol: BioScientifica Ltd, 1999, pp. 75–80.

Ullrey DE, Bernard JB. Vitamin D: Metabolism, sources, unique problems in zoo animals, meeting needs. In: Fowler ME, Miller RE, eds. *Zoo and Wild Animal Medicine, Current Therapy*, vol. 4, Philadelphia: WB Saunders, 1999, pp. 63–78.

CHAPTER 38

Hyposomatotropism in Dogs

Annemarie M.W.Y. Voorbij and Hans S. Kooistra

Pathogenesis

- Congenital hyposomatotropism or pituitary dwarfism occurs most often as an autosomal, recessive inherited disorder in German shepherd dogs or breeds in which German shepherd dogs have been used in the breeding.
- Congenital hyposomatotropism in these breeds is characterized by underdevelopment of the pituitary gland and a deficiency of growth hormone (GH), thyrotropin, prolactin, and gonadotropins, whereas corticotropin secretion is unaffected.
- A mutation of the *Lhx3* gene is the most likely cause of congenital hyposomatotropism.
- Acquired or adult-onset GH deficiency may be caused by damage to the pituitary gland. The exact pathogenesis of other forms of so-called spontaneously acquired hyposomatotropism is not completely clear.

Classical Signs

- Congenital hyposomatotropism is characterized by proportionate growth retardation and retention of the puppy hair coat with concurrent lack of guard hairs and bilaterally symmetrical alopecia.
- Spontaneously acquired hyposomatotropism has been proposed as an explanation for some forms of alopecia.

Diagnosis

- Insufficient GH response to stimulation of the somatotropic cells and low plasma insulin-like growth factor-I (IGF-I) concentration.
- Congenital hyposomatotropism in German shepherd dogs and related breeds can be diagnosed with a specific DNA test.

Treatment

- Porcine GH or progestins.

Clinical Endocrinology of Companion Animals, First Edition. Edited by Jacquie Rand.
© 2013 John Wiley & Sons, Inc. Published 2013 by John Wiley & Sons, Inc.

I. Pathogenesis

A. The **pituitary gland consists of two main parts**: the **adenohypophysis (anterior pituitary)** and the **neurohypophysis (posterior pituitary)**.

B. The **adenohypophysis** contains a functionally diverse population of highly specialized cell types that are classified according to the tropic hormones they produce:

1. Somatotropic cells secrete GH.

2. Lactotropic cells secrete **prolactin.**

3. Gonadotropic cells secrete the **gonadotropins** luteinizing hormone (LH) and follicle-stimulating hormone (FSH).

4. Thyrotropic cells secrete **thyroid-stimulating hormone** (TSH or thyrotropin).

5. Corticotropic cells synthesize the precursor molecule proopiomelanocortin (POMC), which gives rise to **adrenocorticotropic hormone** (ACTH or corticotropin).

C. Congenital hyposomatotropism:

1. The **development of the adenohypophysis** is a highly differentiated process that is **tightly regulated by the coordinated actions of numerous transcription factors.** The individual hormone-secreting cells emerge in a **sequential order.** Of the adenohypophyseal endocrine cells, the corticotropic cells are the first to develop.

2. **Any defect** in adenohypophyseal development may result in **isolated or combined pituitary hormone deficiency.**

3. In dogs, **congenital hyposomatotropism,** that is, congenital GH deficiency or pituitary dwarfism, is the **most striking example** of pituitary hormone deficiency.

4. Congenital hyposomatotropism is known to occur in **different dog breeds,** including the Karelian bear dog, Czechoslovakian wolfhound, and Saarloos wolfhound. However, the condition is encountered most often in **German shepherd dogs.**

5. German shepherd dogs with congenital hyposomatotropism have a **combined deficiency of GH, TSH, prolactin, and the gonadotropins.** In contrast, ACTH secretion is preserved.

6. Originally, **pressure atrophy of the adenohypophysis by cystic enlargement of Rathke's cleft** was thought to cause pituitary dwarfism. But since some pituitary dwarfs have only **very small pituitary cysts** unlikely to cause pressure atrophy and because **ACTH secretion is unaffected** in pituitary dwarfs, **it was concluded that cyst formation could not be the cause of the disorder.**

7. Congenital hyposomatotropism is caused by a **simple, autosomal, recessive genetic** abnormality.

8. Because ACTH secretion is preserved in pituitary dwarfs, it was supposed that a **mutation of a gene encoding a transcription factor that precludes effective expansion of pituitary stem cells after the differentiation of corticotropic cells** is the cause of this disorder.

9. Recent research has revealed that **a mutation of the gene encoding for the transcription factor Lhx3** is the most likely cause of congenital hyposomatotropism in German shepherd dogs and breeds in which German shepherd dogs have been used in the breeding, like Czechoslovakian wolfhounds, Saarloos wolfhounds, and, probably also, Karelian bear dogs.

D. Acquired hyposomatotropism in mature dogs:

1. Damage to the pituitary gland, for example, due to **hypophysectomy** or pituitary **irradiation** as in the treatment of pituitary-dependent hypercortisolism, is an obvious cause of acquired hyposomatotropism. Irradiation will rarely result in clinical signs of GH deficiency.

2. In addition, **spontaneously acquired hyposomatotropism** has been proposed as an explanation for some forms of **alopecia** in certain breeds. Although treatment with heterologous GH is quite often ineffective, the condition has been given names such as **adult-onset GH deficiency and GH-responsive dermatosis.** Uncertainty about the pathogenetic role of GH is illustrated by the coining of alternative names such as **castration-responsive alopecia** and **alopecia X.**

3. In Pomeranians and miniature poodles supposed to have spontaneously acquired hyposomatotropism, the alopecia may actually be the result of **mild hypercortisolism.**

II. Signalment

A. **Congenital hyposomatotropism can be encountered in different dog breeds, including the Karelian bear dog, Czechoslovakian wolfhound, and Saarloos wolfhound. However, the condition has the highest**

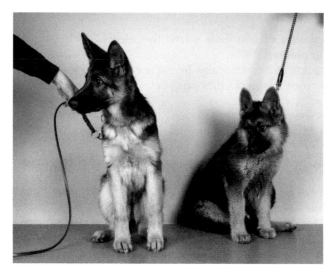

Figure 38.1 A 4-month-old German shepherd dog with congenital hyposomatotropism (right), sitting next to its intact female littermate (left). Note the proportionate growth retardation, the retention of secondary hairs (puppy hair coat), and the lack of primary or guard hairs of the dog with congenital hyposomatotropism.

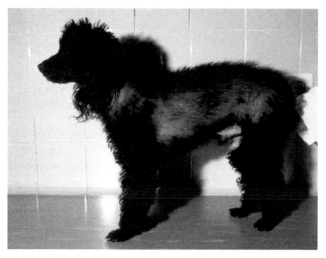

Figure 38.2 A 6-year-old male miniature poodle with progressively worsening truncal alopecia. Basal and GHRH-stimulated plasma GH concentrations were low, consistent with a possible diagnosis of spontaneously acquired hyposomatotropism.

prevalence in German shepherd dogs (Figure 38.1). Because it is an autosomal inherited disorder, there is an equal distribution between males and females.

B. **Spontaneous adult-onset hyposomatotropism** has been reported mainly in breeds such as the **Pomeranian, miniature poodle** (Figure 38.2), **chow chow, and keeshond.** It is reported to occur in **both sexes and at any age, but usually beginning at 1–3 years** of age.

III. Clinical Signs

A. **Congenital hyposomatotropism:**
   1. Congenital hyposomatotropism can lead to a **wide range of clinical manifestations** and not **all dwarfs display the same clinical signs.** An overview of the clinical manifestations and postmortem findings associated with congenital hyposomatotropism is given in Table 38.1.

Table 38.1   Clinical manifestations and postmortem findings associated with congenital hyposomatotropism in dogs.

Musculoskeletal	Dermatologic
Stunted growth	Soft, wooly haircoat
Thin skeleton	Retention of lanugo hairs
Changes in ossification centers	Lack of guard hairs
Delayed closure of growth plates	Isolated patches of guard hair
Delayed dental eruption	Bilateral symmetrical alopecia at trunk, neck, and proximal extremities
Fox-like facial features	Hyperpigmentation of the skin
Muscle atrophy	Thin, fragile skin
	Wrinkles
Reproduction	Scales
Cryptorchidism	Comedones
Flaccid penile sheath	Papules
Failure to have estrus cycles	Pyoderma
	Seborrhea sicca
Other signs	
Shrill, puppy-like bark	**Postmortem findings**
Signs of secondary hypothyroidism	Pituitary cysts
Mental dullness	Atrophy adenohypophysis
Impairment of renal function	Hypoplasia thyroid gland
	Persistent ductus arteriosus

Modified from Nelson, 2003.

2. All dwarfs display a variable degree of **proportionate growth retardation** (Figure 38.3). **During the first weeks of their lives, pituitary dwarfs may be of normal size,** but after this period, they will grow more slowly than their litter mates. **By 3–4 months of age, affected pups are obviously the runts** of their litter and they will never attain full adult dimensions.

3. Another typical clinical sign of canine congenital hyposomatotropism is retention of lanugo or secondary hairs (**puppy hair coat**) with concurrent lack of primary or guard hairs and **bilateral symmetrical alopecia** (Figure 38.4). The alopecia mostly occurs on the **trunk, neck, and proximal extremities**.

4. Most German shepherd dwarfs have a **pointed muzzle,** resembling that of a fox (Figure 38.5).

5. Also **dermatological problems** such as **hyperpigmentation, scaling,** and **bacterial pyoderma** are commonly seen in dogs with congenital hyposomatotropism (Figure 38.4).

6. Male German shepherd dwarfs commonly display **unilateral or bilateral cryptorchidism.** Female dwarfs often have **frequent anovulatory estrous cycles;** anovulatory cycles will not be followed by a luteal phase and, consequently, the bitch will be in heat much more often than usual.

B. **Acquired hyposomatotropism in mature dogs has been proposed** as an explanation for some forms of **alopecia,** mainly involving the trunk, caudal surfaces of the thighs, perineum, and neck.

IV. Diagnosis

A. Although the medical history and clinical manifestations may often be highly suggestive of congenital hyposomatotropism, **other endocrine and nonendocrine causes** of growth retardation have to be **excluded** first.

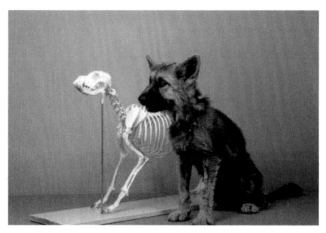

Figure 38.3 A 6-month-old German shepherd dog with congenital hyposomatotropism, sitting next to a skeleton of an adult healthy dog of a small dog breed. The dwarf has the same body proportions as the skeleton.

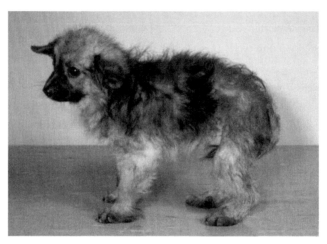

Figure 38.4 A 5-month-old German shepherd dog with congenital hyposomatotropism. Note the retention of secondary hairs (puppy hair coat) and the alopecia.

B. Routine blood work normally does not reveal abnormalities, except that the **plasma creatinine concentration is elevated** in most of the pituitary dwarfs. Since the lack of GH and thyroid hormones may result in maldevelopment of the glomeruli, pituitary dwarfism can be associated with **decreased glomerular filtration**. Although creatinine is typically mildly elevated with a normal BUN and concentrated urine in the early stages, renal failure can develop over time.

C. As expected in secondary hypothyroidism, that is, due to pituitary failure, **the plasma concentrations of thyroxine (T_4) and TSH are usually low.**

D. The function of the somatotropic cells can be evaluated directly by measuring the **circulating GH concentration.** However, since the **basal plasma GH concentration may also be low in healthy dogs**, a stimulation test is required for the diagnosis of GH deficiency.

E. **Definitive diagnosis** of pituitary hormone deficiency should rely on evaluation of pituitary responsiveness to **provocative testing**, that is, challenging the adenohypophyseal cells by **stimulation with releasing hormones**. To determine if a dog has GH deficiency, a stimulation test with **GH-releasing hormone (GHRH)**, in an intravenous dosage of 1 µg/kg body weight, may be used. Alternatively, **α-adrenergic drugs** such as clonidine (10 µg/kg body weight) or xylazine (100 µg/kg body weight) can be used. The plasma GH concentration should be determined before and 20–30 min after intravenous administration of the stimulant. In

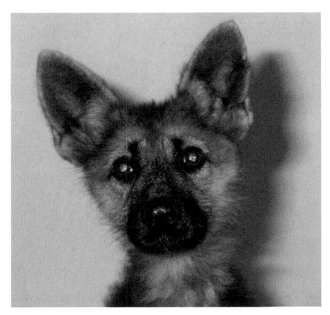

Figure 38.5   German shepherd dwarf with the characteristic pointed muzzle and fox-like facial features, typical of affected dogs.

healthy dogs, plasma GH concentrations should increase at least two- to fourfold after administration of the stimulant. In contrast, there will be **no significant rise in plasma GH concentration** in pituitary dwarfs.

F.   Another test to determine the responsiveness of the somatotropic cells is the **ghrelin stimulation test.** Ghrelin is a potent stimulator of GH release in dogs, and, in young dogs, even more potent than GHRH. Human ghrelin is administrated intravenously at a dose of 2 µg/kg body weight. A post-ghrelin plasma GH concentration of more than 5 µg/L excludes congenital hyposomatotropism.

G.   Unfortunately, **in many countries a commercial canine-specific GH assay is not available.** However, the function of the somatotropic cells can also be evaluated indirectly by measuring the **circulating IGF-I concentration.** Breed and body size have to be taken into account when interpreting the plasma IGF-I concentration. Although the mean plasma IGF-1 concentration of dogs with congenital hyposomatotropism is considerably lower than that of healthy dogs, there may be **some overlap.**

H.   To test the secretory capacity of the other hormone producing pituitary cells, the adenohypophysis can by stimulated with **corticotropin-releasing hormone** (CRH, 1 µg/kg body weight), **thyrotropin-releasing hormone** (TRH, 10 µg/kg body weight), **and gonadotropin-releasing hormone** (GnRH, 10 µg/kg body weight). The results of the combined pituitary anterior lobe function test in healthy dogs and German shepherd dogs with congenital hyposomatotropism are depicted in Figure 38.6.

I.   The morphology of the pituitary gland may be investigated with **computed tomography or magnetic resonance imaging.** In most German shepherd dwarfs, an **intrapituitary cyst** can be identified at a young age (Figure 38.7A), which gradually enlarges during life (Figure 38.7B). Because healthy dogs may have pituitary cysts as well, pituitary dwarfism cannot be diagnosed based upon the presence of a pituitary cyst alone.

J.   The finding that German shepherd dogs with congenital hyposomatotropism have a mutation of the gene encoding the transcription factor **Lhx3** has resulted in the development of a **genetic test.** With this genetic test, not only **dwarfs** but also **carriers** of the mutation can be identified. The test is currently only performed at the **Department of Clinical Sciences of Companion Animals of Utrecht University.**

K.   **Hypophysectomy** leads to a **very low plasma GH concentration** that does **not respond to stimulation** and a **relatively low plasma IGF-I concentration.**

L.   In other forms of so-called **spontaneously acquired hyposomatotropism,** the **GH response to stimulation is less well defined.** In about one-third of the cases, the GH response to stimulation is normal. Furthermore, also in many Pomeranians without alopecia, the circulating GH concentration does not increase significantly after stimulation.

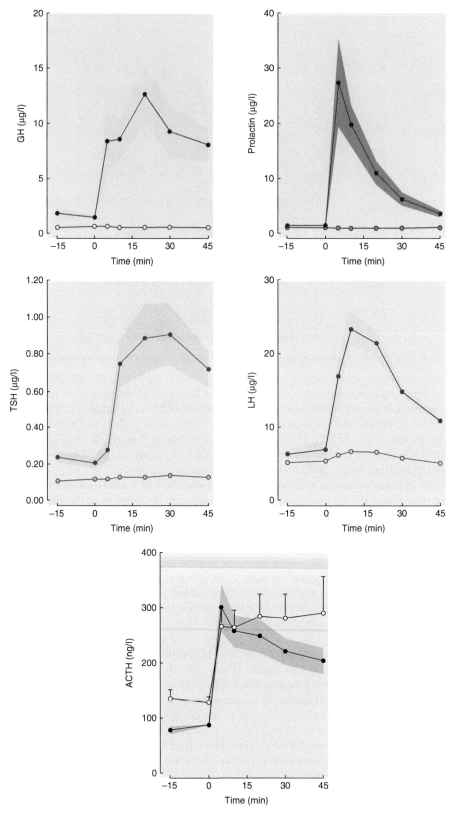

Figure 38.6 Mean (±SEM) plasma concentrations of growth hormone (GH), prolactin, thyrotropin (TSH), luteinizing hormone (LH), and adrenocorticotropic hormone (ACTH) during a combined pituitary anterior lobe function test in eight German shepherd dwarfs (O) and eight healthy beagle dogs (●). Reprinted with permission from Kooistra HS, Voorhout G, Mol JA, Rijnberk A. Combined pituitary hormone deficiency in German shepherd dogs with dwarfism. *Domest Anim Endocrinol* 2000;19:177–190.

(a)

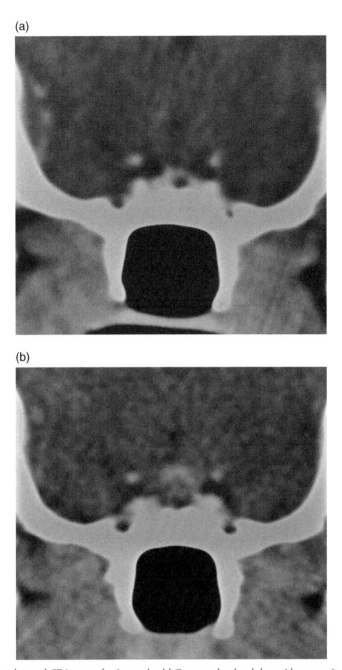

(b)

Figure 38.7   (a) Contrast-enhanced CT image of a 6-month-old German shepherd dog with congenital hyposomatotropism. At the base of the brain, the contrast-enhanced pituitary is visible. The pituitary is of normal size (height 3.6 mm, width 4.3 mm), but contains a radiolucent area due to the presence of a cyst. (b) At the age of 3 years, the pituitary is enlarged (height 6.5 mm, width 5.4 mm). The greater part of the pituitary lacks contrast enhancement due to the presence of the cyst that has increased in size considerably in comparison with 2.5 years earlier.

M. Another reason why it has to be questioned whether true GH deficiency exists in these alopecic dogs with so-called spontaneously acquired hyposomatotropism is that their plasma IGF-I concentrations have been reported to fall within the reference range.

V. Differential Diagnoses

A. Congenital hyposomatotropism:

1. Probably the **most important differential diagnosis** of congenital hyposomatotropism is **congenital hypothyroidism.** In contrast to congenital hyposomatotropism, congenital hypothyroidism leads to disproportionate dwarfism.

2. Other endocrine disorders such as juvenile diabetes mellitus and juvenile hyperparathyroidism should be considered as well.

3. Failure to grow can also be caused by **nonendocrine diseases** like renal disorders, cardiac diseases, chondrodystrophy, hepatic diseases, esophageal obstruction, gastrointestinal disorders, exocrine pancreatic insufficiency, and even malnutrition.

4. Corticosteroid administration at a young age can also lead to significant growth retardation.

5. The possibility that the apparently dwarfed animal is simply **a small individual** should also be considered.

B. Acquired hyposomatotropism in mature dogs:

1. Alopecia in adult dogs may be attributable to **any of the endocrine diseases** known to result in skin atrophy and hair loss (e.g., hypothyroidism, hypercortisolism, and hyperestrogenism due to a testicular tumor).

VI. Treatment

A. GH substitution:

1. Since canine GH is not available for therapeutic use, in the past there have been attempts to treat dogs with hyposomatotropism with human and bovine GH. Unfortunately, formation of antibodies directed against human and bovine GH precludes their use.

2. In more recent years, **porcine GH** has become available for therapeutic use (Figure 38.8). Its administration will not result in the formation of antibodies, because the **amino acid sequence of porcine GH is identical to that of canine GH.**

3. The recommended **subcutaneous starting dose for porcine GH is 0.1–0.3 IU/kg body weight, three times a week.**

B. Progestins:

1. Because progestins are able to induce the expression of the GH gene in the mammary glands, and because mammary GH in dogs is released into the systemic circulation, dogs with hyposomatotropism can also be treated with progestins, such as **medroxyprogesterone acetate (MPA)** (Figure 38.9).

2. MPA should be administered **subcutaneously in doses of 2.5–5 mg/kg body weight,** initially at 3-week intervals (for five times) and subsequently at 6-week intervals.

3. Unfortunately, treatment with MPA does have some quite **undesirable side effects,** such as recurrent periods of pruritic pyoderma, cystic endometrial hyperplasia with mucometra in female animals, and, infrequently, development of mammary tumors. Even though plasma concentrations of GH may not exceed the upper limit of the reference range, some dogs may still develop acromegalic features. This may be reversed by discontinuing treatment for a few months, certainly when the plasma IGF-I concentration approaches 200 µg/L. Endometrial hyperplasia can be prevented by ovariohysterectomy prior to treatment.

C. Treatment with porcine GH or progestins may result in **GH excess** and consequently side effects such as **diabetes mellitus** may develop. Therefore, **monitoring** the plasma concentrations of **GH and glucose** every 3 weeks is recommended. Long-term dose rates should depend on measurements of the plasma concentration of IGF-I.

D. Whether therapy will lead to **linear growth** of a dwarf is dependent on the status of the growth plates at the time treatment is started. If the growth plates have not closed yet, some **linear growth** can be expected in dwarfed animals.

E. A **beneficial response in the skin and hair coat** usually occurs within a few months after the start of therapy. In pituitary dwarfs, the lanugo hairs often regrow, but growth of the guard hairs is variable.

F. Treatment of dogs with congenital hyposomatotropism with either porcine GH or MPA should, in most cases, be accompanied by treatment with **synthetic levothyroxine.** All dogs with pituitary dwarfism due to the Lhx3 gene mutation will have TSH deficiency and, thus, should be treated with L-thyroxine. Other less

(a)

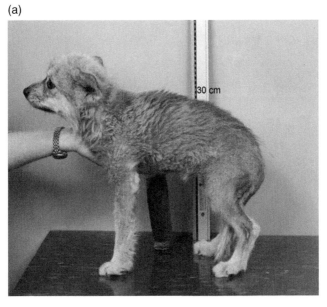

(b)

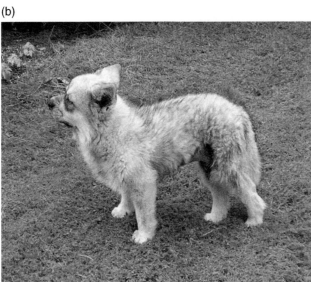

Figure 38.8 A female Saarloos wolfhound with congenital hyposomatotropism before (a) and after treatment with porcine growth hormone and L-thyroxine (b).

common causes of congenital hyposomatotropism may not be accompanied by TSH deficiency. Levothyroxine is administered **orally**, with a **starting dose of 15 µg/kg body weight, twice daily**. The plasma thyroxine concentration should be **monitored closely**, because the absorption and metabolism of levothyroxine is variable. The dosage may have to be adjusted several times before a satisfactory clinical response is reached (see Chapter 25 on Canine hypothyroidism).

G. In some cases of **spontaneously acquired hyposomatotropism**, even if there was a normal GH response to stimulation, **treatment with GH** has been reported to be effective. In others, seemingly unrelated measures such as **castration** or administration of **testosterone** were followed by the appearance of a **new hair coat**.

(a)

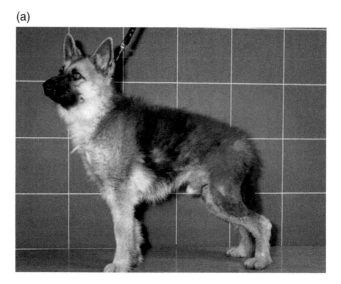

(b)

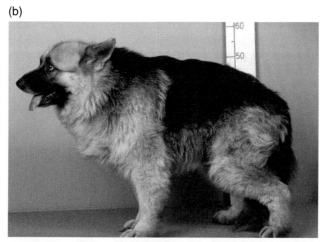

Figure 38.9   A male German shepherd dog with congenital hyposomatotropism before (a) and after treatment with medroxy-progesterone acetate and L-thyroxine (b).

H.   Because the alopecia of miniature poodles and Pomeranians with supposed spontaneously acquired hyposomatotropism may be due to mild hypercortisolism, the **treatment options for hypercortisolism** may also result in regrowth of hairs in these dogs (see Chapter 5 on Canine hyperadrenocorticism).

VII. Prognosis
A.   **Without proper treatment**, the long-term **prognosis of congenital hyposomatotropism is poor**. By the age of 3–5 years, affected dogs usually have become bald, thin, and dull, possibly due to progressive loss of pituitary function, continuing expansion of pituitary cysts, and/or progressive renal failure. At this stage, **owners usually request euthanasia** for their dog, if they have not done so long before this.
B.   Although the **prognosis improves** when dwarfs are **properly treated** with either porcine GH or progestins (and levothyroxine), their prognosis still remains guarded.

VIII. Prevention
A. The identification of the mutation in the ***Lhx3*** **gene** associated with congenital hyposomatotropism in German shepherd dogs (and breeds in which German shepherd dogs have been used in the breeding) has

enabled the development of a **DNA test**. With this DNA test, not only **dwarfs** but also **carriers of the mutation** can be identified. When all potential breeding animals are screened with this DNA test, **eradication** of this form of congenital hyposomatotropism is within reach.

References and Further Readings

Andresen E, Willeberg P. Pituitary dwarfism in German shepherd dogs: Additional evidence of simple autosomal recessive inheritance. *Nord Vet Med* 1976;28:481–486.

Bhatti SFM, De Vliegher SP, Mol JA, Van Ham LML, Kooistra HS. Ghrelin-stimulation test in the diagnosis of canine pituitary dwarfism. *Res Vet Sci* 2006;81:24–30.

Cerundolo R, Lloyd DH, Vaessen MMAR, Mol JA, Kooistra HS, Rijnberk A. Alopecia in pomeranians and miniature poodles in association with high urinary corticoid:creatinine ratios and resistance to glucocorticoid feedback. *Vet Rec* 2007;160:393–397.

Frank LA. Growth hormone-responsive alopecia in dogs. *J Am Vet Med Assoc* 2005;226:1494–1497.

Hamann F, Kooistra HS, Mol JA, Gottschalk S, Bartels T, Rijnberk A. Pituitary function and morphology in two German shepherd dogs with congenital dwarfism. *Vet Rec* 1999;144:644–646.

Kooistra HS. Growth hormone disorders: Acromegaly and pituitary dwarfism. In: Ettinger SJ, Feldman EC, eds. *Textbook of Veterinary Internal Medicine*, 7th edn. St. Louis: Elsevier Saunders, 2010, pp. 1711–1716.

Kooistra HS, Voorhout G, Mol JA, Rijnberk A. Combined pituitary hormone deficiency in German shepherd dogs with dwarfism. *Domest Anim Endocrinol* 2000;19:177–190.

Kooistra HS, Voorhout G, Selman PJ, Rijnberk A. Progestin-induced growth hormone (GH) production in the treatment of dogs with congenital GH deficiency. *Domest Anim Endocrinol* 1998;15:93–102.

Meij BP, Mol JA, Bevers MM, Rijnberk A. Residual pituitary function after transsphenoidal hypophysectomy in dogs with pituitary-dependent hyperadrenocorticism. *J Endocrinol* 1997;155:531–539.

Meij BP, Mol JA, Hazewinkel HAW, Bevers MM, Rijnberk A. Assessment of a combined anterior pituitary function test in beagle dogs: rapid sequential intravenous administration of four hypothalamic releasing hormones. *Domest Anim Endocrinol* 1996;13:161–170.

Nelson RW. Disorders of the hypothalamus and pituitary gland. In: Nelson RW, Couto CG, eds. *Small Animal Internal Medicine*, 3rd edn. St Louis: Mosby, 2003, pp. 660–680.

Rijnberk A, Kooistra HS. Hypothalamus-pituitary system. In: Rijnberk A, Kooistra HS, eds. *Clinical Endocrinology of Dogs and Cats*, 2nd edn. Hannover: Schlütersche Verlagsgesellschaft mbH & Co., 2010, pp. 13–54.

Simmons, DM, Voss JW, Ingraham HA, Holloway JM, Broide RS, Rosenfeld MG, Swanson LW. Pituitary cell phenotypes involve cell-specific Pit-1 mRNA translation and synergistic interactions with other classes of transcription factors. *Genes Dev* 1990;4:695–711.

Voorbij AMWY, Kooistra HS. Pituitary dwarfism in German shepherd dogs. *J Vet Clin Sci* 2009;2:4–11.

Voorbij AMWY, Van Steenbeek FG, Kooistra HS, Leegwater PAJ. Genetic cause of pituitary dwarfism in German shepherd dogs (Abstract). *Proceedings of the 16th ECVIM-CA Congress*, 2006, p. 176.

Zhu X, Gleiberman AS, Rosenfeld MG. Molecular physiology of pituitary development: Signaling and transcriptional networks. *Physiol Rev* 2007;87:933–963.

CHAPTER 39

Hyposomatotropism in Cats

Nicki Reed and Danièlle Gunn-Moore

Pathogenesis

- Primary deficiency of growth hormone as a result of a congenital anomaly.

Classical Signs

- Failure of growth, typically evident from 2–3 months of age.
- Small-statured animals are usually in proportion unless concurrent deficiency is also present in other pituitary hormones, primarily thyroid-stimulating hormone (TSH).

Diagnosis

- Definitive diagnosis requires evidence of lack of increase in growth hormone levels in response to stimulation with xylazine, clonidine, or human growth hormone–releasing hormone (GHRH).
- Presumptive diagnosis may be made by ruling out other causes of small stature and demonstrating low levels of insulin-like growth factor (IGF-1).

Treatment

- Specific treatment requires growth hormone replacement, which is currently unavailable.

I. Pathogenesis
A. **Primary deficiency** of growth hormone:
   1. **Congenital** either due to cystic formation of the pituitary gland, or pituitary hypoplasia. It is thought that cystic changes may develop within the pituitary secondary to abnormal development of the pituitary cells rather than necessarily being the primary defect.
   2. **Acquired** due to destruction of the pituitary gland from inflammatory, neoplastic, traumatic, or vascular disease. This etiology has not been documented in cats.
B. **Secondary deficiency** of growth hormone:
   1. Due to **lack of** GHRH from the hypothalamus. GHRH stimulates release of growth hormone from the anterior pituitary gland.

Clinical Endocrinology of Companion Animals, First Edition. Edited by Jacquie Rand.
© 2013 John Wiley & Sons, Inc. Published 2013 by John Wiley & Sons, Inc.

2. Suppression of growth hormone has been documented in humans with a number of endocrine disorders and in dogs with hyperadrenocorticism; however, this has not been documented in cats.

C. **Peripheral insensitivity** to growth hormone:

1. In these situations, production of growth hormone is adequate, with high levels due to lack of negative feedback, but production of IGF-1 is reduced, possibly due to abnormalities in the growth hormone receptor.

2. This type of abnormality has not been identified in cats.

D. Growth hormone has direct effects on fat and carbohydrate metabolism, causing lipolysis and increased glucose synthesis (see Figure 39.1).

E. Growth hormone stimulates production of IGF-1 which, in conjunction with growth hormone, promotes skeletal growth and protein synthesis (see Figure 39.1).

F. Cases with congenital hyposomatotropism may have concurrent deficiencies in other hormones produced by the anterior pituitary, the most significant of which is TSH. In cases of panhypopituitarism, deficiencies of prolactin, follicle-stimulating hormone, luteinizing hormone, and adrenocorticotrophic hormone may also be present.

II. Signalment

A. In cats, only the congenital form of the disease has been identified, with **kittens typically presenting at 3–6 months of age.**

B. Due to the paucity of reports, no conclusion can be drawn regarding breed or sex predispositions.

III. Clinical Signs

A. **Poor body growth**:

1. Initial growth for the first 1–2 months of life appears normal.

2. At 3–4 months kittens become small, relative to their litter mates.

3. Solitary deficiency of growth hormone leads to "proportionate dwarfism" where the kitten's head and limbs appear in proportion, but the overall stature is reduced.

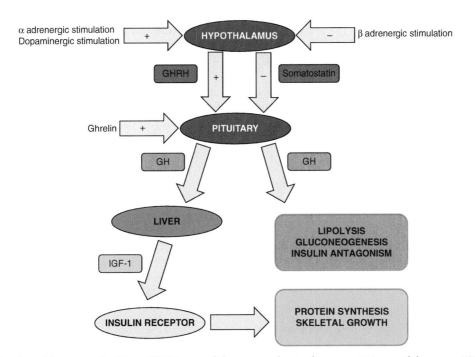

Figure 39.1 Growth hormone physiology. GHRH=growth hormone–releasing hormone, GH=growth hormone, IGF-1= insulin-like growth factor-1, +=positive feedback, −=negative feedback.

4. Concurrent deficiency of TSH will result in "disproportionate dwarfism." These kittens have flat, broad heads, thick tongues, and square limbs. In addition these kittens may appear mentally retarded and suffer from constipation.

5. Radiography of older animals may reveal delayed closure of physeal growth plates. The limb bones are of normal length in hyposomatotropism but are shortened with panhypopituitarism.

B. **Dentition may be slow to erupt,** but is usually normal.

C. **Coat changes** may be apparent:

1. The coat is often soft, due to the absence of primary guard hairs and retention of secondary hairs.

2. Alopecia may develop, as secondary hairs are easily epilated, especially at sites of wear.

D. **Corneal edema** has been reported in association with congenital hyposomatotropism in a kitten.

1. IGF-1 is thought to play a role in maintenance of corneal transparency and proliferation of corneal cells.

IV. Diagnosis

A. **Routine hematology and biochemistry** are often unremarkable. Azotemia may be present and has been attributed to lack of development of glomeruli due to growth hormone deficiency.

B. **Basal growth hormone** concentration is often inconclusive as values may be within reference range, due to the pulsatile nature of growth hormone secretion. In addition, growth hormone has historically been difficult to assay in cats. Recently, a growth hormone assay has been validated in the cat for assessment of acromegaly and this may be of use in investigation of hyposomatotropism.

C. **Growth hormone stimulation tests** assess the capability of the pituitary to secrete growth hormone. While they have been used in dogs, their use has not been reported in cats. The canine protocols are:

1. **Xylazine stimulation test:**

a. Plasma sample obtained before and 15, 30, 45, and 60 min after IV administration of 100 μg/kg xylazine.

b. Plasma GH >10 ng/mL 15–30 min after xylazine administration would be considered normal.

2. **Clonidine stimulation test:**

a. Plasma sample obtained before and 15, 30, 45, and 60 min after IV administration of 10 μg/kg clonidine.

b. Plasma GH >10 ng/mL 15–30 min after clonidine administration would be considered normal.

3. **GHRH stimulation test:**

a. Plasma sample obtained before and 10, 20, 30, 45, and 60 min after IV administration of 1 μg/kg human GHRH.

b. Plasma GH >10 ng/mL 15–30 min after GHRH administration would be considered normal.

4. Side effects from xylazine and clonidine include sedation, vomiting, bradycardia, and hypotension.

5. Side effects from GHRH appear less common, but GHRH may be difficult to source.

D. **IGF-1 assessment:**

1. Measurement of IGF-1 is often easier to perform than growth hormone assays, as it is more stable.

2. Low to undetectable values would be consistent with hyposomatotropism.

E. **Thyrotropin-releasing hormone (TRH) stimulation test:**

1. This is required to rule out concurrent hypothyroidism.

2. Total thyroxine (T_4) and free T_4 may be low in the absence of hypothyroidism due to sick euthyroid syndrome.

3. The lower limit of the TSH assay is not sufficiently sensitive to differentiate TSH deficiency from normal cats.

4. A TSH stimulation test is not appropriate, as the thyroid glands are functional in congenital hypothyroidism. A TRH stimulation test is required to demonstrate inadequate production of TSH.

V. Differential Diagnoses

A. **Small stature, but proportionate appearance:**

1. **Poor nutrition:**

a. Inadequate diet: this should be ascertained from the dietary history.

b. Parasitism: this can be identified readily by fecal analysis.

    c. Exocrine pancreatic insufficiency: a history of diarrhea is likely to be present. Confirmation requires demonstration of low feline trypsin-like immunoreactivity.

   2. Portosystemic vascular anomaly: the history may suggest other signs such as ptyalism (salivation), hyporexia, or evidence of hepatoencephalopathy. Elevated bile acids or ammonia warrants imaging studies to be performed.

   3. Congenital cardiac disease: the history may be suggestive of exercise intolerance, and clinical examination may identify a cardiac murmur, arrhythmia, or cyanosis to support further investigations.

   4. Congenital renal disease is likely to be identified following urinalysis and serum biochemistry. It should be borne in mind that young kittens cannot concentrate their urine as well as adults.

B. **Small stature with disproportionate appearance.**

   1. Endocrine:

    a. Hypothyroidism: see previous discussions and Chapter 26.

   2. Lysosomal storage disorders:

    a. Clinical signs may vary depending on the specific enzyme deficiency, but gangliosidosis, mucopolysaccharidosis, and mucolipidosis typically are associated with stunting of growth.

    b. Concurrent signs may include neurological abnormalities or hepatomegaly.

    c. Radiography may reveal epiphyseal dysplasia.

    d. Urine may be tested for heparin sulfate, chondroitin sulfate, and/or dermatan sulfate by toluidine blue spot test, which may support the diagnosis of mucopolysaccharidosis.

   3. Chondrodystrophy:

    a. This may be a spontaneous mutation or a deliberate breeding policy (e.g., Munchkin cats).

    b. Radiography will confirm joint and limb malformation.

VI. Treatment

A. Specific treatment requires therapy with **growth hormone replacement**:

   1. The use of recombinant human, bovine, or porcine growth hormone has not been reported in the cat.

   2. Use of any of these forms of growth hormone carries the risk of antibody formation, hypersensitivity reactions, or anaphylaxis.

   3. Development of diabetes mellitus could be a theoretic risk from overdose of growth hormone.

B. **Progestogens** have been used successfully in dogs:

   1. Progestogens stimulate production of growth hormone from hyperplastic ductular epithelium in the mammary gland.

   2. The use of progestogens has not been considered of merit in cats as:

    a. A previous study failed to demonstrate an increase in growth hormone following administration of megestrol acetate for 12 months.

    b. Production of growth hormone from the mammary gland has been demonstrated following progestogen administration in cats in association with fibroadenomatous hyperplasia. The complications associated with this condition do not merit the use of progestogens to stimulate growth hormone production.

VII. Prognosis

A. Due to the lack of specific therapy, prognosis remains guarded, with a shortened life expectancy.

B. The coat changes and small stature in themselves are not problematic to the animal.

C. Progressive expansion of the cystic pituitary can lead to development of neurological signs.

VIII. Prevention

A. No known prevention.

References and Further Readings

Donaldson D, Billson FM, Scase TJ, Sparkes AH, McConnell F, Mould JRB, Adams V. Congenital hyposomatotropism in a domestic shorthair cat presenting with congenital corneal oedema. *J Small Anim Pract* 2008;49:306–309.

Feldman EC, Nelson RW. Disorders of growth hormone. In: Feldman EC, Nelson RW, eds. *Canine and Feline Endocrinology and Reproduction*, 3rd edn. St. Louis, Missouri: Saunders, 2004, pp. 45–84.

Jones BR. Hypothyroidism. In: August JR, ed. *Consultations in Feline Internal Medicine 3*. Philadelphia: WB Saunders, 1997, pp. 147–150.

Knottenbelt CM, Herrtage ME. Use of proligestone in the management of three German shepherd dogs with pituitary dwarfism. *J Small Anim Pract* 2002;43:164–170.

Mol JA, van Garderen E, Rutteman GR, Rijnberk A. New insights in the molecular mechanism of progestin-induced proliferation of mammary epithelium: Induction of the local biosynthesis of growth hormone (GH) in the mammary glands of dogs, cats and humans. *J Steroid Biochem Mol Biol* 1996;57(1–2):67–71.

Niessen SJM, Khalid M, Petrie G, Church DB. Validation and application of a radioimmunoassay for ovine growth hormone in the diagnosis of acromegaly in cats. *Vet Rec* 2007;160:902–907.

Ordás J, Millán Y, Espinosa de los Monteros A, Reymundo C, Martín de las Múlas J. Immunohistochemical expression of progesterone receptors, growth hormone and insulin growth factor-I in feline fibroadenomatous change. *Res Vet Sci* 2004;76(3):227–233.

Peterson ME. Effects of megestrol acetate on glucose tolerance and growth hormone secretion in the cat. *Res Vet Sci* 1987;42(3):354–357.

CHAPTER 40

Acromegaly in Dogs

Hans S. Kooistra

Pathogenesis

- Acromegaly is a syndrome of bony and soft tissue overgrowth and insulin resistance due to excessive growth hormone (GH) secretion.
- In most cases, either endogenous progesterone secretion or exogenous progestin administration give rise to acromegaly.
- Rarely primary hypothyroidism or an adenoma of somatotrophs, that is, cells of the pituitary gland that secrete GH, cause acromegaly.

Classical Signs

- Thick skin folds, wide interdental spaces, snoring, and generalized visceromegaly resulting in abdominal enlargement.
- Polyuria and sometimes polyphagia. The polyuria is usually without glucosuria, but overt diabetes mellitus may develop.

Diagnosis

- Hyperglycemia, which in most cases is mild but in some dogs is marked and associated with diabetes mellitus.
- Elevated plasma concentrations of GH and/or insulin-like growth factor-I (IGF-I).

Treatment

- Ovariectomy in case of progesterone-induced acromegaly.
- Withdrawal of progestin administration and/or progesterone receptor blockers in case of progestin-induced acromegaly.

Clinical Endocrinology of Companion Animals, First Edition. Edited by Jacquie Rand.
© 2013 John Wiley & Sons, Inc. Published 2013 by John Wiley & Sons, Inc.

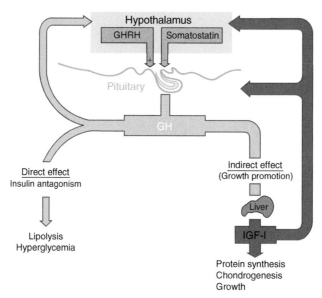

Figure 40.1 Schematic representation of the regulation of pituitary growth hormone (GH) secretion and the main effects of GH. The pituitary GH secretion is under inhibitory (somatostatin) and stimulatory (GHRH) hypothalamic control and is also modulated by negative feedback control of insulin-like growth factor-I (IGF-I) and GH itself. The direct catabolic (diabetogenic) actions of GH are shown on the left side of the figure, and the indirect anabolic actions are shown on the right.

I. Pathogenesis

A. Like the other hormones released by the pituitary gland, **GH is secreted in a pulsatile fashion.**

B. Pituitary GH secretion is regulated mainly by the opposing actions of the stimulatory hypothalamic peptide **GH-releasing hormone (GHRH)** and the inhibitory hypothalamic peptide **somatostatin.** The GH pulses predominantly reflect the pulsatile delivery of GHRH, whereas GH levels between pulses are primarily under somatostatin control (Figure 40.1).

C. **Endogenous progesterone and administration of progestins** may result in elevated plasma GH concentrations and physical changes of GH excess in dogs. **Progesterone/progestin-induced GH is produced in the mammary glands,** indicating that in dogs circulating GH not only originates from the pituitary but also may be of mammary origin.

D. The pulsatile **secretion pattern of GH changes during progression of the luteal phase of healthy bitches,** with higher basal GH secretion and less pulsatile GH secretion during stages with a high plasma progesterone concentration.

E. The effects of circulating GH can be divided into two main categories: **rapid catabolic actions and slow (long-lasting) hypertrophic actions** (Figure 40.1):

 1. The **acute catabolic actions are mainly due to insulin antagonism** and result in enhanced lipolysis, gluconeogenesis, and restricted glucose transport across the cell membrane. The net effect of these catabolic actions is **promotion of hyperglycemia.**

 2. The **slow anabolic effects are mainly mediated via IGF-I.** IGF-I is produced in many different tissues and, in most of these tissues, has a local **growth-promoting effect.** The main source of circulating IGF-I is the liver.

F. Acromegaly is a syndrome of **bony and soft tissue overgrowth** and **insulin resistance** due to excessive GH secretion.

G. As in humans and cats, GH excess can be caused by a **somatotroph adenoma of the pituitary gland,** although this is a very rare disorder in dogs. Much more often, either **endogenous progesterone (luteal phase of the estrous cycle) or exogenous progestins (e.g., used for estrus prevention)** give rise to acromegaly in dogs. Finally, **primary hypothyroidism** is associated with elevated plasma concentrations of GH and IGF-I and physical changes of acromegaly in dogs.

II. Signalment

A. **Mainly middle-aged and elderly female dogs** in the luteal phase of the estrous cycle, typically 3–5 weeks after estrus, or after treatment with progestins for estrus prevention. **Rarely in male dogs** after administration of progestins, for example, for treatment of benign prostatic hyperplasia.

B. Somatotroph adenomas are also found mainly in middle-aged and elderly dogs.

C. Primary hypothyroidism is mainly a condition of young adult to middle-aged dogs (see Chapter 25).

III. Clinical Signs

A. Signs of GH hypersecretion tend to develop slowly and are characterized initially by **soft tissue swelling** of the face and abdomen.

B. In some acromegalic dogs, severe hypertrophy of soft tissues of the mouth, tongue (Figure 40.2), and pharynx causes a **respiratory stridor** and even **dyspnea**.

C. Dogs are often presented with **polyuria** (and sometimes polyphagia). The polyuria is usually without glucosuria, but overt **diabetes mellitus** can develop due to GH-induced **insulin resistance**.

D. Physical examination may reveal thick skin folds, especially in the neck, **prognathism**, and **wide interdental spaces** (Figure 40.2). Prolonged GH excess also leads to generalized visceromegaly resulting in **abdominal enlargement**.

E. **Changes of acromegaly secondary to primary hypothyroidism tend to be much more subtle** than in other types of acromegaly, but dogs with chronically untreated primary hypothyroidism may have physical changes such as some widening of the interdental spaces along with elevated plasma GH and IGF-I concentrations.

IV. Diagnosis

A. Laboratory investigation in acromegalic dogs will often reveal **hyperglycemia** although the elevation is variable and typically below the renal threshold (approximately 216 mg/dL; 12 mmol/L). The plasma glucose concentration may range from within the reference range, to slight hyperglycemia, to severe hyperglycemia, that is, diabetes mellitus is present. Elevated serum alkaline phosphatase activity may also be noted.

B. Radiography and ultrasonography may reveal visceromegaly, but these findings are quite nonspecific.

C. Because of the variation in amino acid sequence of GH in different species, plasma GH concentrations should be determined by a **canine-specific radioimmunoassay**. Unfortunately, in many countries a commercial canine-specific GH assay is not available.

D. **The basal plasma GH concentration in acromegalic dogs often exceeds the upper limit of the reference range.** However, if the disease is mild or just beginning, the basal plasma GH concentration may still be within the reference range. Conversely, a high GH value may be the result of a secretory pulse in a normal dog. The exact sensitivity and specificity of the test remain to be determined.

E. **Nonresponsiveness of normal or elevated plasma GH levels** to stimulation (e.g., by GHRH, in an intravenous dosage of 1 µg/kg body weight) or suppression (e.g., by somatostatin, in an intravenous dosage of 10 µg/kg body weight) may further support the diagnosis. In healthy dogs, circulating GH concentrations should increase at least two- to fourfold following GHRH administration.

F. Being bound to proteins, the plasma IGF-I concentration is much less subject to fluctuation than that of GH. In addition, the amino acid sequence of IGF-I is less species-specific than that of GH and, therefore, **IGF-I can be determined in a heterologous (human) assay**.

G. Thus, **IGF-I measurements can be used as a diagnostic test for acromegaly**. However, there is some overlap in plasma IGF-I concentrations between healthy dogs and individuals with acromegaly. The exact sensitivity and specificity of the test remain to be determined.

H. A strong linear correlation exists between plasma IGF-I concentration and body size. For example, plasma IGF-I concentrations in standard poodles are about six times higher than in toy poodles. **Therefore, breed and body size have to be taken into account with the interpretation of the plasma IGF-I concentration.**

I. It is usually advisable **not to delay treatment of progesterone-induced acromegaly pending the results of GH and/or IGF-I measurements,** for the sooner treatment is started, the greater the chance of **preventing permanent diabetes mellitus.**

J. A pituitary tumor causing hypersecretion of GH can be visualized by computed tomography (CT) or magnetic resonance imaging (MRI).

(a)

(c)

(b)

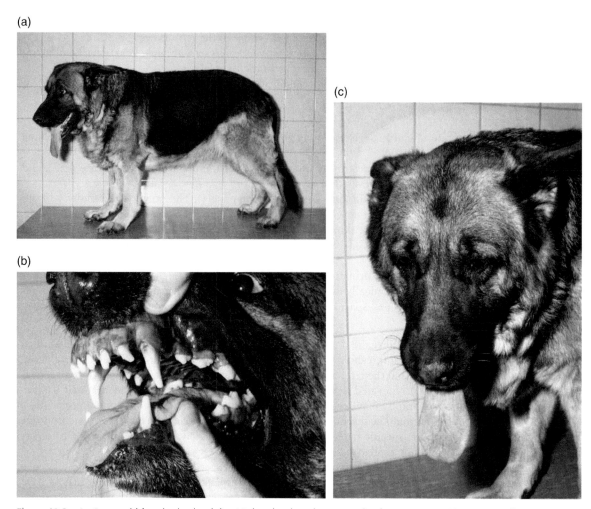

Figure 40.2   An 8-year-old female shepherd dog (a) that developed acromegaly after treatment with progestins for estrus prevention. Note the thick skin folds, especially in the neck, the hyperplasia of the gingiva, the widening of the interdental spaces (b), and the relatively large tongue (c).

V.   Differential Diagnoses

Several other conditions may also be associated with polyuria and increased appetite, such as hypercortisolism and hyperthyroidism. Polyuria during the luteal phase may also be due to pyometra, but in these cases the clinical presentation is usually quite different.

VI.   Treatment

A.   Progesterone-induced acromegaly can be treated effectively by **ovari(ohyster)ectomy**.

In cases in which the GH excess did not lead to complete exhaustion of the pancreatic β cells, elimination of the progesterone source by **ovari(ohyster)ectomy may prevent persistent diabetes mellitus**. If on the day after surgery, fasting blood glucose concentration is >252 mg/dL (>14 mmol/L), insulin therapy for diabetes mellitus should be instituted (see Chapter 15). In insulin-treated dogs, blood glucose concentrations should be closely monitored to prevent iatrogenic hypoglycemia, especially in first 1–3 weeks after surgery when insulin requirements may decrease rapidly as beta cell function recovers. Beta cell function may improve sufficiently to maintain euglycemia once glucotoxicity resolves, especially in dogs with blood glucose concentrations of <290 mg/dL (<16 mmol/L).

C. In dogs with progestin-induced GH excess, progestin administration should be discontinued immediately and for the remainder of the dog's life.

D. Administration of **progesterone receptor blockers** such as aglepristone may help to treat progestin-induced acromegaly. Administration of a weekly dosage of 10 mg/kg subcutaneously resulted in a significant decrease in plasma GH and IGF-I concentrations, but a higher dosage and higher frequency of administration may result in an even better outcome. Unfortunately, the optimal dosage has not been determined.

E. **Treatment with levothyroxine of dogs with primary hypothyroidism** results in normalization of serum concentrations of GH and IGF-I.

F. In dogs with acromegaly due to a somatotroph adenoma, treatment should be directed at the pituitary lesion. In principle, there are three options: medical treatment, radiation therapy, and hypophysectomy:

> **1.** **Medical treatment** with long-acting **somatostatin analogues**, such as octreotide and lanreotide, improves symptoms of acromegaly in most human acromegalic patients, with normalization of plasma concentrations of IGF-I and tumor shrinkage occurring in approximately 50% of cases. There is, however, no experience yet with use of these drugs in dogs with a functional somatotroph adenoma and they are expensive.
>
> **2.** **Radiation therapy** may shrink the pituitary tumor and may improve diabetic control in acromegalic dogs.
>
> **3.** **Transsphenoidal hypophysectomy** has been performed successfully in dogs with hypercortisolism due to a corticotroph adenoma and may also be an effective treatment option for animals with a somatotroph adenoma. Although, like in human medicine, it is probably the method of choice, experience in dogs is limited so far.

VII. Prognosis

A. In general, the **prognosis is good after ovari(ohyster)ectomy** in dogs with progesterone-induced acromegaly, **good after withdrawal of progestin administration** in progestin-induced acromegaly, **and excellent in dogs with primary hypothyroidism treated with levothyroxine, provided that acromegaly did not result in persistent diabetes mellitus**. In case of acromegaly due to a functional somatotroph adenoma, the prognosis depends on the successfulness of the treatment at the pituitary level.

B. **The appearance of the dog may change dramatically after treatment of acromegaly,** due to the reversal of the soft tissue changes. The size of the abdomen decreases, as does the thickening of oropharyngeal soft tissues and thus the associated snoring. The bony changes appear to be irreversible but do not appear to cause clinical problems.

C. In cases in which the GH excess did not lead to complete exhaustion of the pancreatic β cells, the elimination of the progesterone source by ovari(ohyster)ectomy or discontinuation of progestin administration may prevent persistent diabetes mellitus. After diabetes mellitus begins, the sooner insulin therapy is instituted to protect the beta cells from glucotoxicity and surgery is performed, that is, within a few weeks, the higher the chance the diabetes will resolve.

VIII. Prevention

A. No known prevention.

References and Further Readings

Bhatti SFM, Duchateau L, Okkens AC, van Ham LML, Mol JA, Kooistra HS. Treatment of growth hormone excess in dogs with the progesterone receptor antagonist aglépristone. *Theriogenology* 2006;66:797–803.

Diaz-Espineira MM, Mol JA, Rijnberk A, Kooistra HS. Adenohypophyseal function in dogs with primary hypothyroidism and non-thyroidal illness. *J Vet Intern Med* 2009;23:100–107.

Diaz-Espineira MM, Mol JA, van den Ingh TSGAM, van der Vlugt-Meijer RH, Rijnberk A, Kooistra HS. Functional and morphological changes in the adenohypophysis of dogs with induced primary hypothyroidism; loss of TSH hypersecretion, hypersomatotropism, hypoprolactinemia, and pituitary enlargement with transdifferentiation. *Domes Anim Endocrinol* 2008;35:98–111.

Fracassi F, Gandini G, Diana A, Preziosi R, van den Ingh TSGAM, Famigli-Bergamini P, Kooistra HS. Acromegaly due to a somatotroph adenoma in a dog. *Domest Anim Endocrinol* 2007;32:43–54.

Kooistra HS. Acromegaly and pituitary dwarfism. In: Ettinger SJ, Feldman EC, eds. *Textbook of Veterinary Internal Medicine*, 7th edn. St. Louis: Elsevier Saunders, 2010, pp. 1711–1716.

Meij BP, Voorhout G, van den Ingh TSGAM, Hazewinkel HAW, Teske E, Rijnberk A. Results of transsphenoidal hypophyectomy in 52 dogs with pituitary-dependent hyperadrenocorticism. *Vet Surg* 1998;27:246–261.

Rijnberk A, Kooistra HS. Hypothalamus-pituitary system. In: Rijnberk A, Kooistra HS, eds. *Clinical Endocrinology of Dogs and Cats*, 2nd edn. Hannover: Schlütersche Verlagsgesellschaft mbH & Co., 2010, pp. 13–54.

Selman PJ, Mol JA, Rutteman GR, van Garderen E, Rijnberk A. Progestin-induced growth hormone excess in the dog originates in the mammary gland. *Endocrinology* 1994;134:287–292.

CHAPTER 41

Acromegaly in Cats

David Church and Stijn J. M. Niessen

Pathogenesis

- Acromegaly occurs as a result of excessive growth hormone (GH) production.
- Most cases are presumed to be caused by a functional benign pituitary tumor.

Classical Signs

- Most cats are **>6 years of age,** with a median age of 11 years.
- Moderate to marked polyuria/polydipsia due to **uncontrolled diabetes mellitus.**
- **Initial weight loss followed by weight gain,** or weight gain and marked polyphagia.
- Although some show marked physical changes (broad facial features, abdominal [organ] enlargement, prognathia inferior, clubbed paws), **most look like any regular diabetic** cat.

Diagnosis

- **Clinical picture** in combination with **markedly elevated insulin-like growth factor-1 (IGF-1) and/or GH and a pituitary mass** (computed tomography [CT], magnetic resonance imaging [MRI]).

Treatment

- **Conservative treatment** with long-acting insulin to control hyperglycemia, or **definitive** treatment with radiotherapy or hypophysectomy, alongside treatment for acromegaly-induced complications.

I. Pathogenesis
A. **Feline acromegaly** is also called **feline hypersomatotropism.**
B. **The most common** cause of feline acromegaly is a GH-**producing adenoma in the pituitary gland** (micro- or macroadenoma) which disturbs the normally meticulously regulated GH production (Figure 41.1).
C. **Overproduction** of GH has a **range of effects** on a cat, including:
   1. **Direct anabolic and catabolic effects of GH.** Most importantly, GH is a modulator of insulin sensitivity and when present in excess can cause diabetes mellitus. This explains why the great majority of reported acromegalic cats have had concurrent insulin-resistant diabetes mellitus.

Clinical Endocrinology of Companion Animals, First Edition. Edited by Jacquie Rand.
© 2013 John Wiley & Sons, Inc. Published 2013 by John Wiley & Sons, Inc.

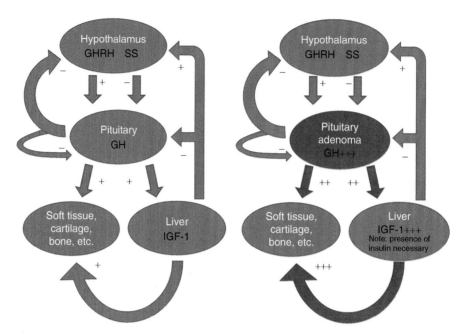

Figure 41.1 Left: Normally GH secretion is finely regulated through stimulation by growth hormone releasing hormone (GHRH) and inhibition by somatostatin (SS) both produced in the hypothalamus, as well as through negative feedback at the level of the pituitary and hypothalamus by GH itself (produced in the pituitary) and IGF-1 (produced predominantly in the liver). Right: In an acromegalic cat, a pituitary adenoma produces excessive GH, resulting in elevated production of IGF-1 if insulin is present in the portal circulation. The pituitary adenoma is not sensitive to negative feedback and the fine regulation is lost.

2. **Indirect anabolic effects of IGF-1.** The excess GH stimulates the production of IGF-1, predominantly by the liver. Insulin has a permissive role in this process—in other words hepatocytes can only produce IGF-1 in the presence of insulin. When IGF-1 is abnormally elevated for extended periods of time, patients can suffer from excessive tissue growth and deformations of internal and/or external organs.

3. **Neurological signs** due to a gradually expanding pituitary tumor (more likely with a macroadenoma). These are however uncommon as the tumors tend to be both benign and slow growing and rarely produce signs referable to an expanding intracranial lesion.

D. **Rare cases of pituitary hyperplasia** are possible.

E. **Progesterone-induced GH overproduction by the mammary gland,** as seen in the dog, has not been described as a clinical problem in the cat.

II. Signalment

A. **Prevalence** of acromegaly among diabetic cats with variable control in North America and the UK was found to be higher than expected; approximately 1:3 to 1:4 diabetic cats. The disease is therefore likely underdiagnosed in poorly controlled diabetic cats; additionally, a **high prevalence** was found **among "insulin-resistant diabetic" cats** in the Netherlands. The prevalence among all newly diagnosed diabetic cats and among nondiabetic cats is currently unknown.

B. **Factors** associated with acromegaly include being middle- to old-aged, male gender and suffering from insulin resistant diabetes mellitus:

1. In a large study of acromegalic cats, **median age was 11 years** (age range: 6–17 years).

2. Like regular diabetic cats, acromegalic cats are more often **male** than female (ratio 8:1).

3. Body condition can range **from normal to overweight** with a median body weight of 5.8 kg (range 3.5–9.2 kg) in a large cohort of acromegalic cats. Acromegalic cats are believed to be less likely to be underweight.

4. **Domestic short-haired** cats seem predominantly affected. A genetic predisposition of certain breeds has not yet been recognized.

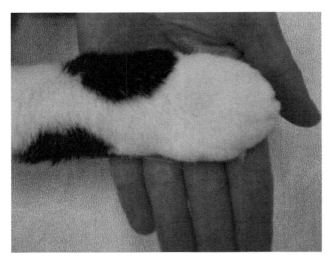

Figure 41.2 Acromegaly can cause a "clubbed" appearance of the lower extremities (previously published in *J Vet Intern Med*, Blackwell-Synergy).

5. The **insulin requirements** of 59 acromegalic diabetic cats were found to be **higher** than in non-acromegalic diabetic cats (median 7 IU q 12 h [range 1–35 IU q 12 h] compared to median 3 IU q 12 h for non-acromegalic diabetic cats).

III. Clinical Signs

A. The earliest witnessed signs tend to be those of unregulated diabetes mellitus: **polyuria and polydipsia**, as well as nocturia and urinary incontinence.

B. **Polyphagia** is often reported and although this also represents a clinical sign commonly associated with uncomplicated primary diabetes mellitus, the excess in GH is likely to play an important role in this phenomenon. This is substantiated by the frequent observation of persistent, and often extreme, polyphagia, despite apparent reasonable control of the diabetes mellitus in acromegalic cats treated with insulin only.

C. **Weight gain** can be seen, but is not always present. However, if present **in an uncontrolled diabetic cat** this should **prompt assessment for acromegaly**.

D. **Changes in physical appearance** may be present but are not always noted by the owner because of their gradual onset. These changes may include:
  1. Weight gain.
  2. Increase in paw size (Figure 41.2).
  3. Broad facial features (Figure 41.3).
  4. Protrusion of the lower jaw (prognathia inferior) (Figure 41.4).
  5. Increased inter-dental space.
  6. Abdominal enlargement.
  7. Large tongue.

E. **Lameness** might occur due to GH- and IGF-1-induced degenerative arthropathy.

F. **Respiratory stridor or "snoring"** has been reported in > 50% of cases and is thought to be due to a GH/IGF-1-induced increase in soft tissue in the oropharyngeal region.

G. **Rear limb weakness or plantigrade posture** (diabetic neuropathy) might be present secondary to uncontrolled diabetes mellitus.

H. Reported possible **central nervous system signs** include lethargy, impaired vision, vocalizing, seizures, vestibular signs, and Horner's syndrome (these though tend to be uncommon in view of the benign and slow growing nature of pituitary tumor).

I. Physical examination can reveal **abdominal organomegaly** (particularly liver and kidneys).

J. Auscultation may reveal a **systolic cardiac murmur** or **gallop rhythm** (reportedly in 24% of cases), hypothesized to be secondary to GH/IGF-1-induced myocardial changes, or respiratory changes due to

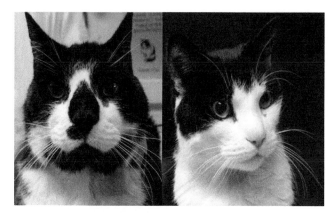

Figure 41.3   The external appearance of an acromegalic cat can vary from classic, including obvious broadening of facial features (left), to undistinguishable from any other diabetic cat (right).

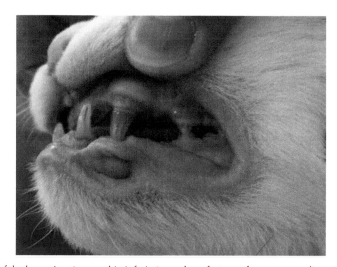

Figure 41.4   Protrusion of the lower jaw (prognathia inferior) may be a feature of an acromegalic cat.

congestive heart failure or referred upper respiratory stridor. However, whether cardiovascular complications are genuinely more common in acromegalic cats compared to age matched controls seems debatable.

K. **Tachypnea or dyspnea** might be witnessed as a consequence of acromegalic-induced congestive heart failure or enlargement of oropharyngeal soft tissue. The latter should produce upper respiratory tract signs while the former produces signs referable to intrathoracic disease.

L. **Poor and unkempt hair coat** may be seen.

M. **Hypertension** has previously been suggested to be prevalent among acromegalic cats and cats can therefore present with hypertension-associated clinical signs, including acute blindness due to ocular hemorrhage. However, in the largest case series of acromegalics reported to date, hypertension was **NOT** more prevalent than would be expected in a group of age-matched control cats. In the authors' opinion, an increased prevalence in acromegalic cats seems unlikely.

N. An acromegalic cat can also present with **diabetic ketoacidosis** due to suboptimal diabetic control or secondary complicating disease.

O. Because the severity of insulin resistance can vary day to day, clinical signs of **hypoglycemia** can occur secondary to exogenous insulin-induced **hypoglycemia** at times of lower insulin resistance. The latter might present as a dazed drunken look, dilated pupils, wobbliness, weakness, head or body tremors, twitching, seizures, or coma.

P. It is important to note that not all of these signs will be consistently present in all cats, especially early in the disease process. Acromegalic cats can be **morphologically indistinguishable from non-acromegalic diabetic cats** at the time of diagnosis, which could account for the possibility of current underdiagnosis of this endocrinopathy (Figure 41.3).

IV. Diagnosis

A. Acromegaly should be considered in **any diabetic cat with insulin resistance**.

B. Unfortunately, no single diagnostic test that is 100% sensitive and specific for acromegaly exists.

C. **It is necessary to combine clinical signs and results of several diagnostic tests to attain a diagnosis with a reasonable level of confidence.**

D. **Circumstantial evidence** might be gathered through:

1. **Routine serum biochemistry:** elevated total protein levels and hematocrit may be evident, in addition to diabetes-associated changes. Anecdotally hyperphosphatemia can also be seen. Nevertheless, in the only study comparing routine clinical pathology in acromegalic versus non-acromegalic diabetic cats, hyperproteinemia was the only genuinely overrepresented parameter among acromegalic cats.

2. **Imaging of the thorax or abdomen:** increased size of liver, kidneys and/or adrenals and pancreatic changes may be seen. An increased size of the cardiac silhouette and signs of congestive heart failure have been reported, although they are not necessarily more prevalent in acromegalic cats than in age-matched controls.

3. **Other radiographic abnormalities** encountered in feline acromegalics can include: increased oropharyngeal soft tissue; degenerative arthropathy with periarticular periosteal activation, osteophytes, soft tissue swelling, and joint space collapse; spinal spondylosis deformans; mandibular enlargement; and hyperostosis of the calvarium.

4. **Echocardiography** might reveal changes similar to those found in hypertrophic cardiomyopathy or might be unremarkable.

E. **Direct evidence** might be provided by:

1. Measuring **serum IGF-1**: a single measurement has proven to be an important and practical screening tool. However, false positive and false negative results have been reported. Therefore:

   a. Documenting an elevated IGF-1 concentration does not constitute a final diagnosis, but merely indicates further testing is indicated.

   b. Documenting a low IGF-1 makes acromegaly less likely, yet does not completely exclude it. Portal insulin is necessary for the production of IGF-1. Therefore, newly diagnosed diabetic cats with acromegaly (that are not yet receiving exogenous insulin) might have lower IGF-1-levels, which will rise into the acromegalic range after initiation of exogenous insulin therapy.

1. **Feline GH** measurement has proven equally useful. Reasonable specificity (95%) and sensitivity (84%) were reported using a particular assay and one particular cutoff concentration. However, in view of the pulsatile secretion of GH in non-acromegalic and acromegalic cats, false positives can be recorded, as well as false negatives.

2. **Combining IGF-1 and GH** determination will significantly increase diagnostic accuracy.

3. Once IGF-1 and/or GH elevation has been established and are suggestive of acromegaly, **intracranial imaging** is indicated. **Contrast-enhanced computed tomography (CT)** and **magnetic resonance imaging (MRI)** are useful to visualize a pituitary abnormality, and, if present, this provides a satisfactory level of confidence in the diagnosis (Figure 41.6).

V. Differential Diagnoses

A. Other common causes of true or apparent insulin-resistant diabetes mellitus need to be excluded, including:

1. **Management associated causes:**

   a. Incorrect insulin administration.

   b. Incorrect insulin storage.

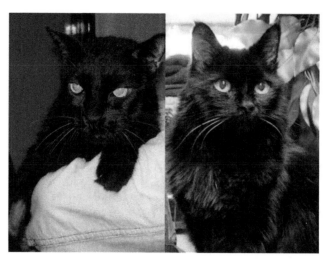

Figure 41.5   Careful observation of the clinical features of these two insulin-resistant diabetic cats suggests acromegaly to be more likely in the cat on the left (broad facial features) and hyperadrenocorticism in the cat on the right (fur color changes; see Chapter 7 for hyperadrenocorticism in the cat). Both diagnoses were subsequently confirmed on the basis of IGF-1, CT, and LDDST, as well as a favorable response to trilostane treatment (latter in right cat only).

      c. Use of inactive insulin preparations.
      d. Underdosing.
      e. Somogyi overswing (hypoglycemia induced hyperglycemia).
      f. Short duration of insulin action.
  2. **Infectious disease** (e.g., urinary tract infection, dental disease).
  3. **Inflammatory disease** (e.g., pancreatitis, inflammatory bowel disease, gingivostomatitis).
  4. **Concurrent endocrinopathies:**
      a. Hyperthyroidism.
      b. Hyperadrenocorticism.
      c. Iatrogenic hormone administration (corticosteroids, megestrol acetate).
  5. **Any other disease** (including obesity, neoplasia, nephropathy, and cardiovascular disease).
  6. **Stress hyperglycemia** mimicking true insulin resistance.

B. **Differentiation of acromegaly from pituitary-dependent hyperadrenocorticism (Chapter 7) is particularly important, since this disease can also cause true insulin-resistant diabetes mellitus, weight gain despite uncontrolled diabetes mellitus and it is potentially associated with adrenomegaly and a pituitary tumor on CT or MRI.** In addition, urine cortisol:creatinine ratios can also be elevated in acromegalic cats. Successful differentiation can often be achieved through:
  1. Careful assessment for specific clinical features which differ between the two diseases:
      a. Acromegaly: broad facial features, clubbed paws, arthropathy, prognathia inferior, particularly severe insulin resistance.
      b. Hyperadrenocorticism: frail skin, fur changes, bruising, less severe insulin resistance (Figure 41.5).
  2. GH and/or IGF-1 determination.
  3. Adrenocorticotropic hormone (ACTH) stimulation test and/or low-dose dexamethasone suppression test (LDDST).

VI. Treatment

A. **The primary goal of therapy** is to achieve a good quality of life through combating the primary disease process and/or secondary complications, and ideally both.

B. Unfortunately, **the ideal treatment protocol to achieve this has yet to be established.**

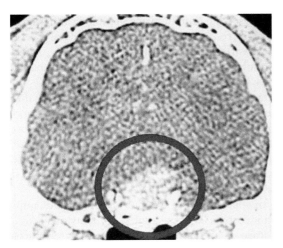 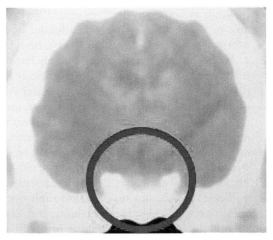

Figure 41.6   CT image of an acromegalic cat with a macroadenoma (indicated with red circle). Radiotherapy has the potential to reduce the size of the pituitary mass, but the effect can be unpredictable both in timing and in nature. Left: at time of diagnosis; right: 6 months after radiotherapy.

C. A conservative or definitive approach can be chosen, alongside addressing acromegaly-associated complications.

D. **Conservative approach**: this involves primarily **treating the diabetes mellitus with insulin**. However, obtaining glycemic control is often difficult, requiring high doses of insulin. Nevertheless, such high-dose insulin treatment can prove acceptable in individual patients and certainly could be attempted if more definitive treatment options are not available:

1. Finding the appropriate dose is an empirical process; dosage increases are implemented until satisfactory clinical improvement is achieved with resolution of clinical signs referable to uncontrolled diabetes, and blood glucose concentrations and/or glycated proteins also improved.

2. **Home monitoring of blood glucose concentrations** and appropriate adjustment of insulin dose according to blood glucose concentrations is particularly useful because of fluctuating insulin resistance. This can assist in reducing clinical hypoglycemic episodes associated with inappropriately high insulin dose relative to the level of hyperglycemia present at the time of the due insulin dose.

3. It is important to remember that some of the clinical signs that might be attributable to poor diabetic control (in particular, the ravenous polyphagia often seen in acromegaly) will not necessarily be reduced with improved diabetic control; thus in a proportion of acromegalics, resolution of polyphagia cannot be used as an indicator of improved diabetic control. In these cats, blood glucose concentrations (especially if measured at home), water drunk, and glycated protein measurements can provide a better indication of diabetic control than improvement in signs of polyphagia.

4. Sometimes, more intense insulin therapy is required to bring the diabetes under control. This could include a period of continuous intravenous insulin infusion or the use of more intense subcutaneous insulin regimes including using combinations of long-acting insulin twice daily and short-acting insulin given two to four times daily with a meal.

E. **Definitive**—this primarily involves trying to decrease the hypersecretion of GH by the pituitary:

1. **Radiotherapy** remains the only currently widely available means of correcting the underlying cause of acromegaly, that is, reducing or stopping autonomous overproduction of GH from the anterior pituitary. The principal aim of radiotherapy is to reduce GH production to levels that are no longer clinically significant, and the secondary goal is to reduce tumor size (Figure 41.6):

a. Unfortunately, radiotherapy is more suited to reducing the size of the tumor than achieving a dramatic reduction in autonomous GH and IGF-1 production.

b. While radiotherapy has been generally effective in resolving or minimizing neurological signs referable to an expanding intracranial lesion, its efficacy in resolving the clinical signs referable to the overproduction of GH and IGF-1 have been far more variable and difficult to predict.

c. While the insulin resistant diabetes mellitus has resolved or become more controllable in some cats, it has remained unchanged in others, despite broadly similar radiotherapy protocols.

d. However, a recent report offers greater encouragement with 13 of 14 insulin-resistant diabetic acromegalic cats responding favorably to the administration of an average total radiation dose of 3700 cGY administered as an incremental, hypofractionated dosage protocol of 10 doses.

e. What is also clear is that serum IGF-1 concentration is not a suitable measure by which remission from the general features of acromegaly or the insulin-resistant diabetes mellitus may be assessed, because concentration does not change substantially during or after radiotherapy regardless of the changes in diabetic control, insulin requirement or GH concentration.

f. While radiotherapy may be a plausible option for some, the need for multiple anesthetics, unpredictable response, limited availability, and significant costs make it unsuitable for many owners.

g. Additionally, as acromegaly is primarily a disease of autonomous endocrine activity it seems counterintuitive to hope a therapeutic modality aimed principally at cell destruction is likely to be the optimum management option. Consequently, efforts to develop alternative treatment methods that are more suited to directly dealing with the hormonal disturbances are an area of active research.

2. **Hypophysectomy/cryohypophysectomy**: hypophysectomy is the treatment of choice for human patients with acromegaly and can result in fast and complete normalization of GH levels:

a. Both experience with and access to transsphenoidal hypophysectomy in acromegalic cats is currently limited.

b. Cryohypophysectomy also requires further evaluation and longer term follow-up before it can be recommended at this stage.

F. **Medical treatment** has so far proven ineffective. The dopamine agonists and somatostatin analogues that have been tested to date have not resulted in detectable clinical improvement:

1. Pegvisomant, a GH-receptor antagonist, effective in most human acromegalics, remains to be tested in cats.

G. **Addressing acromegaly-associated complications and comorbidities:**

1. Analgesia should be provided to palliate **arthropathies**.

2. Any other disease, genuinely or coincidentally associated with the acromegalic state or merely age related, should be assessed and treated appropriately to ensure a good overall health status:

a. For example, if congestive heart failure is present, angiotensin-converting enzyme (ACE) inhibitor, diuretic treatment, and regular veterinary assessments are required. When using these drugs, special attention should be paid to possible electrolyte abnormalities, which can occur more easily in these patients with diabetes-induced osmotic diuresis.

b. Similarly, renal disease or hypertension, whether a specific consequence of acromegaly or merely a comorbidity, will require specific treatment and monitoring (e.g., renal diet, ACE-inhibitors, phosphate binders, calcitriol, etc., in addition to regular assessment of serum biochemistry and urinalysis; amlodipine, regular blood pressure, and retinal evaluation).

H. **Hypoglycemia** represents a genuine danger in acromegalic cats:

1. **Any cat on high-dose insulin therapy is vulnerable to severe clinical hypoglycemia, which can prove fatal if not swiftly and appropriately treated.**

2. Home monitoring of blood glucose and good communication between the attending clinician and owner will be crucial for prevention and early detection of hypoglycemia (see Chapter 16).

3. Cats that have undergone radiotherapy are especially vulnerable to iatrogenic hypoglycemia if a decrease in insulin resistance associated with the onset of treatment effect remains undetected and blood glucose is not measured before each insulin injection.

4. For owners not capable or willing to perform home blood glucose monitoring weekly urine **glucose monitoring** could provide a less optimal yet alternative safety aid for **detecting diabetic remission or improvements** post-radiotherapy:

a. Cats with negative urine glucose should be evaluated immediately. Such evaluation is also indicated when polyuria and polydipsia decline dramatically or resolve.

5. Some authors recommend never giving >2 IU/kg/cat/ dose if the owner is not able to monitor the cat closely for signs of possible hypoglycemia and/or are unable to home monitor blood glucose concentrations. Although conservative dosing helps to avoid life-threatening hypoglycemia, poor diabetic control will substantially impact on the cat's quality of life.

VII. Prognosis

A. Reported survival times of both aggressively and conservatively managed acromegalic cats vary enormously, with some cats surviving for only a few months and others living for many years and dying from causes unlikely to be related to acromegaly.

B. A direct comparison between survival times of both aggressively and conservatively treated cats has never been made.

C. Successful treatment with insulin, while addressing acromegaly-associated complications and/or coincidental comorbidities, can still achieve an acceptable quality of life in a proportion of cats. **Prevention of severe clinical iatrogenic hypoglycemia is essential in achieving a successful outcome.**

D. **A critical assessment of quality of life** should regularly be performed with the owner, regardless of the chosen treatment option. Recently developed standardized and validated quality of life measurement tools for diabetic cats can prove essential in such objective assessment and may stimulate and guide a productive discussion between clinician and owner. This would also ensure that the impact of the cat's acromegaly on the owner's life does not remain unaddressed.

VIII. Prevention

A. There is currently no method to prevent acromegaly.

B. Early detection can prevent unnecessary suffering and the additional costs associated with attempting to achieve good glycemic control of the diabetic cats.

C. Early detection will also allow for an early proactive approach to the possible secondary effects of acromegaly, especially if a definitive treatment option is chosen. However, successful diabetic remission following radiotherapy does not necessarily coincide with remission of other GH- and IGF-1-induced clinical signs.

References and Further Readings

Berg RI, Nelson RW, Feldman EC, Kass PH, Pollard R, Refsal KR. Serum insulin-like growth factor-I concentration in cats with diabetes mellitus and acromegaly. *J Vet Intern Med* 2007;21:892.

Brearley MJ, Polton GA, Littler RM, Niessen SJ. Coarse fractionated radiation therapy for pituitary tumors in cats: a retrospective study of 12 cases. *Vet Comp Oncol* 2006;4:209.

Dunning MD, Lowrie CS, Bexfield NH, Dobson JM, Herrtage ME. Exogenous insulin treatment after hypofractionated radiotherapy in cats with diabetes mellitus and acromegaly. *J Vet Intern Med* 2009;23:243.

Feldman EC, Nelson RW. Disorders of growth hormone. In: Feldman EC, Nelson RW, eds. *Canine and Feline Endocrinology and Reproduction*, 3rd ed. St. Louis: Saunders, 2004, p. 69.

Littler RM, Polton GA, Brearley MJ. Resolution of diabetes mellitus but not acromegaly in a cat with a pituitary macroadenoma treated with hypofractionated radiation. *J Small Anim Pract* 2006;47:392.

Mayer MN, Greco DS, LaRue SM. Outcomes of pituitary tumor irradiation in cats. *J Vet Intern Med* 2006;20:1151.

Niessen SJ. Feline acromegaly: An essential differential diagnosis for the difficult diabetic. *J Feline Med Surg* 2010;12:15–23.

Niessen SJ, Khalid M, Petrie G, Church DB. Validation and application of an ovine radioimmunoassay for the diagnosis of feline acromegaly. *Vet Rec* 2007;160:902–907.

Niessen SJ, Petrie G, Gaudiano F, Khalid M, Church DB. *Routine clinical pathology findings in feline acromegaly. Proceedings of the BSAVA Congress*, Birmingham, UK. 2007, p. 482.

Niessen SJ, Petrie G, Gaudiano F, Khalid M, Smyth JB, Mahoney P, Church DB. Feline acromegaly: An underdiagnosed endocrinopathy? *J Vet Intern Med* 2007;21:899.

Niessen SJ, Powney S, Guitian J, Niessen AP, Pion PD, Shaw JA, Church DB. Evaluation of a quality-of-life tool for cats with diabetes mellitus. *J Vet Intern Med* 2010 Sep-Oct;24(5):1098–1105.

Norman EJ, Mooney CT. Diagnosis and management of diabetes mellitus in five cats with somatotrophic abnormalities. *J Feline Med Surg* 2000;2:183.

Peterson ME, Taylor RS, Greco DS, et al: Acromegaly in 14 cats. *J Vet Intern Med* 1990;4:192.

Slingerland LI, Voorhout G, Rijnberk A, Kooistra HS. Growth hormone excess and the effect of octreotide in cats with diabetes mellitus. *Domest Anim Endocrinol* 2008;35(4):352–361.

CHAPTER 42

Diabetes Insipidus and Polyuria/ Polydipsia in Dogs

Katharine F. Lunn and Katherine M. James

Pathogenesis

- Central diabetes insipidus is due to a lesion in the neurohypophysis (posterior pituitary).
- Nephrogenic diabetes insipidus is due to renal inability to respond to antidiuretic hormone (ADH).
- Nephrogenic diabetes insipidus may be primary (congenital) or secondary (due to one of a large number of diseases that prevent or diminish the renal response to ADH).

Classical Signs

- Polyuria-polydipsia (PUPD).
- Other central nervous system signs are possible with central diabetes insipidus, depending on the underlying cause.
- The myriad disease syndromes that result in nephrogenic diabetes insipidus often have other primary clinical signs, for example, hyperadrenocorticism or renal failure.
- Patients may develop inappropriate urination associated with a high urine volume if they are unable to get outside to void often enough.
- Patients already predisposed may become acutely clinical for incontinence.

Diagnosis

- Investigation of causes of PUPD.
- Central diabetes insipidus is suspected after ruling out nephrogenic diabetes insipidus and primary polydipsia.
- Water deprivation test (WDT) should rarely be necessary.
- Response to synthetic ADH can be used to support a diagnosis of central diabetes insipidus.

Treatment

- Constant access to water is essential in all cases of PUPD except primary polydipsia.

Clinical Endocrinology of Companion Animals, First Edition. Edited by Jacquie Rand.
© 2013 John Wiley & Sons, Inc. Published 2013 by John Wiley & Sons, Inc.

- Synthetic ADH analogues can be used to manage central diabetes insipidus.
- Secondary nephrogenic diabetes insipidus is managed by addressing the primary cause.
- Thiazide diuretics may be used to manage primary nephrogenic diabetes insipidus.
- Nonspecific therapies to reduce urine volume such as reducing solute (e.g., sodium) intake rarely have a significant effect on PUPD.

I. Pathogenesis

A. Normal cellular function requires tight regulation of **plasma osmolality**, which is achieved through regulation of **water balance:**

1. **Normal water balance** depends on an intact thirst mechanism, osmoreceptors in the brain, appropriate release of antidiuretic hormone (vasopressin or ADH) from the posterior pituitary, and renal ability to respond to ADH.

2. In the kidneys, ADH binds to V_2 receptors in the collecting ducts, initiating the insertion of water channels (aquaporin-2) into the apical membranes of the renal tubular epithelial cells.

3. In the presence of a **hypertonic renal medullary interstitium,** water moves by osmosis from the renal collecting ducts into the interstitium.

4. The release of ADH, and thus concentration of urine, will occur in response to an increase in plasma osmolality.

5. Conversely, when plasma osmolality is low, ADH secretion is suppressed and dilute urine is produced.

B. **Polyuria and polydipsia** are the classic signs of **diabetes insipidus:**

1. However, it is important to understand that there are many causes of polyuria/polydipsia and that the term diabetes insipidus can be broadly applied to encompass most of them.

2. In evaluating a patient with polyuria/polydipsia, **it is useful to classify the causes of PUPD as central diabetes insipidus, primary nephrogenic diabetes insipidus, secondary nephrogenic diabetes insipidus, and primary polydipsia.**

3. Primary polydipsia is less common; most patients with PUPD have a primary polyuria.

4. Some patients with polyuria/polydipsia have both a primary polyuria and a primary polydipsia concurrently.

5. Although the distinction between primary polyuria and primary polydipsia may be useful when considering the mechanisms of PUPD, it should be noted that **polyuria and polydipsia almost always occur together,** even when clients may report otherwise. Excess water losses from the gastrointestinal (GI) tract or respiratory tract leading to an appropriate polydipsia without polyuria are detected with a complete history.

C. **Central diabetes insipidus (also termed neurogenic diabetes insipidus)** is an **uncommon or rare** condition, due to a **deficiency of ADH** and may be **total or partial:**

1. **Dogs with complete central diabetes insipidus are unable to concentrate their urine in response to water deprivation;** their urine is persistently hyposthenuric, even in the face of a significant water deficit.

2. **Dogs with partial central diabetes insipidus retain the ability to partially concentrate their urine in response to water deprivation;** the urine may become isosthenuric or slightly more concentrated in response to water deprivation.

3. Dogs with central diabetes insipidus are **capable of responding to exogenous administration of ADH analogues.**

4. Damage to the neurohypophysis causes **central diabetes insipidus.** It may occur at the level of the hypothalamic nuclei (supraoptic and paraventricular) or at the level of the axons that transport ADH to the posterior pituitary. It may result from trauma, surgery, congenital malformations, or primary or metastatic neoplasia.

5. **Many cases** of canine **central diabetes insipidus** appear to be **idiopathic,** with no cause identified on brain imaging or necropsy.

D. **Primary nephrogenic diabetes insipidus** is **rare** in dogs:

1. Primary nephrogenic diabetes insipidus results from a **congenital inability of the renal tubules to respond to ADH.**

2. It could potentially arise from abnormalities in the V_2 receptors, postreceptor signaling mechanisms, or the aquaporin-2 water channels.

E. **Secondary nephrogenic diabetes insipidus accounts for the majority of cases of canine polyuria/polydipsia:**

1. In secondary nephrogenic diabetes insipidus, another disease process interferes with the renal tubular response to ADH, possibly by affecting the binding of ADH to its receptors or disrupting postreceptor mechanisms.

2. Because the movement of water from the renal tubules to the medullary interstitium occurs by osmosis, any decrease in the osmotic gradient will affect the ability of the kidneys to concentrate urine in response to ADH.

3. Thus, renal medullary solute washout and osmotic causes of PUPD also fall within the category of secondary nephrogenic diabetes insipidus.

4. Table 42.1 lists the causes of polyuria/polydipsia in dogs and the suspected mechanism of each. To facilitate diagnostic investigation, the causes of secondary nephrogenic diabetes insipidus are ordered by estimated relative frequency.

II. Signalment

A. The signalment for **central diabetes insipidus depends on the underlying cause:**

1. There is **no particular breed or gender predisposition.**

2. Trauma can occur at any age.

3. Congenital malformations would be expected to manifest in young dogs, and neoplasia is more likely in older animals.

B. **Primary nephrogenic diabetes insipidus** would be expected to occur in **puppies and young dogs:**

1. There are **rare reports** in a variety of breeds.

2. Sex predilection would depend on the mode of inheritance. For example, an X-linked disorder has been described in huskies, in which the V_2 receptors show a low affinity for ADH binding.

C. The signalment for secondary nephrogenic diabetes insipidus **is determined by the underlying cause.** For example, hyperadrenocorticism is typically diagnosed in dogs older than 9 years of age, and there are reported breed predilections for this disorder.

III. Clinical Signs

A. The **cardinal clinical sign of** central diabetes insipidus is polyuria/polydipsia **with hyposthenuria:**

1. In complete central diabetes insipidus, the polyuria/polydipsia is **profound and continuous.** Affected dogs may drink to the exclusion of other activities, and severely affected patients may lose weight as the thirst drive overrides an appetite for food.

2. **Dogs with partial central diabetes insipidus are also polyuric/polydipsic, but less markedly so.**

3. Dogs with central diabetes insipidus will **quickly develop hyperosmolar dehydration** if they do not have constant access to water. They then may even try to drink unexpected liquids, such as their own urine.

B. **Primary nephrogenic diabetes insipidus** also causes **significant** polyuria/polydipsia **and hyposthenuria.** Puppies with renal dysplasia causing primary nephrogenic diabetes insipidus may also have signs of uremia.

C. The **polyuria/polydipsia in secondary nephrogenic diabetes insipidus may vary** from mild to severe:

1. Degree depends on the underlying cause.

2. Patients with secondary nephrogenic diabetes insipidus may have additional signs consistent with the underlying disease. Examples include polyphagia and skin and coat changes in hyperadrenocorticism, mental dullness with liver failure, or weight loss and vomiting with renal failure.

3. However, it is important to recognize that **PUPD can be the first or only apparent clinical sign in some disorders that cause** secondary nephrogenic diabetes insipidus. For example, hypercalcemia of malignancy may cause polyuria/polydipsia before the onset of specific clinical signs of neoplasia, pyelonephritis may cause polyuria/polydipsia in the absence of fever or renal pain, and leptospirosis may present with polyuria/polydipsia as its only sign.

Table 42.1 Causes of polyuria-polydipsia in dogs.

Classification	Disease or disorder	Mechanism(s) of PUPD	Relative frequency as a cause of PUPD	Method of diagnosis
Primary polydipsia	Primary (psychogenic) polydipsia	Abnormal thirst	Uncommon	Exclusion of other causes Entertainment test (see Chapter 44) Rarely WDT
Primary polyuria: CDI	Central diabetes insipidus	Absence or deficiency of ADH	Rare	Exclusion of other causes; Response to DDAVP *Rarely* WDT
Primary polyuria: 1° NDI	Primary (congenital) nephrogenic diabetes insipidus	Renal tubular insensitivity to ADH	Very rare	Exclusion of other causes WDT or lack of response to DDAVP
Primary polyuria: 2° NDI	Chronic renal failure	Osmotic diuresis	Very common	Serum chemistry Urinalysis ±Measurement of GFR
	Diabetes mellitus	Osmotic diuresis	Very common	Serum chemistry Urinalysis Serum fructosamine
	Hyperadrenocorticism	Renal tubular insensitivity to ADH (Partial CDI);* (Psychogenic)	Common	ACTH stimulation test Low-dose dexamethasone suppression test
	Pyelonephritis	Renal tubular insensitivity to ADH Loss of medullary hypertonicity	Common	Urinalysis Urine culture Abdominal ultrasonography Pyelocentesis Contrast radiography
	Polyuric acute renal failure	Osmotic diuresis	Common	Serum chemistry Urinalysis
	Postobstructive diuresis	Osmotic diuresis Downregulation of aquaporin-2	Common	History and PE Serum chemistry
	Hypercalcemia	Renal tubular insensitivity to ADH	Common	Serum calcium (total and ionized)
	Leptospirosis	Renal tubular insensitivity to ADH?	Regionally common	Serology PCR
	Hypoadrenocorticism	Decreased medullary hypertonicity Reduced sodium and water absorption in renal tubules	Uncommon	ACTH stimulation test
	Renal medullary solute washout	Decreased medullary hypertonicity	Uncommon	History Identify underlying cause
	Liver failure	Decreased medullary hypertonicity (Psychogenic)	Uncommon	Serum chemistry Bile acids
	Pyometra	Renal tubular insensitivity to ADH	Uncommon	History and PE Abdominal imaging

(Continued)

Table 42.1 (cont'd)

Classification	Disease or disorder	Mechanism(s) of PUPD	Relative frequency as a cause of PUPD	Method of diagnosis
	Portosystemic shunt	Decreased medullary hypertonicity (Psychogenic) (Increased GFR)	Uncommon	Bile acids Abdominal ultrasonography Computed tomography Transcolonic portal scintigraphy
	Intestinal leiomyosarcoma	Renal tubular insensitivity to ADH	Rare	Abdominal imaging Exploratory surgery
	Chronic partial ureteral obstruction	Downregulation of aquaporin-2	Rare	Abdominal imaging
	Primary renal glycosuria, Fanconi syndrome, and other tubulopathies	Osmotic diuresis	Rare	Urinalysis Urine electrolyte and amino acid analysis
	Hyperthyroidism	Decreased medullary hypertonicity (Psychogenic)	Rare	Serum T4 ± free T4 Thyroid scintigraphy
	Hyponatremia	Decreased medullary hypertonicity	Rare	Serum chemistry
	Pheochromocytoma	Action of catecholamines	Rare	History and PE Abdominal imaging
	Polycythemia	Action of ANP (CDI)	Very rare	CBC
	Hypokalemia	Decreased medullary hypertonicity Downregulation of aquaporin-2	Very rare	Serum chemistry
	Acromegaly	Renal tubular insensitivity to ADH (Partial CDI)	Very rare	History and PE GH or IGF-I levels
	Primary hyperaldosteronism	Renal tubular insensitivity to ADH (CDI)	Very rare	Electrolytes Renin activity Aldosterone levels
Miscellaneous	Diet or drug therapy, e.g., low-protein diet, high salt intake (diet, treats, road salt), anticonvulsants, glucocorticoids, diuretics	Various	Common	History
	Splenomegaly	Unknown	Rare	Abdominal imaging
	Gastrointestinal disease	Unknown	Rare	History and PE Abdominal imaging Endoscopy Exploratory surgery

Classification of the causes of PUPD in dogs, with associated mechanism(s) and methods of diagnosis. Within the category of secondary nephrogenic diabetes insipidus, the causes are ordered by estimated relative frequency.

*Items in parentheses are additional proposed mechanisms for PUPD.

PUPD=polyuria-polydipsia; WDT=water deprivation test; CDI=central diabetes insipidus; ADH=antidiuretic hormone (vasopressin); DDAVP=1-desamino-8-D-arginine vasopressin (desmopressin); 1° NDI=primary nephrogenic diabetes insipidus; 2° NDI=secondary nephrogenic diabetes insipidus; GFR=glomerular filtration rate; ACTH=adrenocorticotropic hormone; PE=physical examination; PCR=polymerase chain reaction; T4=thyroxine; fT4=free thyroxine; ANP=atrial natriuretic peptide; CBC=complete blood count; GH=growth hormone; IGF-I=insulin-like growth factor I; TSH=thyroid-stimulating hormone.

IV. Diagnosis

A. The **hallmark** of diabetes insipidus (whether central or nephrogenic) is polyuria/polydipsia:

1. The diagnosis of polyuria/polydipsia is achieved when the client observes increased urine output or water intake, or both, and/or the clinician consistently detects an inappropriately low urine specific gravity (USG).

2. It is rarely necessary, often difficult, and typically not diagnostically informative to measure urine output or water intake in canine patients in order to confirm that the patient is polyuric/polydipsic. Owner observations in conjunction with measurement of urine specific gravity are usually sufficient to confirm the problem.

3. **Repeated measurement of urine specific gravity can also help** to define whether the patient is truly polyuric/polydipsic. First morning urine specific gravity measurements when the urine is expected to be at its most concentrated are important and may assist in diagnosis of primary polydipsias that only manifest when associated with daytime drinking behaviors.

4. Water should not be deliberately withheld from dogs with polyuria/polydipsia unless primary polydipsia has been confirmed.

B. **When considering urine specific gravity, it is important to consider what is appropriate rather than what is normal:**

1. A low urine specific gravity is expected in patients receiving medical therapy with certain drugs, for example, diuretics or glucocorticoids, and is an expected normal physiological response in a dog that drinks a large amount of water for fun or as a response to stress or boredom.

2. In contrast, a low urine specific gravity is not appropriate in a patient that has been deprived of water and becomes dehydrated.

3. **Terms such as hyposthenuria, isosthenuria, and hypersthenuria are useful in describing urine specific gravity results, but they are not closely correlated with specific diagnoses** (Table 42.2).

C. The **diagnosis of central diabetes insipidus or primary nephrogenic diabetes insipidus** is accomplished through **ruling out other causes of polyuria/polydipsia.** When the differential diagnoses have been narrowed down to central diabetes insipidus, primary nephrogenic diabetes insipidus, and primary polydipsia, a water deprivation test may be considered to differentiate between these conditions. However **because central diabetes insipidus, primary nephrogenic diabetes insipidus, and primary polydipsia are uncommon, the water deprivation test is rarely necessary.**

D. A **staged approach** to the investigation of polyuria/polydipsia will ensure that the more common causes are diagnosed, before potentially performing an unnecessary water deprivation test. This approach also encourages the use of safe, simple, and relatively inexpensive testing, before progressing to tests that are more complex to perform or interpret, more expensive, or associated with more risk to the patient:

1. **Signalment, history, and physical examination** will allow logical ordering of the differential diagnoses for polyuria/polydipsia. For example, primary nephrogenic diabetes insipidus is unlikely in an elderly dog and hyperadrenocorticism is unlikely in a puppy:

a. It is particularly important to review diet and medication history (including those applied topically) and also investigate the possibility of excessive salt ingestion.

b. If in doubt about the drug history, clients can be asked to bring medications to the clinician for inspection.

2. **Serum chemistry profile, complete blood count, and urinalysis** can be used to immediately rule out or rule in many differential diagnoses for polyuria/polydipsia. Serum chemistry and hematology are expected to be **normal in well hydrated dogs with central diabetes insipidus, primary nephrogenic diabetes insipidus (unless accompanied by renal failure), and primary polydipsia.**

3. Particular attention should be paid to **serum sodium concentration ($[Na^+]$)**, which reflects water balance and can sometimes direct the further workup of polyuria/polydipsia:

a. **Elevated $[Na^+]$** is consistent with a water deficit, and therefore supports **primary polyuria** as the cause of polyuria/polydipsia.

b. However, $[Na^+]$ is only expected to be elevated in patients that have an abnormal thirst response or limited access to water. Even **patients with complete central diabetes insipidus can maintain normal $[Na^+]$** if they have continued access to water and the ability to drink.

Table 42.2   Interpretation of urine specific gravity.*

Urine specific gravity	Clinical description	Corresponding urine osmolality (mOsm/kg)	Interpretation
<1.008	Hyposthenuric or dilute urine	<300	Severe PUPD Consistent with CDI, NDI, or primary polydipsia Chronic renal failure *alone* unlikely
1.008–1.012	Isosthenuric or fixed range urine	290–310	Mild to moderate PUPD Complete CDI unlikely May occur with partial CDI, many causes of 2° NDI, or primary polydipsia, depending on water intake
1.012–1.030	Minimally concentrated urine	>310–1000	Mild PUPD Complete CDI ruled out Partial CDI unlikely Consistent with primary polydipsia, depending on water intake May occur with 2° NDI, depending on cause and severity
>1.035	Hypersthenuric or highly concentrated urine	>1500	Obligate PUPD ruled out Primary polydipsia after water restriction or normal animal

Definition and interpretation of urine specific gravity values. PUPD=polyuria-polydipsia; CDI=central diabetes insipidus; NDI=nephrogenic diabetes insipidus; 2°=secondary. Adapted from Lunn and James (2007).
*Clinicians are reminded to obtain several urine specific gravity measurements when attempting to investigate a patient's concentrating ability. Interpretation of a single value can be misleading; repeated measurement of urine specific gravity can more accurately determine the presence and severity of PUPD.

    c. **Decreased [Na⁺]** is consistent with an excess of free water, and this finding would support **primary polydipsia** as the cause of polyuria/polydipsia. However, if renal water excretory mechanisms are intact, [Na⁺] may remain within normal limits.

    d. Thus, **[Na⁺] can help direct further diagnostic testing, but may be normal in many dogs with** polyuria/polydipsia. Hyponatremia may also occur in conditions of decreased effective circulating plasma volume or hypovolemic conditions such as hypoadrenocorticism, excessive renal Na loss, or GI fluid loss. Such patients with hyponatremia may have polyuria/polydipsia, but will also likely have other clinical signs associated with the primary condition.

4. **Urine culture is mandatory** in the evaluation of dogs with polyuria/polydipsia. **Pyelonephritis** is a cause of secondary nephrogenic diabetes insipidus, and many causes of polyuria/polydipsia predispose patients to urinary tract infections:

    a. If pyelonephritis is suspected, it should not be ruled out if a single urine culture is negative.

    b. Further testing should be considered, such as repeated cultures, abdominal ultrasonography, aspiration of one or both renal pelves under ultrasound guidance, or pyelography through the administration of contrast intravenously or by direct injection into the renal pelvis under ultrasound guidance.

5. **Leptospirosis** titers are recommended in dogs with polyuria/polydipsia, unless they live in a desert environment. If clinical signs have been present for <10–14 days, acute and convalescent titers are recommended for the diagnosis of leptospirosis. For patients with a longer duration of signs, single titers may be sufficient, but should be interpreted in conjunction with the vaccination history.

6. **Fasting and postprandial bile acids** are used to test for acquired liver failure or portosystemic shunting.

7. The selection of **endocrine tests** is guided by patient signalment; history; clinical signs; and the results of serum chemistry, hematology, and urinalysis:

    a. **Hyperthyroidism** is rare in dogs, but can be ruled out with measurement of serum thyroxine.

    b. The **ACTH stimulation test** is recommended as the initial screening test for **spontaneous hyperadrenocorticism** as it can also detect **hypoadrenocorticism** and **iatrogenic hyperadrenocorticism**. A **low-dose dexamethasone suppression test** should follow a normal ACTH stimulation test if there is still clinical suspicion of the presence of spontaneous hyperadrenocorticism.

8. **Thoracic and abdominal radiography** and/or **abdominal ultrasonography** are used to screen for a range of causes of polyuria/polydipsia. Examples include neoplasia, splenomegaly, pyometra, adrenal disease, and partial urinary tract obstruction. **Contrast radiography, nuclear medicine, computed tomography (CT), and magnetic resonance imaging** (MRI) might be used to investigate specific differential diagnoses.

9. Measurement of **glomerular filtration rate** is indicated for dogs that are suspected to have chronic renal disease but that have normal blood urea nitrogen (BUN) and serum creatinine concentrations:

    a. Azotemia is expected after the loss of 75% of glomerular filtration rate, but polyuria/polydipsia occurs when approximately 66% of glomerular filtration rate is lost, particularly in nonproteinuric renal disease. Thus, **chronic renal failure can initially manifest as polyuria/polydipsia without azotemia**.

    b. Methods for assessment of glomerular filtration rate include iohexol clearance, exogenous creatinine clearance, and nuclear scintigraphy.

10. **Brain imaging** with CT or MRI is indicated in patients in which acquired **central diabetes insipidus** is suspected.

11. The **water deprivation test is rarely indicated** in the diagnosis of polyuria/polydipsia, because most causes can be diagnosed with the work-up outlined above. The water deprivation test is designed to differentiate between central diabetes insipidus, primary nephrogenic diabetes insipidus, and primary polydipsia:

    a. Primary polydipsia is uncommon, central diabetes insipidus is rare, and primary nephrogenic diabetes insipidus is very rare.

    b. Most patients with polyuria/polydipsia have secondary nephrogenic diabetes insipidus, and the water deprivation test cannot distinguish between primary and secondary nephrogenic diabetes insipidus; thus, the differentiation must be accomplished by a complete diagnostic investigation of all potential causes of secondary nephrogenic diabetes insipidus before a water deprivation test is contemplated.

E. Before performing the water deprivation test, the following must be considered:

   1. **Prerequisites for the water deprivation test:**

    a. All causes of polyuria/polydipsia have been ruled out, except for **central diabetes insipidus, primary nephrogenic diabetes insipidus**, and **primary polydipsia**.

    b. Access to 24-h care with frequent observation of the patient.

    c. Ability to weigh the patient, empty the bladder, and assess urine specific gravity as often as hourly.

    d. Ability to measure electrolytes (particularly sodium), BUN, and creatinine in-house.

    e. The patient is clinically normal, apart from polyuria/polydipsia, and is mentally alert.

   2. **The water deprivation test is contraindicated if:**

    a. All causes of polyuria/polydipsia have not been ruled out, apart from **central diabetes insipidus, primary nephrogenic diabetes insipidus**, and **primary polydipsia**.

    b. 24-h care is unavailable.

    c. Urine specific gravity, serum electrolytes, BUN, and creatinine concentrations cannot be measured in-house.

    d. The patient is clinically sick or mentally dull.

    e. The patient is dehydrated.

    f. The patient is hypernatremic.

    g. The patient is azotemic.

    h. Urine specific gravity >1.030 (this patient has already passed the test).

3. The water deprivation test is particularly dangerous in patients with:
   a. Chronic renal failure.
   b. Pyelonephritis.
   c. Hypoadrenocorticism.
   d. Hypercalcemia.
   e. Leptospirosis.
   f. Liver failure.

   Thus, all attempts must be made to **rule out these diagnoses** before a water deprivation test is considered.

   4. **Modified water deprivation tests in which the client withholds water from the pet overnight,** with the urine specific gravity measured the following morning, are **neither safe nor diagnostically helpful.** It should be remembered that some dogs with polyuria/polydipsia, such as those with complete central diabetes insipidus, have a significant obligate urine production. In these patients, 12 h of water deprivation would be equivalent to a few days of water deprivation in a dog with a normal urine volume and could result in death.

F. The water deprivation test evaluates both the patient's ability to produce endogenous ADH and the kidneys' ability to respond to it. If there is no response to water deprivation, vasopressin or an exogenous ADH analogue (DDAVP; 1-desamino-8-D-arginine vasopressin; desmopressin) is administered. When the modified water deprivation test is performed, renal medullary solute washout is corrected through gradual water deprivation before abrupt water deprivation is initiated:

1. **Predicted response to the water deprivation test:**
   a. **Primary polydipsia:** urine will be concentrated in response to water deprivation.
   b. **Complete central diabetes insipidus:** urine remains hyposthenuric during water deprivation, but specific gravity increases after DDAVP administration.
   c. **Partial central diabetes insipidus:** urine specific gravity may increase into the isosthenuric range (or slightly higher) during water deprivation and will increase further after DDAVP administration.
   d. **Nephrogenic diabetes insipidus:** urine specific gravity does not increase in response to water deprivation or DDAVP administration.

2. **The phases of the modified water deprivation test, with a brief summary of interpretation of results,** are outlined in Table 42.3. If the test is considered necessary, it is strongly recommended that patients be **referred to a specialist** experienced in performing and interpreting the water deprivation test. Although simple in principal, the test is **difficult to perform and interpret,** time consuming, and potentially dangerous.

3. **Complications and caveats in interpreting the water deprivation test:**
   a. Primary nephrogenic diabetes insipidus and secondary nephrogenic diabetes insipidus may be indistinguishable in a water deprivation test; thus, every effort must be made to rule out secondary nephrogenic diabetes insipidus before performing the test.
   b. Depending on the underlying cause, dogs with secondary nephrogenic diabetes insipidus may produce a urine specific gravity in the 1.008–1.020 range in phase 2 (abrupt water deprivation) and be misdiagnosed as having central diabetes insipidus.
   c. Because the polyuria/polydipsia in hyperadrenocorticism may have components of psychogenic polydipsia, partial central diabetes insipidus, and secondary nephrogenic diabetes insipidus, dogs with hyperadrenocorticism can respond in a variety of ways to the water deprivation test.
   d. Dogs with primary polydipsia may produce a urine specific gravity of <1.030 in phase 2 if renal medullary solute washout has not been corrected. This is less likely to occur if phase 1 (gradual water deprivation at home) is incorporated into the water deprivation test.

4. **Serum and urine osmolality in the water deprivation test:**
   a. Osmolality is determined by the number of particles in a solution, whereas specific gravity is also affected by particle size.
   b. Comparison of urine and serum osmolality can more accurately determine urine-concentrating ability during the water deprivation test than measurement of urine specific gravity.
   c. If a specific gravity of 1.030 is not reached, the end of phase 2 of the water deprivation test may be more accurately defined when the urine osmolality reaches a plateau and does not vary by more than 5% over three urine collection periods, 1 h apart.

Table 42.3 The modified water deprivation test.

Phase	Summary	End point	Purpose	Expected response		
				Primary Polydipsia	CDI	NDI
Phase 1	Gradual water deprivation at home, over 3–5 days	Water intake = 100 mL/kg/day Patient lethargic or water seeking	Correct renal medullary solute washout	May concentrate urine (USG >1.030*); if so, test complete	Failure to concentrate	Failure to concentrate
Phase 2	Abrupt water deprivation in the hospital	Loss of >5% body weight Any abnormal clinical signs USG >1.030 Azotemia Hypernatremia	1. Maximally stimulate ADH release 2. Assess renal response to ADH	USG >1.030;* test complete	Complete CDI: USG < 1.008* Partial CDI: USG 1.008–1.020*	1° NDI: USG < 1.008* 2° NDI**: USG <1.008 –1.020*
Phase 3	Response to exogenous ADH with ongoing water deprivation in the hospital	2–12 h (depending on ADH product used)	Assess renal response to ADH	Phase 3 not performed	Increase in USG compared to phase 2	No increase in USG compared to phase 2
Phase 4	Gradual reintroduction of water in the hospital	2 h, if patient clinically normal	Return to normal drinking behavior			

Summary of the phases of the water deprivation test (WDT). This table provides an outline of the test and expected responses. It does **not** provide sufficient detail for **safely** performing a WDT. The reader should consult more detailed texts or refer the patient to a specialist (recommended) if considering the WDT. USG = urine specific gravity.
*Urine specific gravity values are provided here for simplicity, but it is recommended that urine and serum osmolality be evaluated when performing the WDT. See text for further details.
It is important to note that 2° NDI should have been ruled out **before performing the WDT. Therefore, these values are provided for illustrative purposes only. The results of the WDT are **very difficult to interpret** if 2° NDI has not been investigated and ruled out.

d. Osmolality can be approximated by multiplying the last two numbers of the specific gravity by 36; for example, a urine specific gravity of 1.010 is approximately equivalent to an osmolality of 360 mOsm/L.

e. Measurement of osmolality is much less readily available than urine specific gravity. However, urine and serum samples should be frozen and can later be analyzed if it is determined that measurement of osmolality will provide additional diagnostic information.

f. Osmolality measurements are often very valuable in interpreting the results of the water deprivation test, particularly in more difficult cases. Therefore, it is strongly recommended that osmolality be measured whenever possible. This is another reason to recommend referral to a specialist if the water deprivation test is being considered.

G. A **DDAVP response trial** can be used **to confirm a suspected diagnosis of central diabetes insipidus**, thus avoiding a water deprivation test:

  1. **Prerequisites** for a response trial include:
    a. All causes of secondary nephrogenic diabetes insipidus have been ruled out.
    b. Primary polydipsia is considered unlikely, on the basis of signalment, history, serum [Na⁺], repeated urine specific gravity measurements, and absence of response to environmental modification.
    c. The patient can be closely observed and water intake measured. Hospitalization is not necessary, but the patient should not be left unattended at home for more than a few hours when the test is started.

  2. **How to perform the test:**
    a. Measure water intake over 2–3 days.
    b. Measure urine specific gravity prior to starting DDAVP.
    c. Administer DDAVP (intranasal preparation [0.1 mg/mL]: 1–4 drops twice daily in conjunctival sac) for 5–7 days; monitor water intake and urine specific gravity.
    d. Decreased water intake (>50%) or increase in urine specific gravity (>50%) support a diagnosis of central diabetes insipidus.

  3. **A theoretical risk of the DDAVP response trial** is water intoxication and hyponatremia in a patient with primary polydipsia, because the normal renal diluting mechanism will be compromised; however, this appears to be a rare complication in clinical practice.

V. Differential Diagnoses

A. The differential diagnoses for diabetes insipidus **include all the potential causes of** polyuria/polydipsia, which can be broadly divided into primary polydipsia and primary polyuria.

B. **Primary polydipsia is abnormal thirst behavior** resulting in increased water intake, with a compensatory polyuria. In humans, it may be associated with psychiatric disorders:

  1. In dogs, primary polydipsia is **most commonly seen as a behavioral problem** in dogs that are hyperactive, bored, stressed, exercise restricted, or attention seeking.
  2. Dogs with primary polydipsia are **able to concentrate their urine** in response to water deprivation. They may also concentrate their urine in response to environmental changes that cause changes in behavior. For example, a dog that exhibits psychogenic polydipsia when crated at home may cease the behavior at the veterinary clinic or when kept highly entertained (see Chapter 44 for entertainment test).
  3. Primary, or psychogenic, polydipsia may also partially explain the polydipsia that can be associated with hyperthyroidism, hepatic encephalopathy, hypercortisolemia, GI disease, splenomegaly, or, exceptionally rarely, lower urinary tract infection.
  4. A distinction in behavioral polydipsia that is normal versus abnormal is rarely made in veterinary medicine:
    a. Clinically, a dog with polydipsia severe enough to create hyponatremia should clearly be classed as abnormal since the behavior can result in serious self-harm.
    b. Dogs with behavioral polydipsias due to activities like swimming or merely preferring to drink more than most dogs, while they may be noticeably polydipsic to their owners at certain times of day, are not necessarily abnormal.

C. Primary polyuria encompasses all the remaining causes of PUPD, including central diabetes insipidus and all forms of nephrogenic diabetes insipidus.

D. The causes of polyuria/polydipsia, and, therefore, the differential diagnoses for central diabetes insipidus, are listed in Table 42.1. When investigating a patient with polyuria/polydipsia, it can be very useful to start with a complete list of all differential diagnoses, in order to ensure that all possible causes are considered:

  1. The diagnostic plan can be based on clinical suspicion and consideration of the most common causes of polyuria/polydipsia, as outlined in Table 42.1.
  2. Medical problems identified other than polyuria/polydipsia should be pursued concurrently as their investigation may lead to a specific diagnosis more efficiently than the evaluation for polyuria/polydipsia.

Table 42.4   Causes of PUPD in dogs organized by body system.

Endocrine	Renal	Metabolic/hematological	Abdominal	Miscellaneous
Central diabetes insipidus	Primary nephrogenic diabetes insipidus	Hypercalcemia	Liver failure	Primary polydipsia
Diabetes mellitus	Chronic renal failure	Hyponatremia	Pyometra	Renal medullary solute washout
Hyperadrenocorticism	Pyelonephritis	Hypokalemia	Portosystemic shunt	Diet
Hypoadrenocorticism	Polyuric acute renal failure	Polycythemia	Leiomyosarcoma	Medications
Hyperthyroidism	Postobstructive diuresis		Splenomegaly	Excess salt ingestion
Pheochromocytoma	Leptospirosis		Gastrointestinal disease	
Acromegaly	Chronic partial ureteral obstruction			
Primary hyperaldosteronism	Tubulopathies (Fanconi syndrome, primary renal glycosuria)			

3. An alternate diagnostic plan is to consider the differential diagnoses for polyuria/polydipsia using a body systems approach, as outlined in Table 42.4.

4. Finally, the plan can also follow the framework described under "Diagnosis" above.

E. Regardless of the approach used to investigate the patient with polyuria/polydipsia, it is most important that all potential differential diagnoses are considered; safe, simple, and inexpensive tests are prioritized; and the diagnostic plan is modified as results are obtained:

1. The order of testing should ensure that potentially life-threatening disorders are diagnosed as early as possible.

2. Conversely, central diabetes insipidus is not life threatening (as long as affected patients have constant access to water) and, therefore, a water deprivation test or DDAVP trial can, and should, be delayed until all other causes of polyuria/polydipsia have been ruled out.

VI. Treatment

A. **Treatment of central diabetes insipidus is not essential** if the patient has partial central diabetes insipidus and the magnitude of polyuria/polydipsia is tolerable, as long as the patient has constant access to water. Dogs with complete central diabetes insipidus are profoundly polyuric/polydipsic, and most owners will, therefore, elect to treat them. However, if the dog has access to the outdoors for frequent urination and a constant water supply is guaranteed, medical therapy is not essential. The **necessity of a constant water supply cannot be overemphasized.** Dogs with central diabetes insipidus will rapidly become hypernatremic due to their obligate polyuria if deprived of water for any period of time:

1. If medical treatment is elected, partial central diabetes insipidus may respond to administration of thiazide diuretics (see primary nephrogenic diabetes insipidus below).

2. Total or partial central diabetes insipidus may also be managed with **ADH analogues, usually DDAVP.** There are several options available in the United States for administration of DDAVP:

a. Conjunctival: 0.1 mg/mL solution (5 mL) of DDAVP for nasal administration; as most dogs will not tolerate the nasal route, a pharmacist can transfer the solution to a sterile dropper bottle; dose is 1–4 drops in the conjunctival sac once or twice daily; adjust dose for optimal clinical effect.

    b. Nasal: 1.5 mg/mL solution (2.5 mL) for nasal administration; this formulation is not usually used in dogs.

    c. Oral: 0.1 mg and 0.2 mg tablets are available. Starting dose is 0.1 mg (per dog) three times daily. Bioavailability may be low or variable in dogs; adjust dose for optimal clinical effect.

    d. Injectable: 4 μg/mL solution is available in 1-mL ampoules or 10-mL multidose vials. This formulation is expensive; if an injectable product is required (e.g., during the water deprivation test) the 0.1 mg/mL nasal solution can be passed through a filter to create a sterile solution.

    e. All of these options are **relatively expensive.** Clinicians may prefer to begin with conjunctival administration of the 0.1 mg/mL nasal solution. If the patient responds, oral DDAVP can be tried, and may be less expensive in some cases. It may also be possible to target therapy with DDAVP to control polyuria/polydipsia at certain times of the day. For example, therapy could be given only at nighttime for a dog that is outdoors during the day, but sleeps indoors at night.

B.   Dogs with **primary nephrogenic diabetes insipidus** should be managed by **allowing constant free access to water.**

C.   **Thiazide diuretics** (e.g., chlorothiazide) **may reduce polyuria in patients with primary nephrogenic diabetes insipidus and central diabetes insipidus:**

    1. Thiazides inhibit Na reabsorption in the distal convoluted tubule. This leads to hypovolemia, which in turn stimulates proximal tubular reabsorption of Na and water. As a result, delivery of water to the collecting ducts is decreased, with associated reduction in urine output.

    2. The dose of chlorothiazide is 20–40 mg/kg PO twice daily.

    3. Hypokalemia is a potential side effect and serum potassium should be monitored.

D.   **Treatment for secondary nephrogenic diabetes insipidus depends on the underlying cause.** Affected patients should have **continuous access to water.**

E.   **Primary polydipsia** is managed by water restriction and behavioral modification.

F.   **For dogs with a profound primary polyuria, clinicians should consider monitoring serum potassium and magnesium concentrations,** and supplementing as necessary, as urinary losses will be increased. Similarly, it might be anticipated that water-soluble vitamins will be depleted in these patients.

VII. Prognosis

A.   Prognosis for central diabetes insipidus **is good** if there is no associated structural brain disease; otherwise, prognosis is determined by the underlying cause. Polyuria/polydipsia in central diabetes insipidus can be managed medically; however, treatment may be discontinued due to expense.

B.   Prognosis for **primary nephrogenic diabetes insipidus is guarded to poor;** these dogs may develop concurrent signs of uremia.

C.   Prognosis for **secondary nephrogenic diabetes insipidus is dependent on the underlying cause.**

D.   Prognosis for **primary polydipsia is good.**

VIII. Prevention

Prevention is dependent on the underlying cause.

References and Further Readings

Cohen M, Post GS. Nephrogenic diabetes insipidus in a dog with intestinal leiomyosarcoma. *J Am Vet Med Assoc* 1999;215(12):1818–1820.

Cohen M, Post GS. Water transport in the kidney and nephrogenic diabetes insipidus. *J Vet Intern Med* 2002;16(5):510–517.

Cohen M, Post GS, Wright JC. Gastrointestinal leiomyosarcoma in 14 dogs. *J Vet Intern Med* 2003;17(1):107–110.

Couto CG. Lymphadenopathy and splenomegaly. In: Nelson RW, Couto CG, eds. *Small Animal Internal Medicine*, 4th ed. St. Louis: Mosby Elsevier, 2009, pp. 1260–1270.

Deppe TA, Center SA, Simpson KW, et al. Glomerular filtration rate and renal volume in dogs with congenital portosystemic vascular anomalies before and after surgical ligation. *J Vet Intern Med* 1999;13(5):465–471.

DiBartola SP. Disorders of sodium and water: Hypernatremia and hyponatremia. In: DiBartola SP, ed. *Fluid, Electrolyte, and Acid-Base Disorders in Small Animal Practice*, 3rd edn. St. Louis: Saunders, 2006, pp. 47–79.

Feldman EC, Nelson RW. *Canine and Feline Endocrinology and Reproduction*, 3rd edn. St. Louis: Saunders, 2004.

Grauer GF, Pitts RP. Primary polydipsia in three dogs with portosystemic shunts. *J Am Anim Hosp Assoc* 1987;23(2):197–200.

Harb MF, Nelson RW, Feldman EC, et al. Central diabetes insipidus in dogs: 20 cases (1986–1995). *J Am Vet Med Assoc* 1996;209(11):1884–1888.

Henderson SM, Elwood CM. A potential causal association between gastrointestinal disease and primary polydipsia in three dogs. *J Small Anim Pract* 2003;44(6):280–284.

Hoppe A, Karlstam E. Renal dysplasia in boxers and Finnish harriers. *J Small Anim Pract* 2000;41(9):422–426.

James KM, Lunn KF. Normal and abnormal water balance: Hyponatremia and hypernatremia. *Compend Contin Educ Vet* 2007;29(10):589–609.

Lunn KF. Managing the patient with polyuria and polydipsia. In: Bonagura JD, Twedt DC, eds *Kirk's Current Veterinary Therapy XIV*, St. Louis: Saunders Elsevier, 2008, pp. 844–850.

Lunn KF, James KM. Normal and abnormal water balance: Polyuria and polydipsia. *Compend Contin Educ Vet* 2007;29(10):612–624.

Luzius H, Jans DA, Grünbaum EG, Moritz A, Rascher W, Fahrenholz, F. A low affinity vasopressin V2-receptor in inherited nephrogenic diabetes insipidus. *J Recept Res* 1992;12(3):351–368.

Mulnix JA, Rijnberk A, Hendriks HJ. Evaluation of a modified water-deprivation test for diagnosis of polyuric disorders in dogs. *J Am Vet Med Assoc* 1976;169(12):1327–1330.

Nichols R. Clinical use of the vasopressin analogue DDAVP for the diagnosis and treatment of diabetes insipidus. In: Bonagura JD, eds. *Kirk's Current Veterinary Therapy XIII*, 2000, pp. 325–326.

Polzin DJ, Osborne CA, Ross S Chronic kidney disease. In: Ettinger SJ, Feldman EC, eds. *Textbook of Veterinary Internal Medicine*, 6th edn. St. Louis: Elsevier Saunders, 2005, pp. 1756–1785.

Ramsey IK, Dennis R, Herrtage ME. Concurrent central diabetes insipidus and panhypopituitarism in a German shepherd dog. *J Small Anim Pract* 1999;40(6):271–274.

Rijnberk A, Kooistra HS, van Vonderen IK, et al. Aldosteronoma in a dog with polyuria as the leading symptom. *Domest Anim Endocrinol* 2001;20:227–240.

Schwedes CS. Transient diabetes insipidus in a dog with acromegaly. *J Small Anim Pract* 1999;40(8):392–396.

Takemura N. Successful long-term treatment of congenital nephrogenic diabetes insipidus in a dog. *J Small Anim Pract* 1998;39(12):592–594.

Tyler RD, Qualls CW Jr, Heald RD, et al. Renal concentrating ability in dehydrated hyponatremic dogs. *J Am Vet Med Assoc* 1987;191(9):1095–1100.

van Vonderen IK, Meyer HP, Kraus JS, et al. Polyuria and polydipsia and disturbed vasopressin release in 2 dogs with secondary polycythemia. *J Vet Intern Med* 1997;11(5):300–303.

van Vonderen IK, Kooistra HS, Elpetra PM, et al. Disturbed vasopressin release in 4 dogs with so-called primary polydipsia. *J Vet Intern Med* 1999;13(5):419–425.

van Vonderen IK, Kooistra HS, Elpetra PM, et al. Vasopressin response to osmotic stimulation in 18 young dogs with polyuria and polydipsia. *J Vet Intern Med* 2004;18(6):800–806.

CHAPTER 43

Diabetes Insipidus in Cats

Nicki Reed and Danièlle Gunn-Moore

Pathogenesis

- Inadequate production or secretion of antidiuretic hormone (ADH—vasopressin) by the posterior pituitary (central diabetes insipidus), or lack of responsiveness to ADH by the kidney (nephrogenic diabetes insipidus).
- Reported cases in cats have all been central diabetes insipidus.
- Underlying identified etiologies for central diabetes insipidus include congenital anomalies, trauma, and neoplasia, but idiopathic cases are also reported.

Classical Signs

- Marked polyuria due to inability to concentrate urine. The polyuria is accompanied by marked polydipsia, often in excess of 200 mL/kg/q 24 h.
- Urine-specific gravity (USG) is consistently low, usually < 1.010.

Diagnosis

- Diagnosis requires elimination of other causes of polyuria/polydipsia.
- Confirmation of diabetes insipidus requires performance of a water deprivation test; patients with diabetes insipidus are unable to concentrate their urine after 3–5% dehydration.
- Patients with central diabetes insipidus are able to concentrate their urine following administration of synthetic ADH.
- Patients with nephrogenic diabetes insipidus are unable to respond to administration of synthetic ADH.
- Assessment of response to a therapeutic trial with the ADH analogue desmopressin (1-deamino 9-D-arginine vasopressin; DDAVP) is a safer alternative to performance of a water deprivation test.

Treatment

- Treatment of central diabetes insipidus involves treatment with DDAVP, a synthetic analogue of ADH.
- Sodium restriction is beneficial for both central and nephrogenic diabetes insipidus.
- Thiazide diuretics may be considered for nephrogenic diabetes insipidus.
- No therapy is an option, provided continuous access to water is provided.

Clinical Endocrinology of Companion Animals, First Edition. Edited by Jacquie Rand.
© 2013 John Wiley & Sons, Inc. Published 2013 by John Wiley & Sons, Inc.

I. Pathogenesis
A. **All reported cases of feline diabetes insipidus have been central diabetes insipidus (CDI)**, rather than primary nephrogenic diabetes insipidus in origin:
    1. Central diabetes insipidus is due to **failure to synthesize or secrete antidiuretic hormone (ADH— arginine vasopressin) from the posterior pituitary.**
    2. The inability to secrete ADH, in response to increasing plasma osmolarity or decreasing plasma volume, results in an inability of the kidneys to reabsorb water. This inappropriately increases plasma osmolarity further, while urine remains dilute (see Figure 43.1).
B. Central diabetes insipidus may arise as a result of:
    1. **Trauma** resulting in damage to the pituitary gland.
    2. A **congenital or idiopathic anomaly.**
    3. **Neoplasia or an infectious/inflammatory disease process affecting the pituitary gland.**
C. Nephrogenic diabetes insipidus results when the kidney has lost its ability to respond to ADH:

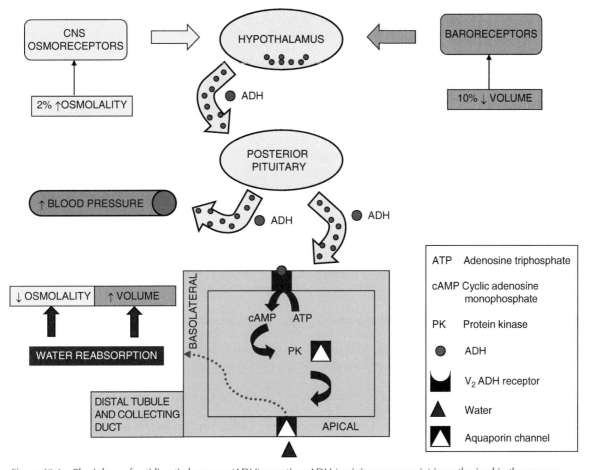

Figure 43.1 Physiology of antidiuretic hormone (ADH) secretion. ADH (arginine vasopressin) is synthesized in the paraventricular and supraoptic nuclei of the hypothalamus in response to increased osmolality or decreased plasma volume. The ADH travels down the hypothalamic-hypophyseal tract and is stored in granules in the posterior pituitary. Neurogenic stimulation causes exocytosis of the granules and release of ADH. ADH binds to the V_1 receptor on blood vessels to cause vasoconstriction, and the V_2 receptor in the distal tubules and collecting ducts of the kidney. Following binding to the V_2 receptor, the second messenger cAMP causes activation of protein kinases. This results in movement of aquaporin channels from their intracellular location to the apical membrane. Insertion of these channels enables water reabsorption, thus increasing plasma volume and decreasing osmolality.

1. **Primary nephrogenic diabetes insipidus** is the result of an **abnormality with the ADH receptor**. This has not been reported in cats.
2. **Secondary nephrogenic diabetes insipidus** may be seen in association with a number of conditions such as **pyelonephritis, hypokalemia, hypercalcemia, hyperadrenocorticism, hepatic insufficiency, and pyometra**, where the production of ADH is adequate, but its action at the receptor is compromised.

II. Signalment
A. Reported cases have varied in age from 8 weeks to 6 years.
B. No sex or breed predilection has been identified.

III. Clinical Signs
A. **Marked polydipsia and polyuria** is reported consistently. Polyuria is the primary problem as these cats are unable to adequately concentrate their urine. The polydipsia is secondary to compensate for the excessive renal fluid loss:
    1. Water consumption will exceed 100 mL/kg/q 24 h, and consumption of 250 mL/kg/q 24 h is not unusual.
    2. Cats may seek water from unusual sources such as dripping taps and toilets.
B. Owners may not be specifically aware of polyuria in cats, especially if litter boxes are used. Polyuria may manifest as:
    1. Litter boxes being required to be changed more frequently.
    2. Litter boxes feeling heavier when changed at regular intervals due to the increased volume of urine.
    3. Cats spending longer time outdoors due to the need to urinate more frequently.
C. Marked polyuria may lead to cats being presented for inappropriate urination out of the litter box. This can lead to investigations for urinary disorders unless the concurrent polydipsia is identified.
D. **Weight loss** may be a feature in some cases due to:
    1. Filling of the stomach with water suppressing appetite.
    2. Calories expended on drinking and urinating.
E. **Neurological signs** may be evident in cases of neoplastic or inflammatory infiltration or where trauma has resulted in damage to the pituitary gland. Mydriasis and proprioceptive deficits have been reported in association with traumatic diabetes insipidus.
F. Physical examination may be unremarkable, other than evidence of dehydration.

IV. Diagnosis
A. Initial investigation should comprise confirmation of polydipsia and polyuria. **Water consumption should be measured and USG assessed.** If water consumption is < 100 mL/kg/q 24 h, or USG > 1.025, then diabetes insipidus should be ruled out.
B. Routine hematology may be within reference range, or the hematocrit may be elevated if the cat is dehydrated.
C. The abnormalities most frequently identified on biochemistry are elevated total protein, urea, and creatinine, attributed to dehydration and elevated sodium, consistent with hyperosmolarity. Biochemistry results may be normal.
D. Urinalysis consistently identifies dilute urine. USG is typically less than 1.010 and urine osmolality is less than plasma osmolality (< 310 mOsm/kg).
E. Plasma osmolality is usually increased (reference range 280–310 mOsm/kg). If osmolality cannot be measured directly, it may be estimated by the following formulas:
    1. $[2(Na^+ + K^+) \, (mEq/L)] + [glucose \, (mg/dL)/18] + [BUN \, (mg/dL)/2.8]$
    2. $[2(Na^+ + K^+) \, (mmol/L)] + [glucose \, (mmol/L)] + [BUN \, (mmol/L)]$
F. Confirmation of diabetes insipidus requires demonstration of an inability to concentrate urine in the face of increased plasma osmolality:
    1. **Causes of secondary nephrogenic diabetes insipidus should be investigated and ruled out before pursuing a diagnosis of diabetes insipidus by means of a water deprivation test.**
    2. **Patients that are clinically dehydrated on presentation should not be subjected to a water deprivation test—they have already failed this test if their urine remains dilute.**

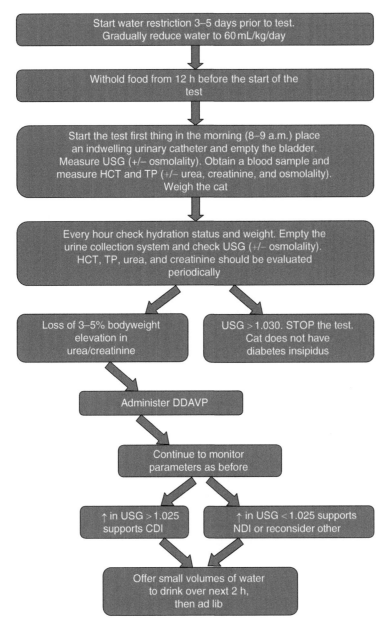

Figure 43.2 Suggested protocol for modified water deprivation test. USG = urine-specific gravity; HCT = hematocrit; TP = total protein; CDI = central diabetes insipidus; NDI = nephrogenic diabetes insipidus; DDx = differential diagnoses.

3. The presence of polyuria/polydipsia can affect the renal concentrating ability due to medullary solute washout. Gradually reducing water consumption for 72 h prior to starting the water deprivation test may be beneficial, as it can restore the medullary concentration gradient:

    a. Water may be reduced by 10% per day for 5–7 days prior to starting the test, to a minimum volume of 60 mL/kg.

    b. Water may be reduced to 120 mL/kg/day, 90 mL/kg/day, and 60 mL/kg/day, 72, 48, and 24 h, respectively, before starting the test.

4. A suggested protocol for the **water deprivation test** is given in Figure 43.2:

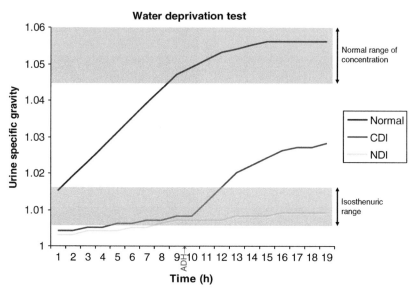

Figure 43.3 Characteristic responses to the water deprivation test in normal patients and those with diabetes insipidus. CDI = central diabetes insipidus; NDI = nephrogenic diabetes insipidus; ADH = administration of exogenous source of antidiuretic hormone.

a. Placement of an indwelling urinary catheter is likely to require sedation or general anesthesia. Alpha 2 agonists should not be used as they can interfere with the release of ADH. Alternatively, the bladder may be emptied by manual expression, but this is less accurate for ensuring complete emptying, and could traumatize the bladder.

b. **The end point of the test** is when the cat has become **3–5% dehydrated**, as assessed by changes in weight, as this indicates maximal stimulation of ADH release. This may also be assumed by failure of urine osmolality to change over three consecutive measurements. Increase in total proteins, hematocrit, or changes in USG are considered less reliable.

c. Normal cats may take 2–3 days to become 5% dehydrated, their USG will increase to 1.047–1.087, and urine osmolality increases to 1581–2984 mOsm/kg. Cats with diabetes insipidus may become **dehydrated within 12 h**, and the **USG remains hyposthenuric (< 1.007)**.

G. **Differentiation between central diabetes insipidus and nephrogenic diabetes insipidus relies on the demonstration of an increased urine concentrating ability in response to administration of extrinsic ADH** (see Figures 43.2 and 43.3):

1. Once the end point of the water deprivation test is reached, an exogenous form of ADH should be administered by one of the following methods:

   a. Desmopressin acetate injection (Minirin® 4 μg/mL, Ferring Pharmaceuticals)—1–2 μg/cat intravenously.

   b. Aqueous vasopressin (Pitressin®, Parke Davis)—0.5 U/kg intramuscularly.

   c. DDAVP intranasal drops (100 μg/mL):

   i. Four drops instilled intranasally or into the conjunctival sac.

   ii. 5 μg by subcutaneous or intravenous injection. This formulation is not sterile, therefore use of a bacterial filter is recommended.

2. The bladder is emptied periodically and USG continues to be monitored:

   a. **Following vasopressin,** the bladder should be emptied every 30 min and USG measured. **An effect is expected after 1–2 h.**

   b. Following desmopressin, the bladder should be emptied every 1–2 h and USG measured. An effect is expected after 2–8 h.

3. An increase in urine osmolality of 50–600% or USG to > 1.020 following administration of ADH is supportive of a diagnosis of central diabetes insipidus.

4. Failure to demonstrate an adequate response to ADH is supportive of a diagnosis of nephrogenic diabetes insipidus.

H. Following completion of the test, water should be gradually reintroduced with small volumes offered for the first 2 h to prevent vomiting from excessive ingestion or water intoxication. Water should also be offered if the cat becomes hypernatremic, azotemic, or shows signs of altered mentation.

I. **Complications that may be associated with the water deprivation test include:**

1. Development of severe hyperosmolality or hypernatremia. Fluid therapy with 0.45% NaCl, or in severe cases, 0.9% NaCl may be required.

2. Requirement to place an indwelling urinary catheter, inaccuracies if it is removed mid-test, and potential for introduction of urinary tract infections.

3. Failure to respond to administration of DDAVP or aqueous vasopressin due to loss of medullary solute concentration gradient or inadequate absorption (particularly if conjunctival route used).

4. Failure to detect an increase in USG due to monitoring for an insufficient period after administration of DDAVP.

5. Water intoxication may occur if free access to large quantities of water is permitted following completion of the test. This can cause cerebral edema.

J. **Due to the problems associated with the water deprivation test, a therapeutic trial may be considered as an alternative method of diagnosing diabetes insipidus.** Other differential diagnoses should be ruled out prior to performing a therapeutic trial:

1. The owner measures the cat's water intake at home for 2–3 days prior to starting the trial. Urine samples are collected to measure USG and/or osmolality.

2. Therapy is then started with DDAVP.

3. After 5–7 days, several urine samples are obtained for measurement of USG (+/– osmolality).

4. A reduction in thirst and increase in urinary concentrating ability (>50%) is supportive of a diagnosis of central diabetes insipidus. Cats with nephrogenic diabetes insipidus would show minimal response.

K. **Imaging of the pituitary region** (MRI or CT) may assist in establishing an underlying etiology, particularly if neoplasia is of concern in an older animal.

V. Differential Diagnoses

A. Other causes of polyuria and polydipsia (PU/PD) should be investigated and ruled out before performing a water deprivation test:

1. **Kidney disease is the most common cause for PU/PD:**

   a. The degree of PU/PD is likely to be more marked with diabetes insipidus than with kidney disease.

   b. The urine concentrating ability is usually fixed in the isosthenuric range (1.007–1.015) in renal disease, or higher.

   c. Azotemia may be present in patients with diabetes insipidus due to dehydration and absent in cats with early kidney disease (IRIS stage I).

   d. If there is any doubt, creatinine clearance tests (endogenous or exogenous) may be performed to assess glomerular filtration rate, **and a water deprivation test should NOT be performed.**

   e. **Urine culture** should be performed to investigate pyelonephritis, but a negative culture does not definitively rule it out.

2. **Diabetes mellitus is another common cause of PU/PD.** Both glycosuria and hyperglycemia will be present (see Chapter 16).

3. **Hyperthyroidism does not typically cause such marked PU/PD as diabetes insipidus.** Assessment of thyroid hormone status, along with other clinical signs, is likely to confirm this diagnosis (see Chapter 29).

4. **Hyperadrenocorticism is a rare cause of PU/PD in cats,** and is likely to be accompanied by other clinical signs such as coat changes, hepatomegaly, and evidence of diabetes mellitus (see Chapter 7).

5. Other systemic causes of PU/PD, for example, hypercalcemia, hypokalemia, and hepatic disease, are likely to have been identified on initial screening blood work.

6. Psychogenic polydipsia is a rare cause of PD/PU in dogs and has not been reported in cats.

VI. Treatment

A. Central diabetes insipidus is managed by replacement of ADH with synthetic analogues.

B. ADH is also known as arginine vasopressin. The 1-desamino-8-D-arginine vasopressin synthetic analogue (DDAVP or desmopressin) is most commonly used to treat this condition. It has reduced effects on systemic blood pressure compared to ADH, but has a greater antidiuretic effect, which is sustained for longer than the natural hormone.

C. **DDAVP** is available in a number of different formulations:

    1. **Nasal drops** (100 µg/mL): whilst these can be administered intranasally, this is not easy in cats so the preferred route of administration is into the conjunctival sac. Typically 1–3 drops are given q 8–12 h; 1 drop is reported to be equivalent to 1.5–4 µg DDAVP.

    2. **Oral tablets** (0.1 mg): oral doses of 25–50 µg q 12 h have been reported to control feline cases of diabetes insipidus.

    3. **Injection** (4 µg/mL): doses of 0.5–2 µg q 12–24 h by subcutaneous injection have been recommended; however, one feline case described in the literature required a dose of 5 µg q 12 h to control clinical signs. As discussed under the diagnosis of diabetes insipidus, the nasal drop formulation may be administered subcutaneously; however, the product is not sterile which may cause some concerns for long-term use.

D. **Response to therapy can be variable, so doses need to be adjusted on an individual basis.**

E. Conjunctival administration can be associated with conjunctival irritation due to the acidic nature of the drops. Drug absorption may be inconsistent.

F. Another synthetic analogue (lysine-8-vasopressin) appears to offer little advantage over DDAVP. It is less potent, with a shorter duration of action, and more expensive. Use of this drug has not been reported in cats.

G. Patients with both central diabetes insipidus and nephrogenic diabetes insipidus should be fed a **low sodium diet**. This encourages sodium avidity in the proximal tubules, which results in passive reabsorption of water. The diet should comprise <0.9 g NaCl/1000 kcal ME.

H. Cases of nephrogenic diabetes insipidus show a minimal response to therapy with DDAVP. Alternative drugs that could be used for this condition are:

    1. **Thiazide diuretics** which work by **decreasing sodium reabsorption** in the **ascending loop of Henle**. This reduces plasma sodium levels in animals that already have a reduced plasma volume. The combination of reduced sodium and extracellular volume promotes sodium retention in the proximal tubule of the kidneys. Water is also passively reabsorbed reducing the volume and increasing the osmolality of the urine produced. Potassium supplementation may be required when treating with thiazide diuretics. Feeding of a **low sodium diet** is necessary if thiazide diuretics are used.

    2. **Chlorpropamide** is a sulfonylurea drug thought to augment the effects of ADH on the kidney, although the exact mechanism of action is unknown. Doses of 10–30 mg/kg/PO q 24 h have been reported, with variable efficacy. As chlorpropamide is used in the management of hyperglycemia, hypoglycemia may be seen with it, unless animals are fed small frequent meals.

I. **No treatment remains an option** provided that the owner can cope with the polyuria. This may be less of an issue with cats than dogs if they have adequate litter tray provision or access outside. Water must be provided at all times, however, as these cats may rapidly become severely dehydrated if unable to replace their fluid losses.

J. **Treatment** of nephrogenic diabetes insipidus includes management of the underlying disease.

VII. Prognosis

A. The prognosis for diabetes insipidus is usually good, particularly if therapy induces remission of clinical signs.

B. Owner compliance and the cost of therapy may result in premature euthanasia of these patients.

C. The prognosis is poorer for cases in which underlying brain pathology has developed than in idiopathic cases.

D. The prognosis for congenital cases may be affected by whether or not concurrent deficiencies of other pituitary hormones exist.

VIII. Prevention

No known prevention.

References and Further Readings

Aroch I, Mazaki-Tovi M, Shemesh O, Sarfaty H, Segev G. Central diabetes insipidus in five cats: Clinical presentation, diagnosis and oral desmopressin therapy. *J Feline Med Surg* 2005;7:333–339.

Burnie AG, Dunn JK. A case of central diabetes insipidus in the cat: Diagnosis and treatment. *J Small Anim Pract* 1982;23:237–241.

Campbell FE, Bredhauer B. Trauma-induced central diabetes insipidus in a cat. *Aust Vet J* 2008;86:102–105.

Court MH, Watson DJ. Idiopathic neurogenic diabetes insipidus in a cat. *Aust Vet J* 1983;60:245–247.

Di Bartola SP. Disorders of sodium and water: Hypernatraemia and hyponatraemia. In: Di Bartola SJ, ed. *Fluid, Electrolyte and Acid-Base Disorders in Small Animal Practice*, 3rd edn. St. Louis, Missouri: Saunders Elsevier, 2006.

Feldman EC, Nelson RW. Water metabolism and diabetes insipidus. In: Feldman EC, Nelson RW, eds. *Canine and Feline Endocrinology and Reproduction*, 3rd edn. St. Louis, Missouri: Saunders, 2004, pp. 2–44.

Green RA, Farrow CS. Diabetes insipidus in a cat. *J Am Vet Med Assoc* 1974;164(5):524–526.

Kraus KH. The use of desmopressin in diagnosis and treatment of diabetes insipidus in cats. *Comp Cont Educ Pract Vet—Small Anim* 1987;9(7):752–756.

Mellanby RJ, Jeffery ND, Gopal MS, Herrtage ME. Secondary hypothyroidism following head trauma in a cat. *J Feline Med Surg* 2005;7:135–139.

Nichols, R. Clinical use of the vasopressin analogue DDAVP for the diagnosis and treatment of diabetes insipidus. In: Bonagura JD, ed. *Kirk's Current Veterinary Therapy XIII*, Philadelphia: W.B. Saunders Company, 2000, pp. 325–326.

Pittari JM. Central diabetes insipidus in a cat. *Feline Pract* 1996;24:18–21

Rogers WA, Valdez H, Anderson BC, Comella C. Partial deficiency of antidiuretic hormone in a cat. *J Am Vet Med Assoc* 1977;170(5):545–547.

Smith JR, Elwood CM. Traumatic partial hypopituitarism in a cat. *J Small Anim Pract* 2004;45:405–409.

Winterbottom, J. Mason KV. Congenital diabetes insipidus in a kitten. *J Small Anim Pract* 1983;24:569–573.

CHAPTER 44

Hyponatremia, SIADH, and Renal Salt Wasting

Katherine M. James

Pathogenesis

- Hyponatremia exists whenever there is an excess of water relative to sodium in the extracellular fluid (ECF).
- Two main causal categories of hyponatremia exist that reflect the mechanisms whereby it develops: translocational and hypoosmolar.
- Pseudohyponatremia is an *in vitro* artifact that may be observed when measuring serum sodium concentration ($[Na^+]$) by flame photometry when plasma lipids or proteins are elevated.

Classical Signs

- Clinical signs of hyponatremia result from the effects of hyponatremia on the central nervous system (CNS). Reduction of the plasma $[Na^+]$ causes water movement from the ECF into cells. Signs result from cerebral edema: lethargy, confusion, nausea, vomiting, seizures, and coma. Development of clinical signs depends both on magnitude of hyponatremia and the rate at which it develops.
- Although severe hyponatremia can itself lead to permanent neurologic damage, too rapid a rate of correction of serum $[Na^+]$ in patients with chronic hyponatremia can result in severe and potentially irreversible neurologic sequelae.
- Polydipsia and polyuria will be present in patients whose hyponatremia is a result of hyperglycemia, primary polydipsia, or obligate polyuria associated with ECF volume depletion in patients who are able to drink (e.g., Addison's disease).

Diagnosis

- Distinguishing between the mechanistic causes of hyponatremia relies heavily on a complete history and an analysis of the patient's other problems.
- Hyponatremia is a water balance problem; the clinician must determine "Why is there too much water?"

Clinical Endocrinology of Companion Animals, First Edition. Edited by Jacquie Rand.
© 2013 John Wiley & Sons, Inc. Published 2013 by John Wiley & Sons, Inc.

Treatment

- Treatment depends on the underlying cause.
- Behavioral therapy is warranted for dogs that have compulsive water drinking behavior to the extent that hyponatremia results.
- Renal salt wasting is managed by salt supplementation.
- Some forms of hyponatremia require careful restriction of water intake.

I. Pathogenesis
A. Normal cellular function requires tight regulation of **plasma osmolality, which is** achieved through regulation of **water balance**:
   1. **Normal water balance** depends on:
      a. An appropriate thirst mechanism.
      b. Osmoreceptors in the brain.
      c. Appropriate release of antidiuretic hormone (vasopressin or ADH) from the posterior pituitary.
      d. Renal ability to regulate water excretion, which includes the ability to:
         1) Conserve sodium.
         2) Respond to ADH by concentrating the urine.
         3) Excrete solute-free water in the absence of ADH by diluting the urine.
   2. Because cell membranes are permeable to water, cells are in osmotic equilibrium with the fluid that surrounds them. Therefore, by stabilizing body fluid tonicity, **osmoregulation controls cell volume, which** is, in turn, critical for normal cell function.
   3. When plasma osmolality (pOsm) is low, ADH release is suppressed and dilute urine should be produced.
   4. **When hypovolemia is present concurrently with low plasma osmolality (pOsm),** however, **ADH will still be released** despite the signal from low pOsm not to release ADH:
      a. ADH release is not as sensitive to hemodynamic stimuli as it is to changes in pOsm.
      b. However, when the hemodynamic stimulus is sufficiently strong, the ADH response will be of greater magnitude than inhibition induced by low pOsm, and ECF volume will be preserved at the expense of further decreased osmolality.
   5. **Plasma sodium concentration is the key determinant of the osmolality of body fluids.** Glucose and urea make minor contributions in normal animals, as reflected in the following equation*:

$$\text{Plasma osmolality} = 2\,[\text{Na}^+]\,(\text{mEq}\,/\,\text{L}) + [\text{glucose}]\,(\text{mg}\,/\,\text{dL})\,/\,18 + [\text{BUN}]\,(\text{mg}\,/\,\text{dL})\,/\,2.8.$$

B. **Water balance is both tightly and briskly regulated:**
   1. Clinicians should become familiar not only with the reference ranges for plasma [Na$^+$] from their laboratory, but also with the mean and variance in the patient population of their practice.
   2. The amount of deviation in the pOsm that would ordinarily alter ADH and thirst in an individual animal is lesser in magnitude than laboratory normal ranges (e.g., a 1–2% change in osmolality is sufficient to induce or suppress thirst).
   3. Because laboratory reference ranges are often wider than differences that are important for **clinical decision-making, trends in [Na$^+$] even while still inside the published range may be important.**
   4. Changes in pOsm result in rapid, that is, within minutes, changes in thirst and ADH secretion.
C. **Hyponatremia is usually, but not exclusively, associated with hypoosmolality. Exceptions are pseudohyponatremia and translocational hyponatremia** secondary to hyperglycemia or the presence of

---

*   This equation is a simplification because it does not account for the fact that plasma is only 93% water, that sodium salts are incompletely dissociated in solution, that some anions are polyvalent, or that Ca^{++}, Mg^{++}, and K$^+$ salts also contribute. However, these factors cancel out numerically, allowing 2 [Na$^+$] to be used as an estimate of the osmotic effect of the plasma ions.

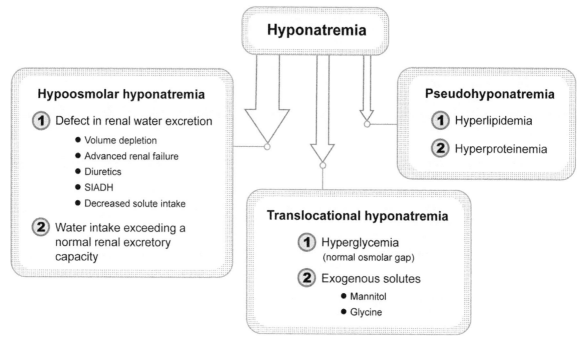

Figure 44.1 Mechanistic localization of hyponatremia (From James KM, Lunn KF. Normal and abnormal water balance: Hyponatremia and hypernatremia. *Comp Cont Educ Pract* 2007;29(10):589–609).

exogenous osmoles, for example, mannitol, in which alternative osmoles are present in large concentration (Figure 44.1):

1. **Normal or elevated effective measured serum osmolality suggests either pseudohyponatremia or translational hyponatremia:**
    a. The distinction of "effective" is used because blood urea nitrogen (BUN) is an ineffective osmole and does not contribute to tonicity.
    b. An effective measured serum osmolality is determined by subtracting serum urea nitrogen, in mmol/L, from measured pOsm. To covert from US units to SI, divide BUN measured in mg/dL by 2.801.
2. **Pseudohyponatremia reflects an *in vitro* artifact** observed when measuring serum [Na+] by flame photometry in the presence of elevated plasma lipid or protein concentration:
    a. In these situations, the measured [Na+] is lower than the true [Na+].
    b. Although newer ion-selective electrodes have largely eliminated this problem in undiluted samples, the terminology persists as a way to distinguish this *in vitro* phenomenon from clinically significant hyponatremia.
3. **Translocational hyponatremia** may be divided into **two categories:**
    a. Conditions in which the measured and calculated serum osmolalities are the same (hyperglycemia).
    b. Conditions in which an osmolar gap is present and measured osmolality is greater than calculated.
        1) In this case, some osmoles are clearly present and are measured, but their identity is not known.
        2) Unidentified osmoles may include mannitol, glycine, and alcohols such as ethanol and ethylene glycol. Only impermeant solutes (e.g., glucose in the absence of insulin, mannitol, glycine) will lead to water translocation from inside to outside cells and cause hyponatremia.
D. For true **hypoosmolar hyponatremia,** two principal pathophysiologic mechanisms exist, which underlie the approach to the problem diagnostically:
    1. **The first mechanism** is impaired renal excretion of free water or, in other words, **impaired diluting ability.** In this situation, the animal is unable to excrete maximally dilute urine (urine osmolality <100 mOsm/L).

2. **Several disease states and conditions can be associated with impaired renal diluting capacity** and impaired free water excretion:

    a. **Hypovolemia** impairs renal diluting ability. It can reflect absolute volume depletion caused by gastrointestinal, skin, or renal losses or, alternatively, be present in high volume edematous states associated with reduced effective plasma volume:

        1) Whenever absolute or effective plasma volume is decreased, the ensuing reduced renal perfusion limits the quantity of glomerular filtrate reaching the diluting segment of the kidneys.

        2) In volume depletion, sodium conservation in the proximal nephrons is enhanced and less sodium reaches the thick ascending limb of Henle's loop.

        3) ADH may also be released in response to volume depletion, overriding the effect of the hypotonicity (which would normally inhibit ADH release), and compounding the defect in water excretion. This override to the control of ADH secretion—where control of hypovolemia and avoidance of shock outranks hyponatremia—occurs in patients with Addison's disease or renal salt wasting.

        4) Similarly, gastrointestinal sodium losses in a patient that is still drinking water will result in hypovolemic hyponatremia.

    b. Another disease state associated with impaired diluting ability is **advanced renal failure, that is, IRIS stage IV or a GFR <10% of normal,** in which the ability to excrete water is approximately 20% of that of normal, healthy kidneys. In early and moderate renal failure, the kidneys retain some tubular function and thus meaningful diluting capacity, albeit somewhat less than normal.

    c. In contrast to hypovolemia, where the ADH elevations are appropriate (i.e., to prevent hypovolemic shock), **the syndrome of inappropriate ADH secretion (SIADH)** refers to conditions in which the ADH elevation leading to hyponatremia is not a consequence of volume depletion:

        1) Urine [Na^+] in SIADH patients is expected to be greater than $20\,mEq/L$, indicating no volume depletion.

        2) SIADH, although well described in humans, is rarely reported in dogs or cats and in some cases may reflect incorrectly diagnosed renal salt wasting (also called cerebral salt wasting).

        3) SIADH in humans may be associated with the following conditions: (1) ectopic ADH production (by certain neoplasms), (2) administration of exogenous ADH or oxytocin, (3) enhanced hypothalamic ADH secretion (due to neuropsychiatric disorders, drugs, or pulmonary disease), or (4) potentiation of ADH effects (due to drugs).

        4) SIADH in dogs has been reported associated with neurological diseases, including hydrocephalus and meningoencephalitis. It has been tentatively diagnosed and reported in other clinical patients, but confirming that these patients were not hypovolemic is difficult.

    d. Certain **diuretics,** such as loop diuretics or thiazides, impair renal water excretion because they decrease sodium transport in the diluting segment of the nephron.

    e. Decreased renal diluting ability is also reported with **highly reduced dietary solute intake:**

        1) One feature that distinguishes this cause of decreased free water excretory capacity from others is that the urine osmolality (uOsm) will be $<100\,mOsm/L$.

        2) This scenario occurs with the practice of "beer potomania" in humans, a syndrome in which individuals consume large quantities of beer (which is hypoosmolar) with inadequate food intake, leading to insufficient dietary solute and impaired ability to excrete free water. Such an occurrence would be highly unexpected in dogs or cats.

3. The **second principal mechanism for development of hypoosmolar hyponatremia,** which is a less common cause of hyponatremia, is when **water intake exceeds maximal renal excretory capacity:**

    a. Renal diluting capacity is adequate in normal circumstances to keep pace with even ardent drinkers. **Thus, most primary polydipsias, including behavioral, do not result in overt hyponatremia.**

    b. In humans, hyponatremia may be seen with the polydipsia that may accompany psychosis.

    c. Perhaps it is valid to make a similar distinction in dogs with so-called **psychogenic polydipsia:**

        1) Those with primary behavioral polydipsia sufficient to cause dilute urine would be judged to have routine behavioral polydipsia.

2) Those with primary polydipsia sufficient to cause the medical complication of hyponatremia would be assessed to have *obsessive polydipsia*. The latter situation is **more common in nervous or hyperactive dogs** that respond to the stress of confinement or boredom by drinking obsessively. Such dogs usually have a hyposthenuric urine-specific gravity (USG) and mild hyponatremia.

4. The **kidneys are ordinarily highly efficient in excreting a water load:**

   a. Thus, patients with primary polydipsia are more likely to have overt hyponatremia when impaired renal water excretion is present concurrently.

   b. It is **important clinically to assess primary polydipsic patients with hyponatremia for concurrent renal diluting defects** such as inappropriate or abnormally regulated ADH secretion before assuming obsessive polydipsia is the sole mechanistic reason for hyponatremia.

II. Signalment

A. There is **no specific signalment associated with hyponatremia itself.** However, some diseases characterized by hyponatremia are overrepresented for certain signalments.

B. Dogs belonging to breeds that require a high level of daily exercise and stimulation may be more prone to boredom and compulsive drinking behavior.

C. Some dog breeds are at higher risk for diabetes mellitus, including females and members of certain breeds (Australian Terriers, Samoyeds, Swedish Elkhounds, and Swedish Lapphunds) and are thus at risk for translational hyponatremia; however, the risk of hyponatremia depends solely on the presence of hyperglycemia.

D. Addison's disease, which is often but not invariably associated with hyponatremia, is overrepresented in certain breeds including West Highland white terriers, standard poodles, great Danes, and bearded collies. Young to middle-aged dogs are predisposed.

III. Clinical Signs

A. The **clinical signs of hyponatremia** arise from its effects on the CNS. Reduction of the plasma [Na$^+$] **causes water to move intracellularly from the ECF.** Signs result from osmotic cerebral edema: **lethargy, confusion, nausea, vomiting, seizures, and coma:**

   1. In contrast to most other types of cerebral edema in which the fluid accumulation is extracellular, hyponatremia results in brain cell swelling.

   2. **Development of clinical signs depends on both the magnitude of hyponatremia and its rate of development; signs of chronic hyponatremia are generally more subtle and nonspecific** than are those of acute hyponatremia.

B. Mild hyponatremia, when not associated with hypovolemia, **may be asymptomatic.**

C. Dogs with obsessive behavioral polydipsia sufficient to cause hyponatremia will have marked polyuria and polydipsia.

D. Patients with hyponatremia may have **myriad other clinical signs depending on their underlying disease.**

IV. Diagnosis

A. As a **first step** in the diagnostic approach to the problem of hyponatremia, pseudohyponatremia and translational hyponatremia should be eliminated from consideration:

   1. **Evaluation of the blood sample** for lipemia and assessment of the plasma protein concentration **can rapidly rule out pseudohyponatremia.**

   2. **Translocational hyponatremia** is easily dismissed by assessment of serum glucose concentration and the absence of a history of administration of an exogenous solute, such as mannitol; it can be confirmed by determining that the effective measured pOsm is not normal or increased.

B. If the above are ruled out, clinicians are then left to answer the question **"Why is there too much water?"** Recalling the mechanisms whereby hyponatremia develops, **clinicians must distinguish primary polydipsia exceeding renal excretory capacity from impaired diluting capacity (impaired water excretion),** although the two may exist simultaneously:

   1. Patients with **primary polydipsia** of sufficient severity to cause hyponatremia are expected to have a **USG less than 1.008.**

   2. It is uncommon for an animal to ingest sufficient water quickly enough to exceed the diluting capacity of healthy kidneys. As soon as pOsm falls, thirst is inhibited. However, **for dogs with obsessive**

behavioral polydipsia, the history is often informative. Upon questioning, the owners may report that the pet is "high strung," easily bored, or left alone for long periods:

    a. Suspicion of obsessive behavioral polydipsia is often easily confirmed by doing an **"entertainment test"** to see whether the USG, particularly the first one of the morning, will become concentrated if the dog is kept very busy and always entertained for a period of a few days:

        1) It is important for such testing that the client always provides the dog something more interesting to do than drink water, but water should always be available.

        2) This method of ruling in primary polydipsia is often easier and far less expensive than a gradual water deprivation test. It **can be done at home by clients using refractometers provided on loan.**

        3) An entertainment test **may also rule in primary behavioral polydipsia in patients whose thirst is not sufficient to cause hyponatremia.**

    b. **Gradual water deprivation tests** can also be done to confirm a suspicion of primary polydipsia:

        1) The author's preferred approach is to measure the daily water intake when the dog is drinking its usual amount.

        2) Then on subsequent days, decrease the volume by 4–5% per day, while maintaining a consistent feeding and exercise schedule.

        3) Each morning of the test, the patient should be weighed and the USG, plasma [Na^+], and BUN measured.

        4) The test is stopped when the dog concentrates the urine to greater than 1.035 (confirms primary polydipsia) or any of monitored parameters suggest ECF volume depletion (diagnosis is the patient has primary polyuria).

        5) **Azotemia is an absolute contraindication** to starting or continuing the test.

3. **Other primary polydipsias,** such as accompany hepatic encephalopathy or Cushing's syndrome (where polyuria and polydipsia can both be simultaneously primary) **rarely cause overt hyponatremia** in the presence of normal renal diluting capacity.

4. The patient should be carefully **assessed for ECF volume depletion on physical examination because the presence or absence of volume depletion will be critical to the choice of therapy:**

    a. ECF volume depletion can exist at a level of up to at least 5% loss of body weight without detectable clinical signs in some animals.

    b. As **clinical estimates of body fluid deficits can be inaccurate,** the patient history should be carefully scrutinized for clues to suggest excess gastrointestinal or urinary fluid loss by asking about whether vomiting, diarrhea, or an increased urine volume are known to be present.

    c. The plasma [Na^+] does not provide any measurement of the total amount of sodium in the ECF, and therefore does not reflect the ECF or total body fluid volume. Thus, the **plasma [Na^+] cannot be used to determine if the patient is hypovolemic. The sodium content, and thus the total fluid volume of the body, can be normal, increased, or decreased with hyponatremia.**

    d. Echocardiography and detection of lower than normal chamber volumes for the patient's size may provide support for the presence of hypovolemia, particularly in cats.

5. For more difficult cases, **laboratory evaluation which includes pOsm, uOsm, and urine [Na^+] may help clinicians to distinguish between impaired water excretion and primary polydipsia:**

    a. Hyponatremic animals with a uOsm > 100 mOsm/L have impaired water excretion.

    b. A decreased pOsm together with a uOsm < 100 mOsm/L suggests primary polydipsia (when polyuria is present) or low solute intake (in which case a recognizable increase in urine volume may be noteworthily absent).

    c. As decreased solute intake is rare in the veterinary setting, **a low uOsm more typically suggests primary polydipsia.**

6. **A low urinary [Na^+]** (< 20 mEq/L in human patients and likely applicable to dogs) **suggests hypovolemia as the cause of hyponatremia.** Patients with SIADH, diuretic-induced hyponatremia, mineralocorticoid deficiency, renal salt-wasting syndrome, or renal failure should have urine [Na^+] > 20 mEq/L.

7. **Determination of plasma ADH concentration is not reliable** to aid in the diagnosis of SIADH due to erratic secretion of excessive ADH in some cases and possible ADH hypersensitivity in others:

    a. Vasopressin assays exist for research purposes but may not be available clinically.

    b. Furthermore, patients with renal salt-wasting syndrome also have elevated ADH due to the presence of hypovolemia. This creates a diagnostic difficulty in distinguishing these two syndromes when the presence of ECF volume depletion is not clearly evident.

V. Differential Diagnoses

A. **Once laboratory error, pseudohyponatremia, and translocational hyponatremia are excluded, the patient must then have some form of hypoosmolar hyponatremia.**

B. **Primary polydipsia** is abnormal thirst behavior resulting in increased water intake with a compensatory polyuria:

    1. Primary polydipsia is **most commonly seen as a behavioral problem in dogs.**

    2. Primary polydipsia may also partially explain the polydipsia that **can be associated with hyperthyroidism, hepatic encephalopathy, hypercortisolemia, gastrointestinal disease, splenomegaly, or, exceptionally rarely, lower urinary tract infection.**

    3. Primary polydipsia is **comparatively less common in cats**, but the differential diagnoses are expected to be similar. Behavioral polydipsia associated with pleasure drinking from faucets or fountains, particularly with the owner present, is observed in cats but would not be expected to be severe enough to cause hyponatremia.

C. **Differential diagnoses for hyponatremia associated with impaired renal diluting capacity** depend on the presence or absence of hypovolemia:

    1. Hypovolemia results from loss of sodium and water in excess of intake. **Once hypovolemia is established, differentials emerge from the analysis of the source of the loss:**

        a. Both primary and secondary gastrointestinal diseases can result in gastrointestinal loss.

        b. Excess loss through skin should be apparent.

        c. Primary renal losses, a diagnosis supported by the presence of polyuria and polydipsia, can exist due to hypoaldosteronism, hypocortisolism, renal failure, renal salt-wasting syndrome, and chronic renal sodium loss due to diuretics (including the diuretic effect of glycosuria in diabetes).

    2. **Patients with decreased effective plasma volume, but elevated true plasma volume, will have edema, ascites, or effusions** associated with congestive heart failure, liver failure, or renal failure most commonly with proteinuria and hypoalbuminemia.

    3. **Patients with impaired renal diluting capacity without hypovolemia or low effective plasma volume have either SIADH or low dietary solute intake**, both of which are rare. The most common cause of SIADH in veterinary patients may be the use of exogenous DDAVP to treat polyuria/polydipsia in patients that do not have central diabetes insipidus.

    4. **The most clinically difficult assessment may involve distinguishing SIADH (no hypovolemia) from renal salt wasting (with hypovolemia)**, because of the difficulty in determining whether ECF volume depletion is present. In human medicine, differences between the two groups with respect to blood uric acid levels and fractional uric acid excretion may aid in distinguishing them, but such comparisons may not apply to dogs or cats.

VI. Treatment

A. **Empirical treatment for hyponatremia depends primarily on the underlying mechanism.** Thus, the patient's volume status must be assessed to determine appropriate fluid therapy:

    1. **Patients with hypovolemia**(i.e., negative sodium balance) require restoration of the ECF sodium content, repletion will return control of ADH secretion and thirst to osmotic factors, and the kidneys will excrete the excess free water once the diluting defect resulting from the hypovolemia is corrected:

        a. Thus, **patients with hypovolemia can initially be treated safely with isotonic (or very mildly hypertonic to the patient's pOsm) fluid replacement.**

        b. Recall that in a hyponatremic patient, a fluid that is truly isotonic would in fact be of lower osmolality than a fluid that is isotonic for a normal patient. Typical balanced electrolyte solutions are actually mildly hypertonic for hyponatremic patients.

        c. **Fluids that are hypotonic to the patient should always be avoided, as should hypertonic saline, unless death from hypovolemic shock is imminent.**

2. If the patient is not severely hyponatremic, **typical fluid rates for ECF volume restoration** (thus dependent on severity) are appropriate even when fluids mildly hypertonic to the patient are used. However, **the general rule for correction of chronic hyponatremia (i.e., present more than 48 h) of not increasing serum [Na⁺] more than 8 mEq/L/24 h should be applied.**

3. Even if isotonic fluids are used, solute-free water will be excreted once hypovolemia is corrected, and this alone could lead to rapid correction of hyponatremia. **Thus, serial monitoring of serum [Na⁺], approximately every 6 h, is essential** in these patients.

4. Since hypovolemia is a result of fluid losses exceeding intake, **provision must be made in the fluid therapy prescription to meet any ongoing losses** in addition to restoration of deficits until the underlying disease (such as Addison's disease or primary gastrointestinal disease) can be resolved with appropriate specific therapy.

B. **Patients with translocational hyponatremia** may have different fluid needs depending on the osmole involved:

1. The most common clinical scenario is unregulated diabetes mellitus, in which hypovolemia is often present and will need to be corrected. Subsequent initiation of insulin therapy will lower plasma glucose concentration and cause excess ECF water to return to its intracellular location.

2. Serum electrolyte concentrations should be monitored with the therapeutic use of mannitol or ethanol so that burgeoning electrolyte disorders are detected early and overt hyponatremia can be prevented.

C. **Patients with edema, pleural effusion, and/or ascites** have excess ECF sodium content and an even greater excess of ECF water:

1. Therapy is more challenging because these patients have a decreased effective plasma volume and renal mechanisms for sodium retention are stimulated.

2. Correction of hyponatremia **generally requires restriction of water intake to below that of urine output,** which can be very difficult because thirst is stimulated.

3. **Therapy for the primary underlying disorder is required** and, thus, specific therapy to correct the hyponatremia prior to diagnostics is generally not indicated.

D. Patients with hyponatremia secondary to **water intoxication** are rare in veterinary medicine; however, they may have clinical signs related to their hypotonicity:

1. Treatment is generally by **water restriction and careful monitoring.** Water restriction is often self-imposed as the patients have sufficient neurologic deficits that they do not drink.

2. **Serial monitoring of plasma [Na⁺] is necessary to adhere to the rule of not increasing [Na⁺] by more than 8 mEq/L/24 h.** Although uncommon, should the plasma [Na⁺] increase more rapidly than 1 mEq/L every 3 h, free water can be given as part of the maintenance fluid or feeding prescriptions. **Using 50% of a maintenance rate and a maintenance solution is a reasonable starting point.**

3. Tube feeding for provision of calories may be problematic if the tube diameter requires the addition of water to get food through the tube.

E. **In all cases, moderation in therapy should be key:**

1. Serum [Na⁺] should be measured frequently and therapy adjusted to ensure that chronic hyponatremia is not corrected by more than 8 mEq/L/day.

2. Although there are no "rules" for how frequently to monitor (and frequency may decrease as severely affected patients improve), **a central venous catheter to allow frequent sampling and monitoring as often as every 3–4 h is recommended initially.**

F. Disease syndromes associated with hyponatremia may have their own primary treatment:

1. Long-term management of dogs with **primary polydipsia** centers on **behavioral modifications. Water restriction may be required in some cases, but must be done judiciously** because the water requirements of dogs can change dramatically depending on heat, humidity, and lifestyle.

2. Vasopressin receptor antagonists have been studied in dogs with **SAIDH** with partial effect. Renal water excretion is improved. However, hyponatremia may not be fully corrected without concurrent water restriction. Oral urea has been used successfully in humans with SIADH.

3. **Hypoadrenocorticism** is treated with mineralocorticoid and/or glucocorticoid replacement therapy.

4. Other forms of renal salt wasting are treated with salt supplementation:

a. Such patients are highly variable in their salt requirements.

b. The author has salted the patient's food (in amounts similar to how a person who likes salt might add salt for taste) and increased the amount based on results of frequent monitoring. Because of the negative effect of salt on appetite and its ability to induce vomiting, small but very frequent dosing is the preferred approach.

VII. Prognosis

A. Prognosis for **mild hyponatremia** is **generally favorable** because the risk for adverse neurological sequelae upon correction is minimal.

B. Prognosis for **severe, symptomatic hyponatremia** is **guarded**; however, some patients can recover normal neurological function if correction of their hyponatremia is done carefully and deliberately.

C. Prognosis in all cases of hyponatremia is **influenced by the presence of associated diseases.**

VIII. Prevention

A. Hyponatremia associated with overzealous use of hypotonic fluid therapy is prevented with careful and appropriate fluid therapy planning and sequential monitoring.

B. Hyponatremia secondary to primary polydipsia is usually prevented with behavioral enrichment and modification:

1. Water restriction is necessary for severe cases but must be done with extreme care.

2. The volume of water a dog must drink to keep up with insensible fluid losses varies greatly with changes in environment conditions and lifestyle.

References and Further Readings

Black RM. Diagnosis and management of hyponatremia. *J Intens Care Med* 1989;4:205–220.

Chastain CB, Panciera D. Syndrome of inappropriate secretion of antidiuretic hormone in a dog with meningoencephalitis. *Sm Anim Clin Endocrinol* 2004;14(1):5–6.

Churcher RK, Watson ADJ, Eaton A. Suspected myelinolysis following rapid correction of hyponatremia in a dog. *JAAHA* 1999;35:493–497.

DiBartola SP. Disorders of sodium and water: Hypernatremia and hyponatremia. In: DiBartola SP, ed. *Fluid, Electrolyte, and Acid-Base Disorders in Small Animal Practice*, 3rd edn. St. Louis: Saunders, 2006, pp. 47–79.

Fall T, Hansson Hamlin H, Hedhammar A, et al. Diabetes mellitus in a population of 180,000 insured dogs: incidence, survival, and breed distribution. *J Vet Intern Med* 2007;21(6):1209–1216.

Fleeman LM, Irwin PJ, Phillips PA, et al. Effects of an oral vasopressin receptor antagonist (OPC-31260) in a dog with syndrome of inappropriate secretion of antidiuretic hormone. *Aust Vet J* 2000;78(12):825–830.

James KM, Lunn KF. Normal and abnormal water balance: Hyponatremia and hypernatremia. *Comp Cont Educ Pract* 2007;29(10):589–609.

Laureno R, Karp BI. Myelinolysis after correction of hyponatremia. *Ann Int Med* 1997;126(1):57–56.

Lunn KF, James KM. Normal and abnormal water balance: Polyuria and polydipsia. Comp Cont Educ Pract 2007; 29(10):612–624.

Milionis HJ, Liamis GL, Elisaf MS. The hyponatremic patient: A systematic approach to laboratory diagnosis. *CMAJ* 2002; 166 (8):1056–1062.

O'Brien DP. CNS effects of sodium imbalances. *Proceedings of the 24th ACVIM Forum*, 2006, pp. 323–324.

O'Brien DP, Kroll RA, Johnson GC, et al. Myelinolysis after correction of hyponatremia in two dogs. *J Vet Int Med* 1994;8(1):40–48.

Shiel RE, Pinilla M, Mooney CT. Syndrome of inappropriate antidiuretic hormone secretion associated with congenital hydrocephalus in a dog. *J Am Anim Hosp Assoc* 2009;45(5):249–252.

Sterns RH, Ocdol H, Schrier RW, et al. (1994) Hyponatremia: pathophysiology, diagnosis, and therapy. In: Narins RG, ed. *Maxwell and Kleeman's Clinical Disorders of Fluid and Electrolyte Metabolism*, New York: McGraw-Hill, 1994, pp. 583–615.

Sterns RH, Spital A, Clark AC. Disorders of water balance. In: Kokko JP, Tannen RL, eds. *Fluids and Electrolytes*, Philadelphia: WB Saunders, 1996, pp. 63–109.

Tyler RD, Qualls CW Jr, Heald RD, et al. Renal concentrating ability in dehydrated hyponatremic dogs. *J Am Vet Med Assoc* 1987;191(9):1095–1100.

CHAPTER 45

Estrogen- and Androgen-Related Disorders

Cheri A. Johnson

Unique Considerations for Correct Assessment of Sex Hormone Excess or Deficiency

A. **Normal reproductive endocrinology** and **physiology vary greatly** according to the **species**, the stage of the estrous **cycle in females,** the presence of one versus two **functional testes in males,** and in both sexes, according to the **neuter status** (sexually intact versus gonadectomy).

B. The **endocrine laboratory** must determine, validate, and provide its **normal ranges** of the **reproductive hormones** for sexually mature animals according to **species,** according to the **stage of the estrous cycle** in females, and according to the **neuter status** in both males and females.

C. **Gonadectomy** is the most common cause of **low concentrations of sex steroid hormones. Primary testicular or ovarian failure** and **hypogonadotropic hypogonadism** are **rarely documented** in dogs and cats.

D. In **dogs and cats, a gonadal source of excess sex steroid hormones is far more likely** than is an **adrenal source.** Exogenous sources, such as **inadvertent exposure to human birth control** or **hormone replacement medications,** should also be considered.

Testicular neoplasia
Ovarian follicular cysts
Ovarian remnant
Vaginal hyperplasia-prolapse
Mammary neoplasia
Benign prostatic hyperplasia
Perineal hernia
Perineal adenoma
Post-spay/neuter effects
Post-spay urinary incontinence

ESTROGEN-RELATED DISORDERS

I. Pathogenesis (General)

A. **All endogenous estrogen** is **synthesized from androgens** (Figure 45.1) via an irreversible reaction catalyzed by aromatase (cytochrome P-450 19).

B. The **primary source of estrogen is the gonads**:

 1. **Females:**

  a. The **ovarian follicular theca cells produce androgens** that are aromatized to estradiol by the follicular granulosa cells.

  b. **Estrogen production** represents the **follicular phase** of the **ovarian cycle.**

  c. **Estrogen actions:**

   1) **Stimulates growth** of **mammary ductal epithelium** and connective tissue.

   2) **Stimulates growth, blood supply,** and water retention in the **uterus, vagina,** and **vulva;** these, in turn, cause the **vulvar swelling and sanguineous discharge** associated with **proestrus and estrus** ("heat" or "season") in bitches.

   3) Causes **cornification** of **vaginal** and preputial **epithelium.**

   4) Causes the **behavioral changes** necessary for breeding, which include increased vocalization (queens), and increased receptivity to males, eventually allowing copulation (bitches and queens).

   5) Estrogens **increase the frequency and magnitude of gonadotropin pulsatility** until the **LH surge occurs.**

   6) **Luteinizing hormone (LH)** causes the **ovarian follicles to ovulate and become corpora lutea (CLs),** which produce progesterone. (This represents the **luteal** phase of the ovarian cycle).

  d. **Estrus:**

   1) **Bitches** typically cycle only **once every 6–8 months.** Heat lasts an average of 18 days (range from 6 to 38 days) and is followed by a luteal phase (progesterone) lasting more than 60 days even in nonpregnant bitches. **The CLs produce progesterone throughout gestation, which averages 63 days.**

   2) **Cats,** being **induced to ovulate by coital stimulation,** have multiple anovulatory cycles lasting about 6 days and occurring every 14–21 days throughout the breeding season (photoperiod of ≥12h of light) if they are not breed. Some cats do ovulate without coital stimulation. **When a cat**

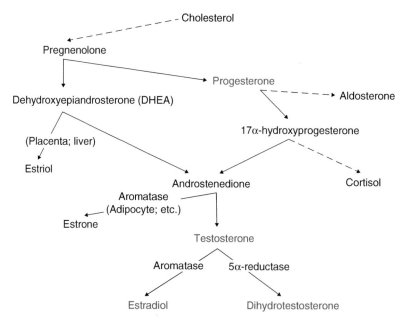

Figure 45.1   Schematic representation of steroidogenesis. Dashed arrows indicate multiple intervening steps.

ovulates but does not conceive, CLs produce **progesterone for only 30–50 days**. The CLs produce progesterone throughout the 65 day gestation.

2. **Males:**

a. In the **testes, Leydig cells (interstitial cells) produce testosterone**, some of which is **aromatized to estradiol by the Sertoli cells**, and/or by the Leydig cells themselves, and/or by the germ cells, depending on the species of animal.

3. **Extra-gonadal estrogen production:**

a. Estrogens (estradiol, estrone, estriol) are also formed by **aromatization of androgens in adrenal, brain, prostate, breast, bone, liver, and adipose tissue.** Aromatase has only intracellular function, converting intracellular androgens to intracellular estrogen. However, the liver and adipocytes contribute **small amounts to systemic estrogen** concentrations as well.

C. **Estrogen receptors (ER):**

1. There are **two estrogen receptors, α and β**, that have both overlapping and distinct functions.

2. Estrogen receptors have **different tissue distribution and binding affinity.** The estrogenic effects may be enhanced in some tissues and suppressed in others. There is also variation among species.

Hyperestrogenism

Pathogenesis

- Hyperestrogenism occurs most commonly as a result of excessive production of estrogen by testicular tumors in male dogs, particularly Sertoli cell tumor, and by ovarian follicular cysts or ovarian remnants in females.
- An adrenal source of estrogen that is the cause of clinical signs of hyperestrogenism has not been documented in dogs or cats.
- Exogenous estrogen could cause similar clinical signs.

Classical Signs

- Bilaterally symmetrical alopecia, hyperpigmentation, and lichenification in male and female dogs. This has not been reported in cats.
- Gynecomastia, pendulous prepuce, testicular mass, atrophy of the contralateral testis, infertility, and signs associated with prostatomegaly in male dogs. This has not been reported in cats.
- Vulvar swelling and sanguineous discharge typical of proestrus/estrus in bitches, and behavioral signs of estrus in both bitches and queens. Persistent estrus and ovulation failure in intact females with cystic follicles. Resumption of estrous cycles in spayed females with ovarian remnant.

Diagnosis

- Clinical signs consistent with estrogenic effects.
- Vaginal or preputial cytology demonstrating cornified epithelial cells.
- Low serum concentrations of LH.
- Testicular tumor found by palpation or ultrasound in male dogs.
- Ovarian remnant or cystic follicles found by ultrasound in female dogs and cats.

Treatment

- Remove the source of estrogen.

I. Pathogenesis

A. The **estrogen source** is the **gonads** in almost all cases:

1. **Males:**

     a. Sertoli cell tumors are the most common cause of hyperestrogenism; however, **neoplastic Leydig cells** (interstitial cell tumor) and **germ cells** (seminoma) occasionally also produce pathologic amounts of estrogen.

     b. Testicular neoplasia is **more common in cryptorchid testes** than in scrotal testes.

     c. Testicular neoplasia is extremely **rare in cats.**

  2. **Females:**

     a. **Ovarian follicular cysts** produce estradiol and cause **persistent heat.**

     b. **"Spayed" bitches** and queens with **ovarian remnants may resume cycling.**

     c. **Ovarian neoplasia is rare in dogs and cats,** and clinical signs are typically not related to excessive hormone production. However, hormone-producing granulosa cell tumors have been reported in ovarian remnants as well as intact ovaries.

B. **Extra-gonadal sources:**

  1. There have been **no conclusive reports of excessive adrenal production of estrogens** that are the **cause of clinical signs of hyperestrogenism** in dogs or cats with adrenal disease.

  2. In normal male and female dogs, intact or neutered, serum concentrations of estradiol remain in the normal basal range in response to adrenocorticotropic hormone (ACTH) administration.

C. **Exogenous estrogens:**

  1. These could cause **similar clinical signs** as endogenous hyperestrogenism, including **persistent estrus in females, but resumption of cyclic estrous activity would be very unlikely.**

  2. Several plant compounds, known as **phytoestrogens,** have estrogenic activity. One group of phytoestrogens, isoflavones, is found in **soybeans,** which are a common ingredient in **commercial dog foods.** Although the concentrations of phytoestrogens in soy-containing dog food are high enough to have biologic effects, clinical hyperestrogenism has yet to be documented.

  3. **Transdermal medications** and **topical creams containing estrogen for birth control** or treatment of postmenopausal symptoms in women have been implicated as an inadvertent source of estrogen for pets.

II. Signalment

A. **Old, intact male dogs with testicular tumors** have a mean **age of about 10 years.** Testicular tumors are extremely **rare in cats.**

B. **Young, intact female dogs and cats with ovarian follicular cysts,** during their **first or second estrous cycle(s).**

C. Female dogs and cats with ovarian remnants are of any age, and any time (weeks to years) after having been spayed.

III. Clinical Signs

A. **Testicular tumors secreting estrogen:**

  1. Most common clinical signs in dogs are **dermatologic** including **bilaterally symmetrical, non-pruritic alopecia, hyperpigmentation, and lichenification,** with signs of "feminization": **gynecomastia and pendulous prepuce.**

  2. On further evaluation, a **testicular mass** with **atrophy of the contralateral testis** and **decreased fertility** are also found. Tumors are **more common in cryptorchid testes than scrotal testes.**

  3. Testicular tumors are extremely **rare in cats.**

B. **Ovarian follicular cysts:**

  1. Most common clinical sign is persistent heat (proestrus + estrus), lasting longer than 35–40 days in bitches or longer than 16 days in queens.

  2. The **cysts are typically anovulatory** but ovulation occasionally occurs and may lead to mammary development typical of luteal activity (i.e., progesterone).

C. **Ovarian remnants in spayed females:**

  1. More common in bitches than in queens.

  2. Most common clinical sign is return to estrous cycling months to years after ovariohysterectomy (range 1 month to 10 years, with a median of 17 months).

  3. Bitches with ovarian remnant may have **dermatologic changes** as do males with hyperestrogenism, with or without return of estrous cycles.

D. **Estrogen-induced bone marrow toxicity in dogs:**

1. Clinical signs associated with estrogen-induced bone marrow toxicity include **pallor, weakness and lethargy (anemia), bleeding (thrombocytopenia), or fever and bacterial infections (neutropenia).**

E. **Less common findings:**

1. **Prostatomegaly** due to estrogen-induced prostatic squamous metaplasia. The most common sign is **tenesmus,** but prostatomegaly may be an asymptomatic incidental finding.
2. **Mammary tumors.**
3. **Cystic endometrial hyperplasia and pyometra:**
    a. Often occurs following **estrogen administration** to prevent pregnancy ("mismating").
    b. May also occur as a result of persistent **estrogen** production from **ovarian follicular cysts or ovarian remnants.**
4. **Vaginal hyperplasia-prolapse.**

IV. Diagnosis

A. The **diagnosis of hyperestrogenism** is suspected on the basis of **history and physical examination findings.**

B. **Males:**

1. Because testicular neoplasia is by far the most likely cause, the next step is to confirm the presence of a **testicular tumor.**
2. If one is not found by **palpation** of the scrotal testes, **testicular ultrasound** can be performed.
3. The possibility of **unrecognized cryptorchidism** should be considered for dogs with classic clinical signs, but lacking a solid history of having had two scrotal testes removed at the time of castration. Careful **palpation of the inguinal-scrotal region** and **abdominal ultrasound** can be used.
4. Hyperestrogenism can cause cornification of the preputial epithelium (see vaginal cytology below); however, negative preputial cytology findings do not exclude hyperestrogenism.

C. **Females:**

1. It is usually important to **confirm that hyperestrogenism exists** and could reasonably be the cause of the clinical signs.
2. This is most easily accomplished with **vaginal cytology** demonstrating a high percentage of **cornified epithelial cells as with proestrus and estrus:**
    a. **Absence of cornification** does **not exclude the possibility of estrogen** as the cause of the clinical signs.
    b. For accurate interpretation, **vaginal cytology** should be performed when cycling females are actually **displaying signs of heat.** Between cycles, estrogen concentrations are low, and the vaginal epithelium will be primarily non-cornified.
    c. Some bitches with hyperestrogenism have **dermatologic signs** but are **not cycling.** Results of **vaginal cytology** are then **variable.**
3. **Abdominal ultrasound:**
    a. **Abdominal ultrasound** is used to **confirm the presence of cystic ovary(ies)** in intact females with persistent estrus.
    b. With skill, ultrasound is also very useful for finding **ovarian remnants** in spayed females.
4. **Serum LH concentrations** can be used to identify females with **ovarian remnants:**
    a. Gonadal sex hormones suppress LH from the pituitary via negative feedback (Figure 45.2).
    b. Therefore, a **finding of low LH concentration confirms** the presence of a **gonad (or, much less likely, exogenous sex hormones).**
    c. In the absence of ovaries and the hormones they produce, there is no negative feedback and **serum LH** concentrations will be **elevated.**
    d. During estrus, the LH surge (i.e., high LH concentrations) induces the ovaries to ovulate.
    e. Thus, a finding of **high LH** indicates either the female has **no ovarian tissue** or she has ovarian tissue, is in heat, and is **about to ovulate.** The latter can be confirmed by physical and behavioral signs of estrus, vaginal cytology, **repeating the LH assay in a day or two, or by measuring** progesterone.
5. **Serum progesterone concentrations:**
    a. **After ovulation,** the ovarian follicles **become CLs and produce progesterone.**
    b. The finding of **serum progesterone concentrations > 3 ng/mL (9 nmol/L)** at least **5–7 days after the signs of heat have abated** confirms the presence of an ovary.

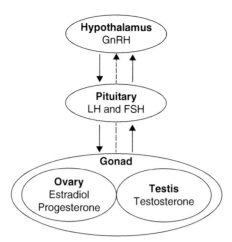

Figure 45.2 Schematic representation of the hypothalamic–pituitary–gonadal axis and feedback loops. Dashed line indicates direct feedback from gonad to hypothalamus.

    c. The advantage of measuring progesterone is that it can be done days or weeks after the female is no longer showing the clinical signs suspected to represent heat:
      1) **In normal bitches,** progesterone may remain elevated for as **long as 60 days,** but by then serum concentrations will be approaching those of anestrus or spayed females.
      2) In **queens, serum progesterone** concentration will **only be increased if ovulation occurred,** which usually requires coital stimulation. If a queen does ovulate, **progesterone** may remain **elevated for 30–40 days** in the absence of pregnancy.
    d. **Low progesterone** concentrations have **no diagnostic significance.** They could represent:
      1) Normal anestrus in an animal with ovaries, or the true absence of ovarian tissue in a spayed animal.
      2) Absence of **sufficient** coital stimulation to cause the LH surge and induce ovulation in a queen.
      3) An ovarian **remnant** that does not respond normally to LH (ovulation failure), or, if it does, corpus luteal function does not continue normally (premature luteolysis).
    e. **Induction of ovulation** to **confirm ovarian remnant** may be attempted during estrus by **administration of gonadotropin releasing hormone (GnRH) or** human **chorionic gonadotropin (hCG):**
      1) They mimic (hCG) or induce (GnRH) LH. Consultation with the endocrinology laboratory is recommended because the dosage and sampling protocols vary among laboratories. **Typically, GnRH, 25 µg per cat,** or **25–100 µg per dog,** (or **2.2 µg/kg), IM, induces ovulation during estrus** in normal females.
      2) **Response to GnRH or hCG varies** according to the stage of the ovarian cycle. For this reason, the **results do not reliably confirm or deny the presence of an ovarian remnant.** When given during estrus, ovulation is expected. When a single dose is given during anestrus, ovulation is unlikely to occur.
      3) If GnRH or hCG **successfully** induce ovulation, **5–7 days later progesterone** concentrations rise above **3 ng/mL (9 nmol/L) and confirm the presence of ovarian tissue.**
      4) **Lack of response** (i.e., low progesterone) could indicate that the female was not actually in estrus when the drug was administered, or any of the explanations for low progesterone concentrations listed above.
D. Measurement of **serum estradiol** concentrations usually is **not helpful to** differentiate **normal from pathologic** conditions in dogs.
E. A **hematology** evaluation should be performed in dogs with hyperestrogenism to evaluate for **estrogen-induced bone marrow suppression.**

V. Differential Diagnoses
A. In male and female dogs, **other causes of alopecia and hyperpigmentation** should be considered.
B. In **female** dogs, other causes of sanguineous vulvar discharge, such as **pyometra,** or **vaginal or uterine neoplasia** can be differentiated on the basis of the following:

1. **If pyometra is present,** neutrophilic inflammation and bacteria will be found on vaginal cytology.
2. **Hemorrhage** (i.e., red blood cells) will typically be the primary cytologic finding with neoplasia because the most common tumor, leiomyoma, does not readily exfoliate.

C. In **female cats, the normal frequent estrous cycles** that occur every 14–21 days might be confused with abnormal persistent estrus caused by cystic ovarian follicles.

D. In female cats, **behavior** such as urinating outside the litter box (suspected marking territory), and increased affectionate behavior or excessive vocalization, which have a variety of potential causes, could be **erroneously attributed to estrus behavior.**

VI. Treatment

A. **Treatment consists of removing the estrogen source.**

B. Ovarian remnant:
   1. Whenever possible, the **suspicion of ovarian remnant** should be supported by endocrine findings such as **cornified vaginal epithelium,** or **low LH,** or **high progesterone,** or confirmed with **ultrasound** before exploratory laparotomy is undertaken.
   2. The ovarian remnant will be located in the **typical location** for **ovaries** and the **ovarian pedicle.** Although experimental studies in normal bitches and queens have demonstrated that ovarian tissue sutured into the mesentery may revascularize, the published evidence from spontaneously occurring clinical cases of spayed bitches and queens with ovarian remnants examined at diagnostic laboratories and in surgical practices shows that the **remnants are in the typical location** for ovaries and are not ectopic:
       a. **Remnant ovaries** may be **unilateral or bilateral.**
       b. Remnants can easily be overlooked if the surgical exposure is inadequate.
       c. The remainder of the **reproductive tract** and the **mammary glands** should be **thoroughly evaluated** because **neoplasia** of the reproductive tract is commonly (33%) found in animals with ovarian remnants.

C. Testicular neoplasia:
   1. **Castration is recommended,** regardless of tumor type and whether or not hyperestrogenism is present. Therefore, confirmation of hyperestrogenism need not be done pre-operatively when a testicular tumor is found.
   2. On the other hand, if a **neoplastic cryptorchid testis** is suspected, its **existence** should be **confirmed** if possible prior to exploratory laparotomy.
   3. Unilateral castration of the affected testis could be considered for a dog that still has value as a stud.
   4. The testicle should be submitted for **histopathologic evaluation.**

D. Ovarian follicular cysts:
   1. May **resolve spontaneously,** but watchful **waiting of persistent estrus** should not continue for very long (perhaps only **2 months**) because of the **adverse effects** of **estrogen on the uterus** increasing susceptibility to **pyometra,** and possibly also on the **bone marrow in bitches.**
   2. **Treatment (GnRH, 2.2 µg/kg, IM, q 24 h for 3 days)** to induce ovulation and interrupt the follicular phase of the cycle has been suggested for bitches, but **results have generally been poor** (effective in 30–50% of cases).
   3. **Ovariohysterectomy is curative:**
       a. Unilateral oophorectomy could be considered for valuable brood stock with unilateral cysts:
           1) Whether the contralateral ovary will then begin normal function will remain to be seen.
           2) Whether **hereditary** factors are involved in the development of cystic ovaries is unknown.

E. Bone marrow suppression:
   1. Should be **treated** with **appropriate supportive care,** such as **blood transfusion** for severe anemia and **prophylactic antibiotic** therapy for severely neutropenic patients.
   2. **Colony-stimulating factor therapy** can also be used. **Lithium** therapy has also been mentioned.

VII. Prognosis

A. **Ovarian remnant:** prognosis for recovery from hyperestrogenism is **excellent** when the **remnant is found and removed. Neoplasia** in other parts of the **reproductive tract** must be addressed.

B. Testicular neoplasia:
   1. Following castration, the prognosis for **recovery from hyperestrogenism** is excellent.

2. If **unilateral castration** is performed in a stud:
   a. **Suppression of gonadotropins** and **spermatogenesis** by the excess estradiol should be **reversible** in an otherwise **healthy dog younger than 10 years of age.**
   b. Older dogs are expected to have an age-related decline in fertility, irrespective of testicular neoplasia.
3. The testicle should be submitted for **histopathologic evaluation:**
   a. If the tumor is **malignant,** staging and appropriate adjunct therapy should be considered in **consultation with a veterinary oncologist.**
   b. Prognosis for malignant testicular tumors is guarded.

C.   **Ovarian follicular cysts causing persistent estrus: prognosis excellent with oophorectomy and poor (50%) for medical management.**

D.   **If bone marrow suppression is present, prognosis is guarded.**

VIII. Prevention

A.   Complete surgical excision of both gonads.

B.   Prevent exposure to exogenous estrogens. For example, transdermal estrogen-containing cream apparently may be transferred from owner's skin to the dog being held in arm or nuzzling face, or by the dog licking owner's skin.

Vaginal Hyperplasia-Prolapse

Pathogenesis

● Vaginal hyperplasia-prolapse in bitches is an unusual response to estrogen that occurs during proestrus or estrus.

Classical Signs

● **Edematous** and/or **hyperplastic mass** protruding from the **vulva of a bitch in heat** (Figure 45.3).

Diagnosis

● Made on the basis of **physical findings** and confirmation that the bitch is in heat.

Differential Diagnoses

● True **vaginal prolapse** that occurs during **parturition.** This would involve the entire vagina.
● **Vaginal neoplasia.** This would not be cyclic in nature.

Treatment

● With rare exceptions, vaginal hyperplasia **resolves spontaneously** within 2 weeks of the end of heat.
● **Ovariohysterectomy is curative.** Vaginal hyperplasia resolves within 7–14 days. Resection of the hyperplastic tissue is usually not necessary.

I.   Pathogenesis

A.   **Vaginal hyperplasia-prolapse** in bitches is an **unusual response to estrogen** that occurs during **proestrus** or **estrus** when **estrogen concentrations are high.**

B.   The **edematous and hyperplastic change** affects a **small portion (1 cm or so)** of the **vaginal floor,** immediately **cranial to the urethral papilla.** Only the edematous, hyperplastic tissues become prolapsed. **The rest of the vagina is normal.**

C.   It occurs during **estrus** and, with rare exceptions, **resolves spontaneously** within days of the end of estrus. Once started, it usually **recurs** during each **subsequent heat.**

D.   Heredity has not been determined, but the condition appears to be familial in nature.

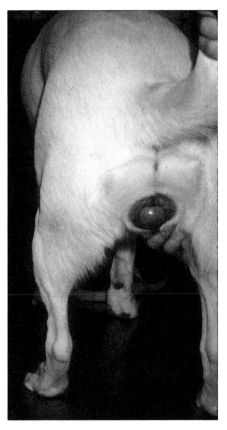

Figure 45.3   Type II vaginal hyperplasia-prolapse in a Labrador retriever.

II.   Signalment
A.   **Young, intact bitch,** usually beginning in **one of her first few cycles** and **recurring** during each **subsequent cycle** thereafter.
B.   **Vaginal hyperplasia has not been reported in queens.**

III.   Clinical Signs
A.   A young bitch that is in heat.
B.   **Type I** is primarily an **edematous smooth mass,** which remains **within the vagina** and **vestibule.** It would likely go unnoticed except that it prevents breeding.
C.   **Type II** is a **large hyperplastic mass protruding** from the **vulva** (Figure 45.3), but arising from a stalk at the same small area of the vaginal floor.
D.   Least often there is **circumferential involvement of the vaginal wall (Type III).**
E.   Although extremely rare, estrogen concentrations may on occasion be sufficiently high at the end of pregnancy that vaginal hyperplasia may recur at that time.

IV.   Diagnosis
A.   Made on the basis of **physical findings** and **confirmation that the bitch is in heat.**

V.   Differential Diagnoses
A.   **True vaginal prolapse** that occurs during **parturition,** not during heat, and involves the entire vagina.
B.   **Vaginal neoplasia,** the appearance of which is **not cyclic in nature.** With the exception of transmissible venereal tumor, vaginal neoplasia is typically a disorder of older bitches.

VI. Treatment

A. With rare exceptions, **vaginal hyperplasia resolves spontaneously within 2 weeks of the end of heat** (estrogen).

B. **Ovariohysterectomy is curative.** Vaginal hyperplasia resolves within 7–14 days unless it has been recurrent for so many cycles that the tissue has also become fibrotic. When that occurs, resection of the hyperplastic tissue in addition to ovariohysterectomy may be necessary.

C. Prolapsed tissue should be protected from trauma and ulceration until regression.

D. In **bitches kept for breeding, artificial insemination** can be used to bypass the hyperplastic tissue, which resolves spontaneously during pregnancy and rarely recurs at parturition.

E. **Surgical excision** of the hyperplastic tissue without ovariohysterectomy **does not prevent recurrence,** but the size during subsequent cycles may be reduced. Excision during estrus requires meticulous hemostasis.

VII. Prognosis

A. **Excellent with ovariohysterectomy.**

B. Left intact, this is **typically a recurrent problem** with subsequent cycles. Due to its recurrent nature, the inconvenience of managing the prolapsed tissue, and a possible genetic basis, affected bitches usually **are not kept in the breeding program.**

VIII. Prevention

A. Ovariectomy.

Mammary Neoplasia

Pathogenesis

- Relative to being intact, ovariohysterectomy (spay) of female dogs and cats prior to 1 year of age is highly protective against future development of mammary neoplasia.
- Mammary neoplasia is rare in males.
- About half of mammary tumors in bitches are benign, whereas in cats they are almost always malignant.
- Malignant mammary tumors metastasize to regional lymph nodes and to the lungs, and may be locally invasive.

Classical Signs

- Nodule or mass in one or more mammary glands, or along the mammary chain, with or without invasion into surrounding tissues.
- Discharge from the nipple.
- Most animals are 10–12 years old and intact, or were spayed after 2 years of age.

Diagnosis

- Highly suspected based on physical findings and signalment. Confirmed by histopathologic evaluation.

Treatment

- Complete surgical excision.
- Adjunct chemotherapy for malignant and metastatic mammary tumors.

I. Pathogenesis

A. **Mammary neoplasia is the most common tumor in female dogs** and the **third most common tumor in queens.**

B. **Estrogen** appears to be the **major hormone involved. Ovariohysterectomy (spay) prior to 1 year of age is highly protective** against future development of mammary neoplasia:

1. The risk of mammary carcinoma is reduced by 91% in cats spayed before 6 months of age, by 86% in cats spayed before 1 year of age, and by 11% in cats spayed between 1 and 2 years of age. After 24 months of age, spaying is not protective.

2. Spaying bitches at or before 1 year of age is significantly protective (odds ration 0.01), and the protective effect diminishes when spayed between 1.1 and 2.5 years of age (odds ratio 0.11) and between 2.6 to 5.0 years of age (odds ratio 0.3).

C. **Treatment** with **exogenous progesterone is a risk factor for mammary carcinoma:**
1. As many as 25% of dogs with mammary tumors are reported to have been treated with progestins. Benign mammary tumors are found in as many as 70% of bitches receiving long-term progestin therapy.
2. Thirty-six percent of male cats with mammary carcinoma had been treated with progestins.

D. In dogs, malignant and benign mammary tumors express estrogen (ER) and progesterone (PR) receptors. A greater proportion of benign tumors express ERα and PR than do malignant tumors. Lack of PR is associated with higher histologic grade, tumor invasion, and metastasis. Conversely, the presence of PR, with or without ERα, is associated with longer 1 year survival after mastectomy. In addition to prognosis, this may have therapeutic implications as it does in women.

E. **Metastasis to local lymph nodes and lungs is common for malignant mammary tumors.**

F. **Feline mammary tumors are usually malignant.**

II. Signalment
A. Most are **females, 10–12 years old.**
B. Most are **intact,** or were **spayed after 2 years of age.**

III. Clinical Signs
A. **Nodule or mass in mammary gland(s) or along mammary chain,** with or without invasion into surrounding tissues.
B. **Discharge from the nipple.**
C. **Local lymph nodes** (axillary, inguinal) may be **enlarged.**
D. Systemic illness or cachexia in animals with advanced cancer.
E. **Inflammatory carcinoma** is characterized by **ulceration** and **extensive invasion into surrounding skin** and soft tissue without distinct nodularity of the mammary tissue.

IV. Diagnosis
A. **Fine needle aspiration** may yield a **cytologic diagnosis of neoplasia.** However, **negative cytologic** evidence for neoplasia **does not exclude the diagnosis.** Inflammation or necrosis may be associated with some tumors, which could lead to a cytologic diagnosis of mastitis should those areas be aspirated.
B. **Histopathologic evaluation** of the mass and its margins is **essential following surgery.**
C. **Evaluation for metastatic disease (local nodes, chest radiographs, abdominal ultrasound).**

V. Differential Diagnoses
A. **Fibroadenomatous mammary hyperplasia** occurs in young, cycling queens and usually affects all glands simultaneously.
B. **Mastitis** causes abnormal milk, and is a postpartum disorder in bitches. Mastitis is extremely rare in queens.

VI. Treatment
A. **Complete surgical excision** of the mass is the mainstay of treatment. Lumpectomy or mastectomy as indicated.
B. **Adjunct chemotherapy for malignant tumors** should be considered in consultation with a veterinary oncologist.
C. **Hormonal therapy** for breast cancer is well established in human medicine. Results vary according to the hormone receptors expressed by the tumor. Many veterinary studies assessing the effects of simultaneous ovariohysterectomy (i.e., hormonal deprivation) and mastectomy lack hormone receptor evaluation of the tumor, making it difficult to draw conclusions regarding efficacy. Therapeutic trials with the selective estrogen-receptor modulator (ERM) tamoxifen have shown undesirable estrogenic effects in dogs.

VII. Prognosis

A. The **prognosis** for **benign mammary tumors following complete excision is excellent.**

B. The **prognosis for malignant tumors** depends upon the size of the tumor, histologic grade, local invasion, and the presence of metastasis.

C. The **prognosis for inflammatory mammary carcinoma is grave.**

VIII. Prevention

A. Ovariectomy prior to first estrous cycle is the most protective against future development of mammary neoplasia.

B. Protective effects of ovariectomy diminish with age as number of estrous cycles experienced increases:
1. By 24 months of age, ovariectomy is no longer protective in queens.
2. By 2.6–5 years of age, the protective effect has decreased to an odds ratio of 0.3 in bitches.

ANDROGEN-RELATED DISORDERS

I. Pathogenesis (General)

A. **Testosterone:**
1. In males, the **primary source of testosterone is the Leydig (interstitial) cells of the testes.**
2. In females, **testosterone is made in the theca cells of the ovarian follicles** and promptly **converted to estradiol in the granulosa cells.**
3. Small amounts are made in the adrenal gland.
4. **Testosterone** is the **obligate precursor** of both **estradiol and dihydrotestosterone:**
   a. Testosterone is converted in the gonad and peripheral tissues to estradiol by aromatase and to dihydrotestosterone by 5 α-reductase (Figure 45.1).
5. Together, **testosterone and dihydrotestosterone** cause the **phenotypic and behavioral characteristics** associated with being **male.**
6. Testosterone feeds back to the hypothalamus for regulation of GnRH. It supports **spermatogenesis and libido, the development of the epididymis and vas deferens, and muscularity.** Testosterone mediates the **inguinal-scrotal phase of testicular descent** by causing regression of the cranial suspensory ligament. The transabdominal phase of testicular descent is androgen-independent.

B. **Dihydrotestosterone causes sexual maturation at puberty, virilization of the external genitalia, and** development of the prostate.

Benign Prostatic Hyperplasia (BPH)

Pathogenesis

- Dihydrotestosterone promotes prostate growth throughout life.
- Prostatomegaly is found in more than 60% of intact male dogs over 5 years of age and in 95% of intact male dogs by 9 years of age.
- Prostatic disease of any kind is rare in cats.

Classical Signs

- Sexually mature, intact male dogs, usually older than 5 or 6 years.
- The most common clinical signs are tenesmus or sanguineous urethral discharge.
- Dogs with benign prostatic hyperplasia are otherwise normal and healthy.
- Many dogs with benign prostatic hyperplasia have no clinical signs. Prostatomegaly is an incidental finding on physical examination or diagnostic imaging.

Diagnosis

- Benign prostatic hyperplasia is highly suspected based on the history and the physical examination findings of nonpainful, symmetrical enlargement of the prostate in an otherwise healthy, mature, intact male dog.
- Radiographs or ultrasound can be used to confirm prostatomegaly.
- Fine needle aspiration or prostatic biopsy can be done to confirm the diagnosis of benign prostatic hyperplasia, but this is usually not necessary.

Treatment

- Treatment is not necessary for asymptomatic dogs with benign prostatic hyperplasia.
- Castration is the treatment of choice because it is curative.
- When castration is not an option for a symptomatic dog, anti-androgen therapy can be used.

I. Pathogenesis
A. **Dihydrotestosterone is the primary hormone** involved with **prostatic development:**
   1. Benign prostatic hyperplasia in dogs is characterized by hyperplasia of the compound tubuloalveolar glandular elements, often with the development of small (few mm) cysts.
   2. After castration, the prostate is comprised mainly of ductal elements, the glandular and stromal elements having atrophied.
B. **Benign prostatic hyperplasia is rare in cats.**

II. Signalment
A. **Sexually mature, intact male dog, usually older than 5 or 6 years:**
   1. **Prostatomegaly** is found in more than **60% of intact male dogs over 5 years of age** and in 95% of intact male dogs **by 9 years of age.**

III. Clinical Signs
A. **Benign prostatic hyperplasia does not cause systemic illness.** Dogs with benign prostatic hyperplasia are otherwise normal and healthy.
B. The most **common clinical signs** are **tenesmus or sanguineous urethral discharge.**
C. Unlike the situation in men, benign prostatic hyperplasia in dogs is rarely associated with urine retention:
   1. When prostatic disease is associated with urine retention in dogs, prostatic neoplasia is a more likely cause.
D. **Many dogs with benign prostatic hyperplasia have no clinical signs.** Prostatomegaly is an incidental finding on physical examination or diagnostic imaging.

IV. Diagnosis
A. Physical examination findings of **nonpainful, symmetrical enlargement of the prostate** in an otherwise **healthy, mature, intact male dog.** The prostate is best examined by simultaneous **abdominal and rectal palpation of the gland:**
   1. When the history and physical findings are typical of benign prostatic hyperplasia, additional diagnostic tests are usually not performed.
B. **Radiographs** can be used to **confirm prostatomegaly,** which has been defined as prostatic diameter greater than 70% of the pelvic canal as seen on the lateral view:
   1. Radiographs are also useful for evaluation of the sublumbar lymph nodes and the boney pelvis and lumbar spine for evidence of metastasis typical of prostatic neoplasia.
C. **Ultrasound of the prostate** will show **homogenous, symmetrical enlargement,** often with **small (mm) anechoic cysts.** The capsule is smooth and intact. The urethra is normal. Local lymph nodes are normal:

1. When these ultrasonographic changes typical of benign prostatic hyperplasia are found in a castrated dog, they should prompt evaluation for unrecognized cryptorchidism.
2. With the exception of unrecognized cryptorchidism, **prostatomegaly in a castrated dog is considered to be neoplastic until proven otherwise.**

D. **Fine needle aspiration or prostatic biopsy** can be done to confirm the diagnosis of benign prostatic hyperplasia, but this is **usually not necessary:**
1. More often, these would be performed when other prostatic disorders, such as prostatitis or neoplasia, are suspected in addition to, or instead of, benign prostatic hyperplasia.
2. Samples should be submitted for culture and cytologic or histopathologic evaluation.

E. The first and third fractions of the **canine ejaculate** are comprised of prostatic fluid. With symptomatic **benign prostatic hyperplasia,** the **prostatic fluid is commonly hemorrhagic,** or it may be normal.

V. Differential Diagnoses
A. **Prostatitis,** with or without concomitant benign prostatic hyperplasia.
B. **Prostatic neoplasia** is the most likely cause of a "normal-" or large-sized prostate in a castrated animal, and should prompt immediate evaluation.
C. **Prostatic abscess and prostatic cysts** are also causes of prostatomegaly, but they are easily **differentiated** from benign prostatic hyperplasia on the basis of the **ultrasonographic finding** of fluid-filled cavities, and on the basis of fluid cytology.

VI. Treatment
A. **Treatment is not necessary for asymptomatic dogs** with benign prostatic hyperplasia. Watchful waiting is a reasonable alternative.
B. **Castration of symptomatic dogs is the treatment of choice because it is curative.** Prostatic size decreases significantly within 7–10 days. Involution is complete by 12 weeks.
C. When **castration is not an option, anti-androgen therapy can be used.** Clinical signs begin to resolve after about a week of treatment. These drugs are **not as effective as castration** in resolution of clinical signs, and the results are temporary, although they often last for many months after the drug has been discontinued:
1. **The progestins megestrol** acetate (0.5 mg/kg, orally, q 24 h, for 10 days to 4 weeks), delmadinone acetate (0.1 mg/kg subcutaneously at 0,1 and 4 weeks), and **medroxyprogesterone** (3 mg/kg subcutaneously, once) have been recommended:
    a. In addition to causing **adrenal suppression** and **insulin resistance,** progestins can **suppress spermatogenesis, spermatozoal motility,** and **serum testosterone concentrations.**
2. **Finasteride** is a drug that inhibits 5-α-reductase, thereby **inhibiting the conversion of testosterone to dihydrotestosterone.** Oral doses of 0.1–0.2 mg/kg q 24 h, **or 5 mg/dog/**day, have been recommended:
    a. **Prostatic size** is **significantly smaller by 8 weeks of treatment.** Other than decrease in semen volume, semen quality and libido are reportedly not affected, but this may not be true for all dogs.
    b. Finasteride is teratogenic and should not be handled by pregnant women.

VII. Prognosis
A. The prognosis for **benign prostatic hyperplasia is excellent.** Many animals are asymptomatic and remain so for years.
B. **Castration** can be performed at any time after the diagnosis of benign prostatic hyperplasia, and it is **curative.**
C. **Medical management** is usually **effective.** There are potential **side effects.**
D. Benign prostatic hyperplasia may **predispose to the development of bacterial prostatitis.** In dogs with bacterial prostatitis, castration hastens the recovery.

VIII. Prevention
A. **Castration** before middle age.
B. **Castration** at any time will resolve benign prostatic hyperplasia and prevent recurrence.
C. **Castration** does not prevent prostatic neoplasia, the other important cause of prostatomegaly in old dogs.

Perineal Hernia

Pathogenesis

● Male dogs and cats account for 98% and 75% of reported cases of perineal hernias, respectively.
● The cause of perineal hernias remains unknown. The majority (83%) of affected dogs are intact but the majority of cats are castrated males.

Classical Signs

● The most common clinical signs are tenesmus, constipation, and bulging of the perineum.

Diagnosis

● The diagnosis is made on the basis of physical examination, rectal palpation, and diagnostic imaging.

Treatment

● Surgical repair is generally more successful than medical management.

I.   Pathogenesis
A.   **The cause of perineal hernias remains unknown.** Nearly all **(98%) the dogs** with **perineal hernias are males** and the majority of them are **intact (83%).** Most **(75%) cats** with perineal hernias are also **males**, but the **majority of them are castrated.**
B.   **No differences in serum concentrations of testosterone and estradiol,** or expression of **relaxin and relaxin-like factor** have been found **between dogs with and without hernia.** However, androgen receptors are lower and relaxin receptors higher in number in the pelvic diaphragm muscles of dogs with perineal hernias than those without.
C.   Contrary to earlier speculation, **prostatomegaly appears not to contribute to the development of perineal hernias in dogs** since it was detected in only 11.5% of the dogs, and of those prostates that were biopsied, 50% were histologically normal.
D.   Concurrent **lower urinary tract disease** or **megacolon** are **identified in 50% of cats with perineal hernia.**

II.   Signalment
A.   **Perineal hernias occur almost exclusively in males.** The average age is **9–10 years.**

III.   Clinical Signs
A.   The most common clinical signs are **tenesmus, constipation, and bulging of the perineum.**
B.   **Retroflexion of the urinary bladder into the hernia** occurs more often in **dogs (20%)** than **cats (2.5%),** and is often associated with **signs of uremia.**

IV.   Diagnosis
A.   The diagnosis is made on the basis of **physical examination, rectal palpation, and diagnostic imaging.**
B.   Diagnostic **imaging** is particularly helpful for assessing the **position of the urinary bladder** and the contents of the hernia.

V.   Differential Diagnoses
A.   **Other causes of tenesmus** such as **colonic or rectal disease,** or **constipation.**
B.   **Other cases of perineal swelling** such as **anal sac disease, neoplasia,** or **abscess of perineal soft tissue or bone.**

VI.   Treatment
A.   **Surgical repair** is generally **more successful** than **medical management** with stool softeners and such.
B.   **Surgical repair is essential if urinary bladder entrapment has occurred.**

VII. Prognosis

A.   In cases **without bladder involvement, the prognosis is fairly good**; however, continuation of some clinical signs and recurrence of hernia and/or peri-incisional cellulitis occur in about 20% of cases.

VIII. Prevention

A.   For dogs, castration before middle age.

B.   For cats, it is unknown if concurrent lower urinary tract disease or megacolon are merely coincidental or if they play a role in the development of perineal hernias.

Perineal Adenomas

Pathogenesis

• Androgen-dependent hepatoid tumors.

Classical Signs

• Somewhat friable, firm, singular, raised masses that occur on the perineal skin or tail near the anus of old intact male dogs. They are occasionally found on the prepuce or inguinal skin.

Diagnosis

• The diagnosis is usually made on the basis of the signalment and physical examination.

Treatment

• Castration, which will cause the mass to regress.
• Surgical excision of the mass is often also performed.

I.   Pathogenesis

A.   **Androgen-dependent hepatoid tumors.**

II.   Signalment

A.   **Geriatric, intact male dog.**

III. Clinical Signs

A.   They are usually somewhat **friable, firm, single, raised masses** that occur on the **perineal skin or tail near the anus.** They are occasionally found on the prepuce or inguinal skin.

B.   Should one occur on a **female or castrated male,** a source of **androgen** should be **investigated.**

C.   **Perineal adenomas** are **rarely,** if ever, seen **in cats.**

IV.   Diagnosis

A.   The diagnosis is made on the basis of the **signalment and physical findings** and confirmed by **cytologic evaluation** of specimens obtained by **fine needle aspiration.**

B.   **Surgical specimens** should be submitted **for histologic** confirmation of the benign nature of the tumor, particularly if they occur on a female or castrated male.

V.   Differential Diagnoses

A.   Other skin tumors.

B.   Malignant hepatoid tumor.

VI.   Treatment

A.   **Castration,** which will cause the mass to regress.

B.   **Surgical excision of the mass** is often also performed.

C.   Adjunct therapy for malignant tumors should be considered in consultation with a veterinary oncologist.

VII. Prognosis

A. The **prognosis is excellent unless castration is not performed** or if the tumor is too large for complete excision.

B. The prognosis for **malignant tumors** is **guarded.**

VIII. Prevention

A. Castration.

Relative Deficiency Of Estrogen And Other Sex Hormones

Pathogenesis

- The gonads are the primary source of the sex hormones. After castration and ovariohysterectomy, serum concentrations are dramatically reduced.
- Hypogonadotropic hypogonadism, and primary ovarian or testicular failure are rarely documented in dogs or cats as causes of sex hormone deficiencies.

Classical Signs

- Occur after castration or ovariohysterectomy in male and female dogs and cats of any age or breed.
- Absence of estrous cycles and sexual behavior in females. Diminished urine marking, roaming, mounting, and fighting in males.
- Decreased odor of urine in male cats.
- Increased body fat.
- Increased risk of urinary incontinence in female dogs, especially those spayed at a young age.

Diagnosis

- Usually based solely on the occurrence of the classical signs in an otherwise healthy, gonadectomized animal.
- Exclusion of other causes of weight gain or urinary incontinence.

Treatment

- None is usually indicated. The behavioral changes are usually desired.
- To maintain optimal body condition, decrease caloric intake to match decreased metabolic rate.
- Post-spay urinary incontinence in female dogs usually responds well to α-adrenergic drugs such as phenylpropanolamine (PPA), or to estrogen, or a combination of the two.

I. Pathogenesis

A. The **gonads are the primary source of the sex hormones.** By far, the most common cause of relative **deficiencies in the sex hormones is gonadectomy.** After castration and ovariohysterectomy, serum concentrations are dramatically reduced.

B. **Diminished concentrations** of **sex hormones** result in a **decreased metabolic rate** in males and females, a **decrease in spontaneous physical activity,** and a **short-term increase in appetite,** which all lead to an **increase in body fat.** This combination of factors can lead to overt **obesity** if caloric intake remains unchanged.

C. **Gonadectomy affects behavior,** but not of all dogs or all cats similarly.

D. A relationship between the development of **urinary incontinence** and spaying has long been recognized because a relative deficiency in estrogen is known to exist, and because **treatment with estrogen improves the condition in spayed female dogs:**

1. There is evidence that **estrogen deficiency is not the sole factor**. In the absence of the negative feedback exerted by the gonadal hormones on the hypothalamus and pituitary gland, serum concentrations of FSH and LH are chronically elevated (Figure 45.2). Differences in expression of LH-, FSH-, and GnRH-receptors in the lower urinary tract and differences in bladder contractility have been demonstrated among intact versus gonadectomized male and female dogs. **The differences are greater in females than in males, greater in spayed females** than in **intact females**, and **greatest in spayed female dogs that are incontinent.**

2. **The risk of developing urinary incontinence is especially increased in female dogs spayed before 3 months of age.**

E. **Hypogonadotropic hypogonadism is rarely documented in dogs and cats.** Lacking normal function of gonadotropic hormones such as GnRH, LH, and/or FSH, there is failure of normal gonadal development:

1. Lacking the gonadal sex hormones, **sexual maturation does not occur.** Affected animals have underdeveloped genitalia, absent or delayed puberty, absence of secondary sex characteristics, and infertility.

F. **Acquired testicular or ovarian failure is uncommon:**

1. In **males, spermatogenesis** is usually **affected** long before androgen production is diminished and therefore the clinical signs are typically limited to **testicular atrophy** and **infertility.** Secondary sex characteristics and behavior, and prostatic development are usually normal.

2. In **females,** the clinical signs **include infrequent or absent heat cycles,** or if cycles occur, **ovulation failure.**

II. Signalment

A. **No specific signalment exists.**

B. Changes can occur in any dog or cat regardless of breed or age at neutering.

III. Clinical Signs

A. **Obesity:**

1. Unless caloric intake is diminished to match the changed metabolic state, males and females will gain weight after gonadectomy.

B. The **odor of the urine of males,** especially tom cats, becomes **less pungent after castration.**

C. The most predictable effect of gonadectomy is on **sexual behavior,** which is **eliminated in females but may persist in males for several months to a year:**

1. Despite the fact that testosterone is metabolized within hours of castration, 20% of male cats and 80% of male dogs continue to display copulatory patterns for weeks after castration, and 60% of male dogs still show the pattern at least occasionally for 1 year.

2. **Roaming, mounting, and urine marking are significantly diminished in the majority of male dogs and cats after castration.**

3. **In cats, fighting with other males is also significantly diminished.**

4. In **dogs, aggression** toward other dogs and toward people, familiar and unfamiliar, is relatively **unchanged by castration.** It is significantly decreased in **fewer** than 20% of male dogs after castration.

5. The effects of castration are not influenced by the duration of the behavior or the amount of behavioral experience prior to castration.

D. In **bitches, a change in coat quality** back to "puppy coat" and a **decrease in the intensity of hair color** has been observed after ovariohysterectomy in some individual animals in a variety of breeds.

E. Urinary incontinence in spayed bitches:

1. Affected bitches had **normal micturition prior to being spayed. Urinary incontinence develops months to years later.**

2. **Incontinence occurs when the animal is sitting or lying, and is relaxed and at rest, most often when she is asleep.** Typically, at all other times, the animal is continent and micturition is normal.

3. **Urethral pressure is diminished.** Detrusor (bladder) muscle function is typically normal, except perhaps at the level of the trigone. For this reason, the condition has been called urethral sphincter mechanism incompetence, or USMI.

4. Reportedly occurs in as many as 20% of spayed bitches.
5. **The risk of developing urinary incontinence is further increased in female dogs spayed before 3 months of age.** In bitches, the increased risk of creating a pet with urinary incontinence should be weighed against any perceived benefit of early spaying.

IV. Diagnosis

A. Diagnosis is made mainly on the basis of **history, clinical signs,** and **physical examination** findings.
B. Measurement of **serum hormone concentrations** is **not helpful** unless there is a **suspicion** that the **animal is not actually neutered.**
C. For urinary incontinence, a urethral pressure profile can confirm the diagnosis of USMI, but the procedure is not widely available and usually is not necessary.

V. Differential Diagnoses

A. Differential diagnoses for **obesity** include **overfeeding** (which, relative to the decreased metabolic state caused by neutering, is the cause of post-neuter weight gain), **insufficient exercise,** and **metabolic diseases** such as **hypothyroidism.**
B. Differential diagnoses for **changes in hair coat quality** or color include **endocrine diseases such as hypothyroidism, hyperadrenocorticism, or hyperestrogenism.**
C. Differential diagnoses for acquired **urinary incontinence** include a wide variety of **urethral, bladder, and neurological disorders.**

VI. Treatment

A. Unless **caloric intake is diminished** to match the changed metabolic state, males and females will gain weight after gonadectomy and obesity can result.
B. For urinary incontinence in bitches caused by USMI, **treatment with α-agonists is very effective (90%), as is treatment with estrogen (60–80%).** The two can also be used in combination, often at reduced doses for each:
  1. **α-agonists:**
     a. PPA, 1.5 mg/kg (**or 12.5–75 mg/dog**), PO, q 8–12 h.
     b. Ephedrine, 1.2 mg/kg PO, q 8 h.
     c. Pseudoephedrine, 0.2–0.4 mg/kg, PO, q 12 h.
     d. **Side effects** include **tachycardia, anxiety, hypertension, anorexia, aggression.**
     e. These are semi-controlled substances.
  2. **Estrogens:**
     a. Diethylstilbestrol (DES), 0.1–1.0 mg/dog, PO, q 24 h for 5–7 days, then weekly as needed (compounding pharmacy; quality depends on source).
     b. Stilbestrol, 0.04–0.06 mg/dog, PO, q 24 h, for 5–7 days then reduced weekly to 0.01–0.02 mg/dog/day.
     c. Premarin® (conjugated estrogens), 0.02 mg/kg, PO, q 24 h for 5–7 days, then q 2–4 days as needed.
     d. **Side effects** include **signs of estrus, behavior change, myelosuppression, pyometra in uterine stump.**
  3. **GnRH analogs:**
     a. Depot leuprolide, 11.25 mg/dog subcut, redose as needed.
     b. Depot deslorelin, 5–10 mg/dog, subcut, redose as needed.
     c. These drugs downregulate chronically elevated LH and FSH. Reportedly **40–90% effective and long duration of control** (70–575 days). **No reported adverse effects.**
  4. **Urethral submucosal bulking agents:**
     a. Reduce urethral luminal size, thereby increasing pressure.
     b. Sixty-eight percent of treated bitches with collagen implants were continent for 1–64 months (mean 17 months).
     c. Limited availability of collagen implant. Other bulking agents are under investigation.
  5. **Additional investigation** into **therapeutic options** for **post-spay urinary incontinence,** such as use of **hydraulic sphincters, is ongoing.**

VII. Prognosis

A. **Prognosis for obesity** is **good** with appropriate exercise and diet management.

B. **Prognosis for spay incontinence:**

1. Response to treatment with α-adrenergic drugs (e.g., PPA), with or without estrogen, is **generally good, but requires life-long therapy.**

2. Urethral bulking agents such as **collagen implants** are also successful, but with time **will require re-treatment.** The availability of collagen is intermittent.

VIII. Prevention

A. Do not remove the gonads. This will maintain sex hormone production and preserve the behavioral and physical manifestations of sexual maturity.

B. Prevent obesity by adjusting caloric intake and exercise.

C. Delay ovariohysterectomy beyond 3 months of age to decrease the risk of urinary incontinence in bitches.

References and Further Readings

Ball R, Birchard S, May L, et al. Ovarian remnant syndrome in dogs and cats: 21 cases (2000–2007). *J Am Vet Med Assoc* 2010;236:548–553.

Belsito K, Vester B, Keel T, et al. Impact of ovariohysterectomy and food intake on body composition, physical activity and adipose gene expression in cats. *J Anim Sci* 2009;87:594–602.

Coit VA, Dowell FJ, Evans NP. Neutering affects mRNA expression levels for the LH- and GnRH-receptors in the canine urinary bladder. *Theriogenology* 2009;71:239–247.

Dorfmann M, Barsanti J. Diseases of the canine prostate gland. *Compend Contin Educ* 1995;17:791–810.

Hart B, Barrett R. Effects of castration on fighting, roaming, and urine spraying in adult male cats. *J Am Vet Med Assoc* 1973;163:290–292.

Hosgood G, Hedland CS, Pechman RD, et al. Perineal herniorrhaphy: perioperative data from 100 dogs. *J Am Anim Hosp Assoc* 1995;31:331–342.

Lane IF, Westropp JL. Urinary incontinence and micturition disorders: Pharmacologic management. In: Bonagura JD, Twedt DC, eds. *Kirk's Current Veterinary Therapy XIV*, St. Louis: Saunders Elsevier, 2009, pp. 955–959.

Löfstedt RM, VanLeeuwen JA. Evaluation of a commercially available luteinizing hormone test to for its ability to distinguish between ovariectomized and sexually intact bitches. *J Am Vet Med Assoc* 2002;220:1331–1335.

Mann FA, Nonneman MS, Pope ER, et al. Androgen receptors in the pelvic diaphragm muscles of dogs with and without perineal hernia. *Am J Vet Res* 1995;56:134–139.

Merlo DD, Pellegrino RC, Ceppi M, et al. Cancer incidence in pet dogs: findings of the animal tumor registry of Genoa, Italy. *J Vet Intern Med* 2008;22:976–984.

Neilson J, Eckstein R, Hart B. Effects of castration on problem behaviors in male dogs with reference to age and duration of behavior. *J Am Vet Med Assoc* 1997;211:180–182.

Olson PN, Mulnix JA, Nett TM. Concentration of luteinizing hormone and follicle-stimulating hormone in the serum of sexually intact and neutered dogs. *Am J Vet Res* 1992;53:762–766.

Overley B, Shofer MH, Goldschmidt MH, et al. Association between ovariohysterectomy and feline mammary carcinoma. *J Vet Intern Med* 2005;19:560–563.

Peréz-Alenza M, Tabanera E, Peña L. Inflammatory mammary carcinoma in dogs: 33 cases (1992–1999). *J Am Vet Med Assoc* 2001;219:1110–1114.

Reichler IM, Jöchle W, Piché CA, et al. Effect of long-acting GnRH analogue or placebo on plasma LH/FSH, urethral pressure profiles and clinical signs of urinary incontinence due to sphincter mechanism incompetence in bitches. *Theriogenology* 2006;66:1227–1236.

Reichler IM, Welle M, Eckrich C, et al. Spaying-induced coat changes: the role of gonadotropins, GnRH and GnRH treatment on the hair cycle of female dogs. *Vet Dermatol* 2008;19:77–87.

Sørenmo KU, Shofer FS, Goldschmidt MH. Effect of spaying and timing of spaying on survival of dogs with mammary carcinoma. *J Vet Intern Med* 2000;14:266–270.

Zoran DL. Anorectal disease. In: Ettinger SJ, Feldman EC, eds. *Textbook of Veterinary Internal Medicine*, 6th edn. St. Louis: Elsevier Saunders, 2000, pp. 1418–1419.

CHAPTER 46

Progesterone and Prolactin-Related Disorders; Adrenal Dysfunction and Sex Hormones

Cheri A. Johnson

Pyometra
Mammary hyperplasia in cats
Hypoluteoidism
Prolactin
Galactorrhea (false pregnancy)
Sex hormones and adrenal disorders

PROGESTERONE-RELATED DISORDERS

I. Pathogenesis (General)
A. The **primary source of progesterone is the corpus luteum of the ovary:**
   1. With ovulation, the follicular theca and granulosa cells luteinize and become the corpora lutea, which produce progesterone.
   2. **Progesterone production** represents the **luteal phase** of the ovarian cycle or **diestrus.**
   3. Progesterone action:
      a. Causes **development** of the **mammary alveoli,** enabling milk production.
      b. Stimulates growth and secretory activity of the **endometrial glands** and **inhibits myometrial contractility.**
      c. In the hypothalamus, **reduces** amplitude and frequency of basal **gonadotropin releasing hormone (GnRH) secretory spikes, prevents the next estrous cycle,** and **inhibits the preovulatory LH surge.**
   4. Elevated concentrations of progesterone **suppress lactation** and, during pregnancy, inhibit the onset of labor.
B. **Progesterone from the corpus luteum is required throughout pregnancy in dogs and cats.** A placental contribution of progesterone, if any, is negligible:
   1. Oophorectomy will terminate pregnancy at any stage.

Clinical Endocrinology of Companion Animals, First Edition. Edited by Jacquie Rand.
© 2013 John Wiley & Sons, Inc. Published 2013 by John Wiley & Sons, Inc.

2. Conversely, the corpus luteum lifespan depends on the presence or absence of pregnancy in the queen, but not the bitch:
   a. The corpus luteum of a queen that was induced to ovulate but did not become pregnant will function for 30–50 days after breeding.
   b. In pregnancy, the corpus luteum function throughout gestation, which averages 65 days in queens.
3. The **corpora lutea of the bitch** are unique in that they **produce progesterone for more than 60 days**, whether or not there is a pregnancy. The average length of gestation in bitches is 63 days after breeding.
C. **Progesterone is an obligate precursor of cortisol** (Figure 45.1).
D. **Progestagins** have been used **therapeutically**:
   1. To suppress estrus in bitches and queens.
   2. For treatment of "false pregnancy" in bitches.
   3. For treatment of a variety of dermatologic conditions in cats.
   4. To suppress aggressive behavior, roaming, urine spraying, and mounting behavior in males.
   5. For treatment of benign prostatic hyperplasia in dogs.
   6. For treatment of hypoluteoidism in bitches.

II. Diagnosis (General)
A. Some considerations for laboratory assessment of progesterone are unique.
B. Sample handling:
   1. **Serum-separator tubes must never be used** for sample collection because progesterone concentrations will be spuriously and significantly decreased.
   2. Because **refrigeration** of canine blood in serum tubes significantly **decreases progesterone** concentration in freshly drawn samples, samples should be held at room temperature and serum separated as soon as possible after clot maturation:
      a. Blood samples that cannot be centrifuged promptly should be held at room temperature for at least 2 h prior to refrigeration.
      b. After 2 h at room temperature, refrigeration of whole blood is no longer harmful.
      c. Some laboratories may accept heparinized plasma. Storage prior to centrifugation of heparinized samples at room temperature (22°C) or refrigerated (4°C) for up to 5 h has no significant effect on plasma progesterone concentrations.
C. Progesterone concentrations are higher in serum than in plasma.
D. Serum progesterone **concentrations** are approximately **1.5 times greater** when measured **by radioimmunoassay than by chemiluminescent immunoassay**.
E. **Stage of the estrous cycle must be taken into account** when interpreting serum concentrations of reproductive hormones. **Endocrine laboratories must determine, validate, and provide their own reference ranges** for the reproductive hormones for sexually mature animals according to:
   1. Species.
   2. Stage of the estrous cycle in females.
   3. Neuter status in both males and females.

UNDUE RESPONSE TO PROGESTERONE

Pyometra

Pathogenesis

- Progesterone increases the number and secretory activity of endometrial glands, which can result in cystic endometrial hyperplasia (CEH).
- Fluid may also accumulate in the uterine lumen causing hydrometra or mucometra.

- Secondary bacterial infection of the CEH-affected uterus causes pyometra.
- Thus, pyometra is seen during diestrus (i.e., usually within 60 days after heat) or after exogenous progestin administration.

Signalment

- Mature, sexually intact, cycling bitches and queens.
- Bitches and queens treated with exogenous progestin therapy.
- Bitches of any age having been given exogenous estrogens.

Classical Signs

- Occurs in mature, sexually intact, cycling bitches and queens.
- Lethargy, anorexia, vomiting.
- Polydipsia/polyuria in bitches.
- Purulent vulvar discharge is present in most, but not all, cases.

Diagnosis

- Highly suspected based on signalment, history, and the physical findings of uterine enlargement and purulent vulvar discharge.
- Abdominal imaging and supporting hematology findings.

Treatment

- Fluids and broad-spectrum antibiotic therapy along with definitive treatment.
- Definitive treatment to remove the infected uterine material includes surgical or medical options.
- Ovariohysterectomy is the treatment of choice, especially for animals not intended for future breeding.
- In animals intended for future breeding, prostaglandin F2α or progesterone-receptor blocker to cause evacuation of uterine contents.

Prognosis

- Good for survival. Mortality rates of 5–28%.
- With medical management, recurrence is likely; however, subsequent pregnancy rates after prostaglandin F2α treatment for open-cervix pyometra are 70–80%.

I. Pathogenesis

A. In dogs and cats, **progesterone initiates endometrial hyperplasia** by increasing the number and secretory function of the endometrial glands.

B. When the **secreted fluid accumulates** in the uterine lumen, **hydrometra or mucometra** result.

C. The abnormal uterus becomes infected, presumably via ascending bacteria from the vagina, causing pyometra:

    1. *E. coli* is the most commonly isolated organism.

    2. The morbidity and mortality associated with pyometra are the result of the bacterial infection.

    3. Pyometra is a **life-threatening** disease.

    4. Sepsis can develop at any time.

D. Pyometra develops during the luteal phase of the cycle when progesterone concentrations are high, **typically within 4–8 weeks of having been in heat:**

    1. It is more common in bitches because of the long (>60 days) duration of diestrus that follows every cycle.

2. Although some queens do ovulate spontaneously, more commonly, queens are only under the influence of progesterone if they are induced by coitus to ovulate.

3. Pyometra is distinctly different from metritis, which is typically a postpartum disorder and is not hormonally mediated.

E. Endometrial hyperplasia can develop as a result of treatment with exogenous progestins.

F. Exogenous estrogens (e.g., estradiol cypionate (ECP) for mismating) can also increase the risk of pyometra, presumably via their effects on progesterone receptors.

G. *E. coli* and its endotoxins cause glomerular and renal tubular damage, that is, azotemia and proteinuria, and unconcentrated urine, respectively.

II. Signalment

A. Mature, sexually intact, cycling bitches and queens. The **mean age** for both species at the time of diagnosis is about **8 years**.

B. Sexually intact bitches and queens of any age treated with **exogenous progestin therapy**.

C. Bitches of any age having been given **exogenous estrogens** to prevent pregnancy following inadvertent breeding. Estrogens are rarely administered to queens.

III. Clinical Signs

A. **Cystic endometrial hyperplasia** alone would likely cause no clinical signs except perhaps **decreased fertility**.

B. **Hydrometra and mucometra:**

1. Clinical signs typically are limited to **uterine enlargement** with or without abdominal distention or mucoid discharge.

2. Lethargy or abdominal discomfort may be present.

3. Queens will also have a **prolonged interestrual interval** because progesterone will suppress the next cycle.

4. The clinical signs could be mistaken for pregnancy.

C. Clinical signs of **pyometra** include **lethargy, anorexia, vomiting, and, in bitches, polydipsia/polyuria:**

1. **Purulent vulvar discharge** is present in most, but not all cases:

   a. The term "open-cervix pyometra" has been used when a vulvar discharge is present.

   b. The term "closed-cervix pyometra" has been used when a vulvar discharge is absent.

2. An **enlarged uterus** and dehydration are found on physical examination.

3. Rectal temperature is usually normal or low. **Fever is uncommon.**

4. **Sepsis and shock often develop quickly.**

IV. Diagnosis

A. Pyometra is highly suspected by finding **uterine enlargement** and purulent/septic **vulvar discharge** on physical examination with a **history of recent heat or treatment with exogenous progestins or estrogen.**

B. Confirmed by **abdominal ultrasound,** which will show echogenic fluid in the uterine lumen and often a thickened uterine wall with endometrial cysts.

C. The pyometra uterus appears as a tubular structure of soft tissue density in the caudal abdomen on **radiographs.** Sometimes the size and radiographic appearance are similar to what would be seen in mid-pregnancy, prior to calcification of fetal skeletons.

D. Laboratory findings:

1. On a hemogram, the most common finding is a **leukocytosis,** which can be profound (50,000–100,000/μL) and is characterized by neutrophilia with a left shift, a monocytosis, and evidence of WBC toxicity:

   a. However, the total WBC is quite variable and there may be a leukopenia with a degenerative left shift.

   b. A mild non-regenerative anemia is usually present.

2. **Unconcentrated urine and proteinuria** are common in bitches but not in queens with pyometra.

3. **Azotemia of prerenal and renal origins** is fairly common in bitches with pyometra.

4. Although not routinely performed, results of vaginal cytology confirm that the discharge is septic (degenerate neutrophils with bacteria).

V. Differential Diagnoses
A. **Pregnancy** with concomitant illness:
1. This is an **important differential** because the drugs (and surgery) used to treat pyometra will terminate pregnancy.
2. Can be differentiated with ultrasound.
B. **Hydrometra or mucometra:**
1. With hydrometra, the uterine fluid seen on ultrasound is typically anechoic.
2. Vaginal cytology findings with mucometra are mucus without bacteria or significant numbers of inflammatory cells.
3. The WBC profile is essentially normal in most cases.
C. **Metritis:**
1. Meritis is distinct from pyometra, is typically a postpartum disorder, and is not hormonally mediated.

VI. Treatment
A. Patients should be hospitalized and receive **fluid therapy**. Intravenous fluid therapy should be prompt and aggressive to correct shock and dehydration, and maintain adequate perfusion.
B. Patients should receive **antibiotic therapy:**
1. Pending culture results, appropriate bactericidal antibiotic likely to be effective against *E. coli*, the **most commonly isolated organism**, should be initiated. Typically these include **enrofloxacin (and other fluoroquinolones), trimethoprim-sulfonamide, and amoxicillin-clavulanate.**
2. **Culture and susceptibility** testing are important:
   a. Almost **40% of the *E. coli*** isolated from dogs with pyometra **are resistant** to multiple drugs.
   b. Organisms other than *E. coli* may be isolated.
C. **Ovariohysterectomy is the treatment of choice** because the results are immediate and it is curative.
D. Because pyometra will eventually recur, **nonsurgical management is usually reserved for relatively healthy animals that will be bred in the future:**
1. The prognosis for achieving another pregnancy (discussed below) is an important factor to consider.
2. Results of **medical management** are better for treatment of **open-cervix** than closed-cervix pyometra.
3. **Medical management of pyometra is not recommended for animals that are critically ill** because results take days to achieve.
E. Medical treatment has focused on the use of luteolytic and uterotonic drugs to decrease progesterone production and to cause myometrial contractions that expel uterine contents, respectively:
1. Options:
   a. **Prostaglandins** have both effects.
   b. **Cabergoline,** a dopamine agonist, suppresses prolactin secretion; in bitches, prolactin is luteotropic.
   c. **Aglepristone,** a competitive antagonist of the progesterone receptor, blocks the effects of progesterone, thus causing cervical dilation and uterine contraction.
2. **These agents will terminate pregnancy, so they should not be handled by pregnant women.**
3. These agents have been used alone or in combination according to a variety of protocols to take advantage of synergistic effects and minimize adverse effects.
4. Adverse effects:
   a. **Prostaglandin F2α:**
      1) Commonly causes **panting, salivation, emesis,** defecation, urination, mydriasis, and nesting behavior.
      2) In queens, it may also cause grooming behavior and vocalization.
      3) Adverse reactions usually occur within 5 minutes of administration and usually resolve within 60 minutes.
      4) Although side effects are common, they are usually not severe. The severity of reaction is directly related to the dosage administered and inversely related to the number of administrations. Reactions tend to become milder with subsequent injections.
   b. **Cloprostenol,** a synthetic prostaglandin, reportedly has fewer side effects, but **gastrointestinal signs** occur in 30–50% of bitches given the drug.

    c. Gastrointestinal signs are the most common side effect of **cabergoline.** (A veterinary preparation is not currently available in the USA.)

    d. **Aglepristone** causes transient pain or swelling at the injection site:

       1) Its ability to cause cervical dilation may make **aglepristone** an attractive treatment option, especially for certain cases with **closed-cervix pyometra.**

F.   Treatment is monitored on the basis of improving clinical condition, increased vulvar discharge indicative of uterine emptying, and improving laboratory parameters:

    1. The efficacy of uterine emptying is **monitored by ultrasound.**

    2. Treatment is "to effect." It is continued until the uterus is empty, which is typically 7–14 days.

    3. From the onset of treatment, the clinical condition of the patient is expected to improve. If this is not the case or **if the clinical condition deteriorates, ovariohysterectomy should be performed.**

G.   Selected protocols for nonsurgical treatment of pyometra:

    1. Bitches and queens: **Prostaglandin F2α** (Lutalyse®, Pfizer) as a single agent; 0.1–0.25 mg/kg, SC, q 12–24 h.

    2. Bitches only (dosages not yet established for cats): **Cloprostenol** (Estrumate®, Schering-Plough) **plus cabergoline** (Dostinex®, Pfizer, compounded to appropriate concentration; Galastop®, Ceva Vetem):

       a. **Cabergoline,** 5 μg/kg, PO, q 24 h, for 7 days, **plus** cloprostenol, 1 μg/kg, SC, q 24 h, for 7 days.

       b. If no response and patient's condition remains stable, cloprostenol may be continued alone (without cabergoline) for 7 more days.

    3. Bitches and queens: **Aglepristone** (Alizine®, Virbac) alone:

       a. 10 mg/kg, SC, one dose on days 1, 2 (or 3), and 8 (or 7).

       b. Reevaluate at day 14; if not resolved and the patient's condition remains stable, one additional dose of 10 mg/kg, SC, may be administered on day 14.

    4. Bitches only: **Aglepristone plus cloprostenol** (dosages not yet established for cats):

       a. Aglepristone, 10 mg/kg, SC, once daily on days 1, 2, and 8, **plus** cloprostenol, 1 μg/kg, SC, q 24 h on days 3 through 7.

       b. Reevaluate on day 14, if not resolved and the patient's condition remains stable, one additional dose of aglepristone, 10 mg/kg, SC, may be administered on day 14.

VII. Prognosis

A.   For animals undergoing **ovariohysterectomy:**

    1. Despite appropriate supportive and surgical management, **morbidity of 3–20%** and **mortality of 5–28%** have been reported.

    2. The majority of cases do survive the perioperative period, and for them the prognosis is excellent.

B.   Data on mortality associated with nonsurgical management is very limited because medical management is usually abandoned and ovariohysterectomy performed whenever a patient's condition deteriorates or does not improve:

    1. However, in one study of 52 bitches with pyometra, 13 failed to respond to treatment with aglepristone with or without cloprostenol:

       a. Ten of them then had ovariohysterectomy.

       b. One was euthanized because of declining health.

       c. One died and one was lost to follow-up, giving at minimum a mortality rate of 8% (1/13).

C.   Success of medical management of pyometra in the bitch has been evaluated in two ways. One is that the bitch herself recovers. The other is by evaluating subsequent pregnancy rates, which has been done for both bitches and queens:

    1. The most significant justification for medical management is to have another litter.

    2. The prognosis for recovery from open-cervix pyometra and subsequent pregnancy during the next 2 years is good following treatment with **prostaglandin F2α:**

       a. **Pregnancy rates of around 80–90%** are reported for bitches and queens with an open cervix.

       b. To date, although the bitches themselves recovered, **pregnancy rates of only 25–34%** are reported for bitches with **closed-cervix pyometra.**

c. There are apparently no reports of pregnancy following medical management of closed-cervix feline pyometra in the English-language literature.

d. Reported **recurrence rates** for animals kept in their breeding programs are **more than 70% for bitches and 15% in queens** in the 2 years following successful treatment with prostaglandin F2α.

3. To date, data on response to **cloprostenol and cabergoline** are somewhat limited:
   a. Five of 29 (17%) bitches failed to respond to treatment and were spayed.
   b. Six of the remaining 24 (25%) had recurrence of pyometra at their first posttreatment estrus.
   c. Only two of the bitches were subsequently bred, and one of them (50%) conceived.

4. To date, data on response to treatment with **aglepristone** are also somewhat limited:
   a. Twelve of 20 (60%) bitches and 9 of 10 (90%) queens recovered after treatment with aglepristone alone.
   b. Pyometra did not recur in the treated queens during the next 2 years. There is no information on subsequent fertility in the queens because none were bred.

5. In different studies, recovery from pyometra occurred in 84% of 32 and 100% of 15 bitches treated with **aglepristone plus cabergoline:**
   a. In the two reported studies, only 6 of the 47 bitches were bred after treatment with aglepristone with or without cloprostenol, and 5 (83%) became pregnant.
   b. Recurrence rate of pyometra in bitches during the first 2 years after treatment was approximately 20%.

D. **Breeding as soon as possible after treatment is important,** especially for bitches because of the long diestrus (period of elevated progesterone concentrations) that follows every estrus:
1. With each cycle, there is a risk of recurrence of pyometra.
2. The goal is to obtain the desired number of puppies before recurrence.

E. The long-term prognosis for fecundity after medical management is relatively poor, particularly in bitches:
1. Pyometra, a potentially life-threatening disease, will eventually recur.
2. Most affected animals are already middle-aged, beyond their reproductive prime.

F. **Recurrent pyometra:**
1. There are a few reports of successful treatment of recurrent pyometra in bitches.
2. However, given the age of the animals and the expected poor fertility under these circumstances, and the confident expectation of yet another recurrence of pyometra, opting for permanent resolution via ovariohysterectomy would be a prudent consideration.

VIII. Prevention
A. Ovariohysterectomy prior to middle age.
B. Ovariohysterectomy will prevent recurrence.
C. Avoid the use of exogenous progestins in sexually intact females.
D. Avoid the use of exogenous estrogens in females during the diestrus stage of ovarian cycle.

Mammary Hyperplasia in Cats

Pathogenesis

- In cats, pathologic fibroadenomatous mammary hyperplasia occasionally develops in response to endogenous or exogenous progestins.

Signalment

- Cycling queens of any age, but it is most common in young cats (≤1 year).
- Intact or spayed female or neutered male cats being treated with exogenous progestins.

Classical Signs

- Rapid, massive enlargement of all mammary glands, which may outgrow the blood supply and begin to ulcerate (Figure 46.1).

Diagnosis

- Physical examination.
- History of recent estrus cycles or progestin therapy.

Differential Diagnosis

- Mammary neoplasia.
- Mastitis.

Treatment

- Remove the progesterone source. This is usually accomplished by a flank approach for ovariohysterectomy.
- Discontinue exogenous progestins.

Prognosis

- Excellent following ovariohysterectomy.

I. Pathogenesis

A. The normal **mammary development induced by progesterone** is evident approximately **30 days after estrus** in bitches and **in queens that ovulate**. This is an expected normal occurrence after ovulation because of the influence of progesterone, whether or not pregnancy exists.

B. In cats, pathologic **fibroadenomatous mammary hyperplasia** occasionally develops in response to endogenous or exogenous **progestins**.

II. Signalment

A. Cycling queens of **any age can** develop fibroadenomatous mammary hyperplasia:
  1. Most common in young **queens (≤ 1 year)**.
  2. Often they are pregnant.

B. Intact or spayed females or neutered male cats being treated with exogenous progestins.

III. Clinical Signs

A. **Rapid, massive enlargement of all glands,** which may outgrow the blood supply and begin to ulcerate (Figure 46.1).

B. Tachycardia is found in some affected cats.

C. Affected cats are usually otherwise healthy, although they may be quite thin, especially if they are also pregnant.

IV. Diagnosis

A. Physical examination.

B. History of recent estrus cycles or progestagin therapy.

V. Differential Diagnoses

A. **Mammary neoplasia:**
  1. Usually does not affect all the glands simultaneously to the same massive extent.
  2. Is not common in young cats.

(a)

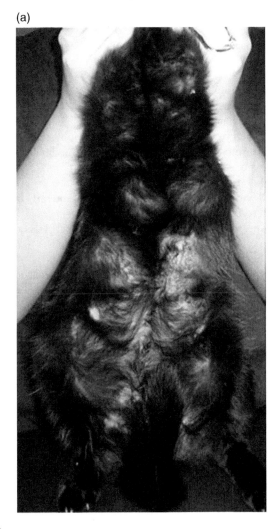

(b)

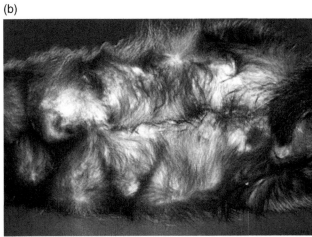

Figure 46.1   (a and b) Feline mammary fibroadenomatous hyperplasia in an 18-month-old queen. Notice the ulceration of the caudal glands. (Courtesy of Dr. Jennifer Simon.)

B. **Mastitis:**
    1. Rarely occurs in queens.
    2. When it does, it is a postpartum disorder.

VI. Treatment
A. Affected cats are **often pregnant**. Owners and veterinarians must be aware that **removing the effect of progesterone, medically or surgically, will terminate the pregnancy**.
B. Remove the source of progesterone:
    1. This is usually accomplished by a flank approach for **ovariohysterectomy**.
    2. The progesterone receptor blocker, **aglepristone**, 20 mg/kg on day 1 (**or** 10 mg/kg on days 1 and 2), SC, once weekly has also been used successfully:
        a. Resolution occurs after 1–4 weeks.
        b. Pregnant cats treated with aglepristone aborted and subsequently developed endometritis, which necessitated ovariohysterectomy.
C. There are reports of a few pregnant queens with mammary hyperplasia that were not treated and had a successful pregnancy:
    1. One was able to nurse her litter.
    2. Others have not nursed, and the kittens were hand-reared or died.
D. Mastectomy could be considered for necrotic or severely ulcerated glands, but this is usually not necessary.
E. Abscesses of the hyperplastic tissue have been managed by surgical drainage and antibiotic therapy.

VII. Prognosis
A. Excellent following ovariohysterectomy or discontinuation of exogenous progestins. **Resolution is expected over 1–4 weeks,** depending upon the severity of the condition.
B. If these fail, aglepristone can be used as described above, and is likely to be effective.

VIII. Prevention
A. Ovariohysterectomy.
B. Avoid exogenous progestin therapy in cats.

OTHER UNDUE RESPONSES TO PROGESTERONE

I. **Progestins induce significant adrenal suppression, especially in cats.**
II. **Progestins cause insulin resistance in both dogs and cats and their administration can cause overt diabetes mellitus (Chapter 15).**
A. In cats, progestin-induced diabetes is reported exclusively with the use of exogenous progestins, not as a result of endogenous progesterone.
B. On rare occasions, diabetes mellitus develops in bitches as a result of endogenous progesterone during normal diestrus or pregnancy:
    1. Assuming that glucose toxicity is controlled with insulin therapy before extensive pancreatic β-cell apoptosis occurs, diabetes will resolve when diestrus ends and progesterone concentrations wane, provided there is no other underlying case of β-cell destruction.
    2. If pancreatic β-cells are still functional, the need for exogenous insulin will abruptly disappear when progesterone concentrations fall.
    3. **Great care must be taken to avoid insulin overdosage and potentially fatal** hypoglycemia at this time.
III. In bitches, progesterone can induce mammary gland production and secretion of growth hormone, which adds to the insulin resistance associated with endogenous progesterone, and results in diabetes mellitus with some features of acromegaly.
IV. Exogenous long-acting progestins can cause a change in coat color at the injection site.
V. Exogenous progestins may promote mammary tumor growth.
VI. Ovarian luteal cysts produce progesterone, which will suppress the next estrous cycle and cause a prolonged interestrual interval.

Progesterone Deficiency

Pathogenesis

- Luteal insufficiency, **hypoluteoidism**, results in serum progesterone concentrations below the reference range.

Signalment

- Pregnant bitches or queens with pregnancy loss.
- Nonpregnant bitches with recurrent, frequent estrus cycles occurring at <5 month intervals.

Classical Signs

- Spontaneous abortion or premature labor in pregnant bitches.
- Short interestrual intervals of less than 4–5 months, and infertility in bitches.

Diagnosis

- Measurement of serum or plasma progesterone concentrations during pregnancy or diestrus.

Differential Diagnosis

- More common causes of pregnancy loss in bitches and queens, such as infection or endometritis.
- In bitches with abnormal cycles, erroneous history of dates of previous estrous cycles.
- In bitches, other causes of infertility.
- Ovulation failure.

Treatment

- In cases where insufficient progesterone is documented, progestin therapy may be helpful to maintain pregnancy.
- Progestin therapy to prolong the interestrual interval in bitches with recurrent short interestrual intervals.
- Ovariohysterectomy in animals not intended for future breeding.

I. Pathogenesis

A. **Luteal insufficiency,** that is, **hypoluteoidism,** results in serum progesterone concentrations below the reference range.

B. The pathophysiology is not understood, but in bitches, prolactin and relaxin, as well as progesterone, may be involved.

C. Hypoluteoidism is an **uncommon cause of pregnancy loss** in dogs and cats:

   1. In bitches, serum progesterone concentrations above 2.0 ng/mL are necessary to support pregnancy.

   2. **A premature drop in progesterone concentration** below 2 ng/mL usually results in **embryonic death** and subsequent resorption, fetal death and subsequent **spontaneous abortion,** or **premature labor,** depending on the stage of gestation at which it occurs.

   3. In bitches, prolactin is the main luteotropic hormone from mid-pregnancy onward:

     a. **Relaxin is synthesized by the placenta** in bitches and queens, beginning as early as day 20 of gestation and continuing throughout pregnancy. It declines rapidly after parturition or abortion:

       1) In pigs, relaxin stimulates prolactin release.

       2) Whether it does so in bitches and queens, and thus might have a luteotropic role, is unknown at this time.

4. Fetal death in bitches and queens may be the cause of declining progesterone concentrations, as well as the result of it.

D. Hypoluteoidism has been reported and studied mainly in bitches, but premature luteolysis and the subsequent decline in progesterone and termination of pregnancy can also occur in queens.

E. In normal nonpregnant bitches, the corpora lutea persist and produce progesterone for a duration of and in concentrations similar to that of pregnancy (i.e., for at least 60 days) after every heat:

1. When the normal duration and concentration of progesterone is diminished by exogenous luteolytic agents such as prostaglandins or if corpus luteum function is spontaneously insufficient, the next estrus cycle usually occurs earlier than normal.

2. When the interval between heat cycles is less than 5 months, bitches are often infertile.

II. Signalment

A. Pregnant bitches or queens with pregnancy loss.

B. Nonpregnant bitches with recurrent, frequent estrus cycles occurring at <5 month intervals. German Shepherds are overrepresented; some of them may have normal fertility.

III. Clinical Signs

A. **Early embryonic death** (which would present as apparent failure to conceive), spontaneous abortion, or premature labor in pregnant bitches or queens.

B. Recurrent short interestrual intervals of less than 4–5 months in bitches, which is usually also associated with infertility.

IV. Diagnosis

A. Documentation of progesterone deficiency by measuring serum or plasma concentrations during pregnancy or diestrus.

B. For animals with apparent pregnancy loss, documentation that pregnancy existed by detecting the pregnancy-specific hormone relaxin in serum and/or by monitoring fetal viability and development with ultrasound. Relaxin is produced by the placenta and therefore its subsequent absence would indicate that pregnancy does not exist.

C. Exclusion of more common causes of embryonic or fetal death or premature labor, such as infection.

D. For infertile animals with short interestrual intervals:

1. Confirmation that other common causes of infertility were not involved.

2. Documentation that ovulation did occur by the finding of serum progesterone concentrations of greater than 10 ng/mL in late estrus or early diestrus.

V. Differential Diagnoses

A. More common causes of pregnancy loss in bitches and queens, such as **infection or endometritis**.

B. In bitches with abnormal cycles, **erroneous history** of dates of previous estrous cycles.

C. In bitches, irrespective of interestrual interval, **other causes of infertility**, such as:

1. Poor semen quality.

2. Insemination during estrus at times other than the optimal fertile period.

3. Only one insemination during the cycle.

4. Lack of intrauterine deposition of frozen-thawed semen.

D. **Ovulation failure,** rather than premature luteolysis, in bitches with short interestrual intervals.

E. Ovulation failure, rather than premature luteolysis, in bitches or queens with presumed, but unconfirmed (by ultrasound or serum concentrations of relaxin) early embryonic death.

VI. Treatment

A. In cases where insufficient progesterone is documented and when more likely causes of embryonic or fetal death, or premature labor, such as infection, have been excluded, progestin therapy may be helpful to maintain pregnancy:

1. Initiation of treatment is based on history of when previous pregnancy loss occurred and by monitoring of serum progesterone concentrations.

2. A variety of **progestins** have been used to treat apparent luteal insufficiency in pregnant bitches. These include:
   a. **Medroxyprogesterone acetate** (MPA) 0.1 mg/kg, orally, once daily.
   b. **Altrenogest**, 0.088 mg/kg, orally, once daily.
   c. **Progesterone** in oil solution, 1–2 mg/kg, IM, every other day.
3. To avoid prolonged gestation:
   a. Orally administered progestins are discontinued several days prior to the expected due date.
   b. Progesterone in oil is discontinued at day 50–55 of gestation.
4. Adverse effects:
   a. In addition to possible prolonged gestation, in people, progestins can cause congenital abnormalities including heart defects, limb-reduction deformities, hypospadias in male fetuses, and mild virilization of the external genitalia of female fetuses, especially when administered during the first 4 months of pregnancy.
   b. Facial deformities were reported in one of four pups in a litter from a bitch treated with MPA for hypoluteoidism.
B. For infertile bitches with **interestrual intervals of** ≤**4 months** that were properly bred to fertile males and are known to have ovulated:
   1. **The next estrus cycle** may be suppressed with either:
      a. **Megestrol acetate**, 2 mg/kg, PO, q 24 h, for 8 days.
      b. **Chlormadinone**, 0.5 mg/kg, PO, q 24 h, for 8 days.
   2. Treatment begins within the first 3 days of the onset of proestrus (first day on which a sanguineous vulvar discharge is observed).
   3. Bitches should be bred to a fertile male using optimal breeding management on the first spontaneous cycle following treatment.

VII. Prognosis
A. The prognosis for maintaining a normal pregnancy in a bitch with suspected hypoluteoidism is somewhat guarded because the diagnosis is difficult to confirm in the first place.
B. However, in animals where other causes of pregnancy loss have been excluded and in which fetal death does not pre-date low serum concentrations of progesterone, treatment has resulted in full-term pregnancies. Litter size, however, has been smaller than normal.
C. The prognosis for achieving normal pregnancy in previously infertile bitches with interestrual intervals of <4–5 months is apparently good when they are bred on the first spontaneous cycle after having had one cycle suppressed.

VIII. Prevention
A. For animals not critical to the breeding program, ovariohysterectomy.
B. In a bitch with normal estrous cycles, avoid estrus induction for the sole purpose of shortening the interestrual interval.

Prolactin

I. Pathogenesis (General)
A. **Prolactin is the hormone that initiates and maintains lactation.**
B. **In bitches,** prolactin is also **luteotropic.**
C. Serum concentrations rise during pregnancy and through the first postpartum week. The **secretion** of prolactin is **mediated by dopamine.**
D. A drop in progesterone concentration, as occurs at parturition in bitches, also stimulates prolactin secretion.
E. Stimulation of the chest wall, mammary gland, and nipple increase prolactin secretion.

Galactorrhea (or so-called False Pregnancy)

Pathogenesis

- Galactorrhea is lactation that is not associated with pregnancy.
- The decrease in serum concentrations of progesterone at the end of diestrus in bitches causes an increase in prolactin secretion.
- Galactorrhea rarely, if ever, occurs in cats.

Classical Signs

- Sexually intact bitch at the end of diestrus (i.e., approximately 60 days after heat).
- Galactorrhea, nesting, and maternal behavior.

Signalment

- Cycling bitches, 60–90 days following estrus.

Diagnosis

- History of recent heat and not having been pregnant.
- Presence of lactation.

Differential Diagnosis

- Pregnancy.
- Mastitis.
- Mammary neoplasia.

Treatment

- None required. Spontaneous recovery occurs, usually in 1–2 weeks.
- Galactorrhea is considered to be normal in bitches.

Prognosis

- Excellent, although frequently recurrent with subsequent cycles.

I.   Pathogenesis
A.   **A decrease in serum progesterone concentrations** stimulates **increased prolactin** concentrations:
   1. In bitches, progesterone concentrations drop at parturition, at the end of normal diestrus, after ovariectomy performed during diestrus, and after discontinuation of exogenous progestin administration.
   2. Sometimes this decline in progesterone concentration is of **sufficient magnitude to cause galactorrhea**, that is, **lactation that is not associated with pregnancy.**
B.   In intact bitches, **galactorrhea, nesting, and maternal behavior occur so commonly at the end of diestrus that they are considered to be normal:**
   1. The condition is usually referred to as *false pregnancy* or *pseudopregnancy*, but these are misnomers because the endocrinologic events (low progesterone, high prolactin), and physiologic manifestations are typical of the immediate postpartum period, not of pregnancy.
   2. Why some bitches and some cycles have overt clinical signs and others do not is unknown, but non-endocrine factors, such as relative over-nutrition, are known to be involved.
C.   Galactorrhea is rare in queens.

II.   Signalment
A.   Cycling bitches, 60–90 days following estrus.

B.   In bitches, shortly after ovariectomy performed during diestrus, or discontinuation of exogenous progestins.

III.   Clinical Signs
A.   **Lactation not associated with pregnancy:**
   1. The quantity and quality of mammary secretions are variable.
   2. They may be minimal and watery to overt dripping of milk.
B.   Nesting and maternal behavior, such as "adopting" toys.

IV.   Diagnosis
A.   Physical examination findings.
B.   History of recent (approximately 60 days ago) heat or discontinuation of progestin administration.

V.   Differential Diagnoses
A.   **Pregnancy:**
   1. It is important to exclude pregnancy as a diagnosis.
   2. If a bitch is pregnant and displaying nesting behavior with lactation, parturition is imminent and immediate preparations should be made.
   3. **Several of the medications used to treat galactorrhea are abortifacient.**
B.   **Mastitis** rarely, if ever, occurs with false pregnancy:
   1. Mastitis, which occurs during postpartum lactation, might be a consideration in a stray bitch with unknown history of recent parturition.
   2. Physical examination would likely find postpartum lochia (vulvar discharge).
C.   **Mammary neoplasia** may cause abnormal secretions from the nipple of the affected gland, but the secretion is not milk.

VI.   Treatment
A.   The clinical signs of false pregnancy typically **resolve spontaneously in 1–2 weeks**. Treatment is not usually necessary.
B.   Medical therapy:
   1. If treatment is desired, typically because of the behavioral signs more so than lactation, options are:
      a. **Cabergoline** (Galastop®, Ceva Vetem; Dostinex®, Pfizer), 5 µg/kg, orally, once daily for 4–7 days.
      b. **Metergoline** (Contralac®, Virbac) 0.1 mg/kg, orally, twice daily for 8 days.
   2. Both are very effective in suppressing lactation.
   3. Both will terminate the pregnancy if one is present and unrecognized.
   4. Side effects are gastrointestinal upset.
   5. Progestins will also suppress lactation, but clinical signs often recur when progestins are discontinued.
C.   Ovariohysterectomy will prevent recurrence.

VII.   Prognosis
A.   Excellent, although recurrence with subsequent cycles is common.
B.   Galactorrhea is not associated with any other reproductive disorders:
   1. To the contrary, it provides strong evidence that the hypothalamic-pituitary-ovarian axis is intact. During the preceding cycle, ovulation occurred, luteal function was sufficient to cause normal mammary development, and prolactin concentrations were adequate to cause lactation.

VIII.   Prevention
A.   Ovariohysterectomy.

Sex Hormones and Adrenal Hyperplasia or Neoplasia

I.   Pathophysiology
A.   **Sex steroid hormones** are **synthesized in the adrenal glands from cholesterol:**
   1. Synthetic pathways are the same as in the gonads.

2. Progesterone and its metabolite 17α-hydroxyprogesterone are obligate precursors of cortisol (Figure 45.1).

B. Corticotropin (ACTH) effectively stimulates production of cortisol and of sex hormones and steroid hormone intermediates of adrenal origin:

　1. This occurs in normal dogs as well as dogs with non-adrenal illness and no evidence of hyperadrenocorticism.

　2. The changes in serum concentrations of sex hormones and steroid hormone intermediates parallel those in cortisol concentrations.

C. Estrogens:

　1. Unlike the situation in ferrets, no reports exist of excessive adrenal production of estrogens causing clinical hyperestrogenism (Chapter 45) in dogs or cats.

　2. In normal male and female dogs, intact or neutered, serum estradiol concentrations do not increase in response to ACTH administration.

　3. A few dogs with hyperadrenocorticism have been reported to have normal basal estradiol concentrations with post-ACTH concentrations above the reference range, but no clinical signs associated with hyperestrogenism were present.

D. Androgens:

　1. An adrenal source of excess testosterone causing pathologic virilization in dogs has not been documented:

　　a. Some dogs with adrenal dysfunction have been reported to have serum testosterone concentrations in the reference range before and after ACTH administration.

　　b. Others have normal basal concentrations with post-ACTH concentrations of testosterone and/or androstenedione above the reference range, but no clinical signs of pathologic virilization, such as the development of benign prostatic hyperplasia in a castrated male or masculinization of external genitalia in a female.

　　c. Recurrent perineal adenomas were reported in a spayed female dog, but the measured serum testosterone, which varied between high and low concentrations, did not correlate with development of the adenomas.

　2. Rarely, an **adrenal source of testosterone** has been documented to cause **clinical signs in cats**:

　　a. An adrenocortical tumor in a 13-year-old neutered male cat without hypercortisolemia but with excess androstenedione and testosterone production caused androgenic clinical signs of pungent urine odor, urine spraying, and an enlarging face.

　　b. Congenital adrenal hyperplasia caused virilization of the external genitalia in a 6-month-old female calico cat.

E. **Progesterone:**

　1. In health, the **adrenal contribution** to systemic progesterone concentrations **is negligible**.

　2. In healthy male and female dogs, intact and neutered, and in healthy neutered and intact female cats, ACTH administration causes a concomitant increase in serum concentrations of progesterone and cortisol:

　　a. This normal response must be taken into account before attributing pathology to the finding of increased serum concentrations of progesterone or 17α-hydroxyprogesterone, especially in animals with hypercortisolemia.

　　b. The correlation between serum concentrations of cortisol and progesterone in response to ACTH is not surprising, given that **progesterone and 17α-hydroxyprogesterone, a metabolite of progesterone, are obligate precursors of cortisol.**

　　c. In healthy bitches during estrus, diestrus, and pregnancy, serum concentrations of 17α-hydroxyprogesterone are higher than in spayed bitches with hyperadrenocorticism.

F. **17α-hydroxyprogesterone:**

　1. Pathologic adrenal production of 17α-hydroxyprogesterone in the absence of hypercortisolemia can cause clinical signs and laboratory abnormalities similar to those seen with classic hyperadrenocorticism (Chapter 5).

2. Because serum cortisol concentrations in these cases are within reference ranges, the situation has been called **atypical hyperadrenocorticism.**
3. To diagnose excessive adrenal 17α-hydroxyprogesterone production:
    a. The initial diagnostic approach is as described for hyperadrenocorticism.
    b. When non-endocrine laboratory and diagnostic results are supportive of a diagnosis of hyperadrenocorticism but cortisol concentrations are within the reference ranges, measuring 17α-hydroxyprogesterone and other sex hormones can be considered.
    c. It is important to first exclude hypercortisolemia because progesterone and/or 17α-hydroxyprogesterone typically parallel the changes in cortisol as described above.

G. Taken together, the studies in dogs and cats suggest that—with the exception of 17α-hydroxyprogesterone, which increases concomitantly with cortisol in normal animals and in animals with adrenal and non-adrenal illness—**an adrenal source of pathologic concentrations of sex hormones causing clinical signs typical of the sex hormone's biologic activity is extremely rare.**

References and Further Readings

Behrend EN, Kemppainen RJ, Boozer AL, et al. Serum 17-α-hydroxyprogesterone and corticosterone concentrations in dogs with nonadrenal neoplasia and dogs with suspected hyperadrenocorticism. *J Am Vet Med Assoc* 2005;227:1762–1767.

Benitah N, Feldman EC, Kass PH, et al. (2005) Evaluation of serum 17α-hydroxyprogesterone concentration after administration of ACTH in dogs with hyperadrenocorticism. *J Am Vet Med Assoc* 2005;227:1095–1101.

Brömel C, Feldman E, Davidson A, et al. Serum 17α-hydroxyprogesterone concentrations during the reproductive cycle in healthy dogs and dogs with hyperadrenocorticism. *J Am Vet Med Assoc* 2010;236:1208–1214.

Burstyn U. Management of mastitis and abscessation of mammary glands secondary to fibroadenomatous hyperplasia in a primiparturient cat. *J Am Vet Med Assoc* 2010;236:326–329.

Corrada Y, Arias D, Rodríguez M, et al. Combination dopamine agonist and prostaglandin agonist treatment of cystic endometrial hyperplasia-pyometra complex in the bitch. *Theriogenology* 2006;66:1557–1559.

Dow SW, Olson PN, Rosychuk RAW, et al. Perineal adenomas and hypertestosteronemia in a spayed bitch with pituitary-dependent hyperadrenocorticism. *J Am vet Med Assoc* 1988;192:1439–1441.

Fieni F. Clinical evaluation of the use of aglepristone, with or without cloprostenol, to treat cystic endometrial hyperplasia-pyometra complex in bitches. *Theriogenology* 2006;66:1550–1556.

Frank L, Rohrbach B, Bailey E, et al. Steroid hormone concentration profiles in healthy intact and neutered dogs before and after cosyntropin administration. *Domest Anim Endocrinol* 2003;24:43–57.

Frank L, Schmeitzel L, Oliver J. Steroidogenic response of adrenal tissue after administration of ACTH to dogs with hypercortisolemia. *J Am Vet Med Assoc* 2001;218:214–216.

Görlinger S, Kooistra HS, van den Brock A, et al. Treatment of fibroadenomatous hyperplasia in cats with aglepristone. *J Vet Intl Med* 2002;16:710–713.

Hill K, Scott-Moncrieff C, Koshko M, et al. Secretion of sex hormones in dogs with adrenal dysfunction. *J Am Vet Med Assoc* 2005;226:556–561.

Johnson CA. High-risk pregnancy and hypoluteoidism in the bitch. *Theriogenology* 2008;70:1424–1430.

Tsutsui T, Kirihara N, Hori T, et al. Plasma progesterone and prolactin concentrations in overtly pseudopregnant bitches: A clinical study. *Theriogenology* 2007;67:1032–1038.

Wanke MM, Loza ME, Rebuelto M. Progestin treatment for infertility in bitches with short interestrous interval. *Theriogenology* 2006;66:1579–1582.

CHAPTER 47

Pathologic Reproductive Endocrinology in Other Species

John Keen and Michelle L. Campbell-Ward

Granulosa-Theca Cell Tumor in the Mare (GTCT)

Pathogenesis

- A benign tumor arising from secretory cells of the ovarian follicle.

Classical Signs

- All ages are affected, but predominantly young adult mares.
- Behavioral changes occur due to hormones released from neoplastic granulosa and/or theca cells.

Diagnosis

- Rectal examination with/without rectal ultrasonography.
- Elevated plasma inhibin and/or other hormones from the GTCT.

Treatment

- Surgical removal.

I. Pathogenesis

A. **GTCT** is caused by a tumor, almost invariably **benign**, arising from the secretory cells of the ovarian follicles, that is, granulosa and/or theca interna layers. It is **often hormonally active**, producing the clinical signs listed below. Production of inhibin by the tumor cells is mainly responsible for the inactive contralateral ovary, by suppressing follicle-stimulating hormone release from the pituitary gland.

II. Signalment

A. All ages are affected but predominantly **young adult mares**. There are no known breed predispositions.

Clinical Endocrinology of Companion Animals, First Edition. Edited by Jacquie Rand.
© 2013 John Wiley & Sons, Inc. Published 2013 by John Wiley & Sons, Inc.

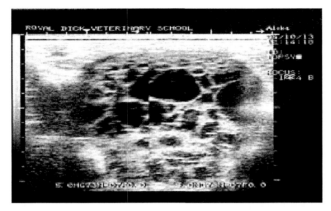

Figure 47.1 Appearance of a granulosa-theca cell tumor per rectum using two-dimensional "B" mode ultrasound. Note the multiple, variably sized, hypoechoic areas separated by thick hyperechoic strands. (Image courtesy of Mr Matt Hanks MRCVS).

III. Clinical Signs

GTCT is the most common hormonally active neoplasm in the equine ovary. Behavioral and reproductive changes are common:

A. **Stallion-like behavior and phenotype:**
   1. Mares may become aggressive and show, for example, mounting behavior.
   2. Some mares may develop a thick nuchal crest or enlarged clitoris.
   3. Stallion-like changes occur when neoplastic thecal cells comprise a significant portion of the tumor (commonly).
B. Mares may be anovulatory, showing a lack of cycling throughout the breeding season.
C. Nymphomania or persistent estrus may occur.
D. Gastrointestinal signs may occur as a complication of usually larger tumors.
   1. Colic and weight loss are the most common signs.
   2. Adhesions, torsion, and hemorrhage of a tumor have also been reported.
E. Some mares may have no clinical signs.

IV. Diagnosis

A. **Rectal examination** reveals a **large ovary, with a small contralateral ovary.** The tumor may or may not be lumpy on palpation.
B. **Per rectum ultrasound examination** usually reveals multiple hypoechoic multiloculated cyst-like structures within affected ovarian tissue, giving a honeycombed appearance (Figure 47.1):
   1. Occasionally GTCTs have solid tissue echogenicity or a single cystic structure is seen.
   2. There should be a small contralateral ovary with little or no follicular activity.
C. **Hormone assays** may be used to aid or confirm a diagnosis of GTCT. One should note that hormone levels released from normal and abnormal ovaries may periodically fluctuate raising the possibility of false-negative or false-positive results:
   1. Inhibin: this hormone is high (>0.7 ng/mL) in most cases (~90%).
   2. Testosterone: often high (>45 pg/mL) (~50–70% of cases):
      a. Normal mares can also have high levels.
      b. Those exhibiting stallion-like behavior are more likely to have high testosterone.
   3. Progesterone levels are usually low. If progesterone is greater than 1 ng/mL, then GTCT is unlikely.
   4. Estradiol is often high, but may be normal.
   5. Anti-Müllerian hormone has recently been suggested to offer potential as a diagnostic test for GTCT but commercial assays are not currently available.
D. **Histopathology** of a surgically removed ovary (Figure 47.2) is required to fully confirm the diagnosis of GTCT.
E. Reevaluation after a specified time period is recommended if doubts over the diagnosis exist.

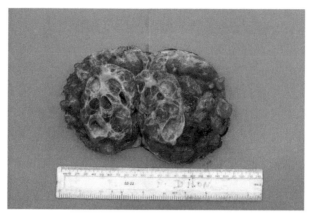

Figure 47.2   Appearance of surgically removed granulosa-theca cell tumor following sectioning. Note the multiple fluid-filled cavities containing serous fluid. (Image courtesy of Miss Safia Barakzai MRCVS).

V.   Differential Diagnoses
A.   Differential diagnoses for the clinical signs include:
    1. Psychological behavioral changes.
    2. Gestation.
    3. Chromosomal abnormalities (intersex).
B.   Differential diagnoses for a palpable and/or ultrasonographically large ovary are:
    1. Transitional period ovary: multiple nondominant follicles.
    2. Gestation: secondary follicular activity may be prominent in the first 2 months of gestation.
    3. Hemorrhagic anovulatory follicle.
    4. Other ovarian neoplastic masses are rare:
      a. Teratoma: these have no effect on behavior, the contralateral ovary, or cycling.
      b. Dysgerminoma: again no effect on behavior, the contralateral ovary, or cycling. These can however metastasize.
      c. Cystic adenoma: little effect on contralateral ovary or cycling but may secrete testosterone.
      d. Lymphoma: no effect on behavior, the contralateral ovary, or cycling.
    5. Ovarian abscessation. This is rare in the absence of prior interventional procedures such as follicular aspiration. The appearance is a thick-walled capsule containing variably hyperechoic material.

VI.   Treatment
A.   Surgical removal is the treatment of choice. Laparotomy (standing or recumbent under general anesthesia) and laparoscopy methods have been described.

VII.   Prognosis
A.   Good. Normal ovarian activity will usually return within 12 months (average 7 months).

VIII.   Prevention
A.   There are no known preventative measures.

Cystic Ovarian Disease in Rodents

Pathogenesis

- Cysts containing clear, serous fluid may develop spontaneously from the rete ovarii in middle-aged to older rodents, especially guinea pigs and gerbils.

Classical Signs

- Non-pruritic bilaterally symmetrical alopecia of the flanks and lumbosacral area.
- Abdominal distension.
- Anorexia, depression, and/or respiratory difficulty.

Diagnosis

- Abdominal palpation.
- Ultrasonographic examination of the ovaries.

Treatment

- Ovariohysterectomy or ovariectomy.

I. Pathogenesis

A. **Cysts containing clear, serous fluid may develop spontaneously from the rete ovarii** in middle-aged to older rodents, especially **guinea pigs and gerbils.** The cysts tend to increase in size over time and can be up to 7 cm in diameter in guinea pigs and up to 5 cm diameter in gerbils. They are usually bilateral, but unilateral disease has been reported. Cysts may be singular or multilobular.

B. Cystic endometrial hyperplasia, mucometra, endometritis, and fibroleiomyomas may occur concurrently.

C. The cysts **may be functional,** that is, cause an increase in serum estrogen or progesterone. Clinical signs often reflect both elevated hormone levels and the space-occupying nature of the cysts.

II. Signalment

A. Cystic ovarian disease is a **common condition** of female **guinea pigs** with a reported incidence of 76%. It is most often diagnosed in guinea pigs **2–4 years of age.**

B. Cystic ovaries also occur commonly in **aged female gerbils** (incidence 20–50%).

C. The incidence in hamsters is 2%.

III. Clinical Signs

A. **Non-pruritic alopecia** (usually bilaterally symmetrical) often over the **flank and lumbosacral area.**

B. **Abdominal distension.**

C. Enlargement of the external genitalia.

D. Failure to breed or reduced litter size.

E. Anorexia or reduced appetite.

F. Depression.

G. Respiratory difficulty in severe cases.

IV. Diagnosis

A. The cysts are usually initially detected during examination via **abdominal palpation.**

B. **Ultrasonography** of the reproductive structures can confirm the diagnosis.

C. **Histopathology** of surgically excised ovaries of affected animals reveals cysts lined by low cuboidal to columnar epithelial cells. Solitary cilia or tufts of cilia are present on the luminal surface of some cells and there may be marked compression of the ovarian tissue. In advanced cases, only remnants of the ovary are found.

V. Differential Diagnoses

A. Alopecia of pregnancy, that is, bilateral non-pruritic flank alopecia seen in guinea pig sows in advanced pregnancy or early lactation.

B. Ovarian or other neoplasia.

C. Ascites.

D. Respiratory disease.

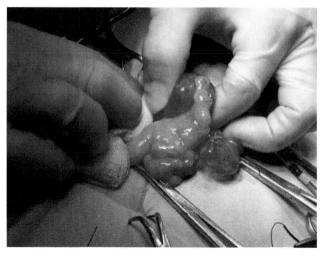

Figure 47.3   Ovariohysterectomy is the treatment of choice for guinea pigs with ovarian cystic disease. Note the large fluid-filled cysts present on both ovaries.

VI.   Treatment

A.   **Surgical removal of the ovaries (ovariohysterectomy or ovariectomy) is the treatment of choice** (Figure 47.3).

B.   Percutaneous drainage of cysts has been reported and may provide immediate relief from the pressure and pain associated with cysts but is not curative.

C.   Temporary improvements in clinical signs have been seen with intramuscular administration of 100 IU human chorionic gonadotropin (once weekly for three doses, or once a fortnight for two doses) in affected guinea pigs.

D.   Alternative adjunctive therapeutic options aimed at suppressing sex steroidogenesis and associated clinical signs in guinea pigs prior to surgery include:

　1.   Leuprolide acetate (30 day depot of 200 μg/guinea pig IM).

　2.   Placement of a 4.7 mg deslorelin implant SC.

E.   Nutritional support and analgesia are critical presurgical considerations.

VII.   Prognosis

A.   The prognosis is **good** in the absence of concurrent disease. A degree of permanent alopecia may remain following surgery.

VIII.   Prevention

A.   **Ovariohysterectomy** or ovariectomy in nonbreeding animals will prevent the condition.

Follicular Stasis in Pet Reptiles

Pathogenesis

● Hormonal disturbances allow ovarian follicles to form without progression to ovulation. Large bunches of follicles can develop to occupy a significant proportion of the coelomic cavity.

● Coelomitis may develop if vitellin/yolk leakage occurs.

Classical signs

● Anorexia.

● Lethargy.

● Coelomic distension (lizards).

> **Diagnosis**
> - Radiography and/or ultrasonography.
>
> **Treatment**
> - Coeliotomy and ovariosalpingectomy.

I. Pathogenesis

A. **Follicular stasis** (sometimes referred to as **preovulatory egg binding**) is a relatively common problem in pet reptiles. Hormonal disturbances allow ovarian follicles to form without progression to ovulation, but the precise etiology is poorly understood. Inappropriate diet and husbandry, lack of hibernation for some species, absence of a male, stress or other medical conditions are thought to contribute.

B. The follicles may become atretic and be resorbed without illness. However, if resorption of follicles does not occur over time, bilateral follicular development can progress to such an extent that a significant proportion of the coelomic cavity is occupied. **The space-occupying nature of the follicles can then cause secondary problems,** such as respiratory difficulty or gastrointestinal obstruction.

C. Additionally, **inflammation of the follicles and ovary frequently develops** and commensal bacteria (e.g., *Salmonella* sp.) may inoculate the yolked follicles during vitellogenesis. Yolk, containing vitellin, may leak out of the follicles into the surrounding tissue and a **severe coelomitis can result.**

II. Signalment

A. Adult female tortoises and lizards isolated from males seem to be particularly prone to this condition.

III. Clinical Signs

A. Anorexia.
B. Lethargy.
C. Coelomic distension (lizards).
D. Early cases may have no clinical signs.

IV. Diagnosis

A. The **history and physical examination** may provide a tentative diagnosis in some patients; for example, in larger lizards the follicles may be palpable.

B. **Radiography and/or ultrasonography** are the preferred noninvasive tools for confirmation of the diagnosis. Ultrasound examination of the ovaries in tortoises is achieved via the prefemoral fossae (immediately in front of the hind limbs).

C. Plasma chemistry may show elevated triglycerides, calcium, phosphorus, and albumin associated with vitellogenesis. If the condition is chronic, hypoalbuminemia from anorexia and hepatic lipidosis may be seen. Hematology will often reveal anemia of chronic disease and leukocytosis associated with inflammation and/or infection.

V. Differential Diagnoses

A. As the clinical signs tend to be nonspecific (anorexia and lethargy), a thorough diagnostic workup including gathering detailed information on husbandry is indicated in most cases.

B. Important differential diagnoses to consider include:
1. Postovulatory egg binding.
2. Traumatic yolk coelomitis.
3. Gastrointestinal impaction.
4. Gastrointestinal parasitism/enteritis.
5. Urolithiasis.

VI. Treatment

A. Improvement of diet and husbandry (including appropriate photoperiod and the ability to thermoregulate properly), ability to have social interaction with a male, and providing a suitable nesting area for non-ill patients with follicular stasis may be sufficient to resolve the problem.

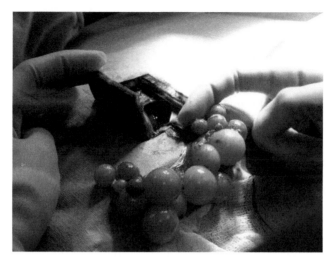

Figure 47.4 Coeliotomy in a Hermann's tortoise for surgical treatment of chronic follicular stasis. Note the large grape-like bunch of yolk-filled follicles.

B. For patients that present with illness, **ovariectomy or ovariosalpingectomy is indicated once stabilized** (Figure 47.4). The coelomic cavity will need to be lavaged copiously during surgery to remove yolk that may have leaked from the friable follicles before or during surgery.

VII. Prognosis

A. In cases in which coelomitis has developed, the prognosis is poor if aggressive medical therapy and surgical correction is not promptly provided.

VIII. Prevention

A. Ensure appropriate husbandry conditions are provided for captive reptiles, including a biologically suitable photoperiod and thermal gradient.

B. Provide a nesting site for females, regardless of whether they are housed with a male or not.

C. Consider ovariosalpingectomy for nonbreeding animals.

References and Further Readings

Bailey MT, Troedsson MHT, Wheaton JE. Inhibin concentrations in mares with granulosa cell tumours. *Theriogenology* 2002;57:1885–1895.

Ball BA, Conley AJ, MacLaughlin DT, et al. Expression of anti-Mullerian hormone in equine granlosa cell tumours and in normal equine ovaries. *Theriogenology* 2008;70:968–977.

Collins BR. Endocrine diseases of rodents. *Vet Clin North Am. Exot. Anim. Pract* 2008;11:153–162.

Eatwell K. Lizards. In: Meredith A, Johnson-Delaney, C, eds. *BSAVA Manual of Exotic Pets*, 5th edn. Gloucester: British Small Animal Veterinary Association, 2010, pp. 273–293.

Johnson JD. Urogenital system. In: Girling, SJ, Raiti, P, eds. *BSAVA Manual of Reptiles*, 2nd edn. Gloucester: British Small Animal Veterinary Association, 2004, pp. 261–272.

Johnson-Delaney C. Guinea pigs, chinchillas, degus and duprasi. In: Meredith A, Johnson-Delaney, C, eds. *BSAVA Manual of Exotic Pets*, 5th edn. Gloucester: British Small Animal Veterinary Association, 2010, pp. 28–62.

Keller LS, Griffith JW, Lang CM. Reproductive failure associated with cystic rete ovarii in guinea pigs. *Vet Pathol* 1987;24:335–339.

McCue PM, Roser JF, Munro CJ, et al. Granulosa cell tumours of the equine ovary. *Vet Clin N Am - Equine* 2006; 22:799–817.

O'Rourke DP. Disease problems of guinea pigs. In: Quesenberry KE, Carpenter JW, eds. *Ferrets, Rabbits and Rodents – Clinical Medicine and Surgery*, 2nd edn. St. Louis: Saunders, 2004, pp. 245–254.

Orr H. Rodents: neoplastic and endocrine disease. In: Keeble E, Meredith A, eds. *BSAVA Manual of Rodents and Ferrets*, Gloucester: British Small Animal Veterinary Association, 2009, pp. 181–192.

Percy DH, Barthold SW. *Pathology of Laboratory Rodents and Rabbits*, 3rd edn. Ames : Blackwell Publishing, 2007.
Sayers I, Smith I. Mice, rats, hamsters and gerbils. In: Meredith A, Johnson-Delaney C, eds. *BSAVA Manual of Exotic Pets*, 5th edn. Gloucester: British Small Animal Veterinary Association, 2010, pp. 1–27.
Yarborough TB. Ovariectomy techniques. In: Robinson NE, Sprayberry KA, eds. *Current Therapy in Equine Medicine 6*, St Louis: WB Saunders, 2009, pp. 781–784.

Index

Note: Page numbers in *italics* refer to Figures; those in **bold** to Tables.

Clinical Endocrinology of Companion Animals, First Edition. Edited by Jacquie Rand.
© 2013 John Wiley & Sons, Inc. Published 2013 by John Wiley & Sons, Inc.

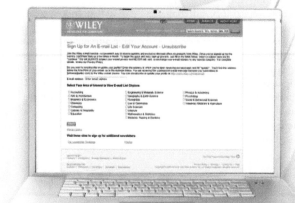
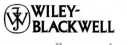